HELPING PARENTS, YOUTH, AND TEACHERS UNDERSTAND MEDICATIONS FOR BEHAVIORAL AND EMOTIONAL PROBLEMS

A Resource Book of Medication Information Handouts

THIRD EDITION

HELPING PARENTS, YOUTH, AND TEACHERS UNDERSTAND MEDICATIONS FOR BEHAVIORAL AND EMOTIONAL PROBLEMS

A Resource Book of Medication Information Handouts

THIRD EDITION

EDITED BY

MINA K. DULCAN, M.D.

CONTRIBUTORS

Thomas Cummins, M.D.

Mina K. Dulcan, M.D.

Anna Ivanenko, M.D.

Poonam Jha, M.D.

Margery Johnson, M.D.

Jeremy Kaplan, M.D.

MaryBeth Lake, M.D.

D. Richard Martini, M.D.

Kathleen McKenna, M.D.

Karen Pierce, M.D.

Sigita Plioplys, M.D.

Department of Child and Adolescent Psychiatry, Children's Memorial Hospital;
Division of Child and Adolescent Psychiatry, Northwestern University Feinberg School of Medicine,
Chicago, Illinois

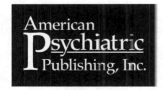

American Psychiatric Publishing, Inc.

Washington, DC
London, England

To buy 25–99 copies of this or any other APPI title, please contact APPI Customer Service at appi@psych.org or 800-368-5777 for a 20% discount. To buy 100 or more copies of the same title, please e-mail bulksales@ psych.org for a price quote.

Copyright © 2007 American Psychiatric Publishing, Inc.
ALL RIGHTS RESERVED

Manufactured in the United States of America on acid-free paper
11   10   09   08   07   5   4   3   2   1
Third Edition

Typeset in Adobe's Janson Text, AG Book Rounded, and Frutiger.

American Psychiatric Publishing, Inc.
1000 Wilson Boulevard
Arlington, VA 22209–3901
www.appi.org

Library of Congress Cataloging-in-Publication Data

Helping parents, youth, and teachers understand medications for behavioral and emotional problems : a resource book of medication information handouts / edited by Mina K. Dulcan ; contributors, Thomas Cummins ... [et al.]. — 3rd ed.
     p. ; cm.
  ISBN 1-58562-253-2 (pbk. : alk. paper)
 1. Pediatric psychopharmacology. 2. Child psychiatry—Differential therapeutics. I. Dulcan, Mina K. II. Cummins, Thomas, M.D.
   [DNLM: 1. Child Behavior Disorders—drug therapy. 2. Adolescent. 3. Child. 4. Psychopharmacology. WS 350.6 H483 2006]

RJ504.7.H44 2006
618.92′8918—dc22
                                                                                          2006014701

British Library Cataloguing in Publication Data

A CIP record is available from the British Library.

Contents

Contributors

Thomas Cummins, M.D.
Medical Director, Inpatient Psychiatry, Department of Child and Adolescent Psychiatry, Children's Memorial Hospital; Assistant Professor of Psychiatry and Behavioral Sciences, Feinberg School of Medicine, Northwestern University, Chicago, Illinois

Mina K. Dulcan, M.D.
Head, Department of Child and Adolescent Psychiatry, and Margaret C. Osterman Professor of Child Psychiatry, Children's Memorial Hospital; Director, Adolescent Psychiatry, Northwestern Memorial Hospital; and Head, Division of Child and Adolescent Psychiatry, Professor of Psychiatry and Behavioral Sciences and Pediatrics, Feinberg School of Medicine, Northwestern University, Chicago, Illinois

Anna Ivanenko, M.D.
Medical Director, Pediatric Sleep Medicine Program, Alexian Brothers Medical Center and Central DuPage Hospital; Assistant Professor, Department of Psychiatry and Behavioral Neurosciences, Loyola University Stritch School of Medicine, Maywood, Illinois

Poonam Jha, M.D.
Attending Physician, Outpatient Psychiatry, Department of Child and Adolescent Psychiatry, Children's Memorial Hospital; Instructor of Psychiatry and Behavioral Sciences, Feinberg School of Medicine, Northwestern University, Chicago, Illinois

Margery Johnson, M.D.
Attending Physician, Outpatient Psychiatry, Department of Child and Adolescent Psychiatry, Children's Memorial Hospital; Assistant Professor of Psychiatry and Behavioral Sciences, Feinberg School of Medicine, Northwestern University, Chicago, Illinois

Jeremy Kaplan, M.D.
Child and Adolescent Psychiatry Chief Resident, Children's Memorial Hospital, McGaw Medical Center, Feinberg School of Medicine, Northwestern University, Chicago, Illinois

MaryBeth Lake, M.D.
Attending Physician, Outpatient Psychiatry, Director of Education in Child and Adolescent Psychiatry, Department of Child and Adolescent Psychiatry, Children's Memorial Hospital; Associate Professor of Psychiatry and Behavioral Sciences, Feinberg School of Medicine, Northwestern University, Chicago, Illinois

D. Richard Martini, M.D.
Clinical Director, Intake and Emergency Services, and Director, Consultation Liaison Services, Department of Child and Adolescent Psychiatry, Children's Memorial Hospital; Associate Professor of Psychiatry and Behavioral Sciences and Pediatrics, Feinberg School of Medicine, Northwestern University, Chicago, Illinois

Kathleen McKenna, M.D.
Director, Psychosis and Special Diagnostic Program, Department of Child and Adolescent Psychiatry, Children's Memorial Hospital; Associate Professor of Psychiatry and Behavioral Sciences, Feinberg School of Medicine, Northwestern University, Chicago, Illinois

Karen Pierce, M.D.
Medical Director, Partial Hospitalization Program, Department of Child and Adolescent Psychiatry, Children's Memorial Hospital; Assistant Professor of Psychiatry and Behavioral Sciences, Feinberg School of Medicine, Northwestern University, Chicago, Illinois

Sigita Plioplys, M.D.
Attending Physician, Outpatient Psychiatry, Department of Child and Adolescent Psychiatry, Children's Memorial Hospital; Assistant Professor of Psychiatry and Behavioral Sciences, Feinberg School of Medicine, Northwestern University, Chicago, Illinois

The following contributors to this book have indicated a financial interest in or other affiliation with a commercial supporter, manufacturer of a commercial product, and/or provider of a commercial service as listed below:

Mina K. Dulcan, M.D.—Member: American Psychiatric Publishing Editorial Advisory Board; Eli Lilly Strattera Global Advisory Board; Consultant: Comprehensive NeuroScience Inc. Editorial Board (a company that develops medication guidelines for managed care and Medicaid)

MaryBeth Lake, M.D.—Research: AstraZeneca, Johnson & Johnson

Kathleen McKenna, M.D.—Research, Consultant: AstraZeneca, Johnson & Johnson

Karen Pierce, M.D.—Speaker: Eli Lilly, Novartis, Shire, McNeil

Sigita Plioplys, M.D.—Speaker: Novartis

Acknowledgments

Thanks are due to the terrific staff at American Psychiatric Publishing, Inc., for all of their support throughout this project, starting with the first edition. Carol Nadelson accepted the original book proposal when no one had seen a book structured in this way and other publishers simply shook their heads. Bob Hales and John McDuffie have worked with us to improve each edition, including the (at the time) innovative use of the CD-ROM.

Dolly Konopka, my intrepid assistant, took on this edition as her first venture in book preparation. It could not have been completed without her organizational efforts, attention to detail, and cheerful patience with many, many edits and changes.

My husband, Richard Wendel, has been, as always, supportive, patient, and tolerant of all the demands on my time.

Mina K. Dulcan, M.D.

July 2006

Introduction for Physicians to the Third Edition

The medication information handouts in this book are intended for use in the context of clinical psychiatric evaluation and treatment of children and adolescents. The purpose of these handouts is to share basic information about medications with parents, teachers, and adolescent patients. The information sheets, especially the ones for youth, do not cover all possible side effects and are not intended for use as informed consent documents. They do not include educational information about disorders. Suggested resources are provided in the pages following this introduction, preceding the medication information sheets. The medication information sheets should be used by prescribing physicians with patients (who are old enough to read and understand them) and families to supplement an ongoing dialogue regarding the indications for medications, medication effects, and side effects. The sheets are not meant to be guides for physicians in prescribing medicine but rather to be used once the decision is made to prescribe a particular medication for a particular patient. The sheets are valuable for teachers (and school nurses) in helping understand the medications used by students. In our clinical practice at Children's Memorial Hospital, nonphysician mental health professionals have found these sheets to be useful when proposing to patients and families an evaluation for possible medication.

Information on each medication in this third edition has been completely updated from the second edition (published in 2003). New medications, such as atomoxetine (Strattera) and aripiprazole (Abilify) have been added. Medications taken off the market, such as pemoline (Cylert) and nefazodone (Serzone), have been removed. New concerns about potential side effects and U.S. Food and Drug Administration (FDA) black box warnings (for antidepressants and stimulants) have been addressed. Coverage of medications used for sleep has been expanded. The book has been entirely restructured, using the format of a combined adult information sheet ("Medication Information for Parents and Teachers") followed by an information sheet specifically for youth. Each medicine now has its own sheet instead of being grouped by drug category as in the second edition. The medications are listed alphabetically by their generic names. The various formulations of stimulant medications have been placed in two sets of group information sheets by the active ingredient, methylphenidate or amphetamine. It is always a dilemma whether to focus on generic names or brand names. In this edition, we have chosen to use the generic names more often, because more medications are going off-patent and have more formulations and also to minimize the commercial focus. As before, we use only U.S. brand names.

New to this edition, appendices list medications typically used for certain indications, in case the clinician wishes to discuss options with the family or to check off which medications have been tried as he or she reviews the patient's medication history with the family. The information on additional mental health resources—books, journals, newsletters, and Internet sites—has been updated.

We have not included some medications (like monoamine oxidase inhibitors or cognitive enhancers) that are virtually never used for youth because of unacceptable side-effect profiles and/or lack of evidence for efficacy. For medications not included in this book, or for more sophisticated and detailed information targeted at highly educated "consumers," an excellent resource is *What Your Patients Need to Know About Psychiatric Medications*, by Hales, Yudofsky, and Chew (American Psychiatric Publishing 2005). The format and intended use are the same as this book, but the target audience is psychiatrists caring for adult patients. Handouts for adults on major psychiatric illnesses, along with information targeted at adult patients and families on groups of psychiatric medications, can be found in *Wyatt's Practical Psychiatric Practice: Forms and Protocols for Clinical Use*, Third Edition, by Wyatt and Chew (American Psychiatric Publishing 2005).

All of the contributors to this book are experienced child and adolescent psychiatrist clinicians who use psychopharmacology as one component of comprehensive mental health treatment of children and adolescents. In the years since the publication of the second edition, we have found that many families have become more sophisticated about psychotropic medications due to increasingly available helpful information from patient–professional advocacy groups and more dramatic but less helpful attention from the media. In response to these developments, we have somewhat increased the complexity of the information sheets. This decision must always be weighed against the reality of different reading levels in order for the information sheets to be accessible to the largest possible audience of patients and families. We hope that we have found the right balance. For brevity and readability, many details and much explanation have been omitted, as well as rare or poorly documented side effects. Each physician is likely to disagree with some aspect of what we have written. The handouts are offered as a resource to those who find them useful, not as a standard for psychopharmacology practice. Only the most common indications are included. If a specific indication has been omitted, that does not necessarily mean that it is inappropriate.

The information provided in these sheets is based on the available scientific literature and the clinical experience of the authors and their colleagues. Unfortunately, most psychopharmacology research is performed on adults, not children and adolescents, although a slight improvement—more research on psychopharmacology for children and adolescents—has occurred in recent years. Many of the indications for medication have not received FDA approval and therefore are not listed in the *Physicians' Desk Reference* (PDR). However, once a drug is approved for any indication, the FDA regulates only the company's advertising of the drug, not what physicians may prescribe. Nearly all psychopharmacological agents and indications (and the majority of the drugs used in pediatrics, as well) lack pediatric labeling and are "unapproved" or "off-label" for use in children. Off-label use may be accepted practice, appropriate, and rational. However, the FDA guidelines as published in the PDR cannot be relied on for appropriate indications, age ranges, or dosages for children. Sources such as the PDR are increasingly available to lay consumers, making the information in this book even more necessary. Lack of FDA approval for an age group or a disorder does not imply improper or illegal use. As a result of pressure from the FDA and new financial incentives (via extending the patent on drugs), pharmaceutical companies have increased their attention to research in children. The Best Pharmaceuticals for Children Act mandates that for any drug that receives pediatric exclusivity (i.e., 6-month extension of patent exclusivity), the manufacturer must submit data to the FDA on all pediatric adverse-event reports for 1 year following the granting of extended exclusivity. This requirement, in addition to applications for new indications, has increased the opportunities for discussion of potential side effects. However, while knowledge of potential risks is clearly beneficial, the resulting FDA hearings and advisory committee meetings have given antipsychiatry groups, such as the Citizens Commission on Human Rights and the Alliance for Human Research Protection, highly visible opportunities for testimony opposing psychiatric medications and even questioning the validity of diagnoses. Unfortunately, this attention to supposed side effects, fueled by attention from the media and plaintiff attorneys, has frightened parents and some physicians and is also likely to dampen industry enthusiasm to pursue needed research in pediatric psychopharmacology. The National Institute of Mental Health budget is unlikely to allow for the large, long-term studies needed to assess efficacy and safety. In the meantime, practitioners must do the best they can to help children and families struggling with mental illness, using the available evidence, good clinical judgment, and appropriate caution.

Selected Additional Reading for Health and Mental Health Professionals

Books

Barkley RA: *Attention-Deficit Hyperactivity Disorder: A Handbook for Diagnosis and Treatment*, 3rd Edition. New York, Guilford, 2006

Bezchlibnyk-Butler KZ, Virani AS (eds): *Clinical Handbook of Psychotropic Drugs for Children and Adolescents*. Cambridge, MA, Hogrefe and Huber, 2004

Dulcan MK, Martini DR, Lake MB: *Concise Guide to Child and Adolescent Psychiatry*, 3rd Edition. Washington, DC, American Psychiatric Publishing, 2003

Green WH: *Child and Adolescent Clinical Psychopharmacology*, 3rd Edition. Philadelphia, PA, Lippincott Williams & Wilkins, 2001

Kutcher SP: *Practical Child and Adolescent Psychopharmacology*. New York, Cambridge University Press, 2002

Journals

Journal of the American Academy of Child and Adolescent Psychiatry, Lippincott Williams & Wilkins; www.jaacap.com

Journal of Child and Adolescent Psychopharmacology, Mary Ann Liebert; www.liebertpub.com/cap

Newsletters

The Brown University Child and Adolescent Psychopharmacology Update, John Wiley & Sons, Wiley Subscription Services, 1-800-825-7550, e-mail: subinfo@wiley.com

Child and Adolescent Psychopharmacology News, Guilford Press, 72 Spring Street, New York, NY 10012, 1-800-365-7006, e-mail: news@guilford.com

Internet

American Psychiatric Association, American Academy of Child and Adolescent Psychiatry: *Physicians Med Guide—The Use of Medication in Treating Childhood and Adolescent Depression: Information for Physicians*. Available at: www.parentsmedguide.org.

Published Resources for Parents and Teachers

Books

American Academy of Child and Adolescent Psychiatry: *Your Child: What Every Parent Needs to Know.* New York, HarperCollins, 1998

American Academy of Child and Adolescent Psychiatry: *Your Adolescent: Emotional, Behavioral and Cognitive Development From Early Adolescence Through the Teen Years.* New York, HarperCollins, 1999

American Academy of Pediatrics: *ADHD: A Complete and Authoritative Guide.* Elk Grove Village, IL, American Academy of Pediatrics, 2004

Barkley RA: *Taking Charge of ADHD: The Complete, Authoritative Guide for Parents.* New York, Guilford, 2000

Barkley RA, Benton CM: *Your Defiant Child.* New York, Guilford, 1998

Bashe PR, Kirby BL: *The OASIS Guide to Asperger Syndrome: Advice, Support, Insights, and Inspiration.* New York, Crown, 2001

Birmaher B: *New Hope for Children and Teens With Bipolar Disorder.* New York, Three Rivers Press, 2004

Braaten E, Felopulos G: *Straight Talk About Psychological Testing for Kids.* New York, Guilford, 2004

Children and Adults With Attention Deficit/Hyperactivity Disorder (CHADD): *The CHADD Information and Resource Guide to AD/HD.* Landover, MD, CHADD, 2000

Clark L: *SOS! Help for Parents: A Practical Guide for Handling Common Everyday Behavior Problems*, 2nd Edition. Berkeley, CA, Parents Press, 1996

Dacey J, Fiore L: *Your Anxious Child.* San Francisco, CA, Jossey-Bass, 2000

Evans DL, Wasmer Andrews L: *If Your Adolescent Has Depression or Bipolar Disorder: An Essential Resource for Parents.* New York, Oxford University Press, 2005

Faraone SV: *Straight Talk About Your Child's Mental Health: What to Do When Something Seems Wrong.* New York, Guilford, 2003

Foa EB, Andrews LW: *If Your Adolescent Has an Anxiety Disorder: An Essential Resource for Parents.* New York, Oxford University Press, 2006

Fristad MA, Arnold JSG: *Raising a Moody Child: How to Cope With Depression and Bipolar Disorder.* New York, Guilford, 2004

Green RW: *The Explosive Child.* New York, HarperCollins, 1998

Gur RE, Johnson AB: *If Your Adolescent Has Schizophrenia: An Essential Resource for Parents.* New York, Oxford University Press, 2006

Jensen P: *Making the System Work for Your Child with ADHD.* New York, Guilford, 2004

Koplewicz HS: *More Than Moody: Recognizing and Treating Adolescent Depression.* New York, Perigee, 2002

Last CG: *Help for Worried Kids: How Your Child Can Conquer Anxiety and Fear.* New York, Guilford, 2006

Lederman J, Fink C: *The Ups and Downs of Raising a Bipolar Child: A Survival Guide for Parents.* New York, Simon & Schuster, 2003

Lock J, LeGrange D: *Help Your Teenager Beat an Eating Disorder.* New York, Guilford, 2005

Manassis K: *Keys to Parenting Your Anxious Child.* Hauppage, NY, Barron's Educational Books, 1996

Manassis K, Levac AM: *Helping Your Teenager Beat Depression: A Problem-Solving Approach for Families.* Bethesda, MD, Woodbine House, 2004

Ozonoff S, Dawson G, McPartland J: *A Parent's Guide to Asperger Syndrome and High-Functioning Autism.* New York, Guilford, 2002

Parker HP: *The ADD Hyperactivity Handbook for Schools.* North Branch, MN, Specialty Press, 1991

Rapee RM, Spence S, Cobham V, et al: *Helping Your Anxious Child: A Step-by-Step Guide for Parents.* Oakland, CA, New Harbinger Publications, 2000

Rapoport JL: *The Boy Who Couldn't Stop Washing: The Experience and Treatment of Obsessive-Compulsive Disorder.* New York, Penguin Books, 1990

Shaw MA: *Your Anxious Child: Raising a Healthy Child in a Frightening World.* Arlington, TX, Tapestry Press, 2003

Szatmari P: *A Mind Apart: Understanding Children With Autism and Asperger Syndrome.* New York, Guilford, 2004

Walsh BT, Cameron VL: *If Your Adolescent Has an Eating Disorder.* New York, Oxford University Press, 2005

Wilens TE: *Straight Talk About Psychiatric Medications for Kids, Revised.* New York, Guilford, 2004

Zeigler Dendy CA: *Teenagers With ADD: A Parents' Guide.* Bethesda, MD, Woodbine House, 1995

Newsletters for Parents

The ADHD Report, Guilford Press, 72 Spring Street, New York, NY 10012; 1-800-365-7006; e-mail: news@guilford.com

Attention! The Magazine for Families and Adults With Attention-Deficit/Hyperactivity Disorder, CHADD, 8181 Professional Place, Suite 150, Landover, MD 20785; 1-301-306-7070; e-mail: attention@chadd.org

Information on the Internet

American Academy of Child and Adolescent Psychiatry (AACAP)
3615 Wisconsin Avenue, NW
Washington, DC 20016-3007
1-202-966-7300
www.aacap.org
Includes "Facts for Families," brief information sheets on a wide variety of topics in child and family development and mental health

American Academy of Pediatrics
www.aap.org

American Psychiatric Association
www.healthyminds.org

Anxiety Disorders Association of America (ADAA)
8730 Georgia Avenue, Suite 600
Silver Spring, MD 20910
1-240-485-1001
www.adaa.org

Autism Society of America
7910 Woodmont Avenue, Suite 300
Bethesda, MD 20814-3067
1-800-3-AUTISM
www.autism-society.org

Center for Mental Health Services (CMHS)
Information on child and adolescent mental health and on family mental health resources
www.mentalhealth.org

Child and Adolescent Bipolar Foundation
1000 Skokie Boulevard, Suite 425
Wilmette, IL 60091
1-847-256-8525
www.bpkids.org

Children and Adults with Attention-Deficit/Hyperactivity Disorder (CHADD)
8181 Professional Place, Suite 150
Landover, MD 20785
1-301-306-7070 (business)
1-800-233-4050 (National Resource Center)
www.chadd.org

Council of Educators for Students With Disabilities
13091 Pond Springs Road, Suite 300
Austin, TX 78729
1-512-219-5043
www.504idea.org

Depression and Bipolar Support Alliance
730 North Franklin Street, Suite 501
Chicago, IL 60610
1-800-826-3632 or 1-312-642-0049
www.dbsalliance.org

National Alliance on Mental Illness (NAMI)
Colonial Place Three
2107 Wilson Boulevard, Suite 300
Arlington, VA 22201
1-703-524-7600
1-800-950-NAMI (Information Helpline)
www.nami.org

National Institute of Mental Health
Public Information and Communications Branch
6001 Executive Boulevard
Room 8184, MSC 9663
Bethesda, MD 20892-9663
1-866-615-6464 or 1-301-443-4513
www.nimh.nih.gov

National Resource Center on AD/HD
A cooperative venture of CHADD and the Centers for Disease Control and Prevention
www.help4adhd.org/library.cfm

Online Asperger Syndrome Information and Support (OASIS)
www.aspergersyndrome.org

Parents Med Guide/Physicians Med Guide
Guides offering practical advice to parents of children and adolescents struggling with depression and information to general practitioners and pediatricians on pediatric depression treatment alternatives and the latest science.
www.ParentsMedGuide.org

The Annenberg Foundation Trust at Sunnylands Adolescent Mental Health Initiative
MindZone—a mental health site for teens
www.CopeCareDeal.org

Tourette Syndrome Association
42-40 Bell Boulevard
Bayside, NY 11361
1-718-224-2999
www.tsa-usa.org

About the CD-ROM

The medication information handouts, resource lists, and appendices are included on the enclosed CD-ROM in Adobe's Portable Document Format (PDF). The PDF files are essentially pictures of the book pages, and they will allow you to view and print the forms exactly as they appear in the book. You need Adobe's Acrobat Reader 5.0.5 or higher to view and print the PDF files; if Acrobat or Adobe Reader is not already installed on your computer, the CD-ROM will prompt you to install this free program. (Adobe Reader 7.0 is included on the CD-ROM.) Please note that you can only view and print the PDF files with the Acrobat Reader; you cannot modify them.

Minimum System Requirements—Adobe® Reader® 7.0

Windows

- Intel® Pentium® processor
- Microsoft® Windows 2000 with Service Pack 2, Windows XP Professional or Home Edition, or Windows XP Tablet PC Edition
- 128MB of RAM
- Up to 90MB of available hard-disk space
- Microsoft Internet Explorer 5 or higher

Macintosh

- PowerPC® G3 processor
- Mac OS X v.10.2.8 or 10.3
- Up to 35MB of RAM
- Up to 125MB of available hard-disk space

Getting Started

Windows

Insert the CD-ROM into your compact disc drive. The disc will AutoRun and will check to see whether Acrobat Reader 5.0.5 or higher, which is needed to open and view the files on the CD-ROM, is already present on your computer. If Acrobat Reader is *not* present, you will be prompted to install Adobe Reader 7.0 (or 6.0 if your system is not compatible with 7.0). If Acrobat or Adobe Reader is present, you'll be presented with four choices:

- **View Main Menu**—Select this option to access the handouts from the CD-ROM. Remember that you'll need to reinsert the CD-ROM each time you want to access the handouts.
- **Continue searching for another version of Acrobat**—Select this option to change the version of Acrobat your system uses, if you are running more than one version.

- **Install Adobe Reader 7.0**—Select this option if AutoRun alerts you that the correct version of Acrobat Reader is not installed on your computer.
- **Install files to hard drive**—Select this option if you would like to install the handouts to your hard drive, instead of accessing them from the CD-ROM. You'll be asked to accept the default subdirectory for the handout files or to change to another subdirectory. Once the files are copied, double-click on **Start.pdf** from the subdirectory you specified to access the handouts.

The CD-ROM uses an AutoRun feature and should start automatically when inserted into your drive. If the disc does not start automatically, or if AutoRun is disabled on your computer, from your Windows Desktop choose **Start,** then **Run,** then type the following command line: x:\autorun.exe, where x represents the drive letter for your CD-ROM drive.

Macintosh OS X

Insert the CD-ROM into your compact disc drive. The disc will open to display four choices (icons):

- **Read Me**—Double-click on this icon to view the installation instructions.
- **Install Adobe Reader 7.0**—Double-click on this icon if Adobe Reader 7.0 or higher is not already installed on your computer.
- **Start.PDF**—Double-click on this icon to access the handouts from the CD-ROM. Remember that you'll need to reinsert the CD-ROM each time you want to access the handouts.
- **Install files to hard drive**—Double-click on this icon if you would like to install the handouts to your hard drive, instead of accessing them from the CD-ROM. You'll be asked to accept the default subdirectory for the handout files or to change to another subdirectory. Once the files are copied, double-click on **Start.pdf** from the subdirectory you specified to access the handouts.

Macintosh OS 9

Insert the CD-ROM into your compact disc drive. The disc will open to display two choices (icons):

- **Read Me**—Double-click on this icon to view the installation instructions.
- **Mac OS Classic**—Double-click on this icon to open the folder with the Mac OS 9 files and indexes.

  The Mac OS Classic folder will list the following two choices (icons):

- **Start.PDF**—Double-click on this icon to access the handouts from the CD-ROM. Remember that you'll need to reinsert the CD-ROM each time you want to access the handouts.
- **Install files to hard drive**—Double-click on this icon if you would like to install the handouts to your hard drive, instead of accessing them from the CD-ROM. You'll be asked to accept the default subdirectory for the handout files or to change to another subdirectory. Once the files are copied, double-click on **Start.pdf** from the subdirectory you specified to access the handouts.

Technical Support

Technical support is available:
  7 A.M. to 1 A.M. (EST) Monday through Friday
  8 A.M. to 8 P.M. (EST) Saturday and Sunday
  Contact:
  Telephone: (888) 266-9544
  E-mail:appisupport@romnet.com

Alprazolam—Xanax, Intensol, Niravam

General Information About Medication

Each child and adolescent is different. No one has exactly the same combination of medical and psychological problems. It is a good idea to talk with the doctor or nurse about the reasons a medicine is being used. It is very important to keep all appointments and to be in touch by telephone if you have concerns. It is important to communicate with the doctor, nurse, or therapist.

It is very important that the medicine be taken exactly as the doctor instructs. However, once in a while, everyone forgets to give a medicine on time. It is a good idea to ask the doctor or nurse what to do if this happens. Do not stop or change a medicine without asking the doctor or nurse first.

If the medicine seems to stop working, it may be because it is not being taken regularly. The youth may be "cheeking" or hiding the medicine or forgetting to take it (especially at school). The doses may be too far apart, or a different dose may be needed. Something at school at home, or in the neighborhood may be upsetting the youth, or he or she may need special help for learning disabilities or tutoring. Please discuss your concerns with the doctor. **Do not just increase the dose.**

All medicines should be kept in a safe place, out of the reach of children, and should be supervised by an adult. If someone takes too much of a medicine, call the doctor, the poison control center, or a hospital emergency room.

Each medicine has a "generic" or chemical name. Just like laundry detergents or paper towels, some medicines are sold by more than one company under different brand names. The same medicine may be available under a generic name and several brand names. The generic medications are usually less expensive than the brand name ones. The generic medications have the same chemical formula, but they may or may not be exactly the same strength as the brand-name medications. Also, some brands of pills contain dye that can cause allergic reactions. It is a good idea to talk to the doctor and the pharmacist about whether it is important to use a specific brand of medicine.

All medicines can cause an allergic reaction. Examples are hives, itching, rashes, swelling, and trouble breathing. Even a tiny amount of a medicine can cause a reaction in patients who are allergic to that medicine. Be *sure* to talk to the doctor before restarting a medicine that has caused an allergic reaction.

Taking more than one medicine at the same time may cause more side effects or cause one of the medicines to not work as well. Always ask the doctor, nurse, or pharmacist before adding another medicine, whether prescription or over-the-counter. Be sure that each doctor knows about *all* of the medicines your child is taking. Also tell the doctor about any vitamins, herbal medicines, or supplements your child may be taking. Some of these may have side effects alone or when taken with this medication.

Everyone taking medicine should have a physical examination at least once a year.

If you suspect the youth is using drugs or alcohol, please tell the doctor right away.

Pregnancy requires special care in the use of medicine. Please tell the doctor immediately if you suspect the teenager is pregnant or might become pregnant.

1

Printed information like this applies to children and adolescents in general. If you have questions about the medicine, or if you notice changes or anything unusual, please ask the doctor or nurse. As scientific research advances, knowledge increases and advice changes. Even experts do not always agree. Many medicines have not been approved by the U.S. Food and Drug Administration (FDA) for use in children. For this reason, use of the medicine for a particular problem or age group often is not listed in the *Physicians' Desk Reference*. This does not necessarily mean that the medicine is dangerous or does not work, only that the company that makes the medicine has not received permission to advertise the medicine for use in children. Companies often do not apply for this permission because it is expensive to do the tests needed to apply for approval for use in children. Once a medication is approved by the FDA for any purpose, a doctor is allowed to prescribe it according to research and clinical experience.

Note to Teachers

It is a good idea to talk with the parent(s) about the reason(s) that a medication is being used. If the parent(s) sign consent to release information, it is often helpful to talk with the doctor. If the parent(s) give permission, the doctor may ask you to fill out rating forms about your experience with the student's behavior, feelings, academic performance, and medication side effects. This information is very useful in selecting and monitoring medication treatment. If you have observations that you think are important, do not hesitate to share these with the student's parent(s) and treating clinicians.

It is very important that the medicine be taken exactly as the doctor instructs. However, everyone forgets to give a medicine on time once in a while. It is a good idea to ask the parent(s) in advance what to do if this happens. Do not stop or change the time you are giving a medicine at school without parental permission. If a medication is to be taken with food, but lunchtime or snack time changes, be sure to notify the parent(s) so appropriate adjustments can be made.

All medicines should be kept in a secure place and should be supervised by an adult. If someone takes too much of a medicine, follow your school procedure for an urgent medical problem.

Taking medicine is a private matter and is best managed discreetly and confidentially. It is important to be sensitive to the student's feelings about taking medicine.

If you suspect that the student is using drugs or alcohol, please tell the parent(s) or a school counselor right away.

Please tell the parent(s) or school nurse if you suspect medication side effects.

Modifications of the classroom environment or assignments may be useful in addition to medication. The student may need to be evaluated for additional help or for an Individualized Education Plan for learning or behavior.

Any expression of suicidal thoughts or feelings or self-harm by a child or adolescent is a clear signal of distress and should be taken seriously. These behaviors should not be dismissed as "attention seeking."

What Is Alprazolam (Xanax, Intensol, Niravam)?

Alprazolam is a *benzodiazepine* or *antianxiety* medicine. It used to be called a *minor tranquilizer*. It is sometimes called an *anxiolytic* or *sedative*. It comes in Xanax brand name and generic immediate-release tablets, Xanax XR extended-release tablets, Intensol liquid, and Niravam orally disintegrating tablets.

How Can This Medicine Help?

Alprazolam can decrease anxiety, nervousness, fears, and excessive worrying. It can help anxious people to be calm enough to learn—with therapy and practice (exposure to feared things or situations)—to understand and tolerate their worries or fears and even to overcome them. People with generalized anxiety disorder, social phobia, posttraumatic stress disorder (PTSD), or panic disorder can be helped by alprazolam. Most often, it is used for a short time when symptoms are very uncomfortable or frightening or when they make it hard to do important things such as go to school. Alprazolam can decrease the severe physical symptoms (rapid heartbeat, trouble breathing, dizziness, sweating) of panic attacks and phobias.

Alprazolam also can be used for sleep problems, such as night terrors (sudden waking up from sleep with great fear) or sleepwalking, when these problems put the youth at risk of an accident or make it impossible for other family members to get enough sleep. Alprazolam can help with insomnia (difficulty falling asleep) when used for a short time along with a behavioral program.

Sometimes alprazolam is used for a few days to treat agitation in mania or psychosis until other medicines start to work.

Occasionally the benzodiazepines are used to reduce the side effects of other medicines.

How Does This Medicine Work?

Alprazolam works by calming the parts of the brain that are too excitable in anxious people. The medicine does this by working on receptors (special places on brain cells) in certain parts of the brain to change the action of GABA—a neurotransmitter—a chemical that the brain makes for brain cells to communicate with each other.

How Long Does This Medicine Last?

Alprazolam usually needs to be taken three times a day. The extended-release tablets may be taken only once a day. For acute symptoms of anxiety or agitation, it can be taken occasionally, as needed. When used for sleep, it is taken at bedtime. There may still be some effects in the morning.

How Will the Doctor Monitor This Medicine?

The doctor will review your child's medical history and physical examination before starting alprazolam. The doctor may order some blood or urine tests or an ECG (electrocardiogram or heart rhythm test) to be sure your child does not have a hidden medical condition. The doctor or nurse may measure your child's height, weight, pulse, and blood pressure before starting alprazolam.

After the medicine is started, the doctor will want to have regular appointments with you and your child to see how the medicine is working, to see if a dose change is needed, to watch for side effects, to see if alprazolam is still needed, and to see if any other treatment is needed. The doctor or nurse may check your child's height, weight, pulse, and blood pressure.

What Side Effects Can This Medicine Have?

Any medicine can have side effects, including an allergy to the medicine. Because each patient is different, the doctor will monitor the youth closely, especially when the medicine is started. The doctor will work with you to increase the positive effects and decrease the negative effects of the medicine. Please tell the doctor if any of the listed side effects appear or if you think that the medicine is causing any other problems. Not all of the rare or unusual side effects are listed.

Side effects are most common after starting the medicine or after a dose increase. Many side effects can be avoided or lessened by starting with a very low dose and increasing it slowly—ask the doctor.

Allergic Reaction

Tell the doctor in a day or two (if possible, before the next dose of medicine):

- Hives
- Itching
- Rash

Stop the medicine and get *immediate* medical care:

- Trouble breathing or chest tightness
- Swelling of lips, tongue, or throat

Alprazolam is usually very safe when used for short periods as the doctor prescribes.

The most common side effect is daytime sleepiness. Alprazolam can also cause dizziness, feeling "spacey," or decreased coordination. If the medicine is causing any of these problems it is very important not to drive a car, ride a bicycle or motorcycle, or operate machinery.

Alprazolam can cause decreased concentration and memory. These problems, along with daytime sleepiness, may decrease learning and performance in school.

People who take alprazolam must not drink alcohol. Severe sleepiness or even loss of consciousness may result.

It is possible to become psychologically and physically dependent on alprazolam, but that is not a common problem for patients who see their doctors regularly. Because some people abuse benzodiazepines, it is illegal to give or sell these medicines to someone other than the patient for whom they were prescribed.

Very rarely, alprazolam causes excitement, irritability, anger, aggression, trouble sleeping, nightmares, uncontrollable behavior, or memory loss. This is called *disinhibition* or a *paradoxical effect*. Stop the medicine and call the doctor if this happens.

Some Interactions With Other Medicines or Food

Please note that the following are only the most likely interactions with food or other medicines.

Alprazolam may be taken with or without food.

Grapefruit juice can increase the levels of alprazolam and increase side effects.

Antibiotics such as erythromycin, oral antifungal agents such as ketoconazole, oral contraceptives (birth control pills), fluoxetine (Prozac), fluvoxamine (Luvox), propranolol (Inderal), valproate (Depakote), and other medicines may increase the levels of alprazolam and increase side effects, especially sedation.

Antacids, carbamazepine (Tegretol), theophylline, and St. John's wort can decrease the positive effects of alprazolam.

It is important not to use other sedatives, tranquilizers, sleeping pills, or antihistamines (such as Benadryl) when taking alprazolam because of greatly increased side effects.

It is better to limit drinks with caffeine (coffee, tea, soft drinks) because caffeine works in the opposite way from this medicine, and the positive effects might be decreased.

What Could Happen If This Medicine Is Stopped Suddenly?

Many medicines cause problems if stopped suddenly. Alprazolam must be decreased slowly (tapered) rather than stopped suddenly. When alprazolam is stopped suddenly, there are withdrawal symptoms that are uncomfortable and may even be dangerous. Problems are more likely in patients taking high doses of alprazolam for 2 months or longer, but even after taking alprazolam for just a few weeks it is important to stop it slowly. Withdrawal symptoms may include anxiety, irritability, shaking, sweating, aches and pains, muscle cramps, vomiting, confusion, and trouble sleeping. If large doses taken for a long time are stopped suddenly, seizures (fits, convulsions), hallucinations (hearing voices or seeing things that are not there), or out-of-control behavior may result.

How Long Will This Medicine Be Needed?

Alprazolam is usually prescribed for only a few weeks to allow the patient to be calm enough to learn new ways to cope with anxiety and to allow the nervous system to become less excitable. Sometimes antianxiety medicines are used for longer periods to treat panic attacks or anxiety that remains after therapy is completed. Each person is unique, and some people may need these medicines for months or years.

What Else Should I Know About This Medicine?

Because benzodiazepines can be abused (especially by people who abuse alcohol or drugs) and can cause psychological dependence or physical dependence (addiction), they are regulated by special state and federal laws as *controlled substances*. These laws place limitations on telephone prescriptions and refills.

Sometimes alprazolam (Xanax) and lorazepam (Ativan) get mixed up; be sure to check the prescription.

People with sleep apnea (breathing stops while they are asleep) should not take alprazolam. Tell the doctor if your child snores very loudly.

Alprazolam should be avoided during pregnancy, especially in the first 3 months, because it may cause birth defects in the baby. If taken regularly at the end of pregnancy, alprazolam may cause withdrawal symptoms in the baby.

Notes

Use this space to take notes or to write down questions you want to ask the doctor.

_____

_____

_____

_____

_____

_____

_____

_____

_____

_____

_____

_____

_____

Medication Information
for Youth

Alprazolam—Xanax, Intensol, Niravam

What the Medicine Is Called and What It Is For

The name of your medicine may be confusing. Most drugs have two names: 1) a scientific name that we call a *generic name* and 2) a trade or *brand name*. The generic name of this medicine is alprazolam. The brand name is Xanax.

Alprazolam is a *benzodiazepine* or *antianxiety* medicine. It works by calming the parts of the brain that are too excitable in anxious people. It can decrease anxiety, nervousness, fears, and excessive worrying. Alprazolam can decrease the physical symptoms (rapid heartbeat, trouble breathing, dizziness, sweating) of panic attacks and phobias. It can help anxious people to be calm enough to learn—with therapy and practice—to understand and tolerate their worries or fears and even to overcome them. Your doctor may have told you that you have a condition such as social phobia, generalized anxiety disorder, separation anxiety disorder, posttraumatic stress disorder (PTSD), or panic disorder. Most often, this medicine is used for a short time when symptoms are very uncomfortable or frightening or when they make it hard to do important things such as go to school.

Alprazolam also can be used for sleep problems, such as night terrors (sudden waking up from sleep with great fear) or sleepwalking. Alprazolam can help with insomnia (difficulty falling asleep) when used for a short time along with routines that help you to relax and fall asleep.

Sometimes alprazolam is used for a few days to treat agitation in mania or psychosis until other medicines start to work.

Occasionally alprazolam is used to reduce the side effects of other medicines.

How You Take the Medicine

It is very important to take the medicine exactly as the doctor or nurse tells you. Do not skip doses or take extra medicine without asking an adult. If you forget a dose, ask your parent(s) what to do.

It is not a good idea to drink a lot of grapefruit juice while on this medicine, because it can increase side effects.

It is better to limit drinks with caffeine (coffee, tea, soft drinks) because caffeine works in the opposite way from this medicine, and the positive effects might be decreased.

This medicine is prescribed only for you. It should never be shared with anyone else.

You do not have to tell others that you are taking this medicine, but it is not something you should feel ashamed or embarrassed about. Many young people are helped by alprazolam. You should talk to your doctor or nurse about any questions you have about the medicine. It is important to remember that the medicine *helps* you. It cannot *make* you do anything or change you as a person.

7

Many medicines cause problems if stopped suddenly. Always ask your doctor before stopping a medicine. Problems are more likely to happen in patients taking high doses of alprazolam for 2 months or longer, but it is important to decrease the medicine slowly (taper) even after a few weeks. If you notice anxiety, irritability, shaking, sweating, aches and pains, muscle cramps, vomiting, or trouble sleeping, you may need to decrease the medicine more slowly. If large doses are stopped suddenly, seizures (fits, convulsions), hallucinations (hearing voices or seeing things that are not there), or out-of-control behavior may result.

How Your Doctor Will Follow Your Progress

Before giving you the medicine, your doctor or nurse will talk with you and your parent(s) and may measure your height, weight, heart rate (pulse), and blood pressure.

Be sure to tell your doctor or nurse about any other medicines or supplements you are taking, including vitamins, herbs, or aids to weight loss or bodybuilding. Also be sure to tell the doctor or nurse if you are using alcohol or drugs. Because many medicines may affect babies, it is very important to tell the doctor if you might be pregnant or if you are at risk of becoming pregnant.

Your teachers may be asked to fill out a form about your grades and behavior in school. A psychologist may give you some tests to see how you learn best.

Most doctors have regular appointments with young people who are taking medicine. You should use these visits to share any concerns you may have about your medicine and to talk about if it has helped you. From time to time, your physician or nurse may measure your height, weight, heart rate (pulse), and blood pressure to be sure that you are in good health while you are taking the medicine. Your doctor also will ask for regular reports from your parent(s) and maybe from your teachers (with your permission) to see how well the medicine is working.

Alprazolam is usually prescribed for only a few weeks to allow you to be calm enough to learn new ways to cope with anxiety and to allow your nervous system to become less excitable. Sometimes antianxiety medicines are used for longer periods to treat panic attacks or anxiety that remain after therapy is completed. Each person is unique, and some people may need these medicines for months or years.

How the Medicine Might Affect You

In addition to the ways the medicine can help you, it may have other effects called *side effects*. Different medicines have different side effects. It is helpful to know about some of the most common side effects of your medicine so that you will understand what they are if they happen. Some people do not have any side effects. Some side effects are just uncomfortable, but others may mean a more serious problem with the medicine. Side effects are most common after starting the medicine or after a dose increase. They may go away with time, or the medicine can be adjusted or changed—ask the doctor.

You could have an allergy to any medicine, which might show up as a rash on your skin, swelling, itching, or trouble breathing.

Please tell your parent(s) and your doctor or nurse about any changes that you notice after taking the medicine. It is especially important to tell a responsible adult if you are feeling depressed or that you may not want to live; if you have thoughts of hurting yourself; or if you begin to feel more irritable, nervous, or restless.

The most common side effect of alprazolam is daytime sleepiness. If this medicine is making you sleepy, it is very important not to drive a car or ride a bicycle or motorcycle. After starting alprazolam or increasing the dose, please be extra careful when driving a car, riding a bike, or using machines until you can tell how the medicine affects your alertness, attention, and coordination.

Sometimes antianxiety medicines seem to work in the opposite way, causing excitement, irritability, anger, aggression, and other problems. If this happens, tell your parent(s) or your doctor.

Drinking alcohol while taking this medicine can cause severe drowsiness or even passing out. **Don't do it!** Do not use marijuana or street drugs while taking this medicine. They can cause serious side effects. Skipping your medicine to take drugs does not work because many medicines can stay in your body for a long time.

Alprazolam can be habit-forming, but that is not a common problem for people who take their medicine as the doctor says.

Notes

Use this space to take notes or to write down questions you want to ask the doctor or nurse.

_____

_____

_____

_____

_____

_____

_____

_____

_____

_____

_____

From Dulcan MK (editor): *Helping Parents, Youth, and Teachers Understand Medications for Behavioral and Emotional Problems: A Resource Book of Medication Information Handouts*, Third Edition. Washington, DC, American Psychiatric Publishing, 2007

Medication Information for Parents and Teachers

Amphetamine—Dexedrine, DextroStat, Adderall

General Information About Medication

Each child and adolescent is different. No one has exactly the same combination of medical and psychological problems. It is a good idea to talk with the doctor or nurse about the reasons a medicine is being used. It is very important to keep all appointments and to be in touch by telephone if you have concerns. It is important to communicate with the doctor, nurse, or therapist.

It is very important that the medicine be taken exactly as the doctor instructs. However, once in a while, everyone forgets to give a medicine on time. It is a good idea to ask the doctor or nurse what to do if this happens. Do not stop or change a medicine without asking the doctor or nurse first.

If the medicine seems to stop working, it may be because it is not being taken regularly. The youth may be "cheeking" or hiding the medicine or forgetting to take it (especially at school). The doses may be too far apart, or a different dose may be needed. Something at school, at home, or in the neighborhood may be upsetting the youth, or he or she may need special help for learning disabilities or tutoring. Please discuss your concerns with the doctor. **Do not just increase the dose.**

All medicines should be kept in a safe place, out of the reach of children, and should be supervised by an adult. If someone takes too much of a medicine, call the doctor, the poison control center, or a hospital emergency room.

Each medicine has a "generic" or chemical name. Just like laundry detergents or paper towels, some medicines are sold by more than one company under different brand names. The same medicine may be available under a generic name and several brand names. The generic medications are usually less expensive than the brand name ones. The generic medications have the same chemical formula, but they may or may not be exactly the same strength as the brand-name medications. Also, some brands of pills contain dye that can cause allergic reactions. It is a good idea to talk to the doctor and the pharmacist about whether it is important to use a specific brand of medicine.

All medicines can cause an allergic reaction. Examples are hives, itching, rashes, swelling, and trouble breathing. Even a tiny amount of a medicine can cause a reaction in patients who are allergic to that medicine. Be *sure* to talk to the doctor before restarting a medicine that has caused an allergic reaction.

Taking more than one medicine at the same time may cause more side effects or cause one of the medicines to not work as well. Always ask the doctor, nurse, or pharmacist before adding another medicine, whether prescription or over-the-counter. Be sure that each doctor knows about *all* of the medicines your child is taking. Also tell the doctor about any vitamins, herbal medicines, or supplements your child may be taking. Some of these may have side effects alone or when taken with this medication.

Everyone taking medicine should have a physical examination at least once a year.

If you suspect the youth is using drugs or alcohol, please tell the doctor right away.

11

Pregnancy requires special care in the use of medicine. Please tell the doctor immediately if you suspect the teenager is pregnant or might become pregnant.

Printed information like this applies to children and adolescents in general. If you have questions about the medicine, or if you notice changes or anything unusual, please ask the doctor or nurse. As scientific research advances, knowledge increases and advice changes. Even experts do not always agree. Many medicines have not been approved by the U.S. Food and Drug Administration (FDA) for use in children. For this reason, use of the medicine for a particular problem or age group often is not listed in the *Physicians' Desk Reference*. This does not necessarily mean that the medicine is dangerous or does not work, only that the company that makes the medicine has not received permission to advertise the medicine for use in children. Companies often do not apply for this permission because it is expensive to do the tests needed to apply for approval for use in children. Once a medication is approved by the FDA for any purpose, a doctor is allowed to prescribe it according to research and clinical experience.

Note to Teachers

It is a good idea to talk with the parent(s) about the reason(s) that a medication is being used. If the parent(s) sign consent to release information, it is often helpful to talk with the doctor. If the parent(s) give permission, the doctor may ask you to fill out rating forms about your experience with the student's behavior, feelings, academic performance, and medication side effects. This information is very useful in selecting and monitoring medication treatment. If you have observations that you think are important, do not hesitate to share these with the student's parent(s) and treating clinicians.

It is very important that the medicine be taken exactly as the doctor instructs. However, everyone forgets to give a medicine on time once in a while. It is a good idea to ask the parent(s) in advance what to do if this happens. Do not stop or change the time you are giving a medicine at school without parental permission. If a medication is to be taken with food, but lunchtime or snack time changes, be sure to notify the parent(s) so appropriate adjustments can be made.

All medicines should be kept in a secure place and should be supervised by an adult. If someone takes too much of a medicine, follow your school procedure for an urgent medical problem.

Taking medicine is a private matter and is best managed discreetly and confidentially. It is important to be sensitive to the student's feelings about taking medicine.

If you suspect that the student is using drugs or alcohol, please tell the parent(s) or a school counselor right away.

Please tell the parent(s) or school nurse if you suspect medication side effects.

Modifications of the classroom environment or assignments may be useful in addition to medication. The student may need to be evaluated for additional help or for an Individualized Education Plan for learning or behavior.

Any expression of suicidal thoughts or feelings or self-harm by a child or adolescent is a clear signal of distress and should be taken seriously. These behaviors should not be dismissed as "attention seeking."

What Is Amphetamine (Dexedrine, DextroStat, Adderall)?

Amphetamine is called a *stimulant*. It is used to treat attention-deficit/hyperactivity disorder (ADHD or ADD), whether the person has hyperactivity (increased moving around) or not. It comes in a generic form and several brand name formulations (see table below). Although all of these medicines have amphetamine as the active ingredient, they are made differently, so that there are many different ways to take amphetamine. This helps the doctor to find just the right form of the medicine for each person.

Generic and brand name formulations

Short-acting, or immediate-release dextroamphetamine (3–5 hours)
    Generic dextroamphetamine
    Dexedrine
    DextroStat
Long-acting dextroamphetamine (6–8 hours)
    Dexedrine Spansule (capsule with particles)
    Dextroamphetamine ER (extended-release)
Mixed amphetamine salts
    Generic mixed amphetamine salts (immediate-release only) (3–5 hours)
    Adderall (immediate-release, short-acting) (3–5 hours)
    Adderall XR (extended-release, very long-acting; capsule with beads—may be sprinkled on food)
        (10–12 hours)

How Can This Medicine Help?

Amphetamine can increase attention and the ability to follow instructions. It can improve attention span, decrease distractibility, increase the ability to finish things, decrease hyperactivity, and improve the ability to think before acting (decrease impulsivity). Handwriting and completion of schoolwork and homework can improve. Amphetamine can improve willingness to follow directions and decrease stubbornness in youngsters with both ADHD and oppositional defiant disorder (ODD).

Many people with Tourette's disorder (chronic motor and vocal tics) also have symptoms of ADHD. Amphetamine may be used cautiously to reduce these symptoms of hyperactivity, impulsivity, and trouble paying attention and usually does not make the tics worse. If the tics get worse, talk with your child's doctor. Lowering the dose or stopping the amphetamine will usually lead to the tics decreasing again. Tics also increase and decrease for a lot of reasons that are not related to medicine.

Medicine may not remove all symptoms in children with ADHD. These children may also need special help in school and behavior modification at home and at school. Some youngsters and families are helped by family therapy or group social skills therapy.

Stimulant medicines last for different amounts of time. ADHD symptoms may come back when the medicine wears off. This does not mean the medicine is not working but that longer coverage may be needed.

Amphetamine is also used to help people with narcolepsy (sudden and uncontrollable episodes of deep sleep) to stay awake.

How Does This Medicine Work?

In people who have ADHD or ADD, parts of the brain are not working as well as they should. An example would be the part that controls impulsive actions ("the brakes"). Amphetamine helps these parts of the brain work better by acting as a stimulant, increasing the activity of neurotransmitters—mostly *dopamine* but also *norepinephrine*. *Neurotransmitters* are the chemicals that the brain makes for the nerve cells to communicate with each other.

Amphetamine is not a tranquilizer or sedative. It works in the same way in children and adults and in people with or without ADHD.

Methylphenidate and amphetamine are both stimulant medicines, but they work in different ways on the neurotransmitters. A person with ADHD might be helped by one stimulant but not the other, so if one is not working, the doctor may try the other one.

How Long Does This Medicine Last?

All types of amphetamine start working in 30–60 minutes after taking them. Different forms last for different lengths of time. The immediate-release or short-acting forms last for 3–5 hours. The long-acting forms of dextroamphetamine last for 6–8 hours. Adderall XR lasts for 10–12 hours. The length of time is different for different people, and the medicine may work longer for some symptoms than for others. An advantage of the longer-acting forms is that they do not have to be given during the school day.

How Will the Doctor Monitor This Medicine?

The doctor will review your child's medical history and physical examination before starting amphetamine. The doctor may order some blood or urine tests to be sure your child does not have a hidden medical condition. Be sure to tell the doctor if your child or anyone in the family has had heart problems, irregular heartbeat (pulse), high blood pressure (hypertension), dizziness, fainting, shortness of breath, or severe tiredness. Tell the doctor if anyone in the family has died suddenly. People who have a history of heart problems generally should not take amphetamine. Also tell the doctor if your child or anyone in the family has had motor or vocal tics (hard-to-control repeated movements or sounds) or Tourette's disorder (also called Tourette's syndrome). The doctor or nurse will measure your child's height, weight, pulse, and blood pressure before starting the medicine. The doctor will usually ask parents and teachers to fill out behavior rating scales (checklists).

After the medicine is started, the doctor will want to have regular appointments with you and your child to see how the medicine is working, to see if a dose change is needed, to watch for side effects, to see if amphetamine is still needed, and to see if any other treatment is needed. The doctor or nurse may check your child's height, weight, pulse, and blood pressure. With parental permission, the doctor will usually ask for reports (rating scale, checklist, testing results, comments) from the teacher(s) to keep track of progress in learning and behavior. Some young people take the medicine three or four times a day, every day. Others need to take it only once or twice a day or only on school days. You and your child's doctor will work out the doses and timing and type of medicine that is best for your child and his or her symptoms and schedule.

What Side Effects Can This Medicine Have?

Any medicine can have side effects, including an allergy to the medicine. Because each patient is different, the doctor will monitor the youth closely, especially when the medicine is started. The doctor will work with you to increase the positive effects and decrease the negative effects of the medicine. Please tell the doctor if any of the listed side effects appear or if you think that the medicine is causing any other problems. Not all of the rare or unusual side effects are listed.

Side effects are most common after starting the medicine or after a dose increase. Many side effects can be avoided or lessened by starting with a very low dose and increasing it slowly—ask the doctor.

Allergic Reaction

Tell the doctor in a day or two (if possible, before the next dose of medicine):

- Hives
- Itching
- Rash

Stop the medicine and get *immediate* medical care:

- Trouble breathing or chest tightness
- Swelling of lips, tongue, or throat

Common Side Effects

If the following side effects do not go away after about 2 weeks, ask the doctor about lowering your child's dose:

- Lack of appetite and weight loss—Encourage your child to eat a good breakfast and afternoon and evening snacks; give medicine during or after meals.
- Insomnia (trouble falling asleep)—This may be the ADHD coming back and not a side effect. Talk with your child's doctor. Changing the time or dose of medicine, starting a bedtime routine, or adding another medicine may help.
- Headaches
- Stomachaches
- Irritability, crankiness, crying, emotional sensitivity
- Loss of interest in friends
- Staring into space
- Rapid pulse rate (heartbeat) or increased blood pressure

Less Common Side Effects

Tell the doctor within a week or two if you notice:

- Rebound—As the medicine wears off, hyperactivity or bad mood may get worse than before the medicine was taken. The doctor can make adjustments to help this problem.
- Slowing of growth—This is why your child's height and weight are checked regularly; if this is a problem, growth usually catches up if the medicine is stopped or the dose is decreased.
- Nervous habits—Examples are picking at skin or biting nails (although these habits are also common in children with ADHD who do not take medicine).
- Stuttering

Rare, but Serious, Side Effects

Call the doctor within a day or two:

- Motor or vocal tics (fast, repeated movements or sounds) or muscle twitches (jerking movements) of parts of the body
- Sadness that lasts more than a few days
- Auditory, visual, or tactile hallucinations (hearing, seeing, or feeling things that are not there)
- Any behavior that is very unusual for your child

Some Interactions With Other Medicines or Food

Please note that the following are only the most likely interactions with food or other medicines.

Caffeine may increase side effects.

Amphetamine may be taken with or without food. Very acid juices (like grapefruit or tomato) or vitamin C may decrease levels of amphetamine so that it does not work as well.

It is not a good idea to combine stimulants with nasal decongestants or cough and cold medicines that contain ingredients such as pseudoephedrine or phenylpropanolamine, because rapid pulse rate (heartbeat) or high blood pressure may develop. If a stuffy nose is really troublesome, it is better to use a nasal spray. Check with the pharmacist before giving an over-the-counter medicine. Also, many children with ADHD become cranky or more hyperactive while taking antihistamines (such as Benadryl). If medicine for allergies is needed, ask your child's doctor.

Using amphetamine together with imipramine (Tofranil) or nortriptyline (Pamelor) may be dangerous because these combinations increase the risk of serious heart problems.

Amphetamine should not be taken at the same time as or even within a month of taking another type of medicine called a *monoamine oxidase inhibitor* (MAOI), such as Eldepryl (selegiline), Nardil (phenelzine), Parnate (tranylcypromine), or Marplan (isocarboxazid). The combination could cause dangerous high blood pressure.

What Could Happen if This Medicine Is Stopped Suddenly?

No medical withdrawal effects occur if amphetamine is stopped suddenly. The ADHD symptoms will come back as soon as the medicine wears off. Some people may have irritability, trouble sleeping, or increased hyperactivity for a day or two if they have been taking the medicine every day for a long time, especially at high doses. It may be better to decrease the medicine slowly (taper) over a week or so.

How Long Will This Medicine Be Needed?

There is no way to know how long a person will need to take amphetamine. The parent(s), the doctor, and the school will work together to determine what is right for each patient. Sometimes the medicine is needed for a few years, but many people need to take medicine for ADHD even as adults.

What Else Should I Know About This Medicine?

Many people have incorrect information about stimulants. If you hear anything that worries you, please check with your doctor.

Unlike methylphenidate, amphetamines are FDA approved for children younger than 6 years old. This is a historical accident that happened as rules changed for approval of medicines. There is actually less research on using amphetamines for ADHD in young children than there is for methylphenidate.

Stimulants do not *cause* drug use or addiction. However, because the patient or other people (especially if they have a history of drug abuse) may abuse these medicines, adult supervision is especially important. Some teenagers may try to sell or share their medicine, so it should be kept in a secure place and given by an adult.

16

Amphetamine will not help people who do not have ADHD to get better grades or do better on tests, but some people think that it will, so they try to take someone else's medicine.

The government considers amphetamine to be a *controlled substance*. There are special rules for how much of this medicine may be prescribed at one time and how soon prescriptions must be filled after they are written. Prescriptions may not have refills and may not be telephoned to the pharmacy. The doctor must write a new prescription for stimulants each time, and prescriptions may not be written with a date in the future. Prescriptions may be mailed or picked up at the doctor's office.

It is important for the child *not* to chew the long-acting tablets because doing so releases too much medicine all at once. For children who cannot swallow pills, the capsule forms may be opened and the tiny beads inside sprinkled onto a spoonful of applesauce. The mixture of applesauce and medicine should be swallowed without chewing. The beads should not be mixed in liquid. The medicine should not be mixed into food and stored.

Some of these medicines have similar names but have different strengths or last different amounts of time (for example, Adderall and Adderall XR). Be sure to check your prescription to be sure you have the correct medicine from the pharmacy.

Questions have been raised after a very small number of people died suddenly while taking amphetamine. Clearly, amphetamine in very high doses can be dangerous. However, the chance of sudden death when taking amphetamine as prescribed by a doctor is not higher than without medication. In most of the deaths, problems in the shape, size, or rhythm of the heart were found that were not related to the amphetamine use. Be sure to tell the doctor if your child or anyone in the family has had heart problems or if a family member died suddenly.

Notes

Use this space to take notes or to write down questions you want to ask the doctor.

_____

_____

_____

_____

_____

_____

_____

_____

_____

_____

_____

_____

_____

Medication Information for Youth

Amphetamine—Dexedrine, DextroStat, Adderall

What the Medicine Is Called and What It Is For

The name of your medicine may be confusing. Most drugs have two names: 1) a scientific name that we call a *generic name* and 2) a trade or *brand name*. The generic name of this medicine is amphetamine. The brand names are Dexedrine, DextroStat, and Adderall.

Amphetamine is called a *stimulant*. It is used to treat attention-deficit/hyperactivity disorder (ADHD or ADD), whether the person has hyperactivity (increased moving around) or not. In people who have ADHD or ADD, parts of the brain are not working as well as they should. An example is the part that controls impulsive actions ("the brakes"). Amphetamine helps these parts of the brain work better. The medicine can help you pay attention at school and at home. It can make it easier for you to listen to and follow directions, to finish more of your schoolwork and homework with fewer mistakes, to think before you act, to sit still for longer periods, and to get into less trouble with adults or other kids.

Although all of these medicines have amphetamine as the active ingredient, they are made differently, so that there are many different ways to take amphetamine. This helps the doctor to find just the right form of the medicine for each person.

How You Take the Medicine

Each of these medicines works for a certain length of time. Your doctor will tell you what times of the day to take the medicine. It is very important that you take it just that way. Sometimes this is at breakfast, lunch, and after school. Long-acting forms may be taken only once a day. Some kids take medicine only on school days, and others take it every day.

Do not skip doses or take extra medicine without asking an adult. If you forget a dose, ask your parent(s) what to do.

Your doctor may talk with you about times that you do not have to take your medicine, such as during school breaks, weekends, and vacations. This is different for each person, so talk to your doctor to be sure you understand this clearly.

This medicine is prescribed only for you. It should never be shared with anyone else.

Do not chew long-acting pills or capsules; you will get too much medicine all at once.

Caffeine (coffee, tea, soft drinks) may increase the side effects of this medicine. Drinking a lot of very acid juices (such as grapefruit or tomato) may decrease levels of amphetamine so that it does not work as well.

19

It is not a good idea to combine stimulants with cold pills or cough medicine because rapid pulse rate (heartbeat) or high blood pressure may develop. If a stuffy nose is really bad, it is better to use a nasal spray.

You do not have to tell others that you are taking this medicine, but it is not something you should feel ashamed or embarrassed about. Many young people are helped by stimulant medicines. This medicine is not habit-forming if taken as your doctor says, and you will not become "hooked" on it. It will not make you into a drug user or an addict. Myths (things that people may believe but that are not true) about these medicines usually are told by people who do not understand ADHD. You should talk to your doctor or nurse about any worries you may have.

It is important to remember that that this medicine cannot change you as a person. Successes that you have in your schoolwork or other areas are *your* achievements, not those of the medicine. The medicine cannot make you do anything; it helps you do what *you* want to do. It helps you to be yourself, only calmer, more efficient, more productive, and more successful.

How Your Doctor Will Follow Your Progress

Before giving you the medicine, your doctor or nurse will talk with you and your parent(s) and may measure your height, weight, heart rate (pulse), and blood pressure. Be sure to tell the doctor if you have had very fast or irregular heartbeat, chest pain, dizziness, fainting, shortness of breath, or severe tiredness, especially when exercising. Also tell the doctor if you have had motor or vocal tics (hard-to-control repeated movements or sounds).

Be sure to tell your doctor or nurse about any other medicines or supplements you are taking, including vitamins, herbs, or aids to weight loss or bodybuilding. Also be sure to tell the doctor or nurse if you are using alcohol or drugs. Because many medicines may affect babies, it is very important to tell the doctor if you might be pregnant or if you are at risk of becoming pregnant.

Your teachers may be asked to fill out a form about your grades and behavior in school. A psychologist may give you some tests to see how you learn best.

Most doctors have regular appointments with young people who are taking medicine. You should use these visits to share any concerns you may have about your medicine and to talk about if it has helped you. From time to time, your physician or nurse will measure your height, weight, heart rate (pulse), and blood pressure to be sure that you are in good health while you are taking the medicine. Your doctor also will ask for regular reports from your parent(s) and maybe from your teachers (with your permission) to see how well the medicine is working.

It is hard to say how long you will need to take this medicine. It is sometimes helpful to people even when they go to college and as they become adults. Your doctor will make that decision with you as he or she watches your progress.

How the Medicine Might Affect You

In addition to the ways the medicine can help you, it may have other effects called *side effects*. Different medicines have different side effects. It is helpful to know about some of the most common side effects of your medicine so that you will understand what they are if they happen. Some people do not have any side effects. Some side effects are just uncomfortable, but others may mean a more serious problem with the medicine. Side effects are most common after starting the medicine or after a dose increase. They may go away with time, or the medicine can be adjusted or changed—ask the doctor.

You could have an allergy to any medicine, which might show up as a rash on your skin, swelling, itching, or trouble breathing.

Please tell your parent(s) and your doctor or nurse about any changes that you notice after taking the medicine. It is especially important to tell a responsible adult if you are feeling depressed or that you may not want to live; if you have thoughts of hurting yourself; or if you begin to feel more irritable, nervous, or restless.

You may have more trouble getting to sleep at night or suddenly have more energy when it is time to go to bed. Your doctor can help you with this problem by changing the time of day that you take your last dose of medicine.

You may not be as hungry as you used to be, and you may not want to eat at mealtimes. Try to eat a good breakfast before taking your medicine. Try to eat something at lunchtime. You also may be more hungry in the evening and want a snack after supper. Eating regularly will help prevent stomachaches and headaches, which are other side effects that some people have. If these feelings do not get better, talk to your doctor. He or she may help you work out a plan to eat many small meals during the day or change the dose of the medicine.

You may feel slower than usual during the day, especially during the first few weeks that you are taking the medicine. This does not mean that you are sick. It is best to do the things you usually do, including sports. This medicine will not hurt your sports ability. Exercising during the day will help you sleep better at night.

If you notice repeated movements of your muscles or your body or that you are making sounds over and over again that are hard to stop ("tics"), be sure to tell your parent(s) and the doctor. This effect is very uncommon and can be helped by adjusting, stopping, or changing your medicine, but your doctor should make this decision.

Tell your parent(s) and the doctor **right away** if you start seeing, hearing, or feeling unusual things or have very fast or irregular heartbeat, chest pain, dizziness, fainting, shortness of breath, or severe tiredness, especially when exercising.

If you feel sad or that nothing is fun for more than a few days, be sure to tell your parent(s) or your doctor.

It is very important not to drink alcohol or use marijuana or street drugs. These could make your ADHD problems worse or increase the side effects of this medicine.

Notes

Use this space to take notes or to write down questions you want to ask the doctor or nurse.

_____

_____

_____

_____

_____

_____

_____

_____

_____

_____

_____

_____

_____

_____

Medication Information for Parents and Teachers

Aripiprazole—Abilify

General Information About Medication

Each child and adolescent is different. No one has exactly the same combination of medical and psychological problems. It is a good idea to talk with the doctor or nurse about the reasons a medicine is being used. It is very important to keep all appointments and to be in touch by telephone if you have concerns. It is important to communicate with the doctor, nurse, or therapist.

It is very important that the medicine be taken exactly as the doctor instructs. However, once in a while, everyone forgets to give a medicine on time. It is a good idea to ask the doctor or nurse what to do if this happens. Do not stop or change a medicine without asking the doctor or nurse first.

If the medicine seems to stop working, it may be because it is not being taken regularly. The youth may be "cheeking" or hiding the medicine or forgetting to take it (especially at school). The doses may be too far apart, or a different dose may be needed. Something at school, at home, or in the neighborhood may be upsetting the youth, or he or she may need special help for learning disabilities or tutoring. Please discuss your concerns with the doctor. **Do not just increase the dose.**

All medicines should be kept in a safe place, out of the reach of children, and should be supervised by an adult. If someone takes too much of a medicine, call the doctor, the poison control center, or a hospital emergency room.

Each medicine has a "generic" or chemical name. Just like laundry detergents or paper towels, some medicines are sold by more than one company under different brand names. The same medicine may be available under a generic name and several brand names. The generic medications are usually less expensive than the brand name ones. The generic medications have the same chemical formula, but they may or may not be exactly the same strength as the brand-name medications. Also, some brands of pills contain dye that can cause allergic reactions. It is a good idea to talk to the doctor and the pharmacist about whether it is important to use a specific brand of medicine.

All medicines can cause an allergic reaction. Examples are hives, itching, rashes, swelling, and trouble breathing. Even a tiny amount of a medicine can cause a reaction in patients who are allergic to that medicine. Be *sure* to talk to the doctor before restarting a medicine that has caused an allergic reaction.

Taking more than one medicine at the same time may cause more side effects or cause one of the medicines to not work as well. Always ask the doctor, nurse, or pharmacist before adding another medicine, whether prescription or over-the-counter. Be sure that each doctor knows about *all* of the medicines your child is taking. Also tell the doctor about any vitamins, herbal medicines, or supplements your child may be taking. Some of these may have side effects alone or when taken with this medication.

Everyone taking medicine should have a physical examination at least once a year.

If you suspect the youth is using drugs or alcohol, please tell the doctor right away.

Pregnancy requires special care in the use of medicine. Please tell the doctor immediately if you suspect the teenager is pregnant or might become pregnant.

23

Printed information like this applies to children and adolescents in general. If you have questions about the medicine, or if you notice changes or anything unusual, please ask the doctor or nurse. As scientific research advances, knowledge increases and advice changes. Even experts do not always agree. Many medicines have not been approved by the U.S. Food and Drug Administration (FDA) for use in children. For this reason, use of the medicine for a particular problem or age group often is not listed in the *Physicians' Desk Reference*. This does not necessarily mean that the medicine is dangerous or does not work, only that the company that makes the medicine has not received permission to advertise the medicine for use in children. Companies often do not apply for this permission because it is expensive to do the tests needed to apply for approval for use in children. Once a medication is approved by the FDA for any purpose, a doctor is allowed to prescribe it according to research and clinical experience.

Note to Teachers

It is a good idea to talk with the parent(s) about the reason(s) that a medication is being used. If the parent(s) sign consent to release information, it is often helpful to talk with the doctor. If the parent(s) give permission, the doctor may ask you to fill out rating forms about your experience with the student's behavior, feelings, academic performance, and medication side effects. This information is very useful in selecting and monitoring medication treatment. If you have observations that you think are important, do not hesitate to share these with the student's parent(s) and treating clinicians.

It is very important that the medicine be taken exactly as the doctor instructs. However, everyone forgets to give a medicine on time once in a while. It is a good idea to ask the parent(s) in advance what to do if this happens. Do not stop or change the time you are giving a medicine at school without parental permission. If a medication is to be taken with food, but lunchtime or snack time changes, be sure to notify the parent(s) so appropriate adjustments can be made.

All medicines should be kept in a secure place and should be supervised by an adult. If someone takes too much of a medicine, follow your school procedure for an urgent medical problem.

Taking medicine is a private matter and is best managed discreetly and confidentially. It is important to be sensitive to the student's feelings about taking medicine.

If you suspect that the student is using drugs or alcohol, please tell the parent(s) or a school counselor right away.

Please tell the parent(s) or school nurse if you suspect medication side effects.

Modifications of the classroom environment or assignments may be useful in addition to medication. The student may need to be evaluated for additional help or for an Individualized Education Plan for learning or behavior.

Any expression of suicidal thoughts or feelings or self-harm by a child or adolescent is a clear signal of distress and should be taken seriously. These behaviors should not be dismissed as "attention seeking."

What Is Aripiprazole (Abilify)?

This medicine is called an *atypical* or *second-generation antipsychotic*. It is sometimes called an *atypical psychotropic agent*, or simply an *atypical*. It comes in brand name Abilify tablets and liquid.

How Can This Medicine Help?

Aripiprazole is used to treat psychosis, such as in schizophrenia, mania, or very severe depression. It can reduce *positive symptoms* such as hallucinations (hearing voices or seeing things that are not there); delusions (troubling beliefs that other people do not share); agitation; and very unusual thinking, speech, and behavior. It is also used to lessen the *negative symptoms* of schizophrenia, such as lack of interest in doing things (apathy), lack of motivation, social withdrawal, and lack of energy.

Aripiprazole may be used as a mood stabilizer in patients with bipolar disorder (manic-depressive illness) or severe mood swings. It can reduce mania and may be able to help maintain a stable mood over the long term.

Sometimes aripiprazole is used to reduce severe aggression or very serious behavioral problems in young people with conduct disorder, mental retardation, autism, or pervasive developmental disorder.

Aripiprazole may be used for behavior problems after a head injury.

This medicine is very powerful and is used to treat very serious problems or symptoms that other medicines do not help. Be patient; the positive effects of this medicine may not appear for 2–3 weeks.

How Does This Medicine Work?

Cells in the brain communicate using chemicals called *neurotransmitters*. Too much or too little of these substances in parts of the brain can cause problems. Aripiprazole works in a different way than other atypicals, by changing the effects of two of these neurotransmitters—dopamine and serotonin—in certain areas of the brain.

How Long Does This Medicine Last?

Aripiprazole can usually be taken only once a day.

How Will the Doctor Monitor This Medicine?

The doctor will review your child's medical history and physical examination before starting aripiprazole. The doctor may order some blood or urine tests to be sure your child does not have a hidden medical condition that would make it unsafe to use this medicine. The doctor or nurse may measure your child's pulse and blood pressure before starting aripiprazole. The doctor may order other tests, such as baseline tests for blood sugar and cholesterol.

Be sure to tell the doctor if anyone in the family has diabetes, high blood pressure, high cholesterol, or heart disease.

Before your child starts taking aripiprazole and every so often afterward, the doctor or nurse may use a test such as the Abnormal Involuntary Movement Scale (AIMS) to check your child's tongue, legs, and arms for unusual movements that could be caused by the medicine.

After the medicine is started, the doctor will want to have regular appointments with you and your child to see how the medicine is working, to see if a dose change is needed, to watch for side effects, to see if aripiprazole is still needed, and to see if any other treatment is needed. The doctor or nurse may check your child's height, weight, pulse, and blood pressure and watch for abnormal movements. Sometimes blood tests are needed to watch for diabetes or increased cholesterol.

What Side Effects Can This Medicine Have?

Any medicine can have side effects, including an allergy to the medicine. Because each patient is different, the doctor will monitor the youth closely, especially when the medicine is started. The doctor will work with you to increase the positive effects and decrease the negative effects of the medicine. Please tell the doctor if any of the listed side effects appear or if you think that the medicine is causing any other problems. Not all of the rare or unusual side effects are listed.

Side effects are most common after starting the medicine or after a dose increase. Many side effects can be avoided or lessened by starting with a very low dose and increasing it slowly—ask the doctor.

Allergic Reaction

Tell the doctor in a day or two (if possible, before the next dose of medicine):

- Hives
- Itching
- Rash

    Stop the medicine and get *immediate* medical care:

- Trouble breathing or chest tightness
- Swelling of lips, tongue, or throat

Common, but Not Usually Serious, Side Effects

Discuss the following side effects with your child's doctor when convenient. These side effects often can be helped by lowering the dose of medicine, changing the times medicine is taken, or adding another medicine.

- Daytime sleepiness or tiredness—Do not allow your child to drive, ride a bicycle or motorcycle, or operate machinery if this happens. This problem may be lessened by taking the medicine at bedtime.
- Insomnia (trouble sleeping)
- Headache
- Nausea
- Vomiting
- Increased appetite
- Weight gain—Seek nutritional counseling; provide your child with low-calorie snacks and encourage regular exercise.

Rare, but Not Usually Serious, Side Effects

Discuss the following side effects with your child's doctor when convenient. These side effects often can be helped by lowering the dose of medicine, changing the times medicine is taken, or adding another medicine.

- Dry mouth—Have your child try using sugar-free gum or candy.
- Dizziness—This side effect is worse when the child stands up quickly, especially when getting out of bed in the morning; try having the child stand up slowly.
- Increased restlessness or inability to sit still

- Shaking of hands and fingers
- Decreased or slowed movement and decreased facial expressions

Very Rare, but Serious, Side Effects

Call the doctor immediately:

- Stiffness of the tongue, jaw, neck, back, or legs
- Seizure (fit, convulsion)—This is more common in people with a history of seizures or head injury.
- Increased thirst, frequent urination (having to go to the bathroom often), lethargy, tiredness, dizziness, and blurred vision—These could be signs of diabetes (especially if your child is overweight or there is a family history of diabetes). **Talk to a doctor within a day.**
- Extreme stiffness or lack of movement, very high fever, mental confusion, irregular pulse rate, or eye pain—**This is a medical emergency. Go to an emergency room right away.**
- Sudden stiffness and inability to breathe or swallow—**Go to an emergency room or call 911. Tell the paramedics, nurses, and doctors that the patient is taking aripiprazole. Other medicines can be used to treat this problem quickly.**

What Else Should I Know About Side Effects?

Most side effects lessen over time. If they are troublesome, talk with your child's doctor. Some side effects can be decreased by taking a smaller dose of medicine, by stopping the medicine, by changing to another medicine, or by adding another medicine.

Sometimes people who take aripiprazole gain weight, although this is less a problem with aripiprazole than with other atypicals. Children seem to have more problems with weight gain than adults. The weight gain may be from increased appetite and from ways that the medicine changes how the body processes food. Aripiprazole may also change the way that the body handles glucose (sugar) and cause high levels (hyperglycemia). People who take aripiprazole, especially those who gain a lot of weight, might be at increased risk of developing diabetes and of having increased fats (lipids—cholesterol and triglycerides) in their blood. Over time, both diabetes and increased fats in the blood may lead to heart disease, stroke, and other complications. The FDA has put warnings on all atypical agents about the increased risks of hyperglycemia, diabetes, and increased blood cholesterol and triglycerides when taking one of these medicines. It is much easier to prevent weight gain than to lose weight later. When your child first starts taking aripiprazole, it is a good idea to be sure that he or she eats a well-balanced diet without "junk food" and with healthy snacks like fruits and vegetables, not sweets or fried foods. He or she should drink water or skim milk, not pop, sodas, soft drinks, or sugary juices. Regular exercise is important for maintaining a healthy weight (and may also help with sleep).

One very rare side effect that may not go away is *tardive dyskinesia* (or TD). Patients with tardive dyskinesia have involuntary movements (movements that they cannot help making) of the body, especially the mouth and tongue. The patient may look as though he or she is making faces over and over again. Jerky movements of the arms, legs, or body may occur. There may be fine, wormlike or sudden repeated movements of the tongue, or the person may appear to be chewing something or smacking or puckering his or her lips. The fingers may look as though they are rolling something. If you notice any unusual movements, be sure to tell the doctor. The doctor may use the AIMS test to look for these movements.

Neuroleptic malignant syndrome is a very rare side effect that can lead to death. The symptoms are severe muscle stiffness, high fever, increased heart rate and blood pressure, irregular heartbeat (pulse), and sweating. It may lead to unconsciousness. If you suspect this, **call 911 or go to an emergency room right away.**

What Medicines Are Used to Treat the Side Effects of Aripiprazole?

The following medicines may be used to treat the movement side effects of aripiprazole. These medicines may have their own side effects as well. Ask the doctor if you suspect a problem.

Brand name	Generic name
Akineton	biperiden
Artane	trihexyphenidyl
Ativan	lorazepam*
Benadryl	diphenhydramine*
Catapres	clonidine*
Cogentin	benztropine mesylate*
Inderal	propranolol*
Klonopin	clonazepam*
Symmetrel	amantadine

*Medicine has its own information sheet in this book.

Some Interactions With Other Medicines or Food

Please note that the following are only the most likely interactions with food or other medicines.

Aripiprazole can be taken with or without food.

Taking aripiprazole together with Prozac (fluoxetine), Tagamet (cimetidine), or Paxil (paroxetine) can increase levels of aripiprazole and increase the risk of side effects.

Taking aripiprazole together with carbamazepine (Tegretol) can decrease the levels of aripiprazole so that it does not work as well.

It is better to limit drinks with caffeine (coffee, tea, soft drinks) because caffeine works in the opposite way from this medicine, and the positive effects might be decreased.

What Could Happen if This Medicine Is Stopped Suddenly?

Involuntary movements, or *withdrawal dyskinesias*, may appear within 1–4 weeks of lowering the dose or stopping the medicine. Usually these go away, but they can last for days to months. If aripiprazole is stopped suddenly, emotional disturbance (such as irritability, nervousness, moodiness, or oppositional behavior) or physical problems (such as stomachache, loss of appetite, nausea, vomiting, diarrhea, sweating, indigestion, trouble sleeping, trembling, or shaking) may appear. These problems usually last only a few days to a few weeks. If they happen, you should tell your child's doctor. The medicine dose may need to be lowered more slowly (tapered). Always check with the doctor before stopping a medicine.

How Long Will This Medicine Be Needed?

How long your child will need to take this medicine depends partly on the reason that it was prescribed. Some problems last for only a few months, whereas others last much longer. It is important to ask the doctor whether medicine is still needed, especially with medicines as powerful as this one. Every few months, you should discuss with your child's doctor the reasons for using the medicine and whether the medicine may be stopped or the dose lowered.

What Else Should I Know About This Medicine?

There are other medicines that are used for the same kinds of problems. If your child is having bad side effects or the medicine does not seem to be working, ask the doctor if another medicine might work as well or better and have fewer side effects for your child. Each person reacts differently to medicines.

Taking this medicine could make overheating or heatstroke more likely. Have your child decrease activity in hot weather, stay out of the sun, and drink water to prevent this.

Notes

Use this space to take notes or to write down questions you want to ask the doctor.

_____

_____

_____

_____

_____

_____

_____

_____

_____

_____

_____

From Dulcan MK (editor): *Helping Parents, Youth, and Teachers Understand Medications for Behavioral and Emotional Problems: A Resource Book of Medication Information Handouts*, Third Edition. Washington, DC, American Psychiatric Publishing, 2007

Medication Information
for Youth

Aripiprazole—Abilify

What the Medicine Is Called and What It Is For

The name of your medicine may be confusing. Most drugs have two names: 1) a scientific name that we call a *generic name* and 2) a trade or *brand name*. The generic name of this medicine is aripiprazole. The brand name is Abilify. It is called an *atypical* medicine.

This medicine helps people who feel very confused and have severe problems thinking clearly. It can lessen hallucinations (seeing or hearing things that are not really there) and delusions (troubling beliefs that other people do not share). The medicine also can improve *negative symptoms*, such as lack of interest in doing things, lack of motivation, loss of interest in friends, and decreased energy. It helps people who have severe depression or mood swings. This medicine also is sometimes used to help young people who have *mania* or who get very angry and hit people or break things.

How You Take the Medicine

It is very important to take the medicine exactly as the doctor or nurse tells you. Do not skip doses or take extra medicine without asking an adult. If you forget a dose, ask your parent(s) what to do.

It is better to limit drinks with caffeine (coffee, tea, soft drinks) because caffeine works in the opposite way from this medicine, and the positive effects might be decreased.

Your doctor will tell you how much medicine to take and how often to take it so that it can help you the most. It is *very important* that you take all the pills you are supposed to take each day. Your doctor will probably recommend that you take your medicine at the same time each day, which may be with meals or at bedtime.

It may be several weeks or longer before you notice the full effect of your medicine. You may feel discouraged and think the medicine is never going to help. You may want to give up and stop taking the medicine. Talk to your doctor and parent(s) about how you feel, but **do not stop** taking your medicine unless your doctor tells you to. It also is important not to take extra pills hoping that you will feel better faster. Doing that could make you very sick.

This medicine is prescribed only for you. It should never be shared with anyone else.

You do not have to tell others that you are taking this medicine, but it is not something you should feel ashamed or embarrassed about. Many young people are helped by aripiprazole. This medicine is not habit-forming, and you cannot become "hooked" on it. You should talk to your doctor or nurse about any questions you have about the medicine. It is important to remember that the medicine *helps* you. It cannot *make* you do anything or change you as a person.

How Your Doctor Will Follow Your Progress

Before giving you the medicine, your doctor or nurse will talk with you and your parent(s) and may measure your height, weight, heart rate (pulse), and blood pressure. There may be other tests, such as blood tests for sugar and cholesterol. Before you start taking the medicine and every so often afterward, the doctor or nurse will look at your tongue, arms, and legs to check for unusual movements. This is called the AIMS (Abnormal Involuntary Movement Scale) test.

Be sure to tell your doctor or nurse about any other medicines or supplements you are taking, including vitamins, herbs, or aids to weight loss or bodybuilding. Also be sure to tell the doctor or nurse if you are using alcohol or drugs. Because many medicines may affect babies, it is very important to tell the doctor if you might be pregnant or if you are at risk of becoming pregnant.

Your teachers may be asked to fill out a form about your grades and behavior in school. A psychologist may give you some tests to see how you learn best.

Most doctors have regular appointments with young people who are taking medicine. You should use these visits to share any concerns you may have about your medicine and to talk about if it has helped you. From time to time, your physician or nurse may measure your height, weight, heart rate (pulse), and blood pressure to be sure that you are in good health while you are taking the medicine. There may be blood tests to watch for diabetes or high cholesterol. Your doctor also will ask for regular reports from your parents and maybe from your teachers (with your permission) to see how well the medicine is working.

If the medicine helps you, your doctor will probably want you to take it for several months to a year. Your doctor will decide how long you will need to take the medicine as he or she watches your progress.

How the Medicine Might Affect You

In addition to the ways the medicine can help you, it may have other effects called *side effects*. Different medicines have different side effects. It is helpful to know about some of the most common side effects of your medicine so that you will understand what they are if they happen. Some people do not have any side effects. Some side effects are just uncomfortable, but others may mean a more serious problem with the medicine. Side effects are most common after starting the medicine or after a dose increase. They may go away with time, or the medicine can be adjusted or changed—ask the doctor.

You could have an allergy to any medicine, which might show up as a rash on your skin, swelling, itching, or trouble breathing.

Please tell your parent(s) and your doctor or nurse about any changes that you notice after taking the medicine. It is especially important to tell a responsible adult if you are feeling depressed or that you may not want to live; if you have thoughts of hurting yourself; or if you begin to feel more irritable, nervous, or restless.

One of the most common side effects of this medicine is feeling tired or sleepy during the day, even if you have had a full night's sleep. If this medicine is making you sleepy, it is very important not to drive a car or ride a bicycle or motorcycle. After starting the medicine or increasing the dose of medicine, please be extra careful when driving a car, riding a bike, or using machines until you can tell how the medicine affects your alertness, attention, and coordination. After you have been taking the medicine for a few weeks, your body will adjust, and this side effect will likely go away. If you had trouble sleeping at night before you started taking the medicine, it can help you sleep better, especially if the doctor tells you to take a dose of medicine in the evening.

Another possible side effect is dry mouth. You may be more thirsty than usual and find that you are drinking more water or other liquids than usual. Sucking on sugar-free hard candy or cough drops usually helps. You also could try chewing sugar-free gum or sucking on ice chips. Do not chew the ice; you could hurt your teeth. Also, using lip balm on your lips will keep them from cracking. It is important to be especially good about brushing your teeth.

If you get very thirsty, have to go to the bathroom a lot, feel very tired, or have dizziness or blurred vision, be sure to tell your parent(s) or doctor.

Taking this medicine could make you more likely to get very sick in hot weather. Be sure to drink plenty of liquids when you go outside in hot weather. Be careful to rest in the shade and not get overheated.

Sometimes teenagers who take aripiprazole gain weight. The weight gain may be from increased appetite and also from ways that the medicine changes how the body processes food. People who take aripiprazole, especially those who gain a lot of weight, might be at increased risk of developing diabetes and of having increased fats (lipids—cholesterol and triglycerides) in their blood. Over time, both diabetes and increased fats in the blood may lead to heart disease, stroke, and other complications. The U.S. Food and Drug Administration has put warnings about these problems on all medicines like aripiprazole. It is much easier to prevent weight gain than to lose weight later. It is a good idea to eat a well-balanced diet without "junk food" and with healthy snacks like fruits and vegetables, not sweets or fried foods. It is better to drink water or skim milk, not pop, sodas, soft drinks, or sugary juices. Regular exercise is important for maintaining a healthy weight (and may also help with sleep).

This is a very powerful medicine. Some side effects include feeling nervous, restless, or shaky or having stiff muscles. They can be helped by adding another medicine or by adjusting or changing the medicine.

Another, more serious, side effect can be longer lasting and more difficult to treat. This very rare side effect is called *tardive dyskinesia* (or TD). A person taking aripiprazole may develop movements of the mouth, tongue, face, arms, legs, or body that are not being made on purpose. This side effect can go away when the medicine is stopped, but in some people it does not go away. Your doctor will explain this effect to you and your parent(s) and how he or she will watch for any signs that you are developing this problem. Be sure to ask your doctor any questions that you may have about this, but do not worry too much about it. It hardly ever happens to teenagers.

You should tell your parent(s) and doctor if you notice anything different or unusual about how you feel once you start taking the medicine. This includes good things, such as feeling less confused, feeling less sad, not hearing voices anymore, or sleeping better at night.

Notes

Use this space to take notes or to write down questions you want to ask the doctor or nurse.

_____

_____

_____

_____

_____

_____

_____

_____

_____

_____

_____

_____

_____

From Dulcan MK (editor): _Helping Parents, Youth, and Teachers Understand Medications for Behavioral and Emotional Problems: A Resource Book of Medication Information Handouts_, Third Edition. Washington, DC, American Psychiatric Publishing, 2007

Medication Information for Parents and Teachers

Atenolol—Tenormin

General Information About Medication

Each child and adolescent is different. No one has exactly the same combination of medical and psychological problems. It is a good idea to talk with the doctor or nurse about the reasons a medicine is being used. It is very important to keep all appointments and to be in touch by telephone if you have concerns. It is important to communicate with the doctor, nurse, or therapist.

It is very important that the medicine be taken exactly as the doctor instructs. However, once in a while, everyone forgets to give a medicine on time. It is a good idea to ask the doctor or nurse what to do if this happens. Do not stop or change a medicine without asking the doctor or nurse first.

If the medicine seems to stop working, it may be because it is not being taken regularly. The youth may be "cheeking" or hiding the medicine or forgetting to take it (especially at school). The doses may be too far apart, or a different dose may be needed. Something at school, at home, or in the neighborhood may be upsetting the youth, or he or she may need special help for learning disabilities or tutoring. Please discuss your concerns with the doctor. **Do not just increase the dose.**

All medicines should be kept in a safe place, out of the reach of children, and should be supervised by an adult. If someone takes too much of a medicine, call the doctor, the poison control center, or a hospital emergency room.

Each medicine has a "generic" or chemical name. Just like laundry detergents or paper towels, some medicines are sold by more than one company under different brand names. The same medicine may be available under a generic name and several brand names. The generic medications are usually less expensive than the brand name ones. The generic medications have the same chemical formula, but they may or may not be exactly the same strength as the brand-name medications. Also, some brands of pills contain dye that can cause allergic reactions. It is a good idea to talk to the doctor and the pharmacist about whether it is important to use a specific brand of medicine.

All medicines can cause an allergic reaction. Examples are hives, itching, rashes, swelling, and trouble breathing. Even a tiny amount of a medicine can cause a reaction in patients who are allergic to that medicine. Be *sure* to talk to the doctor before restarting a medicine that has caused an allergic reaction.

Taking more than one medicine at the same time may cause more side effects or cause one of the medicines to not work as well. Always ask the doctor, nurse, or pharmacist before adding another medicine, whether prescription or over-the-counter. Be sure that each doctor knows about *all* of the medicines your child is taking. Also tell the doctor about any vitamins, herbal medicines, or supplements your child may be taking. Some of these may have side effects alone or when taken with this medication.

Everyone taking medicine should have a physical examination at least once a year.

If you suspect the youth is using drugs or alcohol, please tell the doctor right away.

Pregnancy requires special care in the use of medicine. Please tell the doctor immediately if you suspect the teenager is pregnant or might become pregnant.

35

Printed information like this applies to children and adolescents in general. If you have questions about the medicine, or if you notice changes or anything unusual, please ask the doctor or nurse. As scientific research advances, knowledge increases and advice changes. Even experts do not always agree. Many medicines have not been approved by the U.S. Food and Drug Administration (FDA) for use in children. For this reason, use of the medicine for a particular problem or age group often is not listed in the *Physicians' Desk Reference*. This does not necessarily mean that the medicine is dangerous or does not work, only that the company that makes the medicine has not received permission to advertise the medicine for use in children. Companies often do not apply for this permission because it is expensive to do the tests needed to apply for approval for use in children. Once a medication is approved by the FDA for any purpose, a doctor is allowed to prescribe it according to research and clinical experience.

Note to Teachers

It is a good idea to talk with the parent(s) about the reason(s) that a medication is being used. If the parent(s) sign consent to release information, it is often helpful to talk with the doctor. If the parent(s) give permission, the doctor may ask you to fill out rating forms about your experience with the student's behavior, feelings, academic performance, and medication side effects. This information is very useful in selecting and monitoring medication treatment. If you have observations that you think are important, do not hesitate to share these with the student's parent(s) and treating clinicians.

It is very important that the medicine be taken exactly as the doctor instructs. However, everyone forgets to give a medicine on time once in a while. It is a good idea to ask the parent(s) in advance what to do if this happens. Do not stop or change the time you are giving a medicine at school without parental permission. If a medication is to be taken with food, but lunchtime or snack time changes, be sure to notify the parent(s) so appropriate adjustments can be made.

All medicines should be kept in a secure place and should be supervised by an adult. If someone takes too much of a medicine, follow your school procedure for an urgent medical problem.

Taking medicine is a private matter and is best managed discreetly and confidentially. It is important to be sensitive to the student's feelings about taking medicine.

If you suspect that the student is using drugs or alcohol, please tell the parent(s) or a school counselor right away.

Please tell the parent(s) or school nurse if you suspect medication side effects.

Modifications of the classroom environment or assignments may be useful in addition to medication. The student may need to be evaluated for additional help or for an Individualized Education Plan for learning or behavior.

Any expression of suicidal thoughts or feelings or self-harm by a child or adolescent is a clear signal of distress and should be taken seriously. These behaviors should not be dismissed as "attention seeking."

What Is Atenolol (Tenormin)?

Atenolol is called a *beta-blocker*. It was first used to treat high blood pressure and irregular heartbeat. A newer use is the treatment of emotional and behavioral problems. It is also sometimes used to treat *akathisia*, which is a side effect of some antipsychotic medications. It is used for migraine headaches and a number of other medical conditions.

It comes in generic and brand name Tenormin tablets.

How Can This Medicine Help?

Atenolol can decrease aggressive or violent behavior in children and adolescents. It may be particularly useful for patients who have developmental delays or autism. In addition, atenolol may reduce the aggression and anger that sometimes follow brain injuries. It may reduce some symptoms of anxiety (nervousness) and help children and adolescents who have experienced very frightening events and have posttraumatic stress disorder (PTSD). Atenolol may reduce the severe restlessness resulting from other medicines.

Your child may need to continue taking atenolol for at least 4 weeks before the doctor is able to decide whether the medicine is working.

How Does This Medicine Work?

When atenolol is prescribed for patients with anxiety, aggression, or other behavioral problems, this medicine stops the effect of certain chemicals on nerves in the body and possibly in the brain that are causing the symptoms. For example, atenolol can decrease the physical anxiety symptoms of shaking, sweating, and fast heartbeat.

How Long Does This Medicine Last?

Atenolol is usually taken twice a day.

How Will the Doctor Monitor This Medicine?

The doctor will review your child's medical history and physical examination before starting atenolol. Extreme caution is needed for children and adolescents with asthma, heart disease, diabetes, kidney disease, or thyroid disease. Please be sure to tell the doctor if your child or anyone in the family has one of these problems. The doctor may order some blood or urine tests to be sure your child does not have a hidden medical condition that would make it unsafe to use this medicine. The doctor or nurse will measure your child's height, weight, pulse, and blood pressure before starting atenolol. The doctor may order an ECG (electrocardiogram or heart rhythm test) before starting atenolol.

After the medicine is started, the doctor will want to have regular appointments with you and your child to see how the medicine is working, to see if a dose change is needed, to watch for side effects, to see if atenolol is still needed, and to see if any other treatment is needed. The doctor or nurse will measure pulse rate and blood pressure at each visit, particularly as the dose is increased. Sometimes these measurements are taken while the patient is both sitting or lying down and standing up. If either pulse rate or blood pressure drops too low, a pill may not be given at that time or the regular dose may be decreased.

What Side Effects Can This Medicine Have?

Any medicine can have side effects, including an allergy to the medicine. Because each patient is different, the doctor will monitor the youth closely, especially when the medicine is started. The doctor will work with you

to increase the positive effects and decrease the negative effects of the medicine. Please tell the doctor if any of the listed side effects appear or if you think that the medicine is causing any other problems. Not all of the rare or unusual side effects are listed.

Side effects are most common after starting the medicine or after a dose increase. Many side effects can be avoided or lessened by starting with a very low dose and increasing it slowly—ask the doctor.

Allergic Reaction

Tell the doctor in a day or two (if possible, before the next dose of medicine):

- Hives
- Itching
- Rash

    Stop the medicine and get *immediate* medical care:

- Trouble breathing or chest tightness
- Swelling of lips, tongue, or throat

Occasional Side Effects

Tell the doctor within a week or two:

- Tingling, numbness, cold, or pain in the fingers or toes (Raynaud's phenomenon)
- Tiredness or weakness, especially with exercise
- Slow heartbeat
- Low blood pressure
- Dizziness or light-headedness—When standing up quickly, especially when getting out of bed in the morning; try having the child stand up slowly.

Uncommon Side Effects

Call the doctor within a day or two:

- Sadness or irritability lasting more than a few days
- Nausea
- Trouble sleeping or nightmares
- Diarrhea
- Muscle cramps

Serious Side Effects

Call the doctor *immediately*:

- Wheezing
- Hallucinations (hearing voices or seeing things that are not there)

Some Interactions With Other Medicines or Food

Please note that the following are only the most likely interactions with food or other medicines.

Giving atenolol with food will decrease side effects.

Atenolol interacts with many other medicines. Be sure to tell the doctor about all medicines being taken. A doctor may use atenolol in combination with other medicines to treat a behavioral problem. Talk with your doctor and pharmacist about possible medicine interactions.

What Could Happen if This Medicine Is Stopped Suddenly?

Stopping atenolol suddenly may cause a fast or irregular heartbeat, high blood pressure, or severe emotional problems. Atenolol should be decreased slowly over at least 2 weeks under a doctor's supervision. It is especially important not to miss doses of this medicine, because withdrawal problems may occur. **Be sure not to let the prescription run out!**

How Long Will This Medicine Be Needed?

The length of time atenolol will be needed depends on how well the medicine works for your child, whether any side effects occur, and what condition is being treated. Sometimes medicine is needed for a short time to treat a particular problem. Occasionally a person may require treatment lasting for several months or may need to start the medicine again if symptoms return.

What Else Should I Know About This Medicine?

Atenolol may be confused with albuterol or Tylenol. Tenormin may be confused with Norpramin or thiamine. Be sure to check the prescription when you get it from the pharmacy.

Notes

Use this space to take notes or to write down questions you want to ask the doctor.

_____

_____

_____

_____

_____

_____

_____

_____

_____

_____

_____

_____

_____

_____

_____

From Dulcan MK (editor): _Helping Parents, Youth, and Teachers Understand Medications for Behavioral and Emotional Problems: A Resource Book of Medication Information Handouts,_ Third Edition. Washington, DC, American Psychiatric Publishing, 2007

Medication Information
for Youth

Atenolol—Tenormin

What the Medicine Is Called and What It Is For

The name of your medicine may be confusing. Most drugs have two names: 1) a scientific name that we call a *generic name* and 2) a trade or *brand name*. The generic name of this medicine is atenolol. The brand name is Tenormin.

Atenolol is a *beta-blocker*. These medicines work on parts of your brain and nervous system that control how your body reacts to situations in which you feel frightened, threatened, or angry. Beta-blockers were first used to treat heart and blood pressure problems. Now they are used to help young people who have too much anxiety (nervousness) or posttraumatic stress disorder (PTSD) or who fight or get angry too much. They can decrease shaking, sweating, and fast heartbeat that come from anxiety or anger. They are also sometimes used to treat the side effects (such as restlessness) of other medicines.

How You Take the Medicine

It is very important to take the medicine exactly as the doctor or nurse tells you. Do not skip doses or take extra medicine without asking an adult. If you forget a dose, ask your parent(s) what to do.

It might take as long as 4 weeks before the full effect is noticed. You may feel discouraged and think that the medicine is never going to help. You may want to give up and stop taking the medicine. Talk to your doctor and parent(s) about how you feel, but **do not stop** taking your medicine unless your doctor tells you to. It could be dangerous to stop this medicine suddenly.

This medicine is prescribed only for you. It should never be shared with anyone else.

You do not have to tell others that you are taking this medicine, but it is not something you should feel ashamed or embarrassed about. Many young people are helped by atenolol. This medicine is not habit-forming, and you cannot become "hooked" on it. You should talk to your doctor or nurse about any questions you have about the medicine. It is important to remember that the medicine *helps* you. It cannot *make* you do anything or change you as a person.

How Your Doctor Will Follow Your Progress

Before giving you the medicine, your doctor or nurse will talk with you and your parent(s) and will measure your height, weight, heart rate (pulse), and blood pressure. There may be other tests, such as blood or urine tests, or an ECG (electrocardiogram or heart rhythm test). This test counts your heartbeats through small wires that are taped to your chest. It takes only a few minutes

Be sure to tell your doctor or nurse about any other medicines or supplements you are taking, including vitamins, herbs, or aids to weight loss or bodybuilding. Also be sure to tell the doctor or nurse if you are using alcohol or drugs. Because many medicines may affect babies, it is very important to tell the doctor if you might be pregnant or if you are at risk of becoming pregnant.

Your teachers may be asked to fill out a form about your grades and behavior in school. A psychologist may give you some tests to see how you learn best.

Most doctors have regular appointments with young people who are taking medicine. You should use these visits to share any concerns you may have about your medicine and to talk about if it has helped you. At the appointments, your doctor or nurse will measure your pulse rate (heartbeat) and blood pressure, particularly as the dose is increased. Sometimes these measurements are taken while you are sitting or lying down and then standing up. There may be other tests, such as repeating the ECG. Your doctor also will ask for regular reports from your parents and maybe from your teachers (with your permission) to see how well the medicine is working.

How long you will need to take this medicine depends on how well it works for you, whether there are any side effects, and what problems are being treated. Sometimes medicine is needed for only a short time to treat a particular problem. Some people need it for months or years or may need to start the medicine again if symptoms return.

How the Medicine Might Affect You

In addition to the ways the medicine can help you, it may have other effects called *side effects*. Different medicines have different side effects. It is helpful to know about some of the most common side effects of your medicine so that you will understand what they are if they happen. Some people do not have any side effects. Some side effects are just uncomfortable, but others may mean a more serious problem with the medicine. Side effects are most common after starting the medicine or after a dose increase. They may go away with time, or the medicine can be adjusted or changed—ask the doctor.

You could have an allergy to any medicine, which might show up as a rash on your skin, swelling, itching, or trouble breathing.

Please tell your parent(s) and your doctor or nurse about any changes that you notice after taking the medicine. It is especially important to tell a responsible adult if you are feeling depressed or that you may not want to live; if you have thoughts of hurting yourself; or if you begin to feel more irritable, nervous, or restless.

Some medicines make people feel sleepy or less coordinated. If this medicine is making you sleepy, it is very important not to drive a car or ride a bicycle or motorcycle. After starting a new medicine or increasing the dose of a medicine, please be extra careful when driving a car, riding a bike, or using machines until you can tell how the medicine affects your alertness, attention, and coordination.

You might feel dizzy, tired, or even faint when you stand up fast. Try standing up slowly, especially first thing in the morning when getting out of bed.

You might notice that your fingers or toes feel very cold or tingly, that they look pale, or that they hurt. These are signs of *Raynaud's phenomenon*, which happens when the blood vessels to your fingers or toes tighten. Tell the doctor if you have these symptoms, and the dose of medicine can be adjusted or a different medicine can be used so that the problem will go away.

Other side effects (that hardly ever happen) are hallucinations (hearing voices or seeing things that are not there), upset stomach, nausea, trouble sleeping, nightmares, and sadness or irritability. You should talk to your parent(s) or your doctor if you think you may be having any of these side effects.

If you are having trouble breathing, tell your parent(s) or doctor **right away.**

It is very important not to miss a dose or to stop this medicine suddenly—it could make you very sick.

Notes

Use this space to take notes or to write down questions you want to ask the doctor or nurse.

_____

_____

_____

_____

_____

_____

_____

_____

_____

_____

_____

_____

_____

Medication Information for Parents and Teachers

Atomoxetine—Strattera

General Information About Medication

Each child and adolescent is different. No one has exactly the same combination of medical and psychological problems. It is a good idea to talk with the doctor or nurse about the reasons a medicine is being used. It is very important to keep all appointments and to be in touch by telephone if you have concerns. It is important to communicate with the doctor, nurse, or therapist.

It is very important that the medicine be taken exactly as the doctor instructs. However, once in a while, everyone forgets to give a medicine on time. It is a good idea to ask the doctor or nurse what to do if this happens. Do not stop or change a medicine without asking the doctor or nurse first.

If the medicine seems to stop working, it may be because it is not being taken regularly. The youth may be "cheeking" or hiding the medicine or forgetting to take it (especially at school). The doses may be too far apart, or a different dose may be needed. Something at school, at home, or in the neighborhood may be upsetting the youth, or he or she may need special help for learning disabilities or tutoring. Please discuss your concerns with the doctor. **Do not just increase the dose.**

All medicines should be kept in a safe place, out of the reach of children, and should be supervised by an adult. If someone takes too much of a medicine, call the doctor, the poison control center, or a hospital emergency room.

Each medicine has a "generic" or chemical name. Just like laundry detergents or paper towels, some medicines are sold by more than one company under different brand names. The same medicine may be available under a generic name and several brand names. The generic medications are usually less expensive than the brand name ones. The generic medications have the same chemical formula, but they may or may not be exactly the same strength as the brand-name medications. Also, some brands of pills contain dye that can cause allergic reactions. It is a good idea to talk to the doctor and the pharmacist about whether it is important to use a specific brand of medicine.

All medicines can cause an allergic reaction. Examples are hives, itching, rashes, swelling, and trouble breathing. Even a tiny amount of a medicine can cause a reaction in patients who are allergic to that medicine. Be *sure* to talk to the doctor before restarting a medicine that has caused an allergic reaction.

Taking more than one medicine at the same time may cause more side effects or cause one of the medicines to not work as well. Always ask the doctor, nurse, or pharmacist before adding another medicine, whether prescription or over-the-counter. Be sure that each doctor knows about *all* of the medicines your child is taking. Also tell the doctor about any vitamins, herbal medicines, or supplements your child may be taking. Some of these may have side effects alone or when taken with this medication.

Everyone taking medicine should have a physical examination at least once a year.

If you suspect the youth is using drugs or alcohol, please tell the doctor right away.

Pregnancy requires special care in the use of medicine. Please tell the doctor immediately if you suspect the teenager is pregnant or might become pregnant.

45

Printed information like this applies to children and adolescents in general. If you have questions about the medicine, or if you notice changes or anything unusual, please ask the doctor or nurse. As scientific research advances, knowledge increases and advice changes. Even experts do not always agree. Many medicines have not been approved by the U.S. Food and Drug Administration (FDA) for use in children. For this reason, use of the medicine for a particular problem or age group often is not listed in the *Physicians' Desk Reference*. This does not necessarily mean that the medicine is dangerous or does not work, only that the company that makes the medicine has not received permission to advertise the medicine for use in children. Companies often do not apply for this permission because it is expensive to do the tests needed to apply for approval for use in children. Once a medication is approved by the FDA for any purpose, a doctor is allowed to prescribe it according to research and clinical experience.

Note to Teachers

It is a good idea to talk with the parent(s) about the reason(s) that a medication is being used. If the parent(s) sign consent to release information, it is often helpful to talk with the doctor. If the parent(s) give permission, the doctor may ask you to fill out rating forms about your experience with the student's behavior, feelings, academic performance, and medication side effects. This information is very useful in selecting and monitoring medication treatment. If you have observations that you think are important, do not hesitate to share these with the student's parent(s) and treating clinicians.

It is very important that the medicine be taken exactly as the doctor instructs. However, everyone forgets to give a medicine on time once in a while. It is a good idea to ask the parent(s) in advance what to do if this happens. Do not stop or change the time you are giving a medicine at school without parental permission. If a medication is to be taken with food, but lunchtime or snack time changes, be sure to notify the parent(s) so appropriate adjustments can be made.

All medicines should be kept in a secure place and should be supervised by an adult. If someone takes too much of a medicine, follow your school procedure for an urgent medical problem.

Taking medicine is a private matter and is best managed discreetly and confidentially. It is important to be sensitive to the student's feelings about taking medicine.

If you suspect that the student is using drugs or alcohol, please tell the parent(s) or a school counselor right away.

Please tell the parent(s) or school nurse if you suspect medication side effects.

Modifications of the classroom environment or assignments may be useful in addition to medication. The student may need to be evaluated for additional help or for an Individualized Education Plan for learning or behavior.

Any expression of suicidal thoughts or feelings or self-harm by a child or adolescent is a clear signal of distress and should be taken seriously. These behaviors should not be dismissed as "attention seeking."

What Is Atomoxetine (Strattera)?

Atomoxetine is a medicine developed to treat attention-deficit/hyperactivity disorder (ADHD or ADD) in children, adolescents, and adults. Atomoxetine is not a stimulant (like methylphenidate or amphetamine), and it works in a different way than the stimulant medicines. It is sometimes called a *selective norepinephrine reuptake inhibitor.*

How Can This Medicine Help?

Atomoxetine can increase attention and the ability to follow instructions. It can improve attention span, decrease distractibility, increase the ability to finish things, decrease hyperactivity, and improve the ability to think before acting (decrease impulsivity). Handwriting and completion of schoolwork and homework can improve. Atomoxetine can improve willingness to follow directions and decrease stubbornness in youngsters with both ADHD and oppositional defiant disorder (ODD). Atomoxetine can decrease depression (sadness) and anxiety (nervousness, worrying) in children with ADHD who have these emotional symptoms.

Medicine may not remove all symptoms in people with ADHD. Children may also need special help in school and behavior modification at home and at school. Some youngsters and families are helped by family therapy or group social skills therapy.

How Does This Medicine Work?

Atomoxetine helps certain parts of the brain that control impulsive actions ("the brakes") work better by increasing the activity of the neurotransmitter *norepinephrine*. *Neurotransmitters* are the chemicals that the brain makes for the nerve cells to communicate with each other.

How Long Does This Medicine Last?

When given once a day, atomoxetine works around the clock. It must be taken every day.

How Will the Doctor Monitor This Medicine?

The doctor will review your child's medical history and physical examination before starting atomoxetine. The doctor or nurse may measure your child's height, weight, pulse (heart rate), and blood pressure before starting atomoxetine. The doctor will usually ask parents and teachers to fill out behavior rating scales (checklists).

Unlike most medicines used for behavioral and emotional problems, the correct dose of atomoxetine depends on the youth's weight. The doctor will start with a low dose and increase the dose over several weeks to a "target dose." Often, atomoxetine is started in two divided doses—with breakfast and dinner—to decrease uncomfortable side effects. Once a person is used to the medicine, it can be given once a day, either with breakfast or with dinner. If daytime sleepiness is a problem, it can be given just before or at bedtime.

After the medicine is started, the doctor will want to have regular appointments with you and your child to see how the medicine is working, to see if a dose change is needed, to watch for side effects, to see if atomoxetine is still needed, and to see if any other treatment is needed. The doctor or nurse may check your child's height, weight, pulse, and blood pressure. With parental permission, the doctor will usually ask for reports (rating scale, checklist, testing results, comments) from the teacher(s) to keep track of progress in learning and behavior.

What Side Effects Can This Medicine Have?

Any medicine can have side effects, including an allergy to the medicine. Because each patient is different, the doctor will monitor the youth closely, especially when the medicine is started. The doctor will work with you to increase the positive effects and decrease the negative effects of the medicine. Please tell the doctor if any of the listed side effects appear or if you think that the medicine is causing any other problems. Not all of the rare or unusual side effects are listed.

Side effects are most common after starting the medicine or after a dose increase. Many side effects can be avoided or lessened by starting with a very low dose and increasing it slowly—ask the doctor.

Allergic Reaction

Tell the doctor in a day or two (if possible, before the next dose of medicine):

- Hives
- Itching
- Rash

    Stop the medicine and get *immediate* medical care:

- Trouble breathing or chest tightness
- Swelling of lips, tongue, or throat

Common Side Effects

If the following side effects do not go away after a week or two, ask the doctor about lowering your child's dose:

- Sedation, fatigue, sleepiness—These side effects can be helped by giving more of the medicine with dinner. Do not allow your child to drive, ride a bicycle or motorcycle, or operate machinery if this happens.
- Nausea, upset stomach, stomachache—These side effects can be helped by giving the medicine in two doses a day, with meals.
- Decreased appetite, mild weight loss
- Dizziness
- Headache

Less Common Side Effects

Tell the doctor within a week or two:

- Rapid pulse rate (heartbeat)
- Increased blood pressure
- Motor tics (fast, repeated movements) or muscle twitches (jerking movements)
- Vomiting
- Irritability, jitteriness, nervousness
- Insomnia (trouble sleeping)

- Constipation—Encourage your child to drink more fluids and eat high-fiber foods; if necessary, the doctor may recommend a fiber medicine such as Benefiber or a stool softener such as Colace or mineral oil.
- Dry mouth

Less Common, but More Serious, Side Effects

Call the doctor within a day or two:

- Increased aggression or hostility
- Increased moodiness
- Problems urinating (passing urine)

Rare, but Serious, Side Effects

Call the doctor within a day:

- Any unusual change in behavior
- Thoughts of suicide or hurting himself or herself (very rare)
- Hurting himself or herself on purpose (very rare)
- Increased activity, agitation, rapid speech, feeling "speeded up," decreased need for sleep, being very excited or irritable (cranky)—This is likely to be manic activation. It has been seen only in people who have bipolar disorder together with ADHD.
- Yellowing of skin or eyes, dark urine, pale bowel movements, abdominal pain or fullness, unexplained flu-like symptoms, itchy skin—These side effects are extremely rare but could be signs of liver damage.

Some Interactions With Other Medicines or Food

Please note that the following are only the most likely interactions with food or other medicines.

Atomoxetine may be taken with food.

Caffeine may increase side effects.

Atomoxetine is safe to use together with a stimulant medication (methylphenidate or amphetamine) if neither type of medicine alone works well enough for your child.

Atomoxetine may increase the side effects of albuterol (Ventolin) inhalers; these side effects include palpitations, fast heart rate (pulse), and increased blood pressure.

When atomoxetine is taken together with fluoxetine (Prozac), paroxetine (Paxil), cimetidine (Tagamet), or bupropion (Wellbutrin), the dose of atomoxetine may need to be lowered.

Atomoxetine should not be taken at the same time as or even within a month of taking another type of medicine called a *monoamine oxidase inhibitor* (MAOI), such as Eldepryl (selegiline), Nardil (phenelzine), Parnate (tranylcypromine), or Marplan (isocarboxazid). The combination could cause severe high blood pressure.

What Could Happen if This Medicine Is Stopped Suddenly?

There are no known medical side effects from stopping atomoxetine suddenly. The symptoms of ADHD will gradually come back.

How Long Will This Medicine Be Needed?

There is no way to know how long a person will need to take atomoxetine. The parent(s), the doctor, and the school will work together to determine what is right for each patient. Sometimes the medicine is needed for a few years, but many people need to take medicine for ADHD even as adults.

What Else Should I Know About This Medicine?

Unlike stimulant medicines (methylphenidate or amphetamine), atomoxetine takes several weeks to work (although side effects may show up right away). The full positive effects of a certain dose of atomoxetine may not show for several months, so it helps to be patient.

It is important that the child swallow the capsule whole and not chew it or open it, because the liquid inside can burn the eyes or mouth.

The FDA has required that the label for atomoxetine include a warning regarding possible increased risk of suicidal thinking in children and adolescents being treated with this medicine. The risk of this is very low, but it is important to be careful.

What Should a Parent Do?

1. Be honest with your child about possible risks and benefits of medicine.
2. Talk to your child about whether he or she is having any suicidal thoughts, and tell your child to come to you if he or she is having such thoughts.
3. You, your child, and your child's doctor or nurse should develop a safety plan. Pick adults whom your child can tell if he or she is thinking about suicide.
4. Be sure to tell your child's doctor, nurse, or therapist if you suspect that your child is using alcohol or drugs or if something has happened that might make your child feel worse, such as a family separation, breaking up with a boyfriend or girlfriend, someone close dying or attempting suicide, physical or sexual abuse, or failure in school.
5. Be sure that there are no guns in the home and that all medicines (including over-the-counter medicines like Tylenol) are closely supervised by an adult and kept in a safe place.
6. Watch for new or worse thoughts of suicide, self-harm, depression, anxiety (nerves), feeling very agitated or restless, being angry or aggressive, having more trouble sleeping, or anything else that you see for the first time, seems worse, or worries your child or you. If these appear, contact a mental health professional **right away.** Do not just stop or change the dose of the medicine on your own. If the problems are serious, and you cannot reach one of your clinicians, call a 24-hour psychiatry emergency telephone number or take your child to an emergency room.

The FDA has also required a warning about possible severe liver injury in patients taking atomoxetine. This problem happened only once in more than 3 million patients, but if your child develops itchy skin, yellow skin or eyes, dark urine, abdominal pain or fullness, or unexplained flu-like symptoms, stop the medicine and see the doctor right away. In the one teenager who had this problem, the liver returned to normal after the atomoxetine was stopped.

Notes

Use this space to take notes or to write down questions you want to ask the doctor.

_____

_____

_____

_____

_____

_____

_____

_____

_____

_____

_____

_____

From Dulcan MK (editor): *Helping Parents, Youth, and Teachers Understand Medications for Behavioral and Emotional Problems: A Resource Book of Medication Information Handouts*, Third Edition. Washington, DC, American Psychiatric Publishing, 2007

Medication Information for Youth

Atomoxetine—Strattera

What the Medicine Is Called and What It Is For

The name of your medicine may be confusing. Most drugs have two names: 1) a scientific name that we call a *generic name* and 2) a trade or *brand name*. The generic name of this medicine is atomoxetine. The brand name is Strattera.

Atomoxetine is used to treat attention-deficit/hyperactivity disorder (ADHD or ADD), whether or not the person has hyperactivity (increased moving around). It is different from the stimulant medicines (amphetamine or methylphenidate). In people who have ADHD or ADD, parts of the brain are not working as well as they should. An example is the part that controls impulsive actions ("the brakes"). Atomoxetine helps these parts of the brain work better. The medicine can help you pay attention at school and at home. It can make it easier for you to listen to and follow directions, to finish more of your schoolwork and homework with fewer mistakes, to think before you act, to sit still for longer periods, and to get into less trouble with adults or other kids.

If you have sadness or nervousness along with ADHD (or ADD), atomoxetine may help decrease these uncomfortable feelings as well.

How You Take the Medicine

It is very important to take the medicine exactly as the doctor or nurse tells you. Do not skip doses or take extra medicine without asking an adult. If you forget a dose, ask your parent(s) what to do. The dose of atomoxetine depends on your weight. The doctor will start with a low dose and increase the dose over several weeks. Often, atomoxetine is started in two doses a day—with breakfast and dinner—to decrease side effects. Once you are used to the medicine, it can be given once a day, either with breakfast or with dinner.

It is important to swallow the capsule whole and not chew it or open it, because the liquid inside can burn your eyes or mouth.

This medicine is prescribed only for you. It should never be shared with anyone else.

Some people with ADHD take a stimulant medicine (methylphenidate or amphetamine) along with atomoxetine.

You do not have to tell others that you are taking this medicine, but it is not something you should feel ashamed or embarrassed about. Many young people are helped by atomoxetine. This medicine is not habit-forming, and you cannot become "hooked" on it. You should talk to your doctor or nurse about any questions you have about the medicine.

53

It is important to remember that that this medicine cannot change you as a person. Successes that you have in your schoolwork or other areas are *your* achievements, not those of the medicine. The medicine cannot make you do anything; it helps you do what *you* want to do. It helps you to be yourself, only calmer, more efficient, more productive, and more successful.

How Your Doctor Will Follow Your Progress

Before giving you the medicine, your doctor or nurse will talk with you and your parent(s) and will measure your height, weight, heart rate (pulse), and blood pressure.

Be sure to tell your doctor or nurse about any other medicines or supplements you are taking, including vitamins, herbs, or aids to weight loss or bodybuilding. Also be sure to tell the doctor or nurse if you are using alcohol or drugs. Because many medicines may affect babies, it is very important to tell the doctor if you might be pregnant or if you are at risk of becoming pregnant.

Your teachers may be asked to fill out a form about your grades and behavior in school. A psychologist may give you some tests to see how you learn best.

Most doctors have regular appointments with young people who are taking medicine. You should use these visits to share any concerns you may have about your medicine and to talk about if it has helped you. From time to time, your physician or nurse may measure your height, weight, heart rate (pulse), and blood pressure to be sure that you are in good health while you are taking the medicine. Your doctor also will ask for regular reports from your parents to see how well the medicine is working. With permission from you and your parent, the doctor may ask for reports from your teacher(s) to see if the medicine is helping your grades, learning, and behavior.

There is no way to know ahead of time how long you will need to take atomoxetine. The doctor will work together with you and your parent(s) and teachers to decide what is right for you. Sometimes the medicine is needed for a few years, but some people may need to take medicine for ADHD as they go to college and even as adults.

How the Medicine Might Affect You

Unlike stimulant medicines (methylphenidate or amphetamine), atomoxetine takes several weeks to work (although side effects may show up right away). The full positive effects of a certain dose of atomoxetine may not show for several months, so it helps to be patient.

In addition to the ways the medicine can help you, it may have other effects called *side effects*. Different medicines have different side effects. It is helpful to know about some of the most common side effects of your medicine so that you will understand what they are if they happen. Some people do not have any side effects. Some side effects are just uncomfortable, but others may mean a more serious problem with the medicine. Side effects are most common after starting the medicine or after a dose increase. They may go away with time, or the medicine can be adjusted or changed—ask the doctor.

You could have an allergy to any medicine, which might show up as a rash on your skin, swelling, itching, or trouble breathing.

Please tell your parent(s) and your doctor or nurse about any changes that you notice after taking the medicine. It is especially important to tell a responsible adult right away if you are feeling depressed or that you may not want to live; if you have thoughts of hurting yourself; or if you begin to feel more irritable, nervous, or restless. Also be sure to tell your parent(s) or doctor if you begin to feel more angry or "speeded up" or have trouble sleeping.

This medicine may make you feel sleepy or less coordinated. If this medicine is making you sleepy, it is very important not to drive a car or ride a bicycle or motorcycle. After starting the medicine or increasing the dose, please be extra careful when driving a car, riding a bike, or using machines until you can tell how the medicine affects your alertness, attention, and coordination.

Some people have stomachaches or upset stomach, headache, or feel like eating less. Usually these problems get better after your body is used to the medicine, or with a lower dose. Let the doctor know if these problems do not go away.

Be sure to tell your parent(s) or doctor if you have rapid heartbeat, motor tics (fast, repeated movements) or muscle twitches (jerking movements), vomiting, or if you notice any changes in your urine or bowel movements.

It is very important not to drink alcohol or use marijuana or street drugs. These could make your ADHD problems worse or increase the side effects of this medicine.

Caffeine (in coffee, tea, or soft drinks) may make the side effects of this medicine worse.

Notes

Use this space to take notes or to write down questions you want to ask the doctor or nurse.

_____

_____

_____

_____

_____

_____

_____

_____

From Dulcan MK (editor): _Helping Parents, Youth, and Teachers Understand Medications for Behavioral and Emotional Problems: A Resource Book of Medication Information Handouts_, Third Edition. Washington, DC, American Psychiatric Publishing, 2007

Medication Information for Parents and Teachers

Benztropine—Cogentin

General Information About Medication

Each child and adolescent is different. No one has exactly the same combination of medical and psychological problems. It is a good idea to talk with the doctor or nurse about the reasons a medicine is being used. It is very important to keep all appointments and to be in touch by telephone if you have concerns. It is important to communicate with the doctor, nurse, or therapist.

It is very important that the medicine be taken exactly as the doctor instructs. However, once in a while, everyone forgets to give a medicine on time. It is a good idea to ask the doctor or nurse what to do if this happens. Do not stop or change a medicine without asking the doctor or nurse first.

If the medicine seems to stop working, it may be because it is not being taken regularly. The youth may be "cheeking" or hiding the medicine or forgetting to take it (especially at school). The doses may be too far apart, or a different dose may be needed. Something at school, at home, or in the neighborhood may be upsetting the youth, or he or she may need special help for learning disabilities or tutoring. Please discuss your concerns with the doctor. **Do not just increase the dose.**

All medicines should be kept in a safe place, out of the reach of children, and should be supervised by an adult. If someone takes too much of a medicine, call the doctor, the poison control center, or a hospital emergency room.

Each medicine has a "generic" or chemical name. Just like laundry detergents or paper towels, some medicines are sold by more than one company under different brand names. The same medicine may be available under a generic name and several brand names. The generic medications are usually less expensive than the brand name ones. The generic medications have the same chemical formula, but they may or may not be exactly the same strength as the brand-name medications. Also, some brands of pills contain dye that can cause allergic reactions. It is a good idea to talk to the doctor and the pharmacist about whether it is important to use a specific brand of medicine.

All medicines can cause an allergic reaction. Examples are hives, itching, rashes, swelling, and trouble breathing. Even a tiny amount of a medicine can cause a reaction in patients who are allergic to that medicine. Be *sure* to talk to the doctor before restarting a medicine that has caused an allergic reaction.

Taking more than one medicine at the same time may cause more side effects or cause one of the medicines to not work as well. Always ask the doctor, nurse, or pharmacist before adding another medicine, whether prescription or over-the-counter. Be sure that each doctor knows about *all* of the medicines your child is taking. Also tell the doctor about any vitamins, herbal medicines, or supplements your child may be taking. Some of these may have side effects alone or when taken with this medication.

Everyone taking medicine should have a physical examination at least once a year.

If you suspect the youth is using drugs or alcohol, please tell the doctor right away.

Pregnancy requires special care in the use of medicine. Please tell the doctor immediately if you suspect the teenager is pregnant or might become pregnant.

Printed information like this applies to children and adolescents in general. If you have questions about the medicine, or if you notice changes or anything unusual, please ask the doctor or nurse. As scientific research advances, knowledge increases and advice changes. Even experts do not always agree. Many medicines have not been approved by the U.S. Food and Drug Administration (FDA) for use in children. For this reason, use of the medicine for a particular problem or age group often is not listed in the *Physicians' Desk Reference*. This does not necessarily mean that the medicine is dangerous or does not work, only that the company that makes the medicine has not received permission to advertise the medicine for use in children. Companies often do not apply for this permission because it is expensive to do the tests needed to apply for approval for use in children. Once a medication is approved by the FDA for any purpose, a doctor is allowed to prescribe it according to research and clinical experience.

Note to Teachers

It is a good idea to talk with the parent(s) about the reason(s) that a medication is being used. If the parent(s) sign consent to release information, it is often helpful to talk with the doctor. If the parent(s) give permission, the doctor may ask you to fill out rating forms about your experience with the student's behavior, feelings, academic performance, and medication side effects. This information is very useful in selecting and monitoring medication treatment. If you have observations that you think are important, do not hesitate to share these with the student's parent(s) and treating clinicians.

It is very important that the medicine be taken exactly as the doctor instructs. However, everyone forgets to give a medicine on time once in a while. It is a good idea to ask the parent(s) in advance what to do if this happens. Do not stop or change the time you are giving a medicine at school without parental permission. If a medication is to be taken with food, but lunchtime or snack time changes, be sure to notify the parent(s) so appropriate adjustments can be made.

All medicines should be kept in a secure place and should be supervised by an adult. If someone takes too much of a medicine, follow your school procedure for an urgent medical problem.

Taking medicine is a private matter and is best managed discreetly and confidentially. It is important to be sensitive to the student's feelings about taking medicine.

If you suspect that the student is using drugs or alcohol, please tell the parent(s) or a school counselor right away.

Please tell the parent(s) or school nurse if you suspect medication side effects.

Modifications of the classroom environment or assignments may be useful in addition to medication. The student may need to be evaluated for additional help or for an Individualized Education Plan for learning or behavior.

Any expression of suicidal thoughts or feelings or self-harm by a child or adolescent is a clear signal of distress and should be taken seriously. These behaviors should not be dismissed as "attention seeking."

What Is Benztropine (Cogentin)?

Benztropine is called an *anticholinergic* or *antiparkinson* medicine. It is not used alone, but together with *typical* or *first-generation* antipsychotic medicines, such as haloperidol, fluphenazine, and trifluoperazine. Benztropine comes in brand name Cogentin and generic tablets and Cogentin injections (shots).

How Can This Medicine Help?

Benztropine can reduce some of the movement side effects of the antipsychotic medicines, such as severe restlessness, agitation, and pacing *(akathisia)*; muscle spasms *(dystonia)*; muscle stiffness *(cogwheeling rigidity)*; or trembling. Sometimes these are called *parkinsonian* or *extrapyramidal* symptoms. Benztropine can be given regularly to prevent or treat these problems. If there is a sudden, severe muscle spasm, benztropine may be given as a shot so that it works within 15 minutes.

How Does This Medicine Work?

Benztropine counteracts the effects of the antipsychotic medicines in parts of the brain that control muscle action, but without decreasing the effects of the antipsychotic medicines on thinking and other psychiatric symptoms. It balances the *cholinergic* and *dopamine* systems in the brain.

How Long Does This Medicine Last?

Benztropine is taken two or three times a day.

How Will the Doctor Monitor This Medicine?

The doctor will review your child's medical history and physical examination before starting benztropine. An examination such as the AIMS (Abnormal Involuntary Movement Scale) test may be used to check the child's tongue, legs, and arms for unusual movements that could be helped by the medicine.

After the medicine is started, the doctor will want to have regular appointments with you and your child to see how the medicine is working, to see if a dose change is needed, to watch for side effects, to see if benztropine is still needed, and to see if any other treatment is needed.

What Side Effects Can This Medicine Have?

Any medicine can have side effects, including an allergy to the medicine. Because each patient is different, the doctor will monitor the youth closely, especially when the medicine is started. The doctor will work with you to increase the positive effects and decrease the negative effects of the medicine. Please tell the doctor if any of the listed side effects appear or if you think that the medicine is causing any other problems. Not all of the rare or unusual side effects are listed.

Side effects are most common after starting the medicine or after a dose increase. Many side effects can be avoided or lessened by starting with a very low dose and increasing it slowly—ask the doctor.

59

Allergic Reaction

Tell the doctor in a day or two (if possible, before the next dose of medicine):

- Hives
- Itching
- Rash

  Stop the medicine and get *immediate* medical care:

- Trouble breathing or chest tightness
- Swelling of lips, tongue, or throat

Common Side Effects

Tell the doctor within a week or two:

- Daytime sleepiness—Do not allow your child to drive, ride a bicycle or motorcycle, or operate machinery if this happens.
- Decreased attention or learning in school
- Dry mouth—Have your child try using sugar-free gum or candy.
- Blurred vision
- Constipation—Encourage your child to drink more fluids and eat high-fiber foods; if necessary, the doctor may recommend a fiber medicine such as Benefiber or a stool softener such as Colace or mineral oil.
- Dizziness—When standing up quickly, especially when getting out of bed in the morning; try having the child stand up slowly.
- Loss of appetite, nausea, or upset stomach
- Decreased sweating

Less Common Side Effects

Call the doctor within a day or two:

- Irritability, overactivity
- Rapid heartbeat (pulse) or palpitations
- Difficulty passing urine

Very Rare, but Serious, Side Effects

Call the doctor *immediately*:

- Worsening of asthma or trouble breathing
- Seizure (fit, convulsion)
- Uncontrollable behavior
- Severe confusion, loss of coordination, severe agitation, disorientation

Some Interactions With Other Medicines or Food

Please note that the following are only the most likely interactions with food or other medicines.

Caffeine may increase side effects.

Benztropine may be taken with or without food. Taking it with food may decrease stomach upset.

Tricyclic antidepressants such as imipramine, nortriptyline, or clomipramine also have anticholinergic effects and will increase the side effects of benztropine. Many antipsychotic medications also have anticholinergic effects and increase the side effects of benztropine.

What Could Happen if This Medicine Is Stopped Suddenly?

Stopping benztropine suddenly can cause withdrawal symptoms such as irritability, nausea, vomiting, headache, and trouble sleeping.

How Long Will This Medicine Be Needed?

Sometimes the benztropine will be needed as long as the person is on the antipsychotic medicine, but sometimes it can be carefully tapered (decreased) and stopped if the person has gotten used to the antipsychotic medicine and there are no longer motor side effects.

What Else Should I Know About This Medicine?

Because benztropine decreases sweating, a person may be more likely to get heatstroke or *hyperthermia* (increase in body temperature). Be sure that your child drinks plenty of fluids in hot weather and does not exercise too much in the sun.

Notes

Use this space to take notes or to write down questions you want to ask the doctor.

_____

_____

_____

_____

_____

_____

_____

_____

_____

_____

_____

_____

_____

_____

From Dulcan MK (editor): *Helping Parents, Youth, and Teachers Understand Medications for Behavioral and Emotional Problems: A Resource Book of Medication Information Handouts,* Third Edition. Washington, DC, American Psychiatric Publishing, 2007

Medication Information for Youth

Benztropine—Cogentin

What the Medicine Is Called and What It Is For

The name of your medicine may be confusing. Most drugs have two names: 1) a scientific name that we call a *generic name* and 2) a trade or *brand name*. The generic name of this medicine is benztropine. The brand name is Cogentin.

Benztropine is called an *anticholinergic* or *antiparkinson* medicine. It is not used alone, but only together with antipsychotic medicines. Benztropine can reduce some of the movement side effects of the antipsychotic medicines, such as severe restlessness, agitation, and pacing *(akathisia)*; muscle spasms *(dystonia)*; muscle stiffness *(cogwheeling rigidity)*; or trembling. Sometimes these are called *parkinsonian* or *extrapyramidal* symptoms. Benztropine can be given regularly to prevent or treat these problems. If there is a sudden, severe muscle spasm, benztropine may be given as a shot so that it works within 15 minutes.

How You Take the Medicine

It is very important to take the medicine exactly as the doctor or nurse tells you. Do not skip doses or take extra medicine without asking an adult. If you forget a dose, ask your parent(s) what to do. It is important not to stop taking this medicine suddenly. Talk with your doctor if you want to stop taking it.

If the medicine makes your stomach upset, taking it with food may help.

This medicine is prescribed only for you. It should never be shared with anyone else.

You do not have to tell others that you are taking this medicine, but it is not something you should feel ashamed or embarrassed about. Many young people are helped by benztropine. This medicine is not habit-forming, and you cannot become "hooked" on it. You should talk to your doctor or nurse about any questions you have about the medicine.

How Your Doctor Will Follow Your Progress

Before giving you the medicine, your doctor or nurse will talk with you and your parent(s) and may measure your height, weight, heart rate (pulse), and blood pressure. An examination such as the AIMS (Abnormal Involuntary Movement Scale) test may be used to check your tongue, legs, and arms for unusual movements that could be helped by the medicine.

Be sure to tell your doctor or nurse about any other medicines or supplements you are taking, including vitamins, herbs, or aids to weight loss or bodybuilding. Also be sure to tell the doctor or nurse if you are using alcohol or drugs. Because many medicines may affect babies, it is very important to tell the doctor if you might be pregnant or if you are at risk of becoming pregnant.

Most doctors have regular appointments with young people who are taking medicine. You should use these visits to share any concerns you may have about your medicine and to talk about if it has helped you. Your doctor also will ask for regular reports from your parents and maybe from your teachers (with your permission) to see how well the medicine is working.

Sometimes the benztropine will be needed as long as the person is on the antipsychotic medicine, but sometimes it can be carefully tapered (decreased) and stopped if the person has gotten used to the antipsychotic medicine and there are no longer motor side effects.

How the Medicine Might Affect You

In addition to the ways the medicine can help you, it may have other effects called *side effects*. Different medicines have different side effects. It is helpful to know about some of the most common side effects of your medicine so that you will understand what they are if they happen. Some people do not have any side effects. Some side effects are just uncomfortable, but others may mean a more serious problem with the medicine. Side effects are most common after starting the medicine or after a dose increase. They may go away with time, or the medicine can be adjusted or changed—ask the doctor.

You could have an allergy to any medicine, which might show up as a rash on your skin, swelling, itching, or trouble breathing.

Please tell your parent(s) and your doctor or nurse about any changes that you notice after taking the medicine. It is especially important to tell a responsible adult if you are feeling depressed or that you may not want to live; if you have thoughts of hurting yourself; or if you begin to feel more irritable, nervous, or restless.

Some medicines make people feel sleepy or less coordinated. If this medicine is making you sleepy, it is very important not to drive a car or ride a bicycle or motorcycle. After starting a new medicine or increasing the dose of a medicine, please be extra careful when driving a car, riding a bike, or using machines until you can tell how the medicine affects your alertness, attention, and coordination.

This medicine may cause dry mouth. You may be more thirsty than usual and find that you are drinking more water or other liquids. Sucking on sugar-free hard candy or cough drops usually helps. You could also try chewing sugar-free gum or sucking on ice chips. Do not chew the ice; you could hurt your teeth. Also, using lip balm on your lips will keep them from cracking. It is important to be especially good about brushing your teeth.

Sometimes people taking this medicine notice that their heart is beating faster than normal. Usually this happens within the first few weeks of taking the medicine and gets better or goes away. However, if you notice that your heart is beating very fast for more than a few minutes when you have not been exercising, if you feel light-headed or dizzy when you are sitting or standing still, or if you faint, you should let your parent(s) and doctor know right away.

Some people become constipated (have hard bowel movements) when taking this medicine. Try drinking more water and eating more fruits, vegetables, and whole grains. If that does not help, tell your parent(s) or doctor—you may need a medicine to help with this side effect.

In hot weather, it is very important to drink plenty of water and to not get overheated.

Other side effects happen less often, including not feeling hungry and not wanting to eat much, feeling irritable, having trouble passing urine, or blurred vision. Let your parent(s) and doctor know if you notice anything different or unusual about how you feel once you start taking the medicine.

Caffeine (in coffee, tea, or soft drinks) may make the side effects of this medicine worse.

Notes

Use this space to take notes or to write down questions you want to ask the doctor or nurse.

_____

_____

_____

_____

_____

_____

_____

_____

_____

_____

_____

Medication Information for Parents and Teachers

Bupropion—Wellbutrin, Budeprion

General Information About Medication

Each child and adolescent is different. No one has exactly the same combination of medical and psychological problems. It is a good idea to talk with the doctor or nurse about the reasons a medicine is being used. It is very important to keep all appointments and to be in touch by telephone if you have concerns. It is important to communicate with the doctor, nurse, or therapist.

It is very important that the medicine be taken exactly as the doctor instructs. However, once in a while, everyone forgets to give a medicine on time. It is a good idea to ask the doctor or nurse what to do if this happens. Do not stop or change a medicine without asking the doctor or nurse first.

If the medicine seems to stop working, it may be because it is not being taken regularly. The youth may be "cheeking" or hiding the medicine or forgetting to take it (especially at school). The doses may be too far apart, or a different dose may be needed. Something at school, at home, or in the neighborhood may be upsetting the youth, or he or she may need special help for learning disabilities or tutoring. Please discuss your concerns with the doctor. **Do not just increase the dose.**

All medicines should be kept in a safe place, out of the reach of children, and should be supervised by an adult. If someone takes too much of a medicine, call the doctor, the poison control center, or a hospital emergency room.

Each medicine has a "generic" or chemical name. Just like laundry detergents or paper towels, some medicines are sold by more than one company under different brand names. The same medicine may be available under a generic name and several brand names. The generic medications are usually less expensive than the brand name ones. The generic medications have the same chemical formula, but they may or may not be exactly the same strength as the brand-name medications. Also, some brands of pills contain dye that can cause allergic reactions. It is a good idea to talk to the doctor and the pharmacist about whether it is important to use a specific brand of medicine.

All medicines can cause an allergic reaction. Examples are hives, itching, rashes, swelling, and trouble breathing. Even a tiny amount of a medicine can cause a reaction in patients who are allergic to that medicine. Be *sure* to talk to the doctor before restarting a medicine that has caused an allergic reaction.

Taking more than one medicine at the same time may cause more side effects or cause one of the medicines to not work as well. Always ask the doctor, nurse, or pharmacist before adding another medicine, whether prescription or over-the-counter. Be sure that each doctor knows about *all* of the medicines your child is taking. Also tell the doctor about any vitamins, herbal medicines, or supplements your child may be taking. Some of these may have side effects alone or when taken with this medication.

Everyone taking medicine should have a physical examination at least once a year.

If you suspect the youth is using drugs or alcohol, please tell the doctor right away.

Pregnancy requires special care in the use of medicine. Please tell the doctor immediately if you suspect the teenager is pregnant or might become pregnant.

67

Printed information like this applies to children and adolescents in general. If you have questions about the medicine, or if you notice changes or anything unusual, please ask the doctor or nurse. As scientific research advances, knowledge increases and advice changes. Even experts do not always agree. Many medicines have not been approved by the U.S. Food and Drug Administration (FDA) for use in children. For this reason, use of the medicine for a particular problem or age group often is not listed in the *Physicians' Desk Reference.* This does not necessarily mean that the medicine is dangerous or does not work, only that the company that makes the medicine has not received permission to advertise the medicine for use in children. Companies often do not apply for this permission because it is expensive to do the tests needed to apply for approval for use in children. Once a medication is approved by the FDA for any purpose, a doctor is allowed to prescribe it according to research and clinical experience.

Note to Teachers

It is a good idea to talk with the parent(s) about the reason(s) that a medication is being used. If the parent(s) sign consent to release information, it is often helpful to talk with the doctor. If the parent(s) give permission, the doctor may ask you to fill out rating forms about your experience with the student's behavior, feelings, academic performance, and medication side effects. This information is very useful in selecting and monitoring medication treatment. If you have observations that you think are important, do not hesitate to share these with the student's parent(s) and treating clinicians.

It is very important that the medicine be taken exactly as the doctor instructs. However, everyone forgets to give a medicine on time once in a while. It is a good idea to ask the parent(s) in advance what to do if this happens. Do not stop or change the time you are giving a medicine at school without parental permission. If a medication is to be taken with food, but lunchtime or snack time changes, be sure to notify the parent(s) so appropriate adjustments can be made.

All medicines should be kept in a secure place and should be supervised by an adult. If someone takes too much of a medicine, follow your school procedure for an urgent medical problem.

Taking medicine is a private matter and is best managed discreetly and confidentially. It is important to be sensitive to the student's feelings about taking medicine.

If you suspect that the student is using drugs or alcohol, please tell the parent(s) or a school counselor right away.

Please tell the parent(s) or school nurse if you suspect medication side effects.

- If the student has dry mouth, it helps to allow chewing of sugar-free gum or extra trips to the water fountain.
- The medicine may cause the student to be constipated; allowing the student to drink more fluids and use the bathroom more often may help. The student may need to use a bathroom with more privacy.
- If the medicine gives the student an upset stomach, it may help to take the medicine after a meal or a snack.
- The student may become dizzy when standing up quickly in the classroom or during physical education; suggest that the student stand up more slowly.

Modifications of the classroom environment or assignments may be useful in addition to medication. The student may need to be evaluated for additional help or for an Individualized Education Plan for learning or behavior.

Any expression of suicidal thoughts or feelings or self-harm by a child or adolescent is a clear signal of distress and should be taken seriously. These behaviors should not be dismissed as "attention seeking."

What Is Bupropion (Wellbutrin, Budeprion)?

Bupropion is called an *antidepressant*, but it is used to treat behavioral problems, including attention-deficit/ hyperactivity disorder (ADHD or ADD) and conduct problems, as well as depression. Bupropion comes in immediate-release tablets (Wellbutrin and generic), sustained-release long-acting tablets (Wellbutrin SR, Budeprion SR, and generic), and very long-acting extended-release tablets (Wellbutrin XL). Bupropion also comes in brand names Zyban and Buproban, which are used to help people stop smoking.

How Can This Medicine Help?

Bupropion can decrease symptoms of ADHD, impulsive behavior, depression, and aggression.

How Does This Medicine Work?

Bupropion helps by balancing the levels of certain chemicals that are naturally found in the brain, called *neurotransmitters*. Neurotransmitters are the chemicals that the brain makes for the nerve cells to communicate with each other. Bupropion is sometimes called a *dopamine-norepinephrine reuptake inhibitor*.

How Long Does This Medicine Last?

Immediate-release bupropion must be taken three times a day. The sustained-release form can be taken twice a day, and the extended-release form can be taken only once a day.

How Will the Doctor Monitor This Medicine?

The doctor will review your child's medical history and physical examination before starting bupropion. The doctor may order some tests to be sure your child does not have a hidden medical condition that would make it unsafe to use this medicine. Bupropion should *not* be used if the child has an eating disorder (anorexia nervosa or bulimia) or a brain problem such as seizures (epilepsy), a head injury, or a brain tumor. **Extra caution is needed when using this medicine in children and adolescents with liver or kidney problems.**

The doctor or nurse may measure your child's pulse and blood pressure before starting bupropion.

After the medicine is started, the doctor will want to have regular appointments with you and your child to see how the medicine is working, to see if a dose change is needed, to watch for side effects, to see if bupropion is still needed, and to see if any other treatment is needed. The doctor or nurse may check your child's height, weight, pulse, and blood pressure.

What Side Effects Can This Medicine Have?

Any medicine can have side effects, including an allergy to the medicine. Allergy to bupropion is more common if the patient has had allergic reactions to other medicines. Because each patient is different, the doctor will monitor the youth closely, especially when the medicine is started. The doctor will work with you to increase the positive effects and decrease the negative effects of the medicine. Please tell the doctor if any of the listed side effects appear or if you think that the medicine is causing any other problems. Not all of the rare or unusual side effects are listed.

Side effects are most common after starting the medicine or after a dose increase. Many side effects can be avoided or lessened by starting with a very low dose and increasing it slowly—ask the doctor.

Allergic Reaction

Tell the doctor in a day or two (if possible, before the next dose of medicine):

- Hives
- Itching
- Rash

Stop the medicine and get *immediate* medical care:

- Trouble breathing or chest tightness
- Swelling of lips, tongue, or throat

Common Side Effects

Tell the doctor within a week or two:

- Nervousness or restlessness
- Irritability—Dose may need to be lowered.
- Dry mouth—Have your child try using sugar-free gum or candy.
- Constipation—Encourage your child to drink more fluids and eat high-fiber foods; if necessary, the doctor may recommend a fiber medicine such as Benefiber or a stool softener such as Colace or mineral oil.
- Headache
- Decreased appetite and weight loss
- Nausea—Taking bupropion with food may help.
- Dizziness
- Excessive sweating

Occasional Side Effects

Call the doctor within a day or two if your child experiences any of these side effects:

- Motor tics (fast, repeated movements), muscle twitches (jerking movements), or tremor (shaking)
- Trouble sleeping
- Ringing in the ears

Less Common, but More Serious, Side Effects

Call the doctor *immediately*:

- Vomiting
- Seizures (fits, convulsions), especially if taking more than 400 mg/day or if drinking alcoholic beverages. This is less common with the longer-acting forms.
- Unusual excitement, decreased need for sleep, rapid speech

Some Interactions With Other Medicines or Food

Please note that the following are only the most likely interactions with food or other medicines.

Carbamazepine (Tegretol) may decrease the positive effect of bupropion.

It can be *very dangerous* to take bupropion at the same time as, or even within several weeks of, taking another type of medicine called a *monoamine oxidase inhibitor* (MAOI), such as Eldepryl (selegiline), Nardil (phenelzine), Parnate (tranylcypromine), or Marplan (isocarboxazid). The combination may cause very high fever, high blood pressure, and extreme excitement and agitation.

Caffeine may increase side effects.

What Could Happen if This Medicine Is Stopped Suddenly?

No known medical withdrawal effects occur if bupropion is stopped suddenly. Some people may get a headache as the medicine wears off. If the medicine is stopped, the original problems may come back. Talk to the doctor before stopping the medicine.

How Long Will This Medicine Be Needed?

Bupropion may take up to 4 weeks to reach its full effect. Your child may need to take the medicine for at least several months so that the emotional or behavioral problem does not come back.

What Else Should I Know About This Medicine?

It is *very important* not to chew the sustained-release tablet or to double up doses if one is missed.

Store the medicine away from heat and wetness.

In youth who have bipolar disorder (manic depression) or who are at risk for bipolar disorder, any antidepressant medicine may increase the risk of hypomania or mania (excitement, agitation, increased activity, decreased sleep).

Bupropion is sometimes confused with buspirone. Be sure to check the prescription.

Sometimes the different forms of bupropion are confused. Be sure you know whether the doctor has prescribed the immediate-release, sustained-release, or extended-release form, and check that the pharmacy has dispensed the correct form of medicine. Be sure that the number of "mg" (dose) and the number of times the medicine is taken each day are clear and consistent.

Black Box Antidepressant Warning

In 2004, an advisory committee to the FDA decided that there might be an increased risk of suicidal behavior for some youth taking medicines called *antidepressants*. In the research studies that the committee reviewed, about 3%–4% of youth with depression who took an antidepressant medicine—and 1%–2% of youth with depression who took a placebo (pill without active medicine)—talked about suicidal thoughts (thinking about killing themselves or wishing they were dead) or did something to harm themselves. This means that almost twice as many youth who were taking an antidepressant to treat their depression talked about suicide or had suicidal behavior compared with youth with depression who were taking inactive medicine. There were *no* completed suicides in any of these research studies, which included more than 4,000 children and adolescents. For youth being treated for anxiety, there was no difference in suicidal talking or behavior between those taking antidepressant medication and those taking placebo.

The FDA told drug companies to add a *black box warning* label to all antidepressant medicines. Because of this label, a doctor (or advanced practice nurse) prescribing one of these medicines has to warn youth and their families that there might be more suicidal thoughts and actions in youth taking these medicines.

On the other hand, in places where more youth are taking the newer antidepressant medicines, the number of adolescents who commit suicide has gotten smaller. Also, thinking about or attempting suicide is more common in surveys of teenagers in the community than it is in depressed youth treated in research studies with antidepressant medicine.

If a youth is being treated with this medicine and is doing well, then no changes are needed as a result of this warning. Increased suicidal talk or action is most likely to happen in the first few months of treatment with a medicine. If your child has recently started this medicine, or is about to start, then you and your doctor (or advanced practice nurse) should watch for any changes in behavior. People who are depressed often have suicidal thoughts or actions. It is hard to know whether suicidal thoughts or actions in depressed people are caused by the depression itself or by the medicine. Also, as their depression is getting better, some people talk more about the suicidal thoughts they had before but did not talk about. As young people get better from depression, they might be at higher risk of doing something about suicidal thoughts that they have had for some time, because they have more energy.

What Should a Parent Do?

1. Be honest with your child about possible risks and benefits of medicine.
2. Talk to your child about whether he or she is having any suicidal thoughts, and tell your child to come to you if he or she is having such thoughts.
3. You, your child, and your child's doctor or nurse should develop a safety plan. Pick adults whom your child can tell if he or she is thinking about suicide.
4. Be sure to tell your child's doctor, nurse, or therapist if you suspect that your child is using alcohol or drugs or if something has happened that might make your child feel worse, such as a family separation, breaking up with a boyfriend or girlfriend, someone close dying or attempting suicide, physical or sexual abuse, or failure in school.
5. Be sure that there are no guns in the home and that all medicines (including over-the-counter medicines like Tylenol) are closely supervised by an adult and kept in a safe place.
6. Watch for new or worse thoughts of suicide, self-harm, depression, anxiety (nerves), feeling very agitated or restless, being angry or aggressive, having more trouble sleeping, or anything else that you see for the first time, seems worse, or worries your child or you. If these appear, contact a mental health professional **right away.** Do not just stop or change the dose of the medicine on your own. If the problems are serious, and you cannot reach one of your clinicians, call a 24-hour psychiatry emergency telephone number or take your child to an emergency room.

Youth taking antidepressant medicine should be watched carefully by their parent(s), clinician(s) (doctor, nurse, therapist), and other concerned adults for the first weeks of treatment. It is a good idea to have a visit or telephone call with the doctor, nurse, or therapist weekly for the first month, every 2 weeks for the second month, and after that at least once a month to check for feelings of depression or sadness, thoughts of killing or harming himself or herself, and any problems with the medication. If you have questions, be sure to ask the doctor, nurse, or therapist.

For more information, see http://www.parentsmedguide.org (in English and Spanish).

Notes

Use this space to take notes or to write down questions you want to ask the doctor.

_____

_____

_____

_____

_____

_____

_____

_____

_____

_____

_____

_____

_____

From Dulcan MK (editor): *Helping Parents, Youth, and Teachers Understand Medications for Behavioral and Emotional Problems: A Resource Book of Medication Information Handouts*, Third Edition. Washington, DC, American Psychiatric Publishing, 2007

Medication Information for Youth

Bupropion—Wellbutrin, Budeprion

What the Medicine Is Called and What It Is For

The name of your medicine may be confusing. Most drugs have two names: (1) a scientific name that we call a *generic name* and (2) a trade or *brand name*. The generic name of this medicine is bupropion. The brand names are Wellbutrin and Budeprion. Bupropion is called an *antidepressant*, but it is also used to treat attention-deficit/hyperactivity disorder (ADHD or ADD) and conduct problems. When bupropion is used to help people stop smoking, it comes in forms called Zyban and Buproban.

In people who have ADHD or ADD, parts of the brain are not working as well as they should. An example is the part that controls impulsive actions ("the brakes"). Bupropion helps these parts of the brain work better. The medicine can help you pay attention at school and at home. It can make it easier for you to listen to and follow directions, to finish more of your schoolwork and homework with fewer mistakes, to think before you act, to sit still for longer periods, and to get into less trouble with adults or other kids.

How You Take the Medicine

It is very important to take the medicine exactly as the doctor or nurse tells you. Do not skip doses or take extra medicine without asking an adult. If you forget a dose, ask your parent(s) what to do. When taking a long-acting form of the medicine, swallow it whole. Do not crush or chew it.

This medicine is prescribed only for you. It should never be shared with anyone else.

Caffeine (in coffee, tea, or soft drinks) may make the side effects of this medicine worse.

It is very important not to drink alcohol or use marijuana or street drugs. These could make your ADHD problems worse or increase the side effects of this medicine.

You do not have to tell others that you are taking this medicine, but it is not something you should feel ashamed or embarrassed about. Many young people are helped by bupropion. This medicine is not habit-forming, and you cannot become "hooked" on it. You should talk to your doctor or nurse about any questions you have about the medicine.

It is important to remember that that this medicine cannot change you as a person. Successes that you have in your schoolwork or other areas are your achievements, not those of the medicine. The medicine cannot make you do anything; it helps you do what you want to do. It helps you to be yourself, only calmer, more efficient, more productive, and more successful.

How Your Doctor Will Follow Your Progress

Before giving you the medicine, your doctor or nurse will talk with you and your parent(s) and may measure your height, weight, heart rate (pulse), and blood pressure. Be sure to tell the doctor if you have had motor or vocal tics (hard-to-control repeated movements or sounds). It is very important to tell the doctor if you have had symptoms of an eating disorder (especially severe dieting, vomiting, or use of laxatives). The doctor may do blood or urine tests to be sure that you are in good health before you start taking bupropion.

Be sure to tell your doctor or nurse about any other medicines or supplements you are taking, including vitamins, herbs, or aids to weight loss or bodybuilding. Also be sure to tell the doctor or nurse if you are using alcohol or drugs. Because many medicines may affect babies, it is very important to tell the doctor if you might be pregnant or if you are at risk of becoming pregnant.

Your teachers may be asked to fill out a form about your grades and behavior in school. A psychologist may give you some tests to see how you learn best.

Most doctors have regular appointments with young people who are taking medicine. You should use these visits to share any concerns you may have about your medicine and to talk about if it has helped you. From time to time, your physician or nurse may measure your height, weight, heart rate (pulse), and blood pressure to be sure that you are in good health while you are taking the medicine. Your doctor also will ask for regular reports from your parents and maybe from your teachers (with your permission) to see how well the medicine is working.

It is hard to say how long you will need to take this medicine. It is sometimes helpful to people even when they go to college and as they become adults. Your doctor will make that decision with you as he or she watches your progress.

How the Medicine Might Affect You

Unlike stimulant medicines (like methylphenidate or amphetamine), bupropion takes several weeks to work (although side effects may show up right away). The full positive effects of a certain dose of bupropion may not show for several months, so it helps to be patient.

In addition to the ways the medicine can help you, it may have other effects called *side effects*. Different medicines have different side effects. It is helpful to know about some of the most common side effects of your medicine so that you will understand what they are if they happen. Some people do not have any side effects. Some side effects are just uncomfortable, but others may mean a more serious problem with the medicine. Side effects are most common after starting the medicine or after a dose increase. They may go away with time, or the medicine can be adjusted or changed—ask the doctor.

You could have an allergy to any medicine, which might show up as a rash on your skin, swelling, itching, or trouble breathing.

Please tell your parent(s) and your doctor or nurse about any changes that you notice after taking the medicine. It is especially important to tell a responsible adult if you are feeling depressed or that you may not want to live; if you have thoughts of hurting yourself; or if you begin to feel more irritable, nervous, or restless. Also be sure to tell your parent(s) or your doctor if you begin to feel "speeded up" or have trouble sleeping.

This medicine may cause dry mouth. You may be more thirsty than usual and find that you are drinking more water or other liquids. Sucking on sugar-free hard candy or cough drops usually helps. You also could try chewing sugar-free gum or sucking on ice chips. Do not chew the ice; you could hurt your teeth. Also, using lip balm on your lips will keep them from cracking. It is important to be especially good about brushing your teeth.

Some people become constipated (have hard bowel movements) when taking this medicine. Try drinking more water and eating more fruits, vegetables, and whole grains. If that does not help, tell your parent(s) or doctor—you may need a medicine to help with this side effect.

Other side effects happen less often, including not feeling hungry and not wanting to eat much; headache; motor tics (fast, repeated movements), muscle twitches (jerking movements), or tremor (shaking); or ringing in the ears. Let your parent(s) and doctor know if you notice anything different or unusual about how you feel once you start taking the medicine.

Notes

Use this space to take notes or to write down questions you want to ask the doctor or nurse.

_____

_____

_____

_____

_____

_____

_____

_____

_____

_____

_____

From Dulcan MK (editor): *Helping Parents, Youth, and Teachers Understand Medications for Behavioral and Emotional Problems: A Resource Book of Medication Information Handouts,* Third Edition. Washington, DC, American Psychiatric Publishing, 2007

Medication Information for Parents and Teachers

Buspirone—BuSpar

General Information About Medication

Each child and adolescent is different. No one has exactly the same combination of medical and psychological problems. It is a good idea to talk with the doctor or nurse about the reasons a medicine is being used. It is very important to keep all appointments and to be in touch by telephone if you have concerns. It is important to communicate with the doctor, nurse, or therapist.

It is very important that the medicine be taken exactly as the doctor instructs. However, once in a while, everyone forgets to give a medicine on time. It is a good idea to ask the doctor or nurse what to do if this happens. Do not stop or change a medicine without asking the doctor or nurse first.

If the medicine seems to stop working, it may be because it is not being taken regularly. The youth may be "cheeking" or hiding the medicine or forgetting to take it (especially at school). The doses may be too far apart, or a different dose may be needed. Something at school, at home, or in the neighborhood may be upsetting the youth, or he or she may need special help for learning disabilities or tutoring. Please discuss your concerns with the doctor. **Do not just increase the dose.**

All medicines should be kept in a safe place, out of the reach of children, and should be supervised by an adult. If someone takes too much of a medicine, call the doctor, the poison control center, or a hospital emergency room.

Each medicine has a "generic" or chemical name. Just like laundry detergents or paper towels, some medicines are sold by more than one company under different brand names. The same medicine may be available under a generic name and several brand names. The generic medications are usually less expensive than the brand name ones. The generic medications have the same chemical formula, but they may or may not be exactly the same strength as the brand-name medications. Also, some brands of pills contain dye that can cause allergic reactions. It is a good idea to talk to the doctor and the pharmacist about whether it is important to use a specific brand of medicine.

All medicines can cause an allergic reaction. Examples are hives, itching, rashes, swelling, and trouble breathing. Even a tiny amount of a medicine can cause a reaction in patients who are allergic to that medicine. Be *sure* to talk to the doctor before restarting a medicine that has caused an allergic reaction.

Taking more than one medicine at the same time may cause more side effects or cause one of the medicines to not work as well. Always ask the doctor, nurse, or pharmacist before adding another medicine, whether prescription or over-the-counter. Be sure that each doctor knows about *all* of the medicines your child is taking. Also tell the doctor about any vitamins, herbal medicines, or supplements your child may be taking. Some of these may have side effects alone or when taken with this medication.

Everyone taking medicine should have a physical examination at least once a year.

If you suspect the youth is using drugs or alcohol, please tell the doctor right away.

79

Pregnancy requires special care in the use of medicine. Please tell the doctor immediately if you suspect the teenager is pregnant or might become pregnant.

Printed information like this applies to children and adolescents in general. If you have questions about the medicine, or if you notice changes or anything unusual, please ask the doctor or nurse. As scientific research advances, knowledge increases and advice changes. Even experts do not always agree. Many medicines have not been approved by the U.S. Food and Drug Administration (FDA) for use in children. For this reason, use of the medicine for a particular problem or age group often is not listed in the *Physicians' Desk Reference*. This does not necessarily mean that the medicine is dangerous or does not work, only that the company that makes the medicine has not received permission to advertise the medicine for use in children. Companies often do not apply for this permission because it is expensive to do the tests needed to apply for approval for use in children. Once a medication is approved by the FDA for any purpose, a doctor is allowed to prescribe it according to research and clinical experience.

Note to Teachers

It is a good idea to talk with the parent(s) about the reason(s) that a medication is being used. If the parent(s) sign consent to release information, it is often helpful to talk with the doctor. If the parent(s) give permission, the doctor may ask you to fill out rating forms about your experience with the student's behavior, feelings, academic performance, and medication side effects. This information is very useful in selecting and monitoring medication treatment. If you have observations that you think are important, do not hesitate to share these with the student's parent(s) and treating clinicians.

It is very important that the medicine be taken exactly as the doctor instructs. However, everyone forgets to give a medicine on time once in a while. It is a good idea to ask the parent(s) in advance what to do if this happens. Do not stop or change the time you are giving a medicine at school without parental permission. If a medication is to be taken with food, but lunchtime or snack time changes, be sure to notify the parent(s) so appropriate adjustments can be made.

All medicines should be kept in a secure place and should be supervised by an adult. If someone takes too much of a medicine, follow your school procedure for an urgent medical problem.

Taking medicine is a private matter and is best managed discreetly and confidentially. It is important to be sensitive to the student's feelings about taking medicine.

If you suspect that the student is using drugs or alcohol, please tell the parent(s) or a school counselor right away.

Please tell the parent(s) or school nurse if you suspect medication side effects.

Modifications of the classroom environment or assignments may be useful in addition to medication. The student may need to be evaluated for additional help or for an Individualized Education Plan for learning or behavior.

Any expression of suicidal thoughts or feelings or self-harm by a child or adolescent is a clear signal of distress and should be taken seriously. These behaviors should not be dismissed as "attention seeking."

What Is Buspirone (BuSpar)?

Buspirone is called an *antianxiety* medicine. It comes in BuSpar brand name and generic tablets. It is not chemically related to the *benzodiazepines* (other antianxiety medicines like Valium or Ativan).

How Can This Medicine Help?

Buspirone can decrease anxiety, nervousness, fears, and excessive worrying. It can help anxious people to be calm enough to learn—with therapy and practice—to understand and tolerate their worries or fears and even to overcome them. Most often, it is used for a short time when symptoms are very uncomfortable or frightening or when they make it hard to do important things such as go to school. Occasionally antianxiety medicines are used for longer periods to treat anxiety that remains after therapy is completed.

How Does This Medicine Work?

Buspirone works by calming the parts of the brain that are too excitable in anxious people. It does this by changing the effects of *neurotransmitters*—the chemicals that the brain makes for brain cells to communicate with each other.

Buspirone does not begin to help immediately. The full effect may not appear for 3–4 weeks.

How Long Does This Medicine Last?

Buspirone usually needs to be taken three times a day.

How Will the Doctor Monitor This Medicine?

The doctor will review your child's medical history and physical examination before starting buspirone. The doctor may order some blood or urine tests to be sure your child does not have a hidden medical condition. The doctor or nurse may measure your child's height, weight, pulse, and blood pressure before starting buspirone.

After the medicine is started, the doctor will want to have regular appointments with you and your child to see how the medicine is working, to see if a dose change is needed, to watch for side effects, to see if buspirone is still needed, and to see if any other treatment is needed. The doctor or nurse may check your child's height, weight, pulse, and blood pressure.

What Side Effects Can This Medicine Have?

Any medicine can have side effects, including an allergy to the medicine. Because each patient is different, the doctor will monitor the youth closely, especially when the medicine is started. The doctor will work with you to increase the positive effects and decrease the negative effects of the medicine. Please tell the doctor if any of the listed side effects appear or if you think that the medicine is causing any other problems. Not all of the rare or unusual side effects are listed.

Side effects are most common after starting the medicine or after a dose increase. Many side effects can be avoided or lessened by starting with a very low dose and increasing it slowly—ask the doctor.

Allergic Reaction

Tell the doctor in a day or two (if possible, before the next dose of medicine):

- Hives
- Itching
- Rash

    Stop the medicine and get *immediate* medical care:

- Trouble breathing or chest tightness
- Swelling of lips, tongue, or throat

    Buspirone is usually very safe when used for short periods as the doctor prescribes. Very rarely, buspirone causes excitement, irritability, anger, aggression, nightmares, or uncontrollable behavior. This is called *disinhibition* or a *paradoxical effect*. Stop the medicine and call the doctor if this happens.

    Buspirone may cause dizziness, nervousness, nausea, headache, restlessness, or trouble sleeping but does not cause dependence or sleepiness.

    There are no known long-term side effects of buspirone.

Some Interactions With Other Medicines or Food

Please note that the following are only the most likely interactions with food or other medicines.

    Buspirone may be taken with or without food.

    It is important not to drink alcohol or use other sedatives, tranquilizers, or sleeping pills when taking buspirone.

    Taking buspirone with certain antibiotics (such as erythromycin) may increase levels of buspirone and increase side effects.

    It can be *very dangerous* to take buspirone at the same time as or even within a month of taking another type of medicine called a *monoamine oxidase inhibitor* (MAOI), such as Eldepryl (selegiline), Nardil (phenelzine), Parnate (tranylcypromine), or Marplan (isocarboxazid).

What Could Happen if This Medicine Is Stopped Suddenly?

There are no known problems from stopping buspirone suddenly. There are no withdrawal symptoms, but the anxiety is likely to come back.

How Long Will This Medicine Be Needed?

Buspirone is usually prescribed for only a few weeks to allow the patient to be calm enough to learn new ways to cope with anxiety and to allow the nervous system to become less excitable. Each person is, of course, unique, and some people may need these medicines for months or years.

What Else Should I Know About This Medicine?

Buspirone (BuSpar) is sometimes confused with bupropion (Wellbutrin, an antidepressant medicine). Be sure that you have the correct medicine from the pharmacy.

Notes

Use this space to take notes or to write down questions you want to ask the doctor.

_____

_____

_____

_____

_____

_____

_____

_____

_____

_____

_____

_____

From Dulcan MK (editor): *Helping Parents, Youth, and Teachers Understand Medications for Behavioral and Emotional Problems: A Resource Book of Medication Information Handouts*, Third Edition. Washington, DC, American Psychiatric Publishing, 2007

Medication Information for Youth

Buspirone—BuSpar

What the Medicine Is Called and What It Is For

The name of your medicine may be confusing. Most drugs have two names: 1) a scientific name that we call a *generic name* and 2) a trade or *brand name*. The generic name of this medicine is buspirone. The brand name is BuSpar.

Buspirone is an *antianxiety* medicine. It works by calming the parts of the brain that are too excitable in anxious people. It can decrease anxiety, nervousness, fears, and excessive worrying. It can help anxious people to be calm enough to learn—with therapy and practice—to understand and tolerate their worries or fears and even to overcome them. Your doctor may have told you that you have a condition such as social phobia, generalized anxiety disorder, separation anxiety disorder, or panic disorder. Most often, this medicine is used for a short time when symptoms are very uncomfortable or frightening or when they make it hard to do important things such as go to school.

How You Take the Medicine

It is very important to take the medicine exactly as the doctor or nurse tells you. Do not skip doses or take extra medicine without asking an adult. If you forget a dose, ask your parent(s) what to do.

This medicine is prescribed only for you. It should never be shared with anyone else.

You do not have to tell others that you are taking this medicine, but it is not something you should feel ashamed or embarrassed about. Many young people are helped by buspirone. This medicine is not habit-forming, and you cannot become "hooked" on it. You should talk to your doctor or nurse about any questions you have about the medicine. It is important to remember that the medicine *helps* you. It cannot *make* you do anything or change you as a person.

It is better to limit drinks with caffeine (coffee, tea, soft drinks) because caffeine works in the opposite way from this medicine, and the positive effects might be decreased.

How Your Doctor Will Follow Your Progress

Before giving you the medicine, your doctor or nurse will talk with you and your parent(s) and may measure your height, weight, heart rate (pulse), and blood pressure. There may be other tests to be sure that you are in good health.

Be sure to tell your doctor or nurse about any other medicines or supplements you are taking, including vitamins, herbs, or aids to weight loss or bodybuilding. Also be sure to tell the doctor or nurse if you are using alcohol or drugs. Because many medicines may affect babies, it is very important to tell the doctor if you might be pregnant or if you are at risk of becoming pregnant.

Most doctors have regular appointments with young people who are taking medicine. You should use these visits to share any concerns you may have about your medicine and to talk about if it has helped you. From time to time, your physician or nurse may measure your height, weight, heart rate (pulse), and blood pressure to be sure that you are in good health while you are taking the medicine. Your doctor also will ask for regular reports from your parents and maybe from your teachers (with your permission) to see how well the medicine is working.

Buspirone is usually prescribed for only a few weeks to allow you to be calm enough to learn new ways to cope with anxiety and to allow your nervous system to become less excitable. Sometimes antianxiety medicines are used for longer periods to treat panic attacks or anxiety that remain after therapy is completed. Each person is unique, and some people may need these medicines for months or years.

How the Medicine Might Affect You

Buspirone does not begin to help immediately. The full effect may not appear for 3–4 weeks.

In addition to the ways the medicine can help you, it may have other effects called *side effects*. Different medicines have different side effects. It is helpful to know about some of the most common side effects of your medicine so that you will understand what they are if they happen. Some people do not have any side effects. Some side effects are just uncomfortable, but others may mean a more serious problem with the medicine. Side effects are most common after starting the medicine or after a dose increase. They may go away with time, or the medicine can be adjusted or changed—ask the doctor.

You could have an allergy to any medicine, which might show up as a rash on your skin, swelling, itching, or trouble breathing.

Please tell your parent(s) and your doctor or nurse about any changes that you notice after taking the medicine. It is especially important to tell a responsible adult if you are feeling depressed or that you may not want to live or if you have thoughts of hurting yourself.

Buspirone may cause dizziness, nervousness, upset stomach, headache, restlessness, trouble sleeping, or nightmares.

Very rarely, buspirone seems to work in the opposite way, causing excitement, irritability, anger, aggression, restlessness, and other problems. If this happens, tell your parent(s) or your doctor right away.

Notes

Use this space to take notes or to write down questions you want to ask the doctor or nurse.

_____

_____

_____

_____

_____

_____

_____

_____

_____

_____

From Dulcan MK (editor): _Helping Parents, Youth, and Teachers Understand Medications for Behavioral and Emotional Problems: A Resource Book of Medication Information Handouts,_ Third Edition. Washington, DC, American Psychiatric Publishing, 2007

Medication Information for Parents and Teachers

Carbamazepine—Tegretol, Carbatrol, Epitol, Equetro

General Information About Medication

Each child and adolescent is different. No one has exactly the same combination of medical and psychological problems. It is a good idea to talk with the doctor or nurse about the reasons a medicine is being used. It is very important to keep all appointments and to be in touch by telephone if you have concerns. It is important to communicate with the doctor, nurse, or therapist.

It is very important that the medicine be taken exactly as the doctor instructs. However, once in a while, everyone forgets to give a medicine on time. It is a good idea to ask the doctor or nurse what to do if this happens. Do not stop or change a medicine without asking the doctor or nurse first.

If the medicine seems to stop working, it may be because it is not being taken regularly. The youth may be "cheeking" or hiding the medicine or forgetting to take it (especially at school). The doses may be too far apart, or a different dose may be needed. Something at school, at home, or in the neighborhood may be upsetting the youth, or he or she may need special help for learning disabilities or tutoring. Please discuss your concerns with the doctor. **Do not just increase the dose.**

All medicines should be kept in a safe place, out of the reach of children, and should be supervised by an adult. If someone takes too much of a medicine, call the doctor, the poison control center, or a hospital emergency room.

Each medicine has a "generic" or chemical name. Just like laundry detergents or paper towels, some medicines are sold by more than one company under different brand names. The same medicine may be available under a generic name and several brand names. The generic medications are usually less expensive than the brand name ones. The generic medications have the same chemical formula, but they may or may not be exactly the same strength as the brand-name medications. Also, some brands of pills contain dye that can cause allergic reactions. It is a good idea to talk to the doctor and the pharmacist about whether it is important to use a specific brand of medicine.

All medicines can cause an allergic reaction. Examples are hives, itching, rashes, swelling, and trouble breathing. Even a tiny amount of a medicine can cause a reaction in patients who are allergic to that medicine. Be *sure* to talk to the doctor before restarting a medicine that has caused an allergic reaction.

Taking more than one medicine at the same time may cause more side effects or cause one of the medicines to not work as well. Always ask the doctor, nurse, or pharmacist before adding another medicine, whether prescription or over-the-counter. Be sure that each doctor knows about *all* of the medicines your child is taking. Also tell the doctor about any vitamins, herbal medicines, or supplements your child may be taking. Some of these may have side effects alone or when taken with this medication.

Everyone taking medicine should have a physical examination at least once a year.

If you suspect the youth is using drugs or alcohol, please tell the doctor right away.

Pregnancy requires special care in the use of medicine. Please tell the doctor immediately if you suspect the teenager is pregnant or might become pregnant, because carbamazepine is associated with birth defects.

Printed information like this applies to children and adolescents in general. If you have questions about the medicine, or if you notice changes or anything unusual, please ask the doctor or nurse. As scientific research advances, knowledge increases and advice changes. Even experts do not always agree. Many medicines have not been approved by the U.S. Food and Drug Administration (FDA) for use in children. For this reason, use of the medicine for a particular problem or age group often is not listed in the *Physicians' Desk Reference*. This does not necessarily mean that the medicine is dangerous or does not work, only that the company that makes the medicine has not received permission to advertise the medicine for use in children. Companies often do not apply for this permission because it is expensive to do the tests needed to apply for approval for use in children. Once a medication is approved by the FDA for any purpose, a doctor is allowed to prescribe it according to research and clinical experience.

Note to Teachers

It is a good idea to talk with the parent(s) about the reason(s) that a medication is being used. If the parent(s) sign consent to release information, it is often helpful to talk with the doctor. If the parent(s) give permission, the doctor may ask you to fill out rating forms about your experience with the student's behavior, feelings, academic performance, and medication side effects. This information is very useful in selecting and monitoring medication treatment. If you have observations that you think are important, do not hesitate to share these with the student's parent(s) and treating clinicians.

It is very important that the medicine be taken exactly as the doctor instructs. However, everyone forgets to give a medicine on time once in a while. It is a good idea to ask the parent(s) in advance what to do if this happens. Do not stop or change the time you are giving a medicine at school without parental permission. If a medication is to be taken with food, but lunchtime or snack time changes, be sure to notify the parent(s) so appropriate adjustments can be made.

All medicines should be kept in a secure place and should be supervised by an adult. If someone takes too much of a medicine, follow your school procedure for an urgent medical problem.

Taking medicine is a private matter and is best managed discreetly and confidentially. It is important to be sensitive to the student's feelings about taking medicine.

If you suspect that the student is using drugs or alcohol, please tell the parent(s) or a school counselor right away.

Please tell the parent(s) or school nurse if you suspect medication side effects.

Modifications of the classroom environment or assignments may be useful in addition to medication. The student may need to be evaluated for additional help or for an Individualized Education Plan for learning or behavior.

Any expression of suicidal thoughts or feelings or self-harm by a child or adolescent is a clear signal of distress and should be taken seriously. These behaviors should not be dismissed as "attention seeking."

What Is Carbamazepine (Tegretol, Carbatrol, Epitol, Equetro)?

Carbamazepine was first used to treat seizures (fits, convulsions), so it is sometimes called an *anticonvulsant*. Now it is also used for behavioral problems or bipolar disorder (manic-depressive disorder) whether or not the patient has seizures. It also may be used when the patient has a history of severe mood changes, sometimes called *mood swings*. When used in psychiatry, this medicine is more commonly called a *mood stabilizer*. It is also sometimes used to reduce severe facial nerve pain or nerve pain in people with diabetes.

Carbamazepine comes in brand name and generic tablets, chewable tablets, and liquid. There are also Epitol brand name tablets. Carbamazepine also comes in Tegretol-XR extended-release tablets and Carbatrol and Equetro extended-release capsules.

How Can This Medicine Help?

Carbamazepine can reduce aggression, anger, and severe mood swings. It can treat mania or prevent relapse (mania coming back).

How Does This Medicine Work?

Carbamazepine is thought to work by stabilizing a part of the brain cell (the cell membrane or envelope) and by changing the concentrations of certain *neurotransmitters* (chemicals in the brain) such as *GABA* and *glutamate*.

How Long Does This Medicine Last?

Carbamazepine needs to be taken two to four times a day. Tegretol-XR and Carbatrol may be taken two times a day.

How Will the Doctor Monitor This Medicine?

The doctor will review your child's medical history and physical examination before starting carbamazepine. The doctor may order some blood or urine tests to be sure your child does not have a hidden medical condition that would make it unsafe to use this medicine. The doctor or nurse may measure your child's pulse and blood pressure before starting carbamazepine. The doctor may order a baseline test counting the blood cells.

After the medicine is started, the doctor will want to have regular appointments with you and your child to see how the medicine is working, to see if a dose change is needed, to watch for side effects, to see if carbamazepine is still needed, and to see if any other treatment is needed. The doctor or nurse may check your child's height, weight, pulse, and blood pressure. The doctor will need to order blood tests every month or so to make sure that the medicine is at the right dose and to find any side effects on the blood, such as a decrease in the number of white blood cells (the cells that fight infection) or even in all the kinds of blood cells. To see if the medicine is at the right dose, blood should be drawn first thing in the morning, 10–12 hours after the last dose and before the morning dose. Many things can change the levels of carbamazepine, so tests may be needed every week when the dose of this or other medicines are being changed.

What Side Effects Can This Medicine Have?

Any medicine can have side effects, including an allergy to the medicine. Because each patient is different, the doctor will monitor the youth closely, especially when the medicine is started. The doctor will work with you

to increase the positive effects and decrease the negative effects of the medicine. Please tell the doctor if any of the listed side effects appear or if you think that the medicine is causing any other problems. Not all of the rare or unusual side effects are listed.

Side effects are most common after starting the medicine or after a dose increase. Many side effects can be avoided or lessened by starting with a very low dose and increasing it slowly—ask the doctor.

Allergic Reaction

Tell the doctor in a day or two (if possible, before the next dose of medicine):

- Hives
- Itching
- Rash

Stop the medicine and get *immediate* medical care:

- Trouble breathing or chest tightness
- Swelling of lips, tongue, or throat

General Side Effects

Tell the doctor within a week or two:

The following side effects are more common when first starting the medicine:

- Daytime sleepiness—Do not allow your child to drive, ride a bicycle or motorcycle, or operate machinery if this happens.
- Dizziness
- Clumsiness or decreased coordination
- Nausea or upset stomach—Have your child take medicine with food.

The following side effects are more common at higher doses:

- Double or blurred vision
- Jerky, side-to-side eye movements *(nystagmus)*

Serious Side Effects

Call the doctor within a day or two:

- Anxiety or nervousness
- Agitation or mania
- Impulsive behavior
- Irritability
- Increased aggression
- Hallucinations (hearing voices or seeing things that are not there)
- Motor or vocal tics (fast, repeated movements or sounds)

Very Rare, but Possibly Serious, Side Effects

Call the doctor *immediately:*

- Feeling sick or unusually tired for no reason
- Loss of appetite
- Yellowing of the skin or eyes
- Dark urine or pale bowel movements
- Swelling of the legs or feet
- Greatly increased or decreased frequency of urination
- Unusual bruising or bleeding
- Sore throat or fever
- Mouth ulcers
- Vomiting
- Skin rash, especially with fever
- Severe behavioral problems
- Unsteady gait (wobbling or falling when walking)
- New or worse seizures (convulsions)

Some Interactions With Other Medicines or Food

Please note that the following are only the most likely interactions with food or other medicines.

Caffeine may increase side effects.

A large glass of grapefruit juice may increase levels of carbamazepine and increase side effects.

Carbamazepine interacts with many other medicines. Taking it with another medicine may make one or both not work as well or may cause more side effects. Be sure that each doctor knows about *all* of the medicines your child is taking.

The following medicines (and many others) increase the levels of carbamazepine and increase the risk of serious side effects:

- Tagamet (cimetidine)
- Prozac (fluoxetine)
- Luvox (fluvoxamine)
- Depakote (divalproex)
- Erythromycin and similar antibiotics
- Medicines used to treat fungus infections or tuberculosis (TB)

Carbamazepine may decrease the blood levels of the following medicines (and many others) so that they do not work as well:

- Birth control pills (oral contraceptives)—This combination may lead to accidental pregnancy.
- Theophylline

Carbamazepine should not be taken together with clozapine (Clozaril) because of increased risk of severe decrease in blood cells.

What Could Happen if This Medicine Is Stopped Suddenly?

Stopping carbamazepine suddenly may cause uncomfortable withdrawal symptoms. If the person is taking carbamazepine for epilepsy (seizures), stopping the medicine suddenly could lead to an increase in very dangerous seizures or convulsions.

How Long Will This Medicine Be Needed?

The length of time a person needs to take carbamazepine depends on what problem is being treated. For example, someone with an impulse control disorder usually takes the medicine only until behavioral therapy begins to work. Someone with bipolar disorder may need to take the medicine for many years. Please ask the doctor about the length of treatment needed.

What Else Should I Know About This Medicine?

Carbamazepine increases the risk of sunburn. Be sure that your child wears sunscreen or protective clothing or stays out of the sun.

Taking carbamazepine with food may decrease stomach upset.

Carbamazepine may cause hair loss. The hair usually grows back when the carbamazepine is stopped.

If you are giving the liquid form of carbamazepine, shake it well first and do not give the medicine at the same time as other liquid medicines.

Keep the medicine in a safe place under close supervision. **Carbamazepine is very dangerous in overdose.** Keep the pill container tightly closed and in a dry place, away from bathrooms, showers, and humidifiers. If your home is humid in the summer, do not keep large amounts of carbamazepine and do not use carbamazepine past the expiration date.

Notes

Use this space to take notes or to write down questions you want to ask the doctor.

_____

_____

_____

_____

_____

_____

_____

_____

_____

_____

_____

_____

_____

From Dulcan MK (editor): *Helping Parents, Youth, and Teachers Understand Medications for Behavioral and Emotional Problems: A Resource Book of Medication Information Handouts*, Third Edition. Washington, DC, American Psychiatric Publishing, 2007

Medication Information for Youth

Carbamazepine—Tegretol, Carbatrol, Epitol, Equetro

What the Medicine Is Called and What It Is For

The name of your medicine may be confusing. Most drugs have two names: 1) a scientific name that we call a *generic name* and 2) a trade or *brand name*. The generic name of this medicine is carbamazepine. The brand names are Tegretol, Carbatrol, Epitol, and Equetro.

Carbamazepine was first used to help people with epilepsy (seizures, fits, convulsions), so it is sometimes called an *anticonvulsant*. It is now also called a *mood stabilizer*, because it is used to help people who have severe mood changes, sometimes called *mood swings*, especially in children and adolescents with bipolar disorder (manic-depressive disorder), depression, or trouble controlling anger. Carbamazepine can reduce aggression, anger, and severe mood swings. It can treat mania or prevent relapse (mania coming back). It is thought to work by making brain cells less excitable.

How You Take the Medicine

It is very important to take the medicine exactly as the doctor or nurse tells you. Do not skip doses or take extra medicine without asking an adult. If you forget a dose, ask your parent(s) what to do.

This medicine is prescribed only for you. It should never be shared with anyone else.

You do not have to tell others that you are taking this medicine, but it is not something you should feel ashamed or embarrassed about. Many young people are helped by carbamazepine. This medicine is not habit-forming, and you cannot become "hooked" on it. You should talk to your doctor or nurse about any questions you have about the medicine. It is important to remember that the medicine *helps* you. It cannot *make* you do anything or change you as a person.

If you are taking the long-acting pill (Tegretol-XR or Carbatrol), swallow it whole—do not chew or crush the pill.

If you are taking the liquid, shake the suspension well before taking and do not take other liquid medicines at the same time.

If your stomach is upset, taking the medicine with food may help.

Caffeine (in coffee, tea, or soft drinks) may make you feel worse.

It is better not to drink grapefruit juice, because it can increase the side effects of this medicine.

It is very important not to stop this medicine suddenly—it could be uncomfortable or even dangerous.

How Your Doctor Will Follow Your Progress

Before starting carbamazepine, your doctor or nurse will talk with you and your parent(s) and may measure your height, weight, heart rate (pulse), and blood pressure. The doctor will probably order blood tests to be sure you are healthy before taking the medicine.

Be sure to tell your doctor or nurse about any other medicines or supplements you are taking, including vitamins, herbs, or aids to weight loss or bodybuilding. Also be sure to tell the doctor or nurse if you are using alcohol or drugs. Because carbamazepine may cause birth defects, it is very important to tell the doctor if you might be pregnant or if you are at risk of becoming pregnant. Carbamazepine may make birth control pills not work as well, so it is important to talk to the doctor if you are taking birth control pills.

Your teachers may be asked to fill out a form about your grades and behavior in school. A psychologist may give you some tests to see how you learn best.

Most doctors have regular appointments with young people who are taking medicine. You should use these visits to share any concerns you may have about your medicine and to talk about if it has helped you. From time to time, your physician or nurse may measure your height, weight, heart rate (pulse), and blood pressure to be sure that you are in good health while you are taking the medicine. There will be regular blood tests to be sure that the medicine is at the right dose and to be sure that the medicine is not affecting your blood cells. Your doctor also will ask for regular reports from your parents and maybe from your teachers (with your permission) to see how well the medicine is working.

How the Medicine Might Affect You

In addition to the ways the medicine can help you, it may have other effects called *side effects*. Different medicines have different side effects. It is helpful to know about some of the most common side effects of your medicine so that you will understand what they are if they happen. Some people do not have any side effects. Some side effects are just uncomfortable, but others may mean a more serious problem with the medicine. Side effects are most common after starting the medicine or after a dose increase. They may go away with time, or the medicine can be adjusted or changed—ask the doctor.

You could have an allergy to any medicine, which might show up as a rash on your skin, swelling, itching, or trouble breathing.

Please tell your parent(s) and your doctor or nurse about any changes that you notice after taking the medicine. It is especially important to tell a responsible adult if you are feeling depressed or that you may not want to live; if you have thoughts of hurting yourself; or if you begin to feel more irritable, nervous, or restless. Also be sure to tell your parent(s) or doctor if you begin to feel "speeded up" or have trouble sleeping.

Some medicines make people feel sleepy or less coordinated. If this medicine is making you sleepy, it is very important not to drive a car or ride a bicycle or motorcycle. After starting a new medicine or increasing the dose of a medicine, please be extra careful when driving a car, riding a bike, or using machines until you can tell how the medicine affects your alertness, attention, and coordination.

The most common side effects of carbamazepine are dizziness, daytime sleepiness, unsteadiness, upset stomach, and double or blurred vision. These sometimes go away after you have been taking the medicine for a while or the doctor lowers the dose of medicine you are taking. Your doctor will watch your blood tests closely so that the medicine can be changed if it lowers the number of white blood cells you have to fight colds and infections. Carbamazepine may make you more likely to get sunburned, so cover up or use sunscreen while outside in the sun.

Tell the doctor right away if you notice any change in your urine or bowel movements or if your skin seems to bruise easily.

Notes

Use this space to take notes or to write down questions you want to ask the doctor or nurse.

_____

_____

_____

_____

_____

_____

_____

_____

_____

_____

_____

_____

_____

From Dulcan MK (editor): _Helping Parents, Youth, and Teachers Understand Medications for Behavioral and Emotional Problems: A Resource Book of Medication Information Handouts,_ Third Edition. Washington, DC, American Psychiatric Publishing, 2007

Chlorpromazine—Thorazine, Ormazine

General Information About Medication

Each child and adolescent is different. No one has exactly the same combination of medical and psychological problems. It is a good idea to talk with the doctor or nurse about the reasons a medicine is being used. It is very important to keep all appointments and to be in touch by telephone if you have concerns. It is important to communicate with the doctor, nurse, or therapist.

It is very important that the medicine be taken exactly as the doctor instructs. However, once in a while, everyone forgets to give a medicine on time. It is a good idea to ask the doctor or nurse what to do if this happens. Do not stop or change a medicine without asking the doctor or nurse first.

If the medicine seems to stop working, it may be because it is not being taken regularly. The youth may be "cheeking" or hiding the medicine or forgetting to take it (especially at school). The doses may be too far apart, or a different dose may be needed. Something at school, at home, or in the neighborhood may be upsetting the youth, or he or she may need special help for learning disabilities or tutoring. Please discuss your concerns with the doctor. **Do not just increase the dose.**

All medicines should be kept in a safe place, out of the reach of children, and should be supervised by an adult. If someone takes too much of a medicine, call the doctor, the poison control center, or a hospital emergency room.

Each medicine has a "generic" or chemical name. Just like laundry detergents or paper towels, some medicines are sold by more than one company under different brand names. The same medicine may be available under a generic name and several brand names. The generic medications are usually less expensive than the brand name ones. The generic medications have the same chemical formula, but they may or may not be exactly the same strength as the brand-name medications. Also, some brands of pills contain dye that can cause allergic reactions. It is a good idea to talk to the doctor and the pharmacist about whether it is important to use a specific brand of medicine.

All medicines can cause an allergic reaction. Examples are hives, itching, rashes, swelling, and trouble breathing. Even a tiny amount of a medicine can cause a reaction in patients who are allergic to that medicine. Be *sure* to talk to the doctor before restarting a medicine that has caused an allergic reaction.

Taking more than one medicine at the same time may cause more side effects or cause one of the medicines to not work as well. Always ask the doctor, nurse, or pharmacist before adding another medicine, whether prescription or over-the-counter. Be sure that each doctor knows about *all* of the medicines your child is taking. Also tell the doctor about any vitamins, herbal medicines, or supplements your child may be taking. Some of these may have side effects alone or when taken with this medication.

Everyone taking medicine should have a physical examination at least once a year.

If you suspect the youth is using drugs or alcohol, please tell the doctor right away.

Pregnancy requires special care in the use of medicine. Please tell the doctor immediately if you suspect the teenager is pregnant or might become pregnant.

Printed information like this applies to children and adolescents in general. If you have questions about the medicine, or if you notice changes or anything unusual, please ask the doctor or nurse. As scientific research advances, knowledge increases and advice changes. Even experts do not always agree. Many medicines have not been approved by the U.S. Food and Drug Administration (FDA) for use in children. For this reason, use of the medicine for a particular problem or age group often is not listed in the *Physicians' Desk Reference*. This does not necessarily mean that the medicine is dangerous or does not work, only that the company that makes the medicine has not received permission to advertise the medicine for use in children. Companies often do not apply for this permission because it is expensive to do the tests needed to apply for approval for use in children. Once a medication is approved by the FDA for any purpose, a doctor is allowed to prescribe it according to research and clinical experience.

Note to Teachers

It is a good idea to talk with the parent(s) about the reason(s) that a medication is being used. If the parent(s) sign consent to release information, it is often helpful to talk with the doctor. If the parent(s) give permission, the doctor may ask you to fill out rating forms about your experience with the student's behavior, feelings, academic performance, and medication side effects. This information is very useful in selecting and monitoring medication treatment. If you have observations that you think are important, do not hesitate to share these with the student's parent(s) and treating clinicians.

It is very important that the medicine be taken exactly as the doctor instructs. However, everyone forgets to give a medicine on time once in a while. It is a good idea to ask the parent(s) in advance what to do if this happens. Do not stop or change the time you are giving a medicine at school without parental permission. If a medication is to be taken with food, but lunchtime or snack time changes, be sure to notify the parent(s) so appropriate adjustments can be made.

All medicines should be kept in a secure place and should be supervised by an adult. If someone takes too much of a medicine, follow your school procedure for an urgent medical problem.

Taking medicine is a private matter and is best managed discreetly and confidentially. It is important to be sensitive to the student's feelings about taking medicine.

If you suspect that the student is using drugs or alcohol, please tell the parent(s) or a school counselor right away.

Please tell the parent(s) or school nurse if you suspect medication side effects.

Modifications of the classroom environment or assignments may be useful in addition to medication. The student may need to be evaluated for additional help or for an Individualized Education Plan for learning or behavior.

Any expression of suicidal thoughts or feelings or self-harm by a child or adolescent is a clear signal of distress and should be taken seriously. These behaviors should not be dismissed as "attention seeking."

What Is Chlorpromazine (Thorazine, Ormazine)?

Chlorpromazine is sometimes called a *typical, conventional,* or *first-generation antipsychotic* medicine. It is also called a *neuroleptic* or *phenothiazine.* It used to be called a *major tranquilizer.* It comes in brand name Thorazine and Ormazine generic tablets, liquid, and shots (injections).

How Can This Medicine Help?

Chlorpromazine is used to treat psychosis, such as in schizophrenia, mania, or very severe depression. It can reduce hallucinations (hearing voices or seeing things that are not there) and delusions (troubling beliefs that other people do not share). It can help the patient be less upset and agitated. It can improve the patient's ability to think clearly.

Sometimes chlorpromazine is used for a short time to decrease severe aggression or very serious behavioral problems in young people with mental retardation or autism.

It is sometimes used together with other medicines to help with sleep in people with psychosis.

This medicine is very powerful and should be used to treat very serious problems or symptoms that other medicines do not help.

In medical settings, chlorpromazine is also used to treat severe nausea and vomiting or severe, long-lasting attacks of hiccups.

How Does This Medicine Work?

Cells in the brain (neurons) communicate using chemicals called *neurotransmitters*. Too much or too little of these substances in certain parts of the brain can cause problems. Chlorpromazine reduces the activity of one of these neurotransmitters, dopamine. Blocking the effect of dopamine in certain parts of the brain reduces what have been called *positive symptoms* of psychosis: delusions; hallucinations; disorganized and unusual thinking, speaking, and behavior; excessive activity (agitation); and lack of activity (catatonia). Reducing dopamine action in other parts of the brain may lead to the side effects of this medicine.

How Long Does This Medicine Last?

Chlorpromazine may be taken only once a day, but divided doses are often used to lessen side effects. Sometimes it is used at bedtime only. Sometimes it is used as needed (prn) for immediate agitation or aggression.

How Will the Doctor Monitor This Medicine?

The doctor will review your child's medical history and physical examination before starting chlorpromazine. The doctor may order some blood or urine tests to be sure your child does not have a hidden medical condition. The doctor or nurse may measure your child's pulse and blood pressure before starting chlorpromazine.

Be sure to tell the doctor if anyone in the family is hearing impaired or has had heart problems or died suddenly.

Before starting chlorpromazine and every so often afterward, a test such as the AIMS (Abnormal Involuntary Movement Scale) may be used to check your child's tongue, legs, and arms for unusual movements that could be caused by the medicine.

After the medicine is started, the doctor will want to have regular appointments with you and your child to see how the medicine is working, to see if a dose change is needed, to watch for side effects, to see if chlorpromazine is still needed, and to see if any other treatment is needed. The doctor or nurse may check your child's height, weight, pulse, and blood pressure and watch for abnormal movements.

103

What Side Effects Can This Medicine Have?

Any medicine can have side effects, including an allergy to the medicine. Because each patient is different, the doctor will monitor the youth closely, especially when the medicine is started. The doctor will work with you to increase the positive effects and decrease the negative effects of the medicine. Please tell the doctor if any of the listed side effects appear or if you think that the medicine is causing any other problems. Not all of the rare or unusual side effects are listed.

Side effects are most common after starting the medicine or after a dose increase. Many side effects can be avoided or lessened by starting with a very low dose and increasing it slowly—ask the doctor.

Allergic Reaction

Tell the doctor in a day or two (if possible, before the next dose of medicine):

- Hives
- Itching
- Rash

   Stop the medicine and get *immediate* medical care:

- Trouble breathing or chest tightness
- Swelling of lips, tongue, or throat

Common, but Not Usually Serious, Side Effects

Discuss the following side effects with your child's doctor within a week or two. They often can be helped if the doctor lowers the dose of medicine or changes the times medicine is taken.

- Dry mouth—Have your child try using sugar-free gum or candy.
- Daytime sleepiness or tiredness—Do not allow your child to drive, ride a bicycle or motorcycle, or operate machinery if this happens. This problem may be lessened by taking the medicine at bedtime.
- Constipation—Encourage your child to drink more fluids and eat high-fiber foods; if necessary, the doctor may recommend a fiber medicine such as Benefiber or a stool softener such as Colace or mineral oil.
- Increased risk of sunburn—Have your child wear sunscreen or protective clothing or stay out of the sun.
- Mild trouble urinating
- Blurred vision
- Dizziness—This side effect is worse when the child stands up quickly, especially when getting out of bed in the morning; try having the child stand up slowly.
- Weight gain—Seek nutritional counseling; provide your child with low-calorie snacks and encourage regular exercise.
- Decreased sexual interest or ability
- Changes in menstrual cycle
- Increase in breast size or discharge from the breasts (in both boys and girls)—This may go away with time.

Less Common, but Not Usually Serious, Side Effects

Discuss the following side effects with your child's doctor within a week or two. They often can be helped if the doctor lowers the dose of medicine or changes the times medicine is taken.

- Restlessness or inability to sit still
- Shaking of hands and fingers
- Drooling
- Decreased movement and decreased facial expressions
- Decreased coordination

Less Common, but Potentially Serious, Side Effects

Call the doctor or go to an emergency room *right away:*

- Overheating or heatstroke—Prevent by decreasing activity in hot weather, staying out of the sun, and drinking water.
- Seizure (fit, convulsion)—This is more likely in people with a history of seizures or head injury.
- Severe confusion
- Stiffness of the tongue, jaw, neck, back, or legs

Very Rare, but Serious, Side Effects

- Extreme stiffness or lack of movement, very high fever, mental confusion, irregular pulse rate, or eye pain—**This is a medical emergency. Go to an emergency room *right away*.**
- Sudden stiffness and inability to breathe or swallow—**Go to an emergency room or call 911.** Tell the paramedics, nurses, and doctors that the patient is taking chlorpromazine. Other medicines can be used to treat this problem fast.
- Increased thirst, frequent urination, lethargy, tiredness, dizziness—These could be signs of diabetes (especially if your child is overweight or there is a family history of diabetes). **Talk to a doctor within a day.**
- Yellowing of skin or eyes, dark urine, pale bowel movements, abdominal pain or fullness, unexplained flu-like symptoms, itchy skin (this could be a sign of liver damage—extremely rare). **Talk to a doctor within a day.**

What Else Should I Know About Side Effects?

Most side effects lessen over time. If they are troublesome, talk with your child's doctor. Some side effects can be decreased by taking a smaller dose of medicine, by stopping the medicine, by changing to another medicine, or by adding another medicine.

One side effect that may not go away is *tardive dyskinesia* (or TD). Patients with tardive dyskinesia have involuntary movements of the body, especially the mouth and tongue. The patient may look as though he or she is making faces over and over again. Jerky movements of the arms, legs, or body may occur. There may be fine, wormlike, or sudden repeated movements of the tongue, or the person may appear to be chewing something or smacking or puckering his or her lips. The fingers may look as though they are rolling something. If you notice any unusual movements, be sure to tell the doctor. The doctor may use the AIMS test to look for these movements.

Heart problems are more common if other medicines are also being taken. Be sure to tell all your child's doctors and your pharmacist about all medications your child is taking.

Neuroleptic malignant syndrome is a very rare side effect that can lead to death. The symptoms are severe muscle stiffness, high fever, increased heart rate and blood pressure, irregular heartbeat (pulse), and sweating. It may lead to unconsciousness. If you suspect this, **call 911 or go to an emergency room right away.**

Some Interactions With Other Medicines or Food

Please note that the following are only the most likely interactions with food or other medicines.

Chlorpromazine may be taken with or without food.

Combining chlorpromazine with medicines such as Cogentin, Artane, or Benadryl may increase the side effects of both medicines.

It is better to limit drinks with caffeine (coffee, tea, soft drinks) because caffeine works in the opposite way from this medicine, and the positive effects might be decreased.

What Could Happen if This Medicine Is Stopped Suddenly?

Involuntary movements, or *withdrawal dyskinesias*, may appear within 1–4 weeks of lowering the dose or stopping the medicine. Usually these go away, but they can last for days to months. If chlorpromazine is stopped suddenly, emotional problems, such as irritability, nervousness, or moodiness; behavior problems; or physical problems such as stomachache, loss of appetite, nausea, vomiting, diarrhea, sweating, indigestion, trouble sleeping, trembling, or shaking may appear. These problems usually last only a few days to a few weeks. If they happen, tell your child's doctor. The medicine dose may need to be lowered more slowly (tapered). Always check with the doctor before stopping a medicine!

How Long Will This Medicine Be Needed?

How long your child will need to be on chlorpromazine depends partly on the reason that it was prescribed. Some problems last for only a few months, whereas others last much longer. It is especially important with medicines as powerful as this one to ask the doctor whether it is still needed. Every few months, you should discuss with your child's doctor the reasons for using chlorpromazine and whether it is time to try lowering the dose.

What Else Should I Know About This Medicine?

There are many older and newer medicines that are used for the same kinds of problems. If your child is having bad side effects or the medicine does not seem to be working, ask the doctor if another medicine in this group might work as well or better and have fewer side effects for your child.

Notes

Use this space to take notes or to write down questions you want to ask the doctor.

_____

_____

_____

_____

_____

_____

_____

_____

_____

_____

_____

_____

From Dulcan MK (editor): _Helping Parents, Youth, and Teachers Understand Medications for Behavioral and Emotional Problems: A Resource Book of Medication Information Handouts_, Third Edition. Washington, DC, American Psychiatric Publishing, 2007

Medication Information for Youth

Chlorpromazine—Thorazine, Ormazine

What the Medicine Is Called and What It Is For

The name of your medicine may be confusing. Most drugs have two names: 1) a scientific name that we call a *generic name* and 2) a trade or *brand name*. The generic name of this medicine is chlorpromazine. The brand names are Thorazine and Ormazine.

Chlorpromazine can help people who feel very confused and have severe problems thinking clearly. It can lessen *hallucinations* (seeing or hearing things that are not really there) and *delusions* (troubling beliefs that other people do not share). This medicine also is sometimes used to help young people who have mania or who get very angry and hit people or break things.

How You Take the Medicine

It is very important to take the medicine exactly as the doctor or nurse tells you. Do not skip doses or take extra medicine without asking an adult. If you forget a dose, ask your parent(s) what to do.

It is better to limit drinks with caffeine (coffee, tea, soft drinks) because caffeine works in the opposite way from this medicine, and the positive effects might be decreased.

This medicine is prescribed only for you. It should never be shared with anyone else.

You do not have to tell others that you are taking this medicine, but it is not something you should feel ashamed or embarrassed about. Many young people are helped by chlorpromazine. This medicine is not habit-forming, and you cannot become "hooked" on it. You should talk to your doctor or nurse about any questions you have about the medicine. It is important to remember that the medicine *helps* you. It cannot *make* you do anything or change you as a person.

How Your Doctor Will Follow Your Progress

Before giving you the medicine, your doctor or nurse will talk with you and your parent(s) and may measure your height, weight, heart rate (pulse), and blood pressure. There may be other tests, such as blood tests for sugar and cholesterol. Before you start taking the medicine and every so often afterward, the doctor or nurse will look at your tongue, arms, and legs to check for unusual movements. This is called the AIMS (Abnormal Involuntary Movement Scale) test.

Be sure to tell your doctor or nurse about any other medicines or supplements you are taking, including vitamins, herbs, or aids to weight loss or bodybuilding. Also be sure to tell the doctor or nurse if you are using alcohol or drugs. Because many medicines may affect babies, it is very important to tell the doctor if you might be pregnant or if you are at risk of becoming pregnant.

Your teachers may be asked to fill out a form about your grades and behavior in school. A psychologist may give you some tests to see how you learn best.

Most doctors have regular appointments with young people who are taking medicine. You should use these visits to share any concerns you may have about your medicine and to talk about if it has helped you. From time to time, your physician or nurse may measure your height, weight, heart rate (pulse), and blood pressure to be sure that you are in good health while you are taking the medicine. There may be blood tests, to watch for diabetes or high cholesterol. Your doctor also will ask for regular reports from your parents and maybe from your teachers (with your permission) to see how well the medicine is working.

If the medicine helps you, your doctor will probably want you to take it for several months to a year. Your doctor will decide how long you will need to take the medicine as he or she watches your progress.

How the Medicine Might Affect You

In addition to the ways the medicine can help you, it may have other effects called *side effects*. Different medicines have different side effects. It is helpful to know about some of the most common side effects of your medicine so that you will understand what they are if they happen. Some people do not have any side effects. Some side effects are just uncomfortable, but others may mean a more serious problem with the medicine. Side effects are most common after starting the medicine or after a dose increase. They may go away with time, or the medicine can be adjusted or changed—ask the doctor.

You could have an allergy to any medicine, which might show up as a rash on your skin, swelling, itching, or trouble breathing.

Please tell your parent(s) and your doctor or nurse about any changes that you notice after taking the medicine. It is especially important to tell a responsible adult if you are feeling depressed or that you may not want to live; if you have thoughts of hurting yourself; or if you begin to feel more irritable, nervous, or restless.

One of the most common side effects of this medicine is feeling tired or sleepy during the day, even if you have had a full night's sleep. If this medicine is making you sleepy, it is very important not to drive a car or ride a bicycle or motorcycle. After starting the medicine or increasing the dose of medicine, please be extra careful when driving a car, riding a bike, or using machines until you can tell how the medicine affects your alertness, attention, and coordination. After you have been taking the medicine for a few weeks, your body will adjust, and this side effect will likely go away. If you had trouble sleeping at night before taking the medicine, it can help you sleep better, especially if the doctor tells you to take a dose of medicine in the evening.

You might feel dizzy or light-headed if you stand up fast. Try standing up slowly, especially when getting out of bed in the morning.

Another common side effect is dry mouth. You may be more thirsty than usual and find that you are drinking more water or other liquids than usual. Sucking on sugar-free hard candy or cough drops usually helps. You also could try chewing sugar-free gum or sucking on ice chips. Do not chew the ice; you could hurt your teeth. Also, using lip balm will keep your lips from cracking. It is important to be especially good about brushing your teeth.

Taking this medicine could make you more likely to get badly sunburned or very sick in hot weather. Be sure to drink plenty of liquids and cover up or use sunscreen when you go outside in hot weather. Be careful to rest in the shade and not get overheated.

Sometimes teenagers who take chlorpromazine gain weight. The weight gain may be from increased appetite and also from ways that the medicine changes how the body processes food. It is much easier to prevent weight gain than to lose weight later. It is a good idea to eat a well-balanced diet without "junk food" and with healthy snacks like fruits and vegetables, not sweets or fried foods. It is better to drink water or skim milk, not pop, sodas, soft drinks, or sugary juices. Regular exercise is important for maintaining a healthy weight (and may also help with sleep).

Some people become constipated (have hard bowel movements) when taking this medicine. Try drinking more water and eating more fruits, vegetables, and whole grains. If that does not help, tell your parent(s) or doctor—you may need a medicine to help with this side effect.

This is a very powerful medicine. Some side effects include feeling nervous, restless, or shaky or having stiff muscles. Talk with your doctor about these side effects. They can be helped by adding another medicine, adjusting the dose, or switching to another medicine.

Another more serious side effect can be longer lasting and more difficult to treat. This very rare side effect is called *tardive dyskinesia* (or TD). A person taking chlorpromazine may develop movements of the mouth, tongue, face, arms, legs, or body that are not being made on purpose. This side effect can go away when the medicine is stopped, but in some people it does not go away. Your doctor will explain this effect to you and your parent(s) and how he or she will watch for any signs that you are developing this problem. Be sure to ask your doctor any questions that you may have about this, but do not worry too much about it. It hardly ever happens to teenagers.

You may notice changes in your sexual functioning or in your breasts—it is OK to ask the doctor about this.

You should tell your parent(s) and doctor if you notice anything different or unusual about how you feel once you start taking the medicine. This includes good things, such as feeling less confused, feeling less sad, not hearing voices anymore, or sleeping better at night.

You cannot become addicted to this medicine, but you should not stop it suddenly. Never stop a medicine without talking to the doctor. If chlorpromazine is stopped or decreased suddenly you may notice more moodiness or irritability, stomachaches or upset stomach, trouble sleeping, or trembling or shaking. Let your parent(s) or doctor know if this happens—the medicine may need to be decreased more slowly.

Notes

Use this space to take notes or to write down questions you want to ask the doctor or nurse.

_____

_____

_____

_____

_____

_____

_____

_____

_____

_____

_____

_____

_____

Medication Information for Parents and Teachers

Citalopram—Celexa

General Information About Medication

Each child and adolescent is different. No one has exactly the same combination of medical and psychological problems. It is a good idea to talk with the doctor or nurse about the reasons a medicine is being used. It is very important to keep all appointments and to be in touch by telephone if you have concerns. It is important to communicate with the doctor, nurse, or therapist.

It is very important that the medicine be taken exactly as the doctor instructs. However, once in a while, everyone forgets to give a medicine on time. It is a good idea to ask the doctor or nurse what to do if this happens. Do not stop or change a medicine without asking the doctor or nurse first.

If the medicine seems to stop working, it may be because it is not being taken regularly. The youth may be "cheeking" or hiding the medicine or forgetting to take it (especially at school). The doses may be too far apart, or a different dose may be needed. Something at school, at home, or in the neighborhood may be upsetting the youth, or he or she may need special help for learning disabilities or tutoring. Please discuss your concerns with the doctor. **Do not just increase the dose.**

All medicines should be kept in a safe place, out of the reach of children, and should be supervised by an adult. If someone takes too much of a medicine, call the doctor, the poison control center, or a hospital emergency room.

Each medicine has a "generic" or chemical name. Just like laundry detergents or paper towels, some medicines are sold by more than one company under different brand names. The same medicine may be available under a generic name and several brand names. The generic medications are usually less expensive than the brand name ones. The generic medications have the same chemical formula, but they may or may not be exactly the same strength as the brand-name medications. Also, some brands of pills contain dye that can cause allergic reactions. It is a good idea to talk to the doctor and the pharmacist about whether it is important to use a specific brand of medicine.

All medicines can cause an allergic reaction. Examples are hives, itching, rashes, swelling, and trouble breathing. Even a tiny amount of a medicine can cause a reaction in patients who are allergic to that medicine. Be *sure* to talk to the doctor before restarting a medicine that has caused an allergic reaction.

Taking more than one medicine at the same time may cause more side effects or cause one of the medicines to not work as well. Always ask the doctor, nurse, or pharmacist before adding another medicine, whether prescription or over-the-counter. Be sure that each doctor knows about *all* of the medicines your child is taking. Also tell the doctor about any vitamins, herbal medicines, or supplements your child may be taking. Some of these may have side effects alone or when taken with this medication.

Everyone taking medicine should have a physical examination at least once a year.

If you suspect the youth is using drugs or alcohol, please tell the doctor right away.

113

Pregnancy requires special care in the use of medicine. Please tell the doctor immediately if you suspect the teenager is pregnant or might become pregnant.

Printed information like this applies to children and adolescents in general. If you have questions about the medicine, or if you notice changes or anything unusual, please ask the doctor or nurse. As scientific research advances, knowledge increases and advice changes. Even experts do not always agree. Many medicines have not been approved by the U.S. Food and Drug Administration (FDA) for use in children. For this reason, use of the medicine for a particular problem or age group often is not listed in the *Physicians' Desk Reference*. This does not necessarily mean that the medicine is dangerous or does not work, only that the company that makes the medicine has not received permission to advertise the medicine for use in children. Companies often do not apply for this permission because it is expensive to do the tests needed to apply for approval for use in children. Once a medication is approved by the FDA for any purpose, a doctor is allowed to prescribe it according to research and clinical experience.

Note to Teachers

It is a good idea to talk with the parent(s) about the reason(s) that a medication is being used. If the parent(s) sign consent to release information, it is often helpful to talk with the doctor. If the parent(s) give permission, the doctor may ask you to fill out rating forms about your experience with the student's behavior, feelings, academic performance, and medication side effects. This information is very useful in selecting and monitoring medication treatment. If you have observations that you think are important, do not hesitate to share these with the student's parent(s) and treating clinicians.

It is very important that the medicine be taken exactly as the doctor instructs. However, everyone forgets to give a medicine on time once in a while. It is a good idea to ask the parent(s) in advance what to do if this happens. Do not stop or change the time you are giving a medicine at school without parental permission. If a medication is to be taken with food, but lunchtime or snack time changes, be sure to notify the parent(s) so appropriate adjustments can be made.

All medicines should be kept in a secure place and should be supervised by an adult. If someone takes too much of a medicine, follow your school procedure for an urgent medical problem.

Taking medicine is a private matter and is best managed discreetly and confidentially. It is important to be sensitive to the student's feelings about taking medicine.

If you suspect that the student is using drugs or alcohol, please tell the parent(s) or a school counselor right away.

Please tell the parent(s) or school nurse if you suspect medication side effects.

Modifications of the classroom environment or assignments may be useful in addition to medication. The student may need to be evaluated for additional help or for an Individualized Education Plan for learning or behavior.

Any expression of suicidal thoughts or feelings or self-harm by a child or adolescent is a clear signal of distress and should be taken seriously. These behaviors should not be dismissed as "attention seeking."

What Is Citalopram (Celexa)?

Citalopram (brand name Celexa) is an antidepressant known as a *selective serotonin reuptake inhibitor* (SSRI). It comes in generic and brand name tablets and liquid form.

How Can This Medicine Help?

Citalopram is used to treat depression and anxiety disorders such as obsessive-compulsive disorder (OCD), posttraumatic stress disorder (PTSD), panic disorder, and separation anxiety disorder.

How Does This Medicine Work?

Citalopram increases the amount of a neurotransmitter called *serotonin* in certain parts of the brain. People with emotional and behavioral problems, such as depression and anxiety, may have low levels of serotonin in certain parts of the brain. SSRIs such as citalopram help by increasing the action of brain serotonin to more normal levels.

How Long Does This Medicine Last?

Citalopram can be taken only once a day.

How Will the Doctor Monitor This Medicine?

The doctor will review your child's medical history and physical examination before starting citalopram. The doctor may order some blood or urine tests to be sure your child does not have a hidden medical condition that would make it unsafe to use this medicine. Extra care is needed when using SSRIs in youth with seizures (epilepsy), liver or kidney problems, or diabetes. The doctor or nurse may measure your child's pulse, blood pressure, and weight before starting the medicine.

Be sure to tell the doctor if your child or anyone in the family has bipolar illness (manic-depressive illness) or has tried to kill himself or herself.

After the medicine is started, the doctor will want to have regular appointments with you and your child to see how the medicine is working, to see if a dose change is needed, to watch for side effects, to see if citalopram is still needed, and to see if any other treatment is needed. The doctor or nurse may check your child's height, weight, pulse, and blood pressure.

Before using medicine and at times afterward, the doctor may ask your child to fill out a rating scale about depression to help see how your child is doing.

What Side Effects Can This Medicine Have?

Any medicine can have side effects, including an allergy to the medicine. Because each patient is different, the doctor will monitor the youth closely, especially when the medicine is started. The doctor will work with you to increase the positive effects and decrease the negative effects of the medicine. Please tell the doctor if any of the listed side effects appear or if you think that the medicine is causing any other problems. Not all of the rare or unusual side effects are listed.

Side effects are most common after starting the medicine or after a dose increase. Many side effects can be avoided or lessened by starting with a very low dose and increasing it slowly—ask the doctor.

Allergic Reaction

Tell the doctor in a day or two (if possible, before the next dose of medicine):

- Hives
- Itching
- Rash

  Stop the medicine and get *immediate* medical care:

- Trouble breathing or chest tightness
- Swelling of lips, tongue, or throat

Common Side Effects

Tell the doctor within a week or two:

- Nausea, upset stomach, vomiting
- Diarrhea
- Dry mouth—Have your child try using sugar-free gum or candy.
- Constipation—Encourage your child to drink more fluids and eat high-fiber foods; if necessary, the doctor may recommend a fiber medicine such as Benefiber or a stool softener such as Colace or mineral oil.
- Headache
- Anxiety or nervousness
- Insomnia (trouble sleeping)
- Restlessness, increased activity level
- Daytime sleepiness or tiredness—Do not allow your child to drive, ride a bicycle or motorcycle, or operate machinery if this side effect is present.
- Dizziness—This side effect is worse when the child stands up quickly, especially when getting out of bed in the morning; try having the child stand up slowly.
- Tremor (shakiness)
- Excessive sweating
- Apathy, lack of interest in school or friends—This may happen after a initial good response to treatment.
- Decreased sexual interest, trouble with sexual functioning
- Weight gain
- Weight loss

Less Common, but More Serious, Side Effects

Call the doctor within a day or two:

- Significant suicidal thoughts or self-injurious behavior
- Increased activity, rapid speech, feeling "speeded up," decreased need for sleep, being very excited or irritable (cranky)

Serious Side Effects

Call the doctor *immediately* or go to the nearest emergency room:

- Seizure (fit, convulsion)
- Stiffness, high fever, confusion, tremors (shaking)
- Overheating or heatstroke—Prevent by decreasing activity in hot weather, staying out of the sun, and drinking water.

Serotonin Syndrome

A very serious side effect called *serotonin syndrome* can happen when certain kinds of medicines (including some medicines for migraine headaches—triptans) are taken by the same person. *Very* rarely, it can happen at high doses of just one medicine. The early signs are restlessness, confusion, shaking, skin turning red, sweating, and jerking of muscles. If you see these symptoms, stop the medicine and send or take the youth to an emergency room right away.

Some Interactions With Other Medicines or Food

Please note that the following are only the most likely interactions with food or other medicines.

Citalopram interacts with many other medicines, including some antibiotics and other psychiatric medicines. It is especially important to tell the doctor and pharmacist about all of the medicines your child is taking or has taken in the past few months, including over-the-counter and herbal medicines. Sometimes one medicine can increase or decrease the blood level of another medicine, so that different doses are needed. Generally, citalopram has fewer interactions with other medicines than does fluoxetine, paroxetine, or sertraline. Erythromycin and similar antibiotics, as well as antifungal agents such as ketoconazole, may increase levels of citalopram and increase side effects. Citalopram may increase the heart side effects of pimozide (Orap), so those two medicines should not be taken by the same person. The herbal medicine St. John's wort also increases serotonin and can cause serious side effects if taken with citalopram.

It can be *very dangerous* to take an SSRI at the same time as or even within a month of taking another type of medicine called a *monoamine oxidase inhibitor* (MAOI), such as Eldepryl (selegiline), Nardil (phenelzine), Parnate (tranylcypromine), or Marplan (isocarboxazid).

Citalopram does not usually cause problems when taken with decongestant cold medicines.

Citalopram can be taken with or without food.

Caffeine may increase side effects.

What Could Happen if This Medicine Is Stopped Suddenly?

No known serious medical effects occur if citalopram is stopped suddenly, but there may be uncomfortable feelings, which should be avoided if possible. Your child might have trouble sleeping, nervousness, irritability, dizziness, and flu-like symptoms. Ask the doctor before stopping citalopram or if these symptoms happen while the dose is being decreased.

How Long Will This Medicine Be Needed?

Citalopram may take up to 1–2 months to reach its full effect. If your child has a good response to citalopram, it is a good idea to continue the medicine for at least 6 months.

What Else Should I Know About This Medicine?

In youth who have bipolar disorder (manic depression) or who are at risk for bipolar disorder, any antidepressant medicine may increase the risk of hypomania or mania (excitement, agitation, increased activity, decreased sleep).

In hot weather, make sure your child drinks enough water or other liquids and does not get overheated.

Sometimes, after a person has improved while taking citalopram, he or she loses interest in school or friends or just stops trying. Please tell your child's doctor if this happens—it may be a side effect of the medicine. A lower dose or a different medicine may be needed.

Store the medicine away from sunlight, heat, moisture, and humidity.

Black Box Antidepressant Warning

In 2004, an advisory committee to the FDA decided that there might be an increased risk of suicidal behavior for some youth taking medicines called *antidepressants*. In the research studies that the committee reviewed, about 3%–4% of youth with depression who took an antidepressant medicine—and 1%–2% of youth with depression who took a placebo (pill without active medicine)—talked about suicidal thoughts (thinking about killing themselves or wishing they were dead) or did something to harm themselves. This means that almost twice as many youth who were taking an antidepressant to treat their depression talked about suicide or had suicidal behavior compared with youth with depression who were taking inactive medicine. There were *no* completed suicides in any of these research studies, which included more than 4,000 children and adolescents. For youth being treated for anxiety, there was no difference in suicidal talking or behavior between those taking antidepressant medication and those taking placebo.

The FDA told drug companies to add a *black box warning* label to all antidepressant medicines. Because of this label, a doctor (or advanced practice nurse) prescribing one of these medicines has to warn youth and their families that there might be more suicidal thoughts and actions in youth taking these medicines.

On the other hand, in places where more youth are taking the newer antidepressant medicines, the number of adolescents who commit suicide has gotten smaller. Also, thinking about or attempting suicide is more common in surveys of teenagers in the community than it is in depressed youth treated in research studies with antidepressant medicine.

If a youth is being treated with this medicine and is doing well, then no changes are needed as a result of this warning. Increased suicidal talk or action is most likely to happen in the first few months of treatment with a medicine. If your child has recently started this medicine or is about to start, then you and your doctor (or advanced practice nurse) should watch for any changes in behavior. People who are depressed often have suicidal thoughts or actions. It is hard to know whether suicidal thoughts or actions in depressed people are caused by the depression itself or by the medicine. Also, as their depression is getting better, some people talk more about the suicidal thoughts that they had before but did not talk about. As young people get better from depression, they might be at higher risk of doing something about suicidal thoughts that they have had for some time, because they have more energy.

What Should a Parent Do?

1. Be honest with your child about possible risks and benefits of medicine.

2. Talk to your child about whether he or she is having any suicidal thoughts, and tell your child to come to you if he or she is having such thoughts.

3. You, your child, and your child's doctor or nurse should develop a safety plan. Pick adults whom your child can tell if he or she is thinking about suicide.

4. Be sure to tell your child's doctor, nurse, or therapist if you suspect that your child is using alcohol or drugs or if something has happened that might make your child feel worse, such as a family separation, breaking up with a boyfriend or girlfriend, someone close dying or attempting suicide, physical or sexual abuse, or failure in school.

5. Be sure that there are no guns in the home and that all medicines (including over-the-counter medicines like Tylenol) are closely supervised by an adult and kept in a safe place.

6. Watch for new or worse thoughts of suicide, self-harm, depression, anxiety (nerves), feeling very agitated or restless, being angry or aggressive, having more trouble sleeping, or anything else that you see for the first time, seems worse, or worries your child or you. If these appear, contact a mental health professional **right away.** Do not just stop or change the dose of the medicine on your own. If the problems are serious, and you cannot reach one of your clinicians, call a 24-hour psychiatry emergency telephone number or take your child to an emergency room.

Youth taking antidepressant medicine should be watched carefully by their parent(s), clinician(s) (doctor, nurse, therapist), and other concerned adults for the first weeks of treatment. It is a good idea to have a visit or telephone call with the doctor, nurse, or therapist weekly for the first month, every 2 weeks for the second month, and after that at least once a month to check for feelings of depression or sadness, thoughts of killing or harming himself or herself, and any problems with the medication. If you have questions, be sure to ask the doctor, nurse, or therapist.

For more information, see http://www.parentsmedguide.org/ (in English and Spanish).

Notes

Use this space to take notes or to write down questions you want to ask the doctor.

_____

_____

_____

_____

_____

_____

_____

_____

_____

_____

_____

_____

_____

Medication Information for Youth

Citalopram—Celexa

What the Medicine Is Called and What It Is For

The name of your medicine may be confusing. Most drugs have two names: 1) a scientific name that we call a *generic name* and 2) a trade or *brand name*. The generic name of this medicine is citalopram. The brand name is Celexa.

Citalopram is called an *antidepressant*, or *selective serotonin reuptake inhibitor* (SSRI). Citalopram is used to treat depression and anxiety disorders such as obsessive-compulsive disorder (OCD), posttraumatic stress disorder (PTSD), panic disorder, and separation anxiety disorder. It helps people who feel very sad or depressed, anxious (nervous), or afraid, or who have obsessions (uncomfortable thoughts that will not go away) or compulsions (habits that get in the way of daily life).

How You Take the Medicine

It is very important to take the medicine exactly as the doctor or nurse tells you. Do not skip doses or take extra medicine without asking an adult. If you forget a dose, ask your parent(s) what to do. It is very important that you take all the pills you are supposed to take each day. Your doctor will probably recommend that you take your medicine at the same time each day, which may be with meals or at bedtime.

It may take several weeks before you notice that the medicine is helping. Waiting for the full effect may take even longer. You may feel discouraged and think the medicine is never going to help. You may want to give up and stop taking the medicine. Talk to your doctor and parent(s) about how you feel, but **do not stop** taking the medicine unless your doctor tells you to. It is also important not to take extra pills, hoping that you will feel better faster. Doing that could make you very sick.

Caffeine (in coffee, tea, or soft drinks) may make you feel worse.

This medicine is prescribed only for you. It should never be shared with anyone else.

You do not have to tell others that you are taking this medicine, but it is not something you should feel ashamed or embarrassed about. Many young people are helped by citalopram. This medicine is not habit-forming, and you cannot become "hooked" on it. You should talk to your doctor or nurse about any questions you have about the medicine. It is important to remember that the medicine *helps* you. It cannot *make* you do anything or change you as a person.

How Your Doctor Will Follow Your Progress

Before giving you the medicine, your doctor or nurse will talk with you and your parent(s) and may measure your height, weight, heart rate (pulse), and blood pressure. The doctor may order some blood or urine tests to be sure you are in good health.

Be sure to tell your doctor or nurse about any other medicines or supplements you are taking, including vitamins, herbs, or aids to weight loss or bodybuilding. Also be sure to tell the doctor or nurse if you are using alcohol or drugs. Because many medicines may affect babies, it is very important to tell the doctor if you might be pregnant or if you are at risk of becoming pregnant. Be sure to tell the doctor if you have had thoughts of hurting yourself, have tried to hurt yourself, or sometimes wish that you were not alive.

Your teachers may be asked to fill out a form about your grades and behavior in school. A psychologist may give you some tests to see how you learn best.

Before starting the medicine and afterward, the doctor may ask you to answer questions on paper about depression and anxiety.

Most doctors have regular appointments with young people who are taking medicine. You should use these visits to share any concerns you may have about your medicine and to talk about if it has helped you. From time to time, your physician or nurse may measure your height, weight, heart rate (pulse), and blood pressure to be sure that you are in good health while you are taking the medicine. Your doctor also will ask for regular reports from your parents and maybe from your teachers (with your permission) to see how well the medicine is working.

Some medicines are started at the amount you will take for as long as you are taking that medicine. Other medicines need to be increased or adjusted until your doctor decides you are taking the right amount. Starting at a low dose and increasing it slowly may lessen side effects. If the medicine helps you, your doctor will probably want you to take it for 6 months to a year if you are taking it to treat depression. If you are taking it for another problem, your doctor will decide how long you will need to take the medicine as he or she watches your progress.

It is not dangerous to stop citalopram suddenly, but there might be uncomfortable feelings, such as trouble sleeping, nervousness, irritability, or feeling sick. It is better to decrease it slowly. Do not stop taking a medicine unless the doctor tells you to. If you have any problems after stopping or decreasing this medicine, tell your parent(s) or doctor.

How the Medicine Might Affect You

In addition to the ways the medicine can help you, it may have other effects called *side effects*. Different medicines have different side effects. It is helpful to know about some of the most common side effects of your medicine so that you will understand what they are if they happen. Some people do not have any side effects. Some side effects are just uncomfortable, but others may mean a more serious problem with the medicine. Side effects are most common after starting the medicine or after a dose increase. They may go away with time, or the medicine can be adjusted or changed—ask the doctor.

You could have an allergy to any medicine, which might show up as a rash on your skin, swelling, itching, or trouble breathing.

Please tell your parent(s) and your doctor or nurse about any changes that you notice after taking the medicine. It is especially important to tell a responsible adult if you are feeling depressed or that you may not want to live; if you have thoughts of hurting yourself; or if you begin to feel more irritable, nervous, or restless. Also be sure to tell your parent(s) or doctor if you begin to feel "speeded up" or have trouble sleeping.

Some medicines make people feel sleepy or less coordinated. If this medicine is making you sleepy, it is very important not to drive a car or ride a bicycle or motorcycle. After starting a new medicine or increasing the dose of a medicine, please be extra careful when driving a car, riding a bike, or using machines until you can tell how the medicine affects your alertness, attention, and coordination.

One of the most common side effects of this medicine is feeling tired or sleepy during the day, even if you have had a full night's sleep. After you have been taking the medicine for a few weeks, your body will adjust, and this side effect may go away. If you have had trouble sleeping at night, the medicine can help you sleep better, especially if the doctor tells you to take a dose of medicine in the evening. Other people may feel more restless and excited. Tell your parent(s) or doctor if this is uncomfortable. Sometimes after being on the medicine for a while, people do not care as much about school or friends. Changing the dose or the type of medicine can help this.

This medicine may make your mouth dry. You may be more thirsty than usual and find that you are drinking more water or other liquids. Sucking on sugar-free hard candy or cough drops usually helps. You also could try chewing sugar-free gum or sucking on ice chips. Do not chew the ice; you could hurt your teeth. Also, using lip balm will keep your lips from cracking. It is important to be especially good about brushing your teeth.

Some other side effects that could happen are headache, not feeling hungry and not wanting to eat much, eating more than usual, having an upset stomach, or changes in your bowel movements. You may have a change in your sexual functioning—it is OK to ask the doctor about this. This medicine may make you more likely to get sick if you get overheated, so be sure to drink plenty of liquids and rest in the shade in hot weather.

Please let your parent(s) and doctor know if you notice anything different or unusual about how you feel once you start taking the medicine. This includes good things, such as feeling less sad or less nervous or sleeping better at night.

Notes

Use this space to take notes or to write down questions you want to ask the doctor or nurse.

_____

_____

_____

_____

_____

_____

_____

_____

_____

_____

_____

_____

_____

Medication Information for Parents and Teachers

Clomipramine—Anafranil

General Information About Medication

Each child and adolescent is different. No one has exactly the same combination of medical and psychological problems. It is a good idea to talk with the doctor or nurse about the reasons a medicine is being used. It is very important to keep all appointments and to be in touch by telephone if you have concerns. It is important to communicate with the doctor, nurse, or therapist.

It is very important that the medicine be taken exactly as the doctor instructs. However, once in a while, everyone forgets to give a medicine on time. It is a good idea to ask the doctor or nurse what to do if this happens. Do not stop or change a medicine without asking the doctor or nurse first.

If the medicine seems to stop working, it may be because it is not being taken regularly. The youth may be "cheeking" or hiding the medicine or forgetting to take it (especially at school). The doses may be too far apart, or a different dose may be needed. Something at school, at home, or in the neighborhood may be upsetting the youth, or he or she may need special help for learning disabilities or tutoring. Please discuss your concerns with the doctor. **Do not just increase the dose.**

All medicines should be kept in a safe place, out of the reach of children, and should be supervised by an adult. If someone takes too much of a medicine, call the doctor, the poison control center, or a hospital emergency room.

Each medicine has a "generic" or chemical name. Just like laundry detergents or paper towels, some medicines are sold by more than one company under different brand names. The same medicine may be available under a generic name and several brand names. The generic medications are usually less expensive than the brand name ones. The generic medications have the same chemical formula, but they may or may not be exactly the same strength as the brand-name medications. Also, some brands of pills contain dye that can cause allergic reactions. It is a good idea to talk to the doctor and the pharmacist about whether it is important to use a specific brand of medicine.

All medicines can cause an allergic reaction. Examples are hives, itching, rashes, swelling, and trouble breathing. Even a tiny amount of a medicine can cause a reaction in patients who are allergic to that medicine. Be *sure* to talk to the doctor before restarting a medicine that has caused an allergic reaction.

Taking more than one medicine at the same time may cause more side effects or cause one of the medicines to not work as well. Always ask the doctor, nurse, or pharmacist before adding another medicine, whether prescription or over-the-counter. Be sure that each doctor knows about *all* of the medicines your child is taking. Also tell the doctor about any vitamins, herbal medicines, or supplements your child may be taking. Some of these may have side effects alone or when taken with this medication.

Everyone taking medicine should have a physical examination at least once a year.

If you suspect the youth is using drugs or alcohol, please tell the doctor right away.

Pregnancy requires special care in the use of medicine. Please tell the doctor immediately if you suspect the teenager is pregnant or might become pregnant.

Printed information like this applies to children and adolescents in general. If you have questions about the medicine, or if you notice changes or anything unusual, please ask the doctor or nurse. As scientific research advances, knowledge increases and advice changes. Even experts do not always agree. Many medicines have not been approved by the U.S. Food and Drug Administration (FDA) for use in children. For this reason, use of the medicine for a particular problem or age group often is not listed in the *Physicians' Desk Reference*. This does not necessarily mean that the medicine is dangerous or does not work, only that the company that makes the medicine has not received permission to advertise the medicine for use in children. Companies often do not apply for this permission because it is expensive to do the tests needed to apply for approval for use in children. Once a medication is approved by the FDA for any purpose, a doctor is allowed to prescribe it according to research and clinical experience.

Note to Teachers

It is a good idea to talk with the parent(s) about the reason(s) that a medication is being used. If the parent(s) sign consent to release information, it is often helpful to talk with the doctor. If the parent(s) give permission, the doctor may ask you to fill out rating forms about your experience with the student's behavior, feelings, academic performance, and medication side effects. This information is very useful in selecting and monitoring medication treatment. If you have observations that you think are important, do not hesitate to share these with the student's parent(s) and treating clinicians.

It is very important that the medicine be taken exactly as the doctor instructs. However, everyone forgets to give a medicine on time once in a while. It is a good idea to ask the parent(s) in advance what to do if this happens. Do not stop or change the time you are giving a medicine at school without parental permission. If a medication is to be taken with food, but lunchtime or snack time changes, be sure to notify the parent(s) so appropriate adjustments can be made.

All medicines should be kept in a secure place and should be supervised by an adult. If someone takes too much of a medicine, follow your school procedure for an urgent medical problem.

Taking medicine is a private matter and is best managed discreetly and confidentially. It is important to be sensitive to the student's feelings about taking medicine.

If you suspect that the student is using drugs or alcohol, please tell the parent(s) or a school counselor right away.

Please tell the parent(s) or school nurse if you suspect medication side effects.

Modifications of the classroom environment or assignments may be useful in addition to medication. The student may need to be evaluated for additional help or for an Individualized Education Plan for learning or behavior.

Any expression of suicidal thoughts or feelings or self-harm by a child or adolescent is a clear signal of distress and should be taken seriously. These behaviors should not be dismissed as "attention seeking."

You may notice the following side effects at school:

Common Side Effects

- Dry mouth—Allow the student to chew sugar-free gum or to make extra trips to the water fountain.
- Constipation—Allow the student to drink more fluids or to use the bathroom more often.
- Daytime sleepiness—The student should not drive, ride a bicycle or motorcycle, or operate machinery.
- Dizziness (especially when standing up quickly)—This may happen in the classroom or during physical education). Suggest that the student stand up more slowly.
- Irritability

Occasional Side Effects

- Stuttering
- Increased risk of sunburn (this may be a problem if recess or physical education is outdoors in warm weather)—The student should wear sunscreen or protective clothing or stay out of the sun.

Less Common Side Effects

- Nausea—The student may need to take the medicine after a meal or snack.
- Trouble urinating—The student may need more time in the bathroom.
- Blurred vision—The student may have trouble seeing the blackboard.
- Motor tics (fast, repeated movements) or muscle twitches (jerking movements) of parts of the body
- Increased activity, rapid speech, feeling "speeded up," being very excited or irritable (cranky)
- Skin rash

Rare, but Potentially Serious, Side Effects

Call the parents(s) or follow your school's emergency procedures *immediately* if the student experiences any of the following side effects:

- Seizure (fit, convulsion) **(This is a medical emergency.)**
- Very fast or irregular heartbeat **(This is a medical emergency.)**
- Fainting
- Hallucinations (hearing voices or seeing things that are not there)
- Inability to urinate
- Confusion
- Severe change in behavior

What Is Clomipramine (Anafranil)?

Clomipramine is called a *tricyclic antidepressant*. It is used to treat obsessive-compulsive disorder (OCD) and trichotillomania (compulsive hair pulling). It comes in brand name Anafranil and generic capsules.

How Can This Medicine Help?

Clomipramine can decrease anxiety (nervousness), obsessions and compulsions, or severe habits such as hair pulling (trichotillomania). The medicine may take several weeks to work.

How Does This Medicine Work?

Tricyclic antidepressants affect the natural substances called *neurotransmitters* that are needed for certain parts of the brain to work more normally. These antidepressants increase the activity of the neurotransmitters called *serotonin* and *norepinephrine* to more normal levels in the parts of the brain that regulate concentration, motivation, and mood.

How Long Does This Medicine Last?

Although a dose lasts for a whole day in adults and older teenagers, in younger children several doses a day may be needed.

How Will the Doctor Monitor This Medicine?

The doctor will review your child's medical history and physical examination, paying special attention to pulse rate, blood pressure, weight, and height, before starting clomipramine. These measurements will be taken when the dose is increased and occasionally as long as the medicine is continued. The doctor may order some blood or urine tests to be sure your child does not have a hidden medical condition that would make it unsafe to use this medicine.

Tricyclic antidepressants can slow the speed at which signals move through the heart. This effect is not dangerous if the heart is normal, which is why an ECG (electrocardiogram or heart rhythm test) is done before starting the medicine. The ECG may be repeated as the dose is increased and occasionally while the medicine is being taken. Changes in the heart from the medicine usually can be seen on the ECG before they become a problem, so your child's doctor will order an ECG every so often. To find possible hidden heart risks, it is especially important to tell the doctor if your child or anyone in the family has a history of fainting, palpitations, or irregular heartbeat or if anyone in the family died suddenly.

Be sure to tell the doctor if your child or anyone in the family has bipolar illness (manic-depressive illness) or has tried to kill himself or herself.

Because tricyclic antidepressants may increase the risk of seizures (fits, convulsions), the doctor will want to know whether your child has ever had a seizure or a head injury and if there is any family history of epilepsy. Your child's doctor may want to order an EEG (electroencephalogram or brain wave test) before starting the medicine.

Experts do not agree on whether blood tests are needed to measure the level of this medicine. Blood levels seem to be most useful when your doctor suspects that the dose of medicine is too high or too low. The most accurate level is obtained by drawing blood first thing in the morning, after at least 5 days on the same dose, approximately 12 hours after the evening dose of medicine and before the morning dose.

After the medicine is started, the doctor will want to have regular appointments with you and your child to see how the medicine is working, to see if a dose change is needed, to watch for side effects, to see if clomipramine is still needed, and to see if any other treatment is needed. The doctor or nurse may check your child's height, weight, pulse, and blood pressure or order tests, such as an ECG or blood level.

Before using medicine and at times afterward, the doctor may ask your child to fill out a rating scale about anxiety, to help see how your child is doing.

What Side Effects Can This Medicine Have?

Any medicine can have side effects, including an allergy to the medicine. Because each patient is different, the doctor will monitor the youth closely, especially when the medicine is started. The doctor will work with you to increase the positive effects and decrease the negative effects of the medicine. Please tell the doctor if any of the listed side effects appear or if you think that the medicine is causing any other problems. Not all of the rare or unusual side effects are listed.

Side effects are most common after starting the medicine or after a dose increase. Many side effects can be avoided or lessened by starting with a very low dose and increasing it slowly—ask the doctor.

Allergic Reaction

Tell the doctor in a day or two (if possible, before the next dose of medicine):

- Hives
- Itching
- Rash—This may be caused by an allergy to the medicine or to a dye in the specific brand of pill.

Stop the medicine and get *immediate* medical care:

- Trouble breathing or chest tightness
- Swelling of lips, tongue, or throat

Common Side Effects

Tell the doctor within a week or two:

- Dry mouth—Have your child try using sugar-free gum or candy.
- Constipation—Encourage your child to drink more fluids and eat high-fiber foods; if necessary, the doctor may recommend a fiber medicine such as Benefiber or a stool softener such as Colace or mineral oil.
- Daytime sleepiness—Do not allow your child to drive, ride a bicycle or motorcycle, or operate machinery if this happens.
- Dizziness—This side effect is worse when the child stands up quickly, especially when getting out of bed in the morning; try having the child stand up slowly.
- Weight gain
- Loss of appetite and weight loss
- Irritability
- Acne

Occasional Side Effects

Tell the doctor within a week or two:

- Nightmares
- Stuttering
- Blurred vision
- Increase in breast size, nipple discharge, or both (in girls)
- Increase in breast size (in boys)

Less Common, but More Serious, Side Effects

Call the doctor within a day or two:

- High or low blood pressure
- Nausea
- Trouble urinating
- Motor tics (fast, repeated movements) or muscle twitches (jerking movements)
- Increased activity, rapid speech, feeling "speeded up," decreased need for sleep, being very excited or irritable (cranky)

Rare, but Potentially Serious, Side Effects

Call the doctor *immediately*:

- Seizure (fit, convulsion)—**Go to an emergency room.**
- Very fast or irregular heartbeat—**Go to an emergency room.**
- Fainting
- Hallucinations (hearing voices or seeing things that are not there)
- Inability to urinate
- Confusion
- Severe change in behavior

Some Interactions With Other Medicines or Food

Please note that the following are only the most likely interactions with food or other medicines.

Check with your child's doctor before giving your child decongestants or over-the-counter cold medicine.

Another antidepressant may increase the level of clomipramine and increase side effects.

It can be *very dangerous* to take clomipramine at the same time as or even within a month of taking another type of medicine called a *monoamine oxidase inhibitor* (MAOI), such as Eldepryl (selegiline), Nardil (phenelzine), Parnate (tranylcypromine), or Marplan (isocarboxazid).

Caffeine may worsen side effects on the heart or symptoms of anxiety. It is best not to drink coffee, tea, or soft drinks with caffeine while taking this medicine. A large glass of grapefruit juice may increase the levels and side effects of clomipramine.

What Could Happen if This Medicine Is Stopped Suddenly?

Stopping the medicine suddenly or skipping a dose is not dangerous but can be very uncomfortable. Your child may feel like he or she has the flu—with a headache, muscle aches, stomachache, and upset stomach. Behavioral problems, sadness, nervousness, or trouble sleeping also may occur. If these feelings appear every day, the medicine may need to be given more often during each day.

How Long Will This Medicine Be Needed?

There is no way to know how long a person will need to take this medicine. Parents work together with the doctor to determine what is right for each child. When used to treat obsessive-compulsive disorder, the medicine may be needed for a long time. Some people may need to take the medicine even as adults.

What Else Should I Know About This Medicine?

In youth who have bipolar disorder (manic depression) or who are at risk for bipolar disorder, any antidepressant medicine may increase the risk of hypomania or mania (excitement, agitation, increased activity, decreased sleep).

An overdose by accident or on purpose with tricyclic antidepressants is very dangerous! You must closely supervise the medicine. You may have to lock up the medicine if your child or teenager is suicidal or if young children live in or visit your home.

Tricyclic antidepressants may cause dry mouth, which could increase the chance of tooth decay. Regular brushing of teeth and checkups with the dentist are especially important.

This medicine causes increased risk of sunburn. Be sure that your child wears sunscreen or protective clothing or stays out of the sun.

People who take tricyclic antidepressants must not drink alcohol or use tranquilizers. Severe sleepiness, loss of consciousness, or even death may result.

Black Box Antidepressant Warning

In 2004, an advisory committee to the FDA decided that there might be an increased risk of suicidal behavior for some youth taking medicines called *antidepressants*. In the research studies that the committee reviewed, about 3%–4% of youth with depression who took an antidepressant medicine—and 1%–2% of youth with depression who took a placebo (pill without active medicine)—talked about suicidal thoughts (thinking about killing themselves or wishing they were dead) or did something to harm themselves. This means that almost twice as many youth who were taking an antidepressant to treat their depression talked about suicide or had suicidal behavior compared with youth with depression who were taking inactive medicine. There were *no* completed suicides in any of these research studies, which included more than 4,000 children and adolescents. For youth being treated for anxiety, there was no difference in suicidal talking or behavior between those taking antidepressant medication and those taking placebo.

The FDA told drug companies to add a *black box warning* label to all antidepressant medicines. Because of this label, a doctor (or advanced practice nurse) prescribing one of these medicines has to warn youth and their families that there might be more suicidal thoughts and actions in youth taking these medicines.

On the other hand, in places where more youth are taking the newer antidepressant medicines, the number of adolescents who commit suicide has gotten smaller. Also, thinking about or attempting suicide is more common in surveys of teenagers in the community than it is in depressed youth treated in research studies with antidepressant medicine.

If a youth is being treated with this medicine and is doing well, then no changes are needed as a result of this warning. Increased suicidal talk or action is most likely to happen in the first few months of treatment with a medicine. If your child has recently started this medicine or is about to start, then you and your doctor (or advanced practice nurse) should watch for any changes in behavior. People who are depressed often have suicidal thoughts or actions. It is hard to know whether suicidal thoughts or actions in depressed people are caused by the depression itself or by the medicine. Also, as their depression is getting better, some people talk more about the suicidal thoughts that they had before but did not talk about. As young people get better from depression, they might be at higher risk of doing something about suicidal thoughts that they have had for some time, because they have more energy.

What Should a Parent Do?

1. Be honest with your child about possible risks and benefits of medicine.
2. Talk to your child about whether he or she is having any suicidal thoughts, and tell your child to come to you if he or she is having such thoughts.
3. You, your child, and your child's doctor or nurse should develop a safety plan. Pick adults whom your child can tell if he or she is thinking about suicide.
4. Be sure to tell your child's doctor, nurse, or therapist if you suspect that your child is using alcohol or drugs or if something has happened that might make your child feel worse, such as a family separation, breaking up with a boyfriend or girlfriend, someone close dying or attempting suicide, physical or sexual abuse, or failure in school.
5. Be sure that there are no guns in the home and that all medicines (including over-the-counter medicines like Tylenol) are closely supervised by an adult and kept in a safe place.
6. Watch for new or worse thoughts of suicide, self-harm, depression, anxiety (nerves), feeling very agitated or restless, being angry or aggressive, having more trouble sleeping, or anything else that you see for the first time, seems worse, or worries your child or you. If these appear, contact a mental health professional **right away.** Do not just stop or change the dose of the medicine on your own. If the problems are serious, and you cannot reach one of your clinicians, call a 24-hour psychiatry emergency telephone number or take your child to an emergency room.

Youth taking antidepressant medicine should be watched carefully by their parent(s), clinician(s) (doctor, nurse, therapist), and other concerned adults for the first weeks of treatment. It is a good idea to have a visit or telephone call with the doctor, nurse, or therapist weekly for the first month, every 2 weeks for the second month, and after that at least once a month to check for feelings of depression or sadness, thoughts of killing or harming himself or herself, and any problems with the medication. If you have questions, be sure to ask the doctor, nurse, or therapist.

For more information, see http://www.parentsmedguide.org/ (in English and Spanish).

Notes

Use this space to take notes or to write down questions you want to ask the doctor.

_____

_____

_____

_____

_____

_____

_____

_____

_____

_____

_____

_____

_____

From Dulcan MK (editor): _Helping Parents, Youth, and Teachers Understand Medications for Behavioral and Emotional Problems: A Resource Book of Medication Information Handouts_, Third Edition. Washington, DC, American Psychiatric Publishing, 2007

Medication Information for Youth

Clomipramine—Anafranil

What the Medicine Is Called and What It Is For

The name of your medicine may be confusing. Most drugs have two names: 1) a scientific name that we call a *generic name* and 2) a trade or *brand name*. The generic name of this medicine is clomipramine. The brand name is Anafranil.

Clomipramine is called an *antidepressant* or *tricyclic*. Clomipramine is used to treat obsessive-compulsive disorder (OCD)—when people have obsessions (uncomfortable thoughts that will not go away) or compulsions (habits that get in the way of daily life)—or trichotillomania (hair pulling that you cannot stop).

How You Take the Medicine

It is very important to take the medicine exactly as the doctor or nurse tells you. Do not skip doses or take extra medicine without asking an adult. If you miss a dose, you may feel sick, as though you have the flu. It is very important that you take all the pills you are supposed to take each day. Your doctor will probably recommend that you take your medicine at the same time each day, which may be with meals or at bedtime.

It may take several weeks before you notice that the medicine is helping. Waiting for the full effect may take even longer. You may feel discouraged and think the medicine is never going to help. You may want to give up and stop taking the medicine. Talk to your doctor and parent(s) about how you feel, but **do not stop** taking the medicine unless your doctor tells you to. It is also important not to take extra pills, hoping that you will feel better faster. Doing that could make you very sick.

Stopping the medicine suddenly or skipping a dose can be very uncomfortable. You may feel like you have the flu—with a headache, muscle aches, stomachache, and upset stomach. If these feelings appear every day, the medicine may need to be given more often during each day.

Caffeine (in coffee, tea, or soft drinks) may make you feel worse.

Do not use any other medicines without talking to your doctor first. Do not use alcohol, marijuana, or street drugs while taking this medicine—**it can be very dangerous.** Skipping your medicine to take drugs does not work because many medicines can stay in your body for a long time.

This medicine is prescribed only for you. It should never be shared with anyone else.

You do not have to tell others that you are taking this medicine, but it is not something you should feel ashamed or embarrassed about. Many young people are helped by clomipramine. This medicine is not habit-forming, and you cannot become "hooked" on it. You should talk to your doctor or nurse about any questions you have about the medicine. It is important to remember that the medicine *helps* you. It cannot *make* you do anything or change you as a person.

135

How Your Doctor Will Follow Your Progress

Before giving you the medicine, your doctor or nurse will talk with you and your parent(s) and measure your height, weight, heart rate (pulse), and blood pressure. The doctor may order some blood or urine tests to be sure you are in good health. Be sure to tell the doctor if you have had very fast heartbeat, chest pain, dizziness, or fainting.

Be sure to tell your doctor or nurse about any other medicines or supplements you are taking, including vitamins, herbs, or aids to weight loss or bodybuilding. Also be sure to tell the doctor or nurse if you are using alcohol or drugs. Because many medicines may affect babies, it is very important to tell the doctor if you might be pregnant or if you are at risk of becoming pregnant. Be sure to tell the doctor if you have had thoughts of hurting yourself, have tried to hurt yourself, or sometimes wish that you were not alive.

Before starting clomipramine, at times of increasing the dose, and every 6 months to a year after that, your doctor will ask for an ECG (electrocardiogram or heart rhythm test) to be done. This test counts your heartbeats through small wires that are taped to your chest. It takes only a few minutes. To help make sure that you will not have problems with the medicine, the doctor may ask for an EEG (electroencephalogram or brain wave test) before starting the medicine. This does not tell the doctor anything about what you are thinking or feeling but just shows the rhythms of your brain cells.

Your teachers may be asked to fill out a form about your grades and behavior in school. A psychologist may give you some tests to see how you learn best.

Before starting the medicine and afterward, the doctor may ask you to answer questions on paper about obsessions and compulsions.

Most doctors have regular appointments with young people who are taking medicine. You should use these visits to share any concerns you may have about your medicine and to talk about if it has helped you. From time to time, your physician or nurse may measure your height, weight, heart rate (pulse), and blood pressure to be sure that you are in good health while you are taking the medicine. You may need to have blood tests to see if you are on the right dose of clomipramine. Your doctor also will ask for regular reports from your parents and maybe from your teachers (with your permission) to see how well the medicine is working.

Some medicines are started at the amount you will take for as long as you are taking that medicine. Other medicines need to be increased or adjusted until your doctor decides you are taking the right amount. Starting at a low dose and increasing it slowly may lessen side effects. If the medicine helps you, your doctor will probably want you to take it for a long time, maybe even as an adult.

How the Medicine Might Affect You

In addition to the ways the medicine can help you, it may have other effects called *side effects*. Different medicines have different side effects. It is helpful to know about some of the most common side effects of your medicine so that you will understand what they are if they happen. Some people do not have any side effects. Some side effects are just uncomfortable, but others may mean a more serious problem with the medicine. Side effects are most common after starting the medicine or after a dose increase. They may go away with time, or the medicine can be adjusted or changed—ask the doctor.

You could have an allergy to any medicine, which might show up as a rash on your skin, swelling, itching, or trouble breathing.

Please tell your parent(s) and your doctor or nurse about any changes that you notice after taking the medicine. It is especially important to tell a responsible adult if you are feeling depressed or that you may not want to live; if you have thoughts of hurting yourself; or if you begin to feel more irritable, nervous, or restless. Also be sure to tell your parent(s) or doctor if you begin to feel "speeded up" or have trouble sleeping.

Some medicines make people feel sleepy or less coordinated. If this medicine is making you sleepy, it is very important not to drive a car or ride a bicycle or motorcycle. After starting a new medicine or increasing the dose of a medicine, please be extra careful when driving a car, riding a bike, or using machines until you can tell how the medicine affects your alertness, attention, and coordination.

One of the most common side effects of this medicine is feeling tired or sleepy during the day, even if you have had a full night's sleep. After you have been taking the medicine for a few weeks, your body will adjust, and this side effect may go away. If you have had trouble sleeping at night, the medicine can help you sleep better, especially if the doctor tells you to take a dose of medicine in the evening. Other people may feel more restless and excited. Tell your parent(s) or doctor if this is uncomfortable.

Another common side effect is dry mouth. You may be more thirsty than usual and find that you are drinking more water or other liquids. Sucking on sugar-free hard candy or cough drops usually helps. You also could try chewing sugar-free gum or sucking on ice chips. Do not chew the ice; you could hurt your teeth. Also, using lip balm will keep your lips from cracking. It is important to be especially good about brushing your teeth.

Sometimes people taking clomipramine notice that their heart is beating a little faster than normal. Usually this happens within the first few weeks of taking the medicine and gets better or goes away. However, if you notice that your heart is beating very fast for more than a few minutes when you have not been exercising, if you feel light-headed or dizzy when you are sitting or standing still, or if you faint, you should let your parent(s) and doctor know right away. Some people feel dizzy or light-headed when standing up fast. If this happens, try to get up more slowly, especially first thing in the morning, when getting out of bed.

Some people become constipated (have hard bowel movements). Try drinking more water and eating more fruits, vegetables, and whole grains. If that does not help, tell your parent(s) or doctor—you may need a medicine to help with this side effect.

Some other side effects that could happen are acne, headache, blurred vision, not feeling hungry and not wanting to eat much, eating more than usual, having an upset stomach, changes in your bowel movements, or trouble passing urine. You may have a change in your sexual functioning or in your breasts—it is OK to ask the doctor about this. This medicine may make you more likely to get sick if you get overheated, so be sure to drink plenty of liquids and rest in the shade in hot weather.

Please let your parent(s) and doctor know if you notice anything different or unusual about how you feel once you start taking the medicine. This includes good things, such as feeling less sad or less nervous or sleeping better at night.

Notes

Use this space to take notes or to write down questions you want to ask the doctor or nurse.

_____

_____

_____

_____

_____

_____

_____

_____

From Dulcan MK (editor): _Helping Parents, Youth, and Teachers Understand Medications for Behavioral and Emotional Problems: A Resource Book of Medication Information Handouts,_ Third Edition. Washington, DC, American Psychiatric Publishing, 2007

Medication Information for Parents and Teachers

Clonazepam—Klonopin

General Information About Medication

Each child and adolescent is different. No one has exactly the same combination of medical and psychological problems. It is a good idea to talk with the doctor or nurse about the reasons a medicine is being used. It is very important to keep all appointments and to be in touch by telephone if you have concerns. It is important to communicate with the doctor, nurse, or therapist.

It is very important that the medicine be taken exactly as the doctor instructs. However, once in a while, everyone forgets to give a medicine on time. It is a good idea to ask the doctor or nurse what to do if this happens. Do not stop or change a medicine without asking the doctor or nurse first.

If the medicine seems to stop working, it may be because it is not being taken regularly. The youth may be "cheeking" or hiding the medicine or forgetting to take it (especially at school). The doses may be too far apart, or a different dose may be needed. Something at school, at home, or in the neighborhood may be upsetting the youth, or he or she may need special help for learning disabilities or tutoring. Please discuss your concerns with the doctor. **Do not just increase the dose.**

All medicines should be kept in a safe place, out of the reach of children, and should be supervised by an adult. If someone takes too much of a medicine, call the doctor, the poison control center, or a hospital emergency room.

Each medicine has a "generic" or chemical name. Just like laundry detergents or paper towels, some medicines are sold by more than one company under different brand names. The same medicine may be available under a generic name and several brand names. The generic medications are usually less expensive than the brand name ones. The generic medications have the same chemical formula, but they may or may not be exactly the same strength as the brand-name medications. Also, some brands of pills contain dye that can cause allergic reactions. It is a good idea to talk to the doctor and the pharmacist about whether it is important to use a specific brand of medicine.

All medicines can cause an allergic reaction. Examples are hives, itching, rashes, swelling, and trouble breathing. Even a tiny amount of a medicine can cause a reaction in patients who are allergic to that medicine. Be *sure* to talk to the doctor before restarting a medicine that has caused an allergic reaction.

Taking more than one medicine at the same time may cause more side effects or cause one of the medicines to not work as well. Always ask the doctor, nurse, or pharmacist before adding another medicine, whether prescription or over-the-counter. Be sure that each doctor knows about *all* of the medicines your child is taking. Also tell the doctor about any vitamins, herbal medicines, or supplements your child may be taking. Some of these may have side effects alone or when taken with this medication.

Everyone taking medicine should have a physical examination at least once a year.

If you suspect the youth is using drugs or alcohol, please tell the doctor right away.

Pregnancy requires special care in the use of medicine. Please tell the doctor immediately if you suspect the teenager is pregnant or might become pregnant.

Printed information like this applies to children and adolescents in general. If you have questions about the medicine, or if you notice changes or anything unusual, please ask the doctor or nurse. As scientific research advances, knowledge increases and advice changes. Even experts do not always agree. Many medicines have not been approved by the U.S. Food and Drug Administration (FDA) for use in children. For this reason, use of the medicine for a particular problem or age group often is not listed in the *Physicians' Desk Reference*. This does not necessarily mean that the medicine is dangerous or does not work, only that the company that makes the medicine has not received permission to advertise the medicine for use in children. Companies often do not apply for this permission because it is expensive to do the tests needed to apply for approval for use in children. Once a medication is approved by the FDA for any purpose, a doctor is allowed to prescribe it according to research and clinical experience.

Note to Teachers

It is a good idea to talk with the parent(s) about the reason(s) that a medication is being used. If the parent(s) sign consent to release information, it is often helpful to talk with the doctor. If the parent(s) give permission, the doctor may ask you to fill out rating forms about your experience with the student's behavior, feelings, academic performance, and medication side effects. This information is very useful in selecting and monitoring medication treatment. If you have observations that you think are important, do not hesitate to share these with the student's parent(s) and treating clinicians.

It is very important that the medicine be taken exactly as the doctor instructs. However, everyone forgets to give a medicine on time once in a while. It is a good idea to ask the parent(s) in advance what to do if this happens. Do not stop or change the time you are giving a medicine at school without parental permission. If a medication is to be taken with food, but lunchtime or snack time changes, be sure to notify the parent(s) so appropriate adjustments can be made.

All medicines should be kept in a secure place and should be supervised by an adult. If someone takes too much of a medicine, follow your school procedure for an urgent medical problem.

Taking medicine is a private matter and is best managed discreetly and confidentially. It is important to be sensitive to the student's feelings about taking medicine.

If you suspect that the student is using drugs or alcohol, please tell the parent(s) or a school counselor right away.

Please tell the parent(s) or school nurse if you suspect medication side effects.

Modifications of the classroom environment or assignments may be useful in addition to medication. The student may need to be evaluated for additional help or for an Individualized Education Plan for learning or behavior.

Any expression of suicidal thoughts or feelings or self-harm by a child or adolescent is a clear signal of distress and should be taken seriously. These behaviors should not be dismissed as "attention seeking."

What Is Clonazepam (Klonopin)?

Clonazepam is a *benzodiazepine*. It comes in brand name Klonopin and generic tablets and Klonopin rapid-dissolving tablets.

How Can This Medicine Help?

Clonazepam was most commonly used in the treatment of epilepsy (seizures, convulsions) and panic disorder. It can also help decrease anxiety in social anxiety disorder or posttraumatic stress disorder (PTSD). It can help calm people who have mania or acute psychosis. The rapid-dissolving tablets can be held in the mouth and work very fast.

How Does This Medicine Work?

Clonazepam works on special places *(receptors)* in brain cells to increase the action of the brain chemical *GABA* (a *neurotransmitter*) in parts of the brain.

How Long Does This Medicine Last?

Clonazepam needs to be taken two or three times a day if taken regularly. The rapid-dissolving tablet may be taken as needed to prevent or stop a panic attack.

How Will the Doctor Monitor This Medicine?

The doctor will review your child's medical history and physical examination before starting clonazepam. The doctor may order some blood or urine tests to be sure your child does not have a hidden medical condition. The doctor or nurse may measure your child's pulse and blood pressure before starting clonazepam. Blood tests are not usually needed before starting clonazepam.

After the medicine is started, the doctor will want to have regular appointments with you and your child to see how the medicine is working, to see if a dose change is needed, to watch for side effects, to see if clonazepam is still needed, and to see if any other treatment is needed. The doctor or nurse may check your child's height, weight, pulse, and blood pressure.

What Side Effects Can This Medicine Have?

Any medicine can have side effects, including an allergy to the medicine. Because each patient is different, the doctor will monitor the youth closely, especially when the medicine is started. The doctor will work with you to increase the positive effects and decrease the negative effects of the medicine. Please tell the doctor if any of the listed side effects appear or if you think that the medicine is causing any other problems. Not all of the rare or unusual side effects are listed.

Side effects are most common after starting the medicine or after a dose increase. Many side effects can be avoided or lessened by starting with a very low dose and increasing it slowly—ask the doctor.

141

Allergic Reaction

Tell the doctor in a day or two (if possible, before the next dose of medicine):

- Hives
- Itching
- Rash

    Stop the medicine and get *immediate* medical care:

- Trouble breathing or chest tightness
- Swelling of lips, tongue, or throat

Common Side Effects

The following side effects are more common when first starting the medicine:

    Tell the doctor within a week or two:

- Difficulty with balance
- Daytime drowsiness or sleepiness—Do not allow your child to drive, ride a bicycle or motorcycle, or operate machinery if this happens.

Behavioral and Emotional Side Effects

Call the doctor within a day or two:

- Irritability
- Excitement
- Increased anger or aggression
- Severe change in behavior
- Trouble sleeping or nightmares
- Decreased concentration
- Memory loss
- Feeling "spacey"

Serious Side Effects

- **Call the doctor or go to an emergency room immediately if your child exhibits uncontrollable behavior.**
- **People who take clonazepam must not drink alcohol. Severe sleepiness, loss of consciousness, or even death may result.**

Some Interactions With Other Medicines or Food

Please note that the following are only the most likely interactions with food or other medicines.

Clonazepam may be taken with or without food.

Taking clonazepam with alcohol and/or other sedative medicines or antihistamines (such as Benadryl) increases sleepiness, decreases muscle coordination, and may even decrease breathing.

It is better to limit drinks with caffeine (coffee, tea, soft drinks) because caffeine works in the opposite way from this medicine, and the positive effects might be decreased.

What Could Happen if This Medicine Is Stopped Suddenly?

Stopping clonazepam suddenly could cause seizures (fits, convulsions), especially if your child is being treated for seizures. Other symptoms caused by stopping suddenly could be headache, vomiting, decreased concentration, confusion, tremor (shaking), and muscle cramps.

How Long Will This Medicine Be Needed?

When being used for anxiety, agitation, or mania, clonazepam is usually used for a relatively short time, until other medications and/or behavioral treatments can start to work.

What Else Should I Know About This Medicine?

Because benzodiazepines can be abused (especially by people who abuse alcohol or drugs) and can cause psychological dependence or physical dependence (addiction), they are regulated by special state and federal laws as *controlled substances*. These laws place limitations on telephone prescriptions and refills.

Use of clonazepam for a long time may lead to dependence on the medicine.

People with sleep apnea (breathing stops while they are asleep) should not take clonazepam. Tell the doctor if your child snores very loudly.

Clonazepam should be avoided during pregnancy, especially in the first 3 months, because it may cause birth defects in the baby.

Klonopin may be confused with clonidine. Be sure to check the prescription when you get it from the pharmacy.

Notes

Use this space to take notes or to write down questions you want to ask the doctor.

_____

_____

_____

_____

_____

_____

_____

_____

_____

_____

_____

From Dulcan MK (editor): _Helping Parents, Youth, and Teachers Understand Medications for Behavioral and Emotional Problems: A Resource Book of Medication Information Handouts_, Third Edition. Washington, DC, American Psychiatric Publishing, 2007

Medication Information for Youth

Clonazepam—Klonopin

What the Medicine Is Called and What It Is For

The name of your medicine may be confusing. Most drugs have two names: 1) a scientific name that we call a *generic name* and 2) a trade or *brand name*. The generic name of this medicine is clonazepam. The brand name is Klonopin.

Clonazepam is a *benzodiazepine*. It works by calming the parts of the brain that are too excitable in anxious people. It can decrease anxiety, nervousness, fears, and excessive worrying. Clonazepam can decrease the physical symptoms (rapid heartbeat, trouble breathing, dizziness, sweating) of panic attacks and fears. It can help anxious people to be calm enough to learn—with therapy and practice—to understand and tolerate their worries or fears and even to overcome them. Your doctor may have told you that you have a condition such as social phobia (social anxiety disorder), posttraumatic stress disorder (PTSD), or panic disorder.

Sometimes clonazepam is used for a few days to treat agitation in mania or psychosis until other medicines start to work.

How You Take the Medicine

It is very important to take the medicine exactly as the doctor or nurse tells you. Do not skip doses or take extra medicine without asking an adult. If you forget a dose, ask your parent(s) what to do.

The rapid-dissolving tablets can be held in the mouth and work very fast.

It is better to limit drinks with caffeine (coffee, tea, soft drinks) because caffeine works in the opposite way from this medicine, and the positive effects might be decreased.

This medicine is prescribed only for you. It should never be shared with anyone else.

You do not have to tell others that you are taking this medicine, but it is not something you should feel ashamed or embarrassed about. Many young people are helped by clonazepam. You should talk to your doctor or nurse about any questions you have about the medicine. It is important to remember that the medicine *helps* you. It cannot *make* you do anything or change you as a person.

Many medicines cause problems if stopped suddenly. Always ask your doctor before stopping a medicine. Problems are more likely to happen in patients taking high doses of clonazepam for 2 months or longer, but it is important to decrease the medicine slowly (taper) even after a few weeks. If you notice anxiety, irritability, shaking, sweating, aches and pains, muscle cramps, vomiting, or trouble sleeping, you may need to decrease the medicine more slowly. If large doses are stopped suddenly, seizures (fits, convulsions), hallucinations (hearing voices or seeing things that are not there), or out-of-control behavior may result.

How Your Doctor Will Follow Your Progress

Before giving you the medicine, your doctor or nurse will talk with you and your parent(s) and may measure your height, weight, heart rate (pulse), and blood pressure. There may be other tests to be sure that you are in good health.

Be sure to tell your doctor or nurse about any other medicines or supplements you are taking, including vitamins, herbs, or aids to weight loss or bodybuilding. Also be sure to tell the doctor or nurse if you are using alcohol or drugs. Because many medicines may affect babies, it is very important to tell the doctor if you might be pregnant or if you are at risk of becoming pregnant.

Your teachers may be asked to fill out a form about your grades and behavior in school. A psychologist may give you some tests to see how you learn best.

Most doctors have regular appointments with young people who are taking medicine. You should use these visits to share any concerns you may have about your medicine and to talk about if it has helped you. From time to time, your physician or nurse may measure your height, weight, heart rate (pulse), and blood pressure to be sure that you are in good health while you are taking the medicine. Your doctor also will ask for regular reports from your parents and maybe from your teachers (with your permission) to see how well the medicine is working.

Clonazepam is usually prescribed for only a few weeks to allow you to be calm enough to learn new ways to cope with anxiety and to allow your nervous system to become less excitable. Sometimes it is used for longer periods to treat panic attacks or anxiety that remain after therapy is completed. Each person is unique, and some people may need these medicines for months or years.

How the Medicine Might Affect You

In addition to the ways the medicine can help you, it may have other effects called *side effects*. Different medicines have different side effects. It is helpful to know about some of the most common side effects of your medicine so that you will understand what they are if they happen. Some people do not have any side effects. Some side effects are just uncomfortable, but others may mean a more serious problem with the medicine. Side effects are most common after starting the medicine or after a dose increase. They may go away with time, or the medicine can be adjusted or changed—ask the doctor.

You could have an allergy to any medicine, which might show up as a rash on your skin, swelling, itching, or trouble breathing.

Please tell your parent(s) and your doctor or nurse about any changes that you notice after taking the medicine. It is especially important to tell a responsible adult if you are feeling depressed or that you may not want to live; if you have thoughts of hurting yourself; or if you begin to feel more irritable, nervous, or restless.

The most common side effect of clonazepam is daytime sleepiness. If this medicine is making you sleepy, it is very important not to drive a car or ride a bicycle or motorcycle. After starting clonazepam or increasing the dose, please be extra careful when driving a car, riding a bike, or using machines until you can tell how the medicine affects your alertness, attention, and coordination.

Sometimes clonazepam seems to work in the opposite way, causing excitement, irritability, anger, aggression, and other problems. If this happens, tell your parent(s) or your doctor.

Drinking alcohol while taking this medicine can cause severe drowsiness or even passing out. **Don't do it!** Do not use marijuana or street drugs while taking this medicine. They can cause serious side effects. Skipping your medicine to take drugs does not work because many medicines can stay in your body for a long time.

Clonazepam can be habit-forming, but that is not a common problem for people who take their medicine as the doctor says.

Notes

Use this space to take notes or to write down questions you want to ask the doctor or nurse.

_____

_____

_____

_____

_____

_____

_____

_____

_____

_____

_____

_____

_____

From Dulcan MK (editor): _Helping Parents, Youth, and Teachers Understand Medications for Behavioral and Emotional Problems: A Resource Book of Medication Information Handouts,_ Third Edition. Washington, DC, American Psychiatric Publishing, 2007

Medication Information for Parents and Teachers

Clonidine—Catapres

General Information About Medication

Each child and adolescent is different. No one has exactly the same combination of medical and psychological problems. It is a good idea to talk with the doctor or nurse about the reasons a medicine is being used. It is very important to keep all appointments and to be in touch by telephone if you have concerns. It is important to communicate with the doctor, nurse, or therapist.

It is very important that the medicine be taken exactly as the doctor instructs. However, once in a while, everyone forgets to give a medicine on time. It is a good idea to ask the doctor or nurse what to do if this happens. Do not stop or change a medicine without asking the doctor or nurse first.

If the medicine seems to stop working, it may be because it is not being taken regularly. The youth may be "cheeking" or hiding the medicine or forgetting to take it (especially at school). The doses may be too far apart, or a different dose may be needed. Something at school, at home, or in the neighborhood may be upsetting the youth, or he or she may need special help for learning disabilities or tutoring. Please discuss your concerns with the doctor. **Do not just increase the dose.**

All medicines should be kept in a safe place, out of the reach of children, and should be supervised by an adult. If someone takes too much of a medicine, call the doctor, the poison control center, or a hospital emergency room.

Each medicine has a "generic" or chemical name. Just like laundry detergents or paper towels, some medicines are sold by more than one company under different brand names. The same medicine may be available under a generic name and several brand names. The generic medications are usually less expensive than the brand name ones. The generic medications have the same chemical formula, but they may or may not be exactly the same strength as the brand-name medications. Also, some brands of pills contain dye that can cause allergic reactions. It is a good idea to talk to the doctor and the pharmacist about whether it is important to use a specific brand of medicine.

All medicines can cause an allergic reaction. Examples are hives, itching, rashes, swelling, and trouble breathing. Even a tiny amount of a medicine can cause a reaction in patients who are allergic to that medicine. Be *sure* to talk to the doctor before restarting a medicine that has caused an allergic reaction.

Taking more than one medicine at the same time may cause more side effects or cause one of the medicines to not work as well. Always ask the doctor, nurse, or pharmacist before adding another medicine, whether prescription or over-the-counter. Be sure that each doctor knows about *all* of the medicines your child is taking. Also tell the doctor about any vitamins, herbal medicines, or supplements your child may be taking. Some of these may have side effects alone or when taken with this medication.

Everyone taking medicine should have a physical examination at least once a year.

If you suspect the youth is using drugs or alcohol, please tell the doctor right away.

149

Pregnancy requires special care in the use of medicine. Please tell the doctor immediately if you suspect the teenager is pregnant or might become pregnant.

Printed information like this applies to children and adolescents in general. If you have questions about the medicine, or if you notice changes or anything unusual, please ask the doctor or nurse. As scientific research advances, knowledge increases and advice changes. Even experts do not always agree. Many medicines have not been approved by the U.S. Food and Drug Administration (FDA) for use in children. For this reason, use of the medicine for a particular problem or age group often is not listed in the *Physicians' Desk Reference*. This does not necessarily mean that the medicine is dangerous or does not work, only that the company that makes the medicine has not received permission to advertise the medicine for use in children. Companies often do not apply for this permission because it is expensive to do the tests needed to apply for approval for use in children. Once a medication is approved by the FDA for any purpose, a doctor is allowed to prescribe it according to research and clinical experience.

Note to Teachers

It is a good idea to talk with the parent(s) about the reason(s) that a medication is being used. If the parent(s) sign consent to release information, it is often helpful to talk with the doctor. If the parent(s) give permission, the doctor may ask you to fill out rating forms about your experience with the student's behavior, feelings, academic performance, and medication side effects. This information is very useful in selecting and monitoring medication treatment. If you have observations that you think are important, do not hesitate to share these with the student's parent(s) and treating clinicians.

It is very important that the medicine be taken exactly as the doctor instructs. However, everyone forgets to give a medicine on time once in a while. It is a good idea to ask the parent(s) in advance what to do if this happens. Do not stop or change the time you are giving a medicine at school without parental permission. If a medication is to be taken with food, but lunchtime or snack time changes, be sure to notify the parent(s) so appropriate adjustments can be made.

All medicines should be kept in a secure place and should be supervised by an adult. If someone takes too much of a medicine, follow your school procedure for an urgent medical problem.

Taking medicine is a private matter and is best managed discreetly and confidentially. It is important to be sensitive to the student's feelings about taking medicine.

If you suspect that the student is using drugs or alcohol, please tell the parent(s) or a school counselor right away.

Please tell the parent(s) or school nurse if you suspect medication side effects.

Modifications of the classroom environment or assignments may be useful in addition to medication. The student may need to be evaluated for additional help or for an Individualized Education Plan for learning or behavior.

Any expression of suicidal thoughts or feelings or self-harm by a child or adolescent is a clear signal of distress and should be taken seriously. These behaviors should not be dismissed as "attention seeking."

What Is Clonidine (Catapres)?

Clonidine was first used to treat high blood pressure, so it is sometimes called an *antihypertensive*. Now it is being used to treat symptoms of Tourette's disorder, chronic tics (fast, repeated movements), and attention-deficit/hyperactivity disorder (ADHD) and to reduce symptoms of withdrawal from cigarettes and narcotics. It is sometimes used to treat aggression, posttraumatic stress disorder (PTSD), anxiety (nervousness), or panic disorder in children and adolescents. It is used at bedtime to treat severe sleep problems in youth with ADHD, mental retardation, or autism. It comes in brand name Catapres and generic tablets and a skin patch (transdermal form, Catapres-TTS) that releases medicine slowly for 5 days.

How Can This Medicine Help?

Clonidine can decrease symptoms of hyperactivity, impulsivity, anxiety, irritability, temper tantrums, explosive anger, and tics. It can increase patience and frustration tolerance as well as improve self-control and cooperation with adults. Clonidine is sometimes used together with a stimulant medication (methylphenidate or amphetamine) for ADHD or with an atypical or pimozide (Orap) for Tourette's disorder. The positive effects usually do not start for 2 weeks after a stable dose is reached. The full benefit may not be seen for 2–4 months.

How Does This Medicine Work?

Clonidine works by decreasing the level of excitement in parts of the brain. It is sometimes called an *alpha-adrenergic agonist*. It affects the levels of *norepinephrine*, one of the *neurotransmitters* (chemicals that the brain makes for nerve cells to communicate with each other). This effect helps people with tic disorders to stop moving or making noises when they do not want to and helps people with ADHD to slow down and think before doing something. It calms parts of the brain that are too excited in people with severe anxiety. This medicine is chemically different from sedatives or tranquilizers, even though it may make your child sleepy when he or she first starts taking it.

How Long Does This Medicine Last?

When children take clonidine for problems with emotions or behavior, it must be taken three to four times a day. When clonidine is taken for high blood pressure, a single dose lasts for 6–10 hours. When taken for sleep, it may be used at bedtime only. Sometimes the sleepiness lasts into the next day. Sometimes the clonidine effect does not last the whole night, and the youth wakes up in the middle of the night.

How Will the Doctor Monitor This Medicine?

The doctor will review your child's medical history and physical examination before starting clonidine. The doctor may order some blood or urine tests to be sure your child does not have a hidden medical condition. Be sure to tell the doctor if your child or anyone in the family has high blood pressure, heart disease, or diabetes. The doctor also may want to obtain an ECG (electrocardiogram or heart rhythm test) before starting the medicine. The doctor or nurse will measure your child's height, weight, pulse, and blood pressure before starting clonidine.

After the medicine is started, the doctor will want to have regular appointments with you and your child to see how the medicine is working, to see if a dose change is needed, to watch for side effects, to see if clonidine is still needed, and to see if any other treatment is needed. The doctor or nurse will check your child's height, weight, pulse, and blood pressure.

What Side Effects Can This Medicine Have?

Any medicine can have side effects, including an allergy to the medicine. Because each patient is different, the doctor will monitor the youth closely, especially when the medicine is started. The doctor will work with you to increase the positive effects and decrease the negative effects of the medicine. Please tell the doctor if any of the listed side effects appear or if you think that the medicine is causing any other problems. Not all of the rare or unusual side effects are listed.

Side effects are most common after starting the medicine or after a dose increase. Many side effects can be avoided or lessened by starting with a very low dose and increasing it slowly—ask the doctor.

Allergic Reaction

Tell the doctor in a day or two (if possible, before the next dose of medicine):

- Hives
- Itching
- Rash

  Stop the medicine and get *immediate* medical care:

- Trouble breathing or chest tightness
- Swelling of lips, tongue, or throat

Common, but Usually Mild, Side Effects

The following side effects are more common when starting clonidine or when the dose is increased. If these effects do not go away after a week or two, ask the doctor about lowering the dose.

- Daytime sleepiness, especially when bored or not doing anything—This is usually worst in the first 2–4 weeks. Do not allow your child to drive, ride a bicycle or motorcycle, or operate machinery if this happens.
- Fatigue or tiredness
- Low blood pressure (rarely a serious problem)
- Dizziness or light-headedness—This side effect is worse when the child stands up quickly, especially when getting out of bed in the morning; try having the child stand up slowly.
- Headache
- Stomachache

  If one of the following side effects appears, call the doctor within a day or two:

- Slow pulse rate (heartbeat)
- Temporary worsening of tics in Tourette's disorder
- Insomnia (trouble sleeping)—This may be caused by the medicine wearing off.
- Ringing in the ears
- Redness and itching under the skin patch

Less Common Side Effects

Call the doctor within a day or two:

* Depression or increased irritability
* Confusion
* Bed-wetting
* Muscle cramps
* Itching
* Runny nose

Less Common, but Serious, Side Effects

Call the doctor *immediately*:

* Severe or increased dizziness or light-headedness
* Sleepiness that worsens or returns after the initial sleepiness has stopped from getting used to the current dose of the medicine.

Very Rare, but Serious, Side Effects

Call the doctor *immediately*:

* Fainting
* Irregular heartbeat
* Trouble breathing
* Decreased frequency of urination; rapid, puffy swelling of the body (especially the legs and feet); sudden headaches with nausea and vomiting—These could be signs of kidney failure.

Side Effects Reported in Adults but Rare in Children

Tell the doctor within a week:

* Dry mouth—Have your child try using sugar-free gum or candy.
* Constipation—Encourage your child to drink more fluids and eat high-fiber foods; if necessary, the doctor may recommend a fiber medicine such as Benefiber or a stool softener such as Colace or mineral oil.
* Low blood pressure
* Weakness
* Nightmares
* Increased blood sugar (mainly in persons with diabetes)
* Sensation of cold or pain in fingers or toes
* Weight gain

Some Interactions With Other Medicines or Food

Please note that the following are only the most likely interactions with food or other medicines.

Increased sleepiness will occur in combination with medications for anxiety (sedatives or tranquilizers), sleep (hypnotics), allergy or colds (antihistamines), psychosis, or seizures (anticonvulsants).

What Could Happen if This Medicine Is Stopped Suddenly?

It is important not to stop clonidine suddenly but to decrease it slowly (taper) as directed by the doctor. Stopping clonidine suddenly may result in

- Very high blood pressure, even if blood pressure was normal before starting the medicine (rebound hypertension)
- Temporary worsening of behavioral problems or tics
- Nervousness or anxiety
- Rapid or irregular heartbeat
- Chest pain
- Headache
- Stomach cramps, nausea, vomiting
- Trouble sleeping

It is also very important not to miss a dose of clonidine, because withdrawal symptoms such as heart or blood pressure problems may occur. **Be sure not to let the prescription run out!** It is especially important not to miss any clonidine doses if methylphenidate is also being taken.

How Long Will This Medicine Be Needed?

There is no way to know how long a person will need to take clonidine. The parent(s), the doctor, and the school will work together to determine what is right for each patient. Some people need the medicine for a few years; some people may need it longer.

What Else Should I Know About This Medicine?

If a child is sleepy from the clonidine, something active or interesting to do will help the child to stay awake. Sleeping extra hours will not help. Sleepiness usually decreases as the child gets used to the medicine. If the youth is still sleepy in the daytime after 4 weeks at the same dose, a lower dose or a different medicine may be needed.

If the skin patch is being used, it should be applied on an area of the body without hair that is difficult for the child to reach. First, wash the skin with soap and water, then dry. The patch is applied like an adhesive bandage. The child can take a shower or bath with the patch on, but the patch may need to be replaced after swimming or heavy sweating. A protective cover may be placed on top of the patch, but the cover may worsen skin irritation. The patch may contain conducting metal (such as aluminum), so remove the patch before getting an MRI (magnetic resonance imaging).

Clonidine may be confused with clonazepam, clozapine, Klonopin, or quinidine. Be sure to check the prescription when you get it from the pharmacy.

Notes

Use this space to take notes or to write down questions you want to ask the doctor.

_____

_____

_____

_____

_____

_____

_____

_____

_____

_____

_____

_____

_____

From Dulcan MK (editor): *Helping Parents, Youth, and Teachers Understand Medications for Behavioral and Emotional Problems: A Resource Book of Medication Information Handouts*, Third Edition. Washington, DC, American Psychiatric Publishing, 2007

Medication Information
for Youth

Clonidine—Catapres

What the Medicine Is Called and What It Is For

The name of your medicine may be confusing. Most drugs have two names: 1) a scientific name that we call a *generic name* and 2) a trade or *brand name*. The generic name of this medicine is clonidine. The brand name is Catapres.

Clonidine was first used to treat high blood pressure, so it is sometimes called an *antihypertensive*. Now it is also used to help children and teenagers who have trouble sitting still, are too active ("hyperactive") or impulsive, have a bad temper, are hitting people or breaking things, are feeling scared and worried, are feeling too anxious (nervous), are having trouble sleeping, or have tics (fast, repeated movements or sounds that are hard to control). Your doctor may have told you that you have attention-deficit/hyperactivity disorder (ADHD) or Tourette's disorder. Clonidine is sometimes used to help posttraumatic stress disorder (PTSD) or panic disorder. It can be used at bedtime to treat severe problems falling asleep.

How You Take the Medicine

It is very important to take the medicine exactly as the doctor or nurse tells you. Do not skip doses or take extra medicine without asking an adult. If you forget a dose, ask your parent(s) what to do.

Clonidine comes as a pill and also as a skin patch called the Catapres-TTS (TTS stands for transdermal therapeutic system), which looks like a square adhesive bandage. The medicine is actually in the patch and goes right into your body through your skin so you do not have to take pills. The skin patch should be applied on a part of your body that does not have hair on it. First, wash the skin with soap and water, then dry. The patch is applied like an adhesive bandage. You can take a shower or bath with the patch on, but the patch may need to be replaced after swimming or sweating a lot. Your doctor will tell you how many days to leave the patch on before changing to a new one.

If you are taking the medicine as pills, it is very important that you take *all* the pills you are supposed to take each day. Your doctor will probably recommend that you take your medicine at the same time each day, which may be with meals and at bedtime or at bedtime only.

You may notice some help from the medicine within the first few weeks. However, clonidine does not take full effect until as long as 2–4 months after you start taking it. You may feel discouraged and think it is not really helping you. You may want to give up and stop taking the medicine. Talk to your doctor and parent(s) about how you feel, but **do not stop** taking your medicine unless your doctor tells you to. It can be **very dangerous** to stop this medicine suddenly.

Do not use any other medicines without talking to your doctor first. Some people with ADHD or Tourette's disorder will take clonidine together with another medicine because the doctor tells them to.

Do not use alcohol, marijuana, or street drugs while taking clonidine. They can cause serious side effects. Skipping your medicine to take drugs does not work because the medicine stays in your body for a long time.

This medicine is prescribed only for you. It should never be shared with anyone else.

You do not have to tell others that you are taking this medicine, but it is not something you should feel ashamed or embarrassed about. Many young people are helped by clonidine. This medicine is not habit-forming, and you cannot become "hooked" on it. You should talk to your doctor or nurse about any questions you have about the medicine. It is important to remember that the medicine *helps* you. It cannot *make* you do anything or change you as a person.

How Your Doctor Will Follow Your Progress

Before giving you the medicine, your doctor or nurse will talk with you and your parent(s) and may measure your height, weight, heart rate (pulse), and blood pressure. You also may need to take a test called an ECG (electrocardiogram or heart rhythm test). This simple test counts your heartbeats through small wires that are taped to your chest. It takes only a few minutes. This test may need to be repeated at some time while you are taking the medicine. It is important to tell the doctor if you have ever had a very fast heartbeat, chest pain, dizziness, or fainting.

Be sure to tell your doctor or nurse about any other medicines or supplements you are taking, including vitamins, herbs, or aids to weight loss or bodybuilding. Also be sure to tell the doctor or nurse if you are using alcohol or drugs. Because many medicines may affect babies, it is very important to tell the doctor if you might be pregnant or if you are at risk of becoming pregnant.

Your teachers may be asked to fill out a form about your grades and behavior in school. A psychologist may give you some tests to see how you learn best.

You will probably start by taking one pill or part of a pill each day. Your doctor will tell you if and when you should start taking more medicine. He or she will watch your progress and decide when you are taking the right amount and how long you need to take the medicine.

Most doctors have regular appointments with young people who are taking medicine. You should use these visits to share any concerns you may have about your medicine and to talk about if it has helped you. From time to time, your physician or nurse may measure your height, weight, heart rate (pulse), and blood pressure to be sure that you are in good health while you are taking the medicine. Your doctor also will ask for regular reports from your parents and maybe from your teachers (with your permission) to see how well the medicine is working.

How the Medicine Might Affect You

In addition to the ways the medicine can help you, it may have other effects called *side effects*. Different medicines have different side effects. It is helpful to know about some of the most common side effects of your medicine so that you will understand what they are if they happen. Some people do not have any side effects. Some side effects are just uncomfortable, but others may mean a more serious problem with the medicine. Side effects are most common after starting the medicine or after a dose increase. They may go away with time, or the medicine can be adjusted or changed—ask the doctor.

You could have an allergy to any medicine, which might show up as a rash on your skin, swelling, itching, or trouble breathing.

Please tell your parent(s) and your doctor or nurse about any changes that you notice after taking the medicine. It is especially important to tell a responsible adult if you are feeling depressed or that you may not want to live; if you have thoughts of hurting yourself; or if you begin to feel more irritable, nervous, or restless.

Some medicines make people feel sleepy or less coordinated. If this medicine is making you sleepy, it is very important not to drive a car or ride a bicycle or motorcycle. After starting a new medicine or increasing the dose of a medicine, please be extra careful when driving a car, riding a bike, or using machines until you can tell how the medicine affects your alertness, attention, and coordination.

One of the most common side effects of clonidine is feeling tired or sleepy during the day, especially if things are boring. After you have been taking the medicine for a few weeks, your body will adjust, and you should not feel as sleepy during the day. If you do not stop feeling sleepy during the day, or if you start to feel more sleepy than you did before, let your parent(s) and your doctor know. If you have had trouble sleeping at night or have had problems with nightmares, the medicine can help you sleep better. If you wake up in the middle of the night and have trouble going back to sleep or have nightmares, be sure to tell the doctor.

If you become very sad while taking clonidine, let your doctor know how you are feeling. Your medicine may need to be changed.

Because clonidine can lower blood pressure, you may have problems if your blood pressure gets too low. If you become dizzy or light-headed or if you faint, let your parent(s) and doctor know right away. It will help if you get up slowly in the morning instead of jumping right out of bed.

A common side effect of the Catapres skin patch is itching of the skin under the patch. Your doctor may be able to give you some cream to help this. You should remember that even if the patch becomes *really* itchy or if you are bothered by some side effect of the pills, you should not just pull off the patch or stop taking the pills. Doing that could cause you to feel very nervous and anxious and also could cause your blood pressure to go very high. If you have any side effects that make you so uncomfortable that you want to stop taking the medicine, talk to your doctor. **Do not just stop taking it!**

Other side effects that people sometimes have from clonidine are headache or stomachache.

You should tell your parent(s) and doctor if you notice anything different or unusual about how you feel once you start taking the medicine. This includes good things such as feeling less nervous or sleeping better at night.

Notes

Use this space to take notes or to write down questions you want to ask the doctor or nurse.

_____

_____

_____

_____

_____

_____

_____

_____

_____

_____

_____

_____

_____

Medication Information for Parents and Teachers

Clozapine—Clozaril, FazaClo

General Information About Medication

Each child and adolescent is different. No one has exactly the same combination of medical and psychological problems. It is a good idea to talk with the doctor or nurse about the reasons a medicine is being used. It is very important to keep all appointments and to be in touch by telephone if you have concerns. It is important to communicate with the doctor, nurse, or therapist.

It is very important that the medicine be taken exactly as the doctor instructs. However, once in a while, everyone forgets to give a medicine on time. It is a good idea to ask the doctor or nurse what to do if this happens. Do not stop or change a medicine without asking the doctor or nurse first.

If the medicine seems to stop working, it may be because it is not being taken regularly. The youth may be "cheeking" or hiding the medicine or forgetting to take it (especially at school). The doses may be too far apart, or a different dose may be needed. Something at school, at home, or in the neighborhood may be upsetting the youth, or he or she may need special help for learning disabilities or tutoring. Please discuss your concerns with the doctor. **Do not just increase the dose.**

All medicines should be kept in a safe place, out of the reach of children, and should be supervised by an adult. If someone takes too much of a medicine, call the doctor, the poison control center, or a hospital emergency room.

Each medicine has a "generic" or chemical name. Just like laundry detergents or paper towels, some medicines are sold by more than one company under different brand names. The same medicine may be available under a generic name and several brand names. The generic medications are usually less expensive than the brand name ones. The generic medications have the same chemical formula, but they may or may not be exactly the same strength as the brand-name medications. Also, some brands of pills contain dye that can cause allergic reactions. It is a good idea to talk to the doctor and the pharmacist about whether it is important to use a specific brand of medicine.

All medicines can cause an allergic reaction. Examples are hives, itching, rashes, swelling, and trouble breathing. Even a tiny amount of a medicine can cause a reaction in patients who are allergic to that medicine. Be *sure* to talk to the doctor before restarting a medicine that has caused an allergic reaction.

Taking more than one medicine at the same time may cause more side effects or cause one of the medicines to not work as well. Always ask the doctor, nurse, or pharmacist before adding another medicine, whether prescription or over-the-counter. Be sure that each doctor knows about *all* of the medicines your child is taking. Also tell the doctor about any vitamins, herbal medicines, or supplements your child may be taking. Some of these may have side effects alone or when taken with this medication.

Everyone taking medicine should have a physical examination at least once a year.

If you suspect the youth is using drugs or alcohol, please tell the doctor right away.

161

Pregnancy requires special care in the use of medicine. Please tell the doctor immediately if you suspect the teenager is pregnant or might become pregnant.

Printed information like this applies to children and adolescents in general. If you have questions about the medicine, or if you notice changes or anything unusual, please ask the doctor or nurse. As scientific research advances, knowledge increases and advice changes. Even experts do not always agree. Many medicines have not been approved by the U.S. Food and Drug Administration (FDA) for use in children. For this reason, use of the medicine for a particular problem or age group often is not listed in the *Physicians' Desk Reference*. This does not necessarily mean that the medicine is dangerous or does not work, only that the company that makes the medicine has not received permission to advertise the medicine for use in children. Companies often do not apply for this permission because it is expensive to do the tests needed to apply for approval for use in children. Once a medication is approved by the FDA for any purpose, a doctor is allowed to prescribe it according to research and clinical experience.

Note to Teachers

It is a good idea to talk with the parent(s) about the reason(s) that a medication is being used. If the parent(s) sign consent to release information, it is often helpful to talk with the doctor. If the parent(s) give permission, the doctor may ask you to fill out rating forms about your experience with the student's behavior, feelings, academic performance, and medication side effects. This information is very useful in selecting and monitoring medication treatment. If you have observations that you think are important, do not hesitate to share these with the student's parent(s) and treating clinicians.

It is very important that the medicine be taken exactly as the doctor instructs. However, everyone forgets to give a medicine on time once in a while. It is a good idea to ask the parent(s) in advance what to do if this happens. Do not stop or change the time you are giving a medicine at school without parental permission. If a medication is to be taken with food, but lunchtime or snack time changes, be sure to notify the parent(s) so appropriate adjustments can be made.

All medicines should be kept in a secure place and should be supervised by an adult. If someone takes too much of a medicine, follow your school procedure for an urgent medical problem.

Taking medicine is a private matter and is best managed discreetly and confidentially. It is important to be sensitive to the student's feelings about taking medicine.

If you suspect that the student is using drugs or alcohol, please tell the parent(s) or a school counselor right away.

Please tell the parent(s) or school nurse if you suspect medication side effects.

Modifications of the classroom environment or assignments may be useful in addition to medication. The student may need to be evaluated for additional help or for an Individualized Education Plan for learning or behavior.

Any expression of suicidal thoughts or feelings or self-harm by a child or adolescent is a clear signal of distress and should be taken seriously. These behaviors should not be dismissed as "attention seeking."

What Is Clozapine (Clozaril, FazaClo)?

Clozapine is called an *atypical* or *second-generation antipsychotic*. It is sometimes called an *atypical psychotropic agent*, or simply an *atypical*. It comes in brand name Clozaril and generic tablets and FazaClo orally disintegrating (dissolves in the mouth) tablets.

How Can This Medicine Help?

Clozapine is used to treat psychosis, such as in schizophrenia, mania, or very severe depression, if other anti-psychotic medicines have not helped enough. It can reduce *positive symptoms* such as hallucinations (hearing voices or seeing things that are not there); delusions (troubling beliefs that other people do not share); agitation; and very unusual thinking, speech, and behavior. It is also used to lessen the *negative symptoms* of schizophrenia, such as lack of interest in doing things (apathy), lack of motivation, social withdrawal, and lack of energy.

This medicine is very powerful and is used to treat very serious problems or symptoms that other medicines do not help. Be patient; the positive effects of this medicine may not appear for 4–6 weeks, and the full positive effect may not be seen for 6–12 months.

How Does This Medicine Work?

Cells in the brain communicate using chemicals called *neurotransmitters*. Too much or too little of these substances in parts of the brain can cause problems. Clozapine works by blocking the action of two of these neurotransmitters—*dopamine* and *serotonin*—in certain areas of the brain.

How Long Does This Medicine Last?

Clozapine can usually be taken only once a day, although at higher doses, dividing into two doses may be needed to decrease side effects.

How Will the Doctor Monitor This Medicine?

The doctor will review your child's medical history and physical examination before starting clozapine. The doctor may order some blood or urine tests to be sure your child does not have a hidden medical condition that would make it unsafe to use this medicine. The doctor or nurse may measure your child's pulse and blood pressure before starting clozapine. The doctor may order other tests, such as baseline tests for blood sugar and cholesterol. A blood test to count the different kinds of blood cells must be done before starting clozapine. An EEG (electroencephalogram or brain wave test) may be done before starting clozapine to see if there is an increased risk of seizures (convulsions).

Be sure to tell the doctor if anyone in the family has diabetes, high blood pressure, high cholesterol, or heart disease.

After the medicine is started, the doctor will want to have regular appointments with you and your child to see how the medicine is working, to see if a dose change is needed, to watch for side effects, to see if clozapine is still needed, and to see if any other treatment is needed. The doctor or nurse will check your child's height, weight, pulse, and blood pressure, and watch for abnormal movements. The FDA has a required schedule of blood tests to watch for a decrease in the number of white blood cells (see "What Else Should I Know About Side Effects?"). Sometimes blood tests are needed to watch for diabetes or increased cholesterol.

What Side Effects Can This Medicine Have?

Any medicine can have side effects, including an allergy to the medicine. Because each patient is different, the doctor will monitor the youth closely, especially when the medicine is started. The doctor will work with you to increase the positive effects and decrease the negative effects of the medicine. Please tell the doctor if any of the listed side effects appear or if you think that the medicine is causing any other problems. Not all of the rare or unusual side effects are listed.

Side effects are most common after starting the medicine or after a dose increase. Many side effects can be avoided or lessened by starting with a very low dose and increasing it slowly—ask the doctor.

Allergic Reaction

Tell the doctor in a day or two (if possible, before the next dose of medicine):

- Hives
- Itching
- Rash

    Stop the medicine and get *immediate* medical care:

- Trouble breathing or chest tightness
- Swelling of lips, tongue, or throat

Common, but Not Usually Serious, Side Effects

Discuss the following side effects with your child's doctor when convenient. These side effects often can be helped by lowering the dose of medicine, changing the times medicine is taken, or adding another medicine.

- Daytime sleepiness or tiredness—Do not allow your child to drive, ride a bicycle or motorcycle, or operate machinery if this happens. This problem may be lessened by taking the medicine at bedtime.
- Dry mouth—Have your child try using sugar-free gum or candy.
- Trouble urinating
- Constipation—Encourage your child to drink more fluids and eat high-fiber foods; if necessary, the doctor may recommend a fiber medicine such as Benefiber or a stool softener such as Colace or mineral oil.
- Blurred vision
- Dizziness—This side effect is worse when the child stands up quickly, especially when getting out of bed in the morning; try having the child stand up slowly.
- Increased appetite
- Weight gain—Seek nutritional counseling; provide your child with low-calorie snacks and encourage regular exercise.
- Nausea
- Vomiting
- Stomach pain
- Headache
- Bed-wetting

Very Rare, but Not Usually Serious, Side Effects

Discuss the following side effects with your child's doctor when convenient. These side effects often can be helped by lowering the dose of medicine, changing the times medicine is taken, or adding another medicine.

- Drooling
- Increased restlessness or inability to sit still
- Shaking of hands and fingers
- Decreased or slowed movement and decreased facial expressions

Less Common, but Potentially Serious, Side Effects

Call the doctor *immediately*:

- Stiffness of the tongue, jaw, neck, back, or legs
- Seizure (fit, convulsion)—This is more common in people with a history of seizures or head injury and at higher doses of clozapine.

   Talk to a doctor within a day:

- Increased thirst, frequent urination (having to go to the bathroom often), lethargy, tiredness, dizziness, and blurred vision—These could be signs of diabetes (especially if your child is overweight or there is a family history of diabetes).
- Fast or irregular heartbeat (pulse)

Very Rare, but Serious, Side Effects

- Fever, chills, sore throat, or skin bruising or small spots—This may mean a decrease in the number of blood cells. **Call the doctor within a day or two.**
- Extreme stiffness or lack of movement, very high fever, mental confusion, irregular pulse rate, or eye pain—**This is a medical emergency. Go to an emergency room *right away.***
- Sudden stiffness and inability to breathe or swallow—**Go to an emergency room or call 911.** Tell the paramedics, nurses, and doctors that the patient is taking clozapine. Other medicines can be used to treat this problem fast.
- Heart problems have been reported in adults taking clozapine. If your child is extremely tired all of the time, has changes in breathing, a rapid heartbeat, or chest pain, **call the doctor right away.**

What Else Should I Know About Side Effects?

Most side effects lessen over time. If they are troublesome, talk with your child's doctor. Some side effects can be decreased by taking a smaller dose of medicine, by stopping the medicine, by changing to another medicine, or by adding another medicine. Clozapine is often increased very slowly to reduce the risk of side effects.

   Most people who take clozapine gain weight. Children seem to have more problems with this than adults. The weight gain may be from increased appetite and from ways that the medicine changes how the body processes food. Clozapine may also change the way that the body handles glucose (sugar) and may cause high levels *(hyperglycemia)*. People who take clozapine, especially those who gain a lot of weight, are at increased risk of developing *diabetes* and of having increased fats *(lipids—cholesterol* and *triglycerides)* in their blood. Over time, both diabetes and increased fats in the blood may lead to heart disease, stroke, and other complications. The FDA has put warnings on all atypical agents about the increased risks of hyperglycemia, diabetes, and increased blood cholesterol and triglycerides when taking one of these medicines. It is much easier to prevent weight gain than to lose weight later. When your child first starts taking clozapine, it is a good idea to be sure that he or she eats a well-balanced diet without "junk food" and with healthy snacks like fruits and vegetables, not sweets or fried foods. He or she should drink water or skim milk, not pop, sodas, soft drinks, or sugary juices. Regular exercise is important for maintaining a healthy weight (and may also help with sleep).

Because clozapine may cause a rare but very dangerous decrease in the white blood cells (*agranulocytosis*), people taking this medicine must be registered by the pharmacy to be sure that the white cells in the blood are measured as required. The pharmacy is allowed to dispense the medicine only after being sure that the white blood cell count (WBC) is normal. This must be done every week for the first 6 months, then every 2 weeks for 6 months, and then once a month for as long as clozapine is taken.

One very rare side effect that may not go away is *tardive dyskinesia* (or TD). Patients with tardive dyskinesia have involuntary movements (movements that they cannot help making) of the body, especially the mouth and tongue. The patient may look as though he or she is making faces over and over again. Jerky movements of the arms, legs, or body may occur. There may be fine, wormlike, or sudden repeated movements of the tongue, or the person may appear to be chewing something or smacking or puckering his or her lips. The fingers may look as though they are rolling something. If you notice any unusual movements, be sure to tell the doctor. The doctor may use the AIMS test to look for these movements. Clozapine is less likely than other antipsychotic medicines to cause tardive dyskinesia and may even decrease the symptoms of tardive dyskinesia that are caused by other antipsychotic medicines.

Neuroleptic malignant syndrome is a very rare side effect that can lead to death. The symptoms are severe muscle stiffness, high fever, increased heart rate and blood pressure, irregular heartbeat (pulse), and sweating. It may lead to unconsciousness. If you suspect this, **call 911 or go to an emergency room right away.**

Some Interactions With Other Medicines or Food

Please note that the following are only the most likely interactions with food or other medicines.

Clozapine may be taken with or without food.

It is better to limit drinks with caffeine (coffee, tea, soft drinks) because caffeine works in the opposite way from clozapine, may increase the side effects of the medicine, and might decrease the positive effects.

Carbamazepine (Tegretol) should not be taken with clozapine because of increased risk of decreased white blood cells.

Antidepressants (selective serotonin reuptake inhibitors or SSRIs) such as Prozac (fluoxetine), Celexa (citalopram), Luvox (fluvoxamine), Zoloft (sertraline), and Paxil (paroxetine); antibiotics such as erythromycin; and antifungal agents such as ketoconazole may increase blood levels of clozapine.

What Could Happen if This Medicine Is Stopped Suddenly?

Involuntary movements, or *withdrawal dyskinesias*, may appear within 1–4 weeks of lowering the dose or stopping the medicine. Usually these go away, but they can last for days to months. If this medicine is stopped suddenly, emotional disturbance (such as irritability, nervousness, moodiness, or oppositional behavior) or physical problems (such as stomachache, loss of appetite, nausea, vomiting, diarrhea, sweating, indigestion, trouble sleeping, trembling, or shaking) may appear. These problems usually last only a few days to a few weeks. If they happen, you should tell your child's doctor. The medicine dose may need to be lowered more slowly (tapered). Always check with the doctor before stopping a medicine.

How Long Will This Medicine Be Needed?

How long your child will need to take this medicine depends partly on the reason that it was prescribed. Some problems last for only a few months, whereas others last much longer. It is important to ask the doctor whether medicine is still needed, especially with medicines as powerful as this one. Every few months, you should discuss with your child's doctor the reasons for using the medicine and whether the medicine may be stopped or the dose lowered.

What Else Should I Know About This Medicine?

There are other medicines that are used for the same kinds of problems. If your child is having bad side effects or the medicine does not seem to be working, ask the doctor if another medicine might work as well or better and have fewer side effects for your child. Each person reacts differently to medicines.

The orally disintegrating tablet should be removed from the package by peeling apart, just before use. The tablet should be melted in the mouth and swallowed with saliva. If the tablet needs to be split, throw away the part not taken.

Notes

Use this space to take notes or to write down questions you want to ask the doctor.

_____

_____

_____

_____

_____

_____

_____

_____

_____

_____

_____

_____

_____

From Dulcan MK (editor): _Helping Parents, Youth, and Teachers Understand Medications for Behavioral and Emotional Problems: A Resource Book of Medication Information Handouts_, Third Edition. Washington, DC, American Psychiatric Publishing, 2007

Medication Information for Youth

Clozapine—Clozaril, FazaClo

What the Medicine Is Called and What It Is For

The name of your medicine may be confusing. Most drugs have two names: 1) a scientific name that we call a *generic name* and 2) a trade or *brand name*. The generic name of this medicine is clozapine. The brand name is Clozaril. It is called an *atypical* medicine.

This medicine helps people who feel very confused and have severe problems thinking clearly. It can lessen hallucinations (seeing or hearing things that are not really there) and delusions (troubling beliefs that other people do not share). The medicine also can improve *negative symptoms*, such as lack of interest in doing things, lack of motivation, loss of interest in friends, and decreased energy. Clozapine can help people who were not helped by other medicines.

How You Take the Medicine

It is very important to take the medicine exactly as the doctor or nurse tells you. Do not skip doses or take extra medicine without asking an adult. If you forget a dose, ask your parent(s) what to do.

Your doctor will tell you how much medicine to take and how often to take it so that it can help you the most.

It may be a month or longer before you notice that clozapine is helping. The full effect may take 6–12 months to appear. You may feel discouraged and think the medicine is never going to help. You may want to give up and stop taking the medicine. Talk to your doctor and parent(s) about how you feel, but **do not stop** taking your medicine unless your doctor tells you to. If you stop the medicine suddenly, there may be uncomfortable feelings.

Caffeine (in coffee, tea, or soft drinks) could make you feel worse.

This medicine is prescribed only for you. It should never be shared with anyone else.

You do not have to tell others that you are taking this medicine, but it is not something you should feel ashamed or embarrassed about. Many young people are helped by clozapine. This medicine is not habit-forming, and you cannot become "hooked" on it. You should talk to your doctor or nurse about any questions you have about the medicine. It is important to remember that the medicine *helps* you. It cannot *make* you do anything or change you as a person.

If you take the tablet that melts in your mouth, peel the foil away to get the pill out of the package; do not push it through. Let the pill dissolve in your mouth and swallow, without drinking anything.

How Your Doctor Will Follow Your Progress

Before giving you the medicine, your doctor or nurse will talk with you and your parent(s) and will measure your height, weight, heart rate (pulse), and blood pressure. There will be other tests, such as blood tests for sugar and cholesterol and to count the number of your blood cells. To help make sure that you will not have problems with the medicine, the doctor may ask for an EEG (electroencephalogram or brain wave test) before starting the medicine. This does not tell the doctor anything about what you are thinking or feeling but just shows the rhythms of your brain cells.

Be sure to tell your doctor or nurse about any other medicines or supplements you are taking, including vitamins, herbs, or aids to weight loss or bodybuilding. Also be sure to tell the doctor or nurse if you are using alcohol or drugs. Because many medicines may affect babies, it is very important to tell the doctor if you might be pregnant or if you are at risk of becoming pregnant.

Your teachers may be asked to fill out a form about your grades and behavior in school. A psychologist may give you some tests to see how you learn best.

Most doctors have regular appointments with young people who are taking medicine. You should use these visits to share any concerns you may have about your medicine and to talk about if it has helped you. From time to time, your physician or nurse will measure your height, weight, heart rate (pulse), and blood pressure to be sure that you are in good health while you are taking the medicine. There will be blood tests every week for a while to count the number of your blood cells. There will be other blood tests to watch for signs of diabetes or high cholesterol. Your doctor also will ask for regular reports from your parents and maybe from your teachers (with your permission) to see how well the medicine is working.

If the medicine helps you, your doctor will probably want you to take it for at least a year. Your doctor will decide how long you will need to take the medicine as he or she watches your progress.

How the Medicine Might Affect You

Clozapine is a very powerful medicine. In addition to the ways the medicine can help you, it may have other effects called *side effects*. Different medicines have different side effects. It is helpful to know about some of the most common side effects of your medicine so that you will understand what they are if they happen. Some people do not have any side effects. Some side effects are just uncomfortable, but others may mean a more serious problem with the medicine. Side effects are most common after starting the medicine or after a dose increase. They may go away with time, or the medicine can be adjusted or changed—ask the doctor.

You could have an allergy to any medicine, which might show up as a rash on your skin, swelling, itching, or trouble breathing.

Please tell your parent(s) and your doctor or nurse about any changes that you notice after taking the medicine. It is especially important to tell a responsible adult if you are feeling depressed or that you may not want to live; if you have thoughts of hurting yourself; or if you begin to feel more irritable, nervous, or restless.

One of the most common side effects of this medicine is feeling tired or sleepy during the day, even if you have had a full night's sleep. If this medicine is making you sleepy, it is very important not to drive a car or ride a bicycle or motorcycle. After starting the medicine or increasing the dose of medicine, please be extra careful when driving a car, riding a bike, or using machines until you can tell how the medicine affects your alertness, attention, and coordination. After you have been taking the medicine for a few weeks, your body will adjust, and this side effect will likely go away. If you had trouble sleeping at night before taking the medicine, it can help you sleep better, especially if the doctor tells you to take a dose of medicine in the evening.

You might feel dizzy, tired, or even faint when you stand up fast. Try standing up slowly, especially first thing in the morning when getting out of bed.

Another common side effect is dry mouth. You may be more thirsty than usual and find that you are drinking more water or other liquids than usual. Sucking on sugar-free hard candy or cough drops usually helps. You also could try chewing sugar-free gum or sucking on ice chips. Do not chew the ice; you could hurt your teeth. Also, using lip balm will keep your lips from cracking. It is important to be especially good about brushing your teeth. Some people have too much saliva (spit) when taking this medicine. If this is a big problem, another medicine can be added to help with this.

Sometimes people taking this medicine notice that their heart is beating faster than normal. Usually this happens within the first few weeks of taking the medicine and gets better or goes away. However, if you notice that your heart is beating very fast for more than a few minutes when you have not been exercising, if you feel light-headed or dizzy when you are sitting or standing still, or if you faint, you should let your parent(s) and doctor know right away.

Some people become constipated (have hard bowel movements) when taking this medicine. Try drinking more water and eating more fruits, vegetables, and whole grains. If that does not help, tell your parent(s) or doctor—you may need a medicine to help with this side effect

Other side effects that some people get from clozapine are having trouble passing urine, blurred vision, stomachache, upset stomach, or headache.

Many teenagers who take clozapine gain weight. The weight gain may be from increased appetite and also from ways that the medicine changes how the body processes food. People who take clozapine, especially those who gain a lot of weight, might be at increased risk of developing *diabetes* and of having increased fats (*lipids—cholesterol* and *triglycerides*) in their blood. Over time, both diabetes and increased fats in the blood may lead to heart disease, stroke, and other complications. The U.S. Food and Drug Administration (FDA) has put warnings about these problems on all medicines like clozapine. It is much easier to prevent weight gain than to lose weight later. It is a good idea to eat a well-balanced diet without "junk food" and with healthy snacks like fruits and vegetables, not sweets or fried foods. It is better to drink water or skim milk, not pop, sodas, soft drinks, or sugary juices. Regular exercise is important for maintaining a healthy weight (and may also help with sleep).

If you get very thirsty, have to go to the bathroom a lot, feel *very* tired, or have dizziness or blurred vision, be sure to tell your parent(s) or doctor.

Some side effects include feeling nervous, restless, or shaky or having stiff muscles. These effects can be helped by adding another medicine or by adjusting or changing this medicine.

Another, more serious, side effect can be longer lasting and more difficult to treat. This very rare side effect is called *tardive dyskinesia* (or TD). A person taking clozapine may develop movements of the mouth, tongue, face, arms, legs, or body that are not being made on purpose. This side effect can go away when the medicine is stopped, but in some people it does not go away. Your doctor will explain this effect to you and your parent(s) and how he or she will watch for any signs that you are developing this problem. Be sure to ask your doctor any questions that you may have about this, but do not worry too much about it. It hardly ever happens to teenagers taking this medicine.

You should tell your parent(s) and doctor if you notice anything different or unusual about how you feel once you start taking the medicine. This includes good things, such as feeling less confused, feeling less sad, not hearing voices anymore, or sleeping better at night.

Notes

Use this space to take notes or to write down questions you want to ask the doctor or nurse.

_____

_____

_____

_____

_____

_____

_____

_____

_____

_____

_____

_____

From Dulcan MK (editor): *Helping Parents, Youth, and Teachers Understand Medications for Behavioral and Emotional Problems: A Resource Book of Medication Information Handouts,* Third Edition. Washington, DC, American Psychiatric Publishing, 2007

Medication Information for Parents and Teachers

Cyproheptadine—Periactin

General Information About Medication

Each child and adolescent is different. No one has exactly the same combination of medical and psychological problems. It is a good idea to talk with the doctor or nurse about the reasons a medicine is being used. It is very important to keep all appointments and to be in touch by telephone if you have concerns. It is important to communicate with the doctor, nurse, or therapist.

It is very important that the medicine be taken exactly as the doctor instructs. However, once in a while, everyone forgets to give a medicine on time. It is a good idea to ask the doctor or nurse what to do if this happens. Do not stop or change a medicine without asking the doctor or nurse first.

If the medicine seems to stop working, it may be because it is not being taken regularly. The youth may be "cheeking" or hiding the medicine or forgetting to take it (especially at school). The doses may be too far apart, or a different dose may be needed. Something at school, at home, or in the neighborhood may be upsetting the youth, or he or she may need special help for learning disabilities or tutoring. Please discuss your concerns with the doctor. **Do not just increase the dose.**

All medicines should be kept in a safe place, out of the reach of children, and should be supervised by an adult. If someone takes too much of a medicine, call the doctor, the poison control center, or a hospital emergency room.

Each medicine has a "generic" or chemical name. Just like laundry detergents or paper towels, some medicines are sold by more than one company under different brand names. The same medicine may be available under a generic name and several brand names. The generic medications are usually less expensive than the brand name ones. The generic medications have the same chemical formula, but they may or may not be exactly the same strength as the brand-name medications. Also, some brands of pills contain dye that can cause allergic reactions. It is a good idea to talk to the doctor and the pharmacist about whether it is important to use a specific brand of medicine.

All medicines can cause an allergic reaction. Examples are hives, itching, rashes, swelling, and trouble breathing. Even a tiny amount of a medicine can cause a reaction in patients who are allergic to that medicine. Be *sure* to talk to the doctor before restarting a medicine that has caused an allergic reaction.

Taking more than one medicine at the same time may cause more side effects or cause one of the medicines to not work as well. Always ask the doctor, nurse, or pharmacist before adding another medicine, whether prescription or over-the-counter. Be sure that each doctor knows about *all* of the medicines your child is taking. Also tell the doctor about any vitamins, herbal medicines, or supplements your child may be taking. Some of these may have side effects alone or when taken with this medication.

Everyone taking medicine should have a physical examination at least once a year.

If you suspect the youth is using drugs or alcohol, please tell the doctor right away.

Pregnancy requires special care in the use of medicine. Please tell the doctor immediately if you suspect the teenager is pregnant or might become pregnant.

Printed information like this applies to children and adolescents in general. If you have questions about the medicine, or if you notice changes or anything unusual, please ask the doctor or nurse. As scientific research advances, knowledge increases and advice changes. Even experts do not always agree. Many medicines have not been approved by the U.S. Food and Drug Administration (FDA) for use in children. For this reason, use of the medicine for a particular problem or age group often is not listed in the *Physicians' Desk Reference*. This does not necessarily mean that the medicine is dangerous or does not work, only that the company that makes the medicine has not received permission to advertise the medicine for use in children. Companies often do not apply for this permission because it is expensive to do the tests needed to apply for approval for use in children. Once a medication is approved by the FDA for any purpose, a doctor is allowed to prescribe it according to research and clinical experience.

Note to Teachers

It is a good idea to talk with the parent(s) about the reason(s) that a medication is being used. If the parent(s) sign consent to release information, it is often helpful to talk with the doctor. If the parent(s) give permission, the doctor may ask you to fill out rating forms about your experience with the student's behavior, feelings, academic performance, and medication side effects. This information is very useful in selecting and monitoring medication treatment. If you have observations that you think are important, do not hesitate to share these with the student's parent(s) and treating clinicians.

It is very important that the medicine be taken exactly as the doctor instructs. However, everyone forgets to give a medicine on time once in a while. It is a good idea to ask the parent(s) in advance what to do if this happens. Do not stop or change the time you are giving a medicine at school without parental permission. If a medication is to be taken with food, but lunchtime or snack time changes, be sure to notify the parent(s) so appropriate adjustments can be made.

All medicines should be kept in a secure place and should be supervised by an adult. If someone takes too much of a medicine, follow your school procedure for an urgent medical problem.

Taking medicine is a private matter and is best managed discreetly and confidentially. It is important to be sensitive to the student's feelings about taking medicine.

If you suspect that the student is using drugs or alcohol, please tell the parent(s) or a school counselor right away.

Please tell the parent(s) or school nurse if you suspect medication side effects.

Modifications of the classroom environment or assignments may be useful in addition to medication. The student may need to be evaluated for additional help or for an Individualized Education Plan for learning or behavior.

Any expression of suicidal thoughts or feelings or self-harm by a child or adolescent is a clear signal of distress and should be taken seriously. These behaviors should not be dismissed as "attention seeking."

What Is Cyproheptadine (Periactin)?

Cyproheptadine is called an *antihistamine*. Antihistamines were developed to treat allergies. Cyproheptadine is sometimes used to treat anxiety (nervousness) or insomnia (difficulty falling asleep). It may be used to increase appetite in people who do not eat enough food and to prevent cluster and migraine headaches. Cyproheptadine comes in generic and Periactin brand tablets and syrup.

How Can This Medicine Help?

Cyproheptadine may decrease nervousness. When used for anxiety, it works best when used for a short time along with psychotherapy. Cyproheptadine can help with insomnia when used for a short time along with a behavioral program, such as regular soothing routines at bedtime and increased exercise in the daytime. In people who are not eating enough and are too thin, it can increase appetite and help to gain weight.

How Does This Medicine Work?

Cyproheptadine can help decrease anxiety and help falling asleep because of its sedative effect—that is, it makes people a little sleepy so that they feel less nervous and fall asleep more easily. It works on the *serotonin* system as well as the *cholinergic* and *histamine* systems.

How Long Does This Medicine Last?

Cyproheptadine lasts for 4–7 hours.

How Will the Doctor Monitor This Medicine?

The doctor will review your child's medical history and physical examination before starting cyproheptadine. Be sure to tell the doctor if your child or anyone in the family has a history of asthma or of heart rhythm problems, palpitations, or fainting. The doctor or nurse may measure your child's height, weight, pulse, and blood pressure before starting the medicine. An examination such as the AIMS (Abnormal Involuntary Movement Scale) test may be used to check your child's tongue, legs, and arms for unusual movements that could be helped by the medicine.

After the medicine is started, the doctor will want to have regular appointments with you and your child to see how the medicine is working, to see if a dose change is needed, to watch for side effects, to see if cyproheptadine is still needed, and to see if any other treatment is needed. The doctor or nurse may check your child's height, weight, pulse, and blood pressure.

What Side Effects Can This Medicine Have?

Any medicine can have side effects, including an allergy to the medicine. Because each patient is different, the doctor will monitor the youth closely, especially when the medicine is started. The doctor will work with you to increase the positive effects and decrease the negative effects of the medicine. Please tell the doctor if any of the listed side effects appear or if you think that the medicine is causing any other problems. Not all of the rare or unusual side effects are listed.

Side effects are most common after starting the medicine or after a dose increase. Many side effects can be avoided or lessened by starting with a very low dose and increasing it slowly—ask the doctor.

Allergic Reaction

Tell the doctor in a day or two (if possible, before the next dose of medicine):

- Hives
- Itching
- Rash

Stop the medicine and get *immediate* medical care:

- Trouble breathing or chest tightness
- Swelling of lips, tongue, or throat

Common Side Effects

Tell the doctor within a week or two:

- Daytime sleepiness—Do not allow your child to drive, ride a bicycle or motorcycle, or operate machinery if this happens.
- Decreased attention, memory, or learning in school
- Increased appetite and weight gain
- Dry mouth—Have your child try using sugar-free gum or candy.
- Headache
- Blurred vision
- Constipation—Encourage your child to drink more fluids and eat high-fiber foods; if necessary, the doctor may recommend a fiber medicine such as Benefiber or a stool softener such as Colace or mineral oil.
- Trouble passing urine
- Dizziness or light-headedness—This side effect is worse when the child stands up quickly, especially when getting out of bed in the morning; try having the child stand up slowly.
- Nausea or upset stomach

Less Common Side Effects

Call the doctor within a day or two:

- Poor coordination
- Motor tics (fast, repeated movements)
- Unusual muscle movements
- Irritability, overactivity
- Waking up after sleeping for a short time and being unable to get back to sleep
- Exposure to sunlight may cause severe sunburn, skin rash, redness, or itching; have the child stay out of the sun or use sunscreen or protective clothing.

Very Rare, but Serious, Side Effects

Call the doctor *immediately:*

- Worsening of asthma or trouble breathing
- Seizure (fit, convulsion)
- Uncontrollable behavior
- Hallucinations (seeing things that are not really there)
- Severe muscle stiffness
- Irregular heartbeat (pulse), fainting, palpitations

Some Interactions With Other Medicines or Food

Please note that the following are only the most likely interactions with food or other medicines.

If other medicines that can cause sleepiness are taken with cyproheptadine, severe sleepiness can result.

It can be *very dangerous* to take cyproheptadine at the same time as or even within a month of taking another type of medicine called a *monoamine oxidase inhibitor* (MAOI), such as Eldepryl (selegiline), Nardil (phenelzine), Parnate (tranylcypromine), or Marplan (isocarboxazid).

What Could Happen if This Medicine Is Stopped Suddenly?

Stopping this medicine suddenly does not usually cause problems, but diarrhea or feeling sick may result if it has been taken for a long time. The problem being treated may come back. Always ask the doctor whether a medicine can be stopped suddenly or must be decreased slowly (tapered).

How Long Will This Medicine Be Needed?

When used for nervousness or sleep, cyproheptadine is usually prescribed for a very short time to allow the patient to be calm enough to learn new ways to cope. If the person needs treatment for a longer time, another medicine is usually prescribed.

What Else Should I Know About This Medicine?

The medicine should be given with milk or food.

People who take cyproheptadine must not drink alcohol. Severe sleepiness or even loss of consciousness may result.

Notes

Use this space to take notes or to write down questions you want to ask the doctor.

_____

_____

_____

_____

_____

_____

_____

_____

_____

_____

_____

_____

From Dulcan MK (editor): _Helping Parents, Youth, and Teachers Understand Medications for Behavioral and Emotional Problems: A Resource Book of Medication Information Handouts_, Third Edition. Washington, DC, American Psychiatric Publishing, 2007

Medication Information for Youth

Cyproheptadine—Periactin

What the Medicine Is Called and What It Is For

The name of your medicine may be confusing. Most drugs have two names: 1) a scientific name that we call a *generic name* and 2) a trade or *brand name*. The generic name of this medicine is cyproheptadine. The brand name is Periactin.

Cyproheptadine is called an *antihistamine*, a type of medicine first used to treat allergies. Cyproheptadine is sometimes used to treat anxiety (nervousness) or insomnia (difficulty falling asleep). It can help anxious people to be calm enough to learn—with therapy and practice—to understand and tolerate their worries or fears and even to overcome them. Most often, this medicine is used for a short time when symptoms are very uncomfortable or frightening or when they make it hard to do important things such as go to school. Cyproheptadine can help people with insomnia when used for a short time along with calming routines that help them to fall asleep. In people who are not eating enough and are too thin, it can increase appetite and help to gain weight.

How You Take the Medicine

It is very important to take the medicine exactly as the doctor or nurse tells you. Do not skip doses or take extra medicine without asking an adult. If you forget a dose, ask your parent(s) what to do. It is best to take this medicine with milk or food.

Do not use any other medicines without talking to your doctor first. Do not use alcohol, marijuana, or street drugs while taking this medicine. They can cause serious side effects. Skipping your medicine to take drugs does not work because many medicines can stay in your body for a long time.

Caffeine (in coffee, tea, or soft drinks) could make you feel worse.

This medicine is prescribed only for you. It should never be shared with anyone else.

You do not have to tell others that you are taking this medicine, but it is not something you should feel ashamed or embarrassed about. Many young people are helped by cyproheptadine. This medicine is not habit-forming, and you cannot become "hooked" on it. You should talk to your doctor or nurse about any questions you have about the medicine. It is important to remember that the medicine *helps* you. It cannot *make* you do anything or change you as a person.

If you stop the medicine suddenly it might cause you to feel sick, or the problem being treated may come back. Do not stop the medicine unless the doctor tells you to.

How Your Doctor Will Follow Your Progress

Before giving you the medicine, your doctor or nurse will talk with you and your parent(s) and may measure your height, weight, heart rate (pulse), and blood pressure.

Be sure to tell your doctor or nurse about any other medicines or supplements you are taking, including vitamins, herbs, or aids to weight loss or bodybuilding. Also be sure to tell the doctor or nurse if you are using alcohol or drugs. Because many medicines may affect babies, it is very important to tell the doctor if you might be pregnant or if you are at risk of becoming pregnant.

Your teachers may be asked to fill out a form about your grades and behavior in school. A psychologist may give you some tests to see how you learn best.

Most doctors have regular appointments with young people who are taking medicine. You should use these visits to share any concerns you may have about your medicine and to talk about if it has helped you. From time to time, your physician or nurse may measure your height, weight, heart rate (pulse), and blood pressure to be sure that you are in good health while you are taking the medicine. Your doctor also will ask for regular reports from your parents and maybe from your teachers (with your permission) to see how well the medicine is working.

How the Medicine Might Affect You

In addition to the ways the medicine can help you, it may have other effects called *side effects*. Different medicines have different side effects. It is helpful to know about some of the most common side effects of your medicine so that you will understand what they are if they happen. Some people do not have any side effects. Some side effects are just uncomfortable, but others may mean a more serious problem with the medicine. Side effects are most common after starting the medicine or after a dose increase. They may go away with time, or the medicine can be adjusted or changed—ask the doctor.

You could have an allergy to any medicine, which might show up as a rash on your skin, swelling, itching, or trouble breathing.

Please tell your parent(s) and your doctor or nurse about any changes that you notice after taking the medicine. It is especially important to tell a responsible adult if you are feeling depressed or that you may not want to live; if you have thoughts of hurting yourself; or if you begin to feel more irritable, nervous, or restless.

The most common side effect of cyproheptadine is daytime sleepiness. If this medicine is making you sleepy, it is very important not to drive a car or ride a bicycle or motorcycle. After starting cyproheptadine or increasing the dose, please be extra careful when driving a car, riding a bike, or using machines until you can tell how the medicine affects your alertness, attention, and coordination.

Drinking alcohol while taking this medicine can cause severe drowsiness or even passing out. **Don't do it!**

Tell your parent(s) or the doctor if you wake up at night after sleeping for a short time and cannot get back to sleep.

Sometimes cyproheptadine seems to work in the opposite way, causing excitement, irritability, anger, aggression, and other problems. If this happens, tell your parent(s) or your doctor.

You might feel dizzy, tired, or even faint when you stand up fast. Try standing up slowly, especially first thing in the morning when getting out of bed.

Another common side effect is dry mouth. You may be more thirsty than usual and find that you are drinking more water or other liquids than usual. Sucking on sugar-free hard candy or cough drops usually helps. You also could try chewing sugar-free gum or sucking on ice chips. Do not chew the ice; you could hurt your teeth. Also, using lip balm will keep your lips from cracking. It is important to be especially good about brushing your teeth.

Some people become constipated (have hard bowel movements) when taking this medicine. Try drinking more water and eating more fruits, vegetables, and whole grains. If that does not help, tell your parent(s) or doctor—you may need a medicine to help with this side effect.

Taking this medicine could make you more likely to get badly sunburned or very sick in hot weather. Be sure to drink plenty of liquids and cover up or use sunscreen when you go outside in hot weather. Be careful to rest in the shade and not get overheated.

Other side effects that some people get from cyproheptadine are having trouble passing urine, blurred vision, stomachache, upset stomach, or headache.

Serious side effects hardly ever happen when taking this medicine. You should tell your parent(s) and doctor if you notice anything different or unusual about how you feel once you start taking the medicine, especially if you are having trouble breathing or your body seems to be moving differently than usual.

Notes

Use this space to take notes or to write down questions you want to ask the doctor or nurse.

_____

_____

_____

_____

_____

_____

_____

_____

_____

From Dulcan MK (editor): _Helping Parents, Youth, and Teachers Understand Medications for Behavioral and Emotional Problems: A Resource Book of Medication Information Handouts_, Third Edition. Washington, DC, American Psychiatric Publishing, 2007

Medication Information for Parents and Teachers

Desipramine—Norpramin

General Information About Medication

Each child and adolescent is different. No one has exactly the same combination of medical and psychological problems. It is a good idea to talk with the doctor or nurse about the reasons a medicine is being used. It is very important to keep all appointments and to be in touch by telephone if you have concerns. It is important to communicate with the doctor, nurse, or therapist.

It is very important that the medicine be taken exactly as the doctor instructs. However, once in a while, everyone forgets to give a medicine on time. It is a good idea to ask the doctor or nurse what to do if this happens. Do not stop or change a medicine without asking the doctor or nurse first.

If the medicine seems to stop working, it may be because it is not being taken regularly. The youth may be "cheeking" or hiding the medicine or forgetting to take it (especially at school). The doses may be too far apart, or a different dose may be needed. Something at school, at home, or in the neighborhood may be upsetting the youth, or he or she may need special help for learning disabilities or tutoring. Please discuss your concerns with the doctor. **Do not just increase the dose.**

All medicines should be kept in a safe place, out of the reach of children, and should be supervised by an adult. If someone takes too much of a medicine, call the doctor the poison control center, or a hospital emergency room.

Each medicine has a "generic" or chemical name. Just like laundry detergents or paper towels, some medicines are sold by more than one company under different brand names. The same medicine may be available under a generic name and several brand names. The generic medications are usually less expensive than the brand name ones. The generic medications have the same chemical formula, but they may or may not be exactly the same strength as the brand-name medications. Also, some brands of pills contain dye that can cause allergic reactions. It is a good idea to talk to the doctor and the pharmacist about whether it is important to use a specific brand of medicine.

All medicines can cause an allergic reaction. Examples are hives, itching, rashes, swelling, and trouble breathing. Even a tiny amount of a medicine can cause a reaction in patients who are allergic to that medicine. Be *sure* to talk to the doctor before restarting a medicine that has caused an allergic reaction.

Taking more than one medicine at the same time may cause more side effects or cause one of the medicines to not work as well. Always ask the doctor, nurse, or pharmacist before adding another medicine, whether prescription or over-the-counter. Be sure that each doctor knows about *all* of the medicines your child is taking. Also tell the doctor about any vitamins, herbal medicines, or supplements your child may be taking. Some of these may have side effects alone or when taken with this medication.

Everyone taking medicine should have a physical examination at least once a year.

If you suspect the youth is using drugs or alcohol, please tell the doctor right away.

Pregnancy requires special care in the use of medicine. Please tell the doctor immediately if you suspect the teenager is pregnant or might become pregnant.

Printed information like this applies to children and adolescents in general. If you have questions about the medicine, or if you notice changes or anything unusual, please ask the doctor or nurse. As scientific research advances, knowledge increases and advice changes. Even experts do not always agree. Many medicines have not been approved by the U.S. Food and Drug Administration (FDA) for use in children. For this reason, use of the medicine for a particular problem or age group often is not listed in the *Physicians' Desk Reference*. This does not necessarily mean that the medicine is dangerous or does not work, only that the company that makes the medicine has not received permission to advertise the medicine for use in children. Companies often do not apply for this permission because it is expensive to do the tests needed to apply for approval for use in children. Once a medication is approved by the FDA for any purpose, a doctor is allowed to prescribe it according to research and clinical experience.

Note to Teachers

It is a good idea to talk with the parent(s) about the reason(s) that a medication is being used. If the parent(s) sign consent to release information, it is often helpful to talk with the doctor. If the parent(s) give permission, the doctor may ask you to fill out rating forms about your experience with the student's behavior, feelings, academic performance, and medication side effects. This information is very useful in selecting and monitoring medication treatment. If you have observations that you think are important, do not hesitate to share these with the student's parent(s) and treating clinicians.

It is very important that the medicine be taken exactly as the doctor instructs. However, everyone forgets to give a medicine on time once in a while. It is a good idea to ask the parent(s) in advance what to do if this happens. Do not stop or change the time you are giving a medicine at school without parental permission. If a medication is to be taken with food, but lunchtime or snack time changes, be sure to notify the parent(s) so appropriate adjustments can be made.

All medicines should be kept in a secure place and should be supervised by an adult. If someone takes too much of a medicine, follow your school procedure for an urgent medical problem.

Taking medicine is a private matter and is best managed discreetly and confidentially. It is important to be sensitive to the student's feelings about taking medicine.

If you suspect that the student is using drugs or alcohol, please tell the parent(s) or a school counselor right away.

Please tell the parent(s) or school nurse if you suspect medication side effects.

Modifications of the classroom environment or assignments may be useful in addition to medication. The student may need to be evaluated for additional help or for an Individualized Education Plan for learning or behavior.

Any expression of suicidal thoughts or feelings or self-harm by a child or adolescent is a clear signal of distress and should be taken seriously. These behaviors should not be dismissed as "attention seeking."

You may notice the following side effects at school:

Common Side Effects

- Dry mouth—Allow the student to chew sugar-free gum or to make extra trips to the water fountain.
- Constipation—Allow the student to drink more fluids or to use the bathroom more often.
- Daytime sleepiness—The student should not drive, ride a bicycle or motorcycle, or operate machinery.
- Dizziness (especially when standing up quickly)—This may happen in the classroom or during physical education). Suggest that the student stand up more slowly.
- Irritability

Occasional Side Effects

- Stuttering
- Increased risk of sunburn (this may be a problem if recess or physical education is outdoors in warm weather)—The student should wear sunscreen or protective clothing or stay out of the sun.

Less Common Side Effects

- Nausea—The student may need to take the medicine after a meal or snack.
- Trouble urinating—The student may need more time in the bathroom.
- Blurred vision—The student may have trouble seeing the blackboard.
- Motor tics (fast, repeated movements) or muscle twitches (jerking movements) of parts of the body
- Increased activity, rapid speech, feeling "speeded up," being very excited or irritable (cranky)
- Skin rash

Rare, but Potentially Serious, Side Effects

Call the parents(s) or follow your school's emergency procedures *immediately* if the student experiences any of the following side effects:

- Seizure (fit, convulsion) **(This is a medical emergency.)**
- Very fast or irregular heartbeat **(This is a medical emergency.)**
- Fainting
- Hallucinations (hearing voices or seeing things that are not there)
- Inability to urinate
- Confusion
- Severe change in behavior

What Is Desipramine (Norpramin)?

Desipramine is called a *tricyclic antidepressant*. It was first used to treat depression but is now used to treat attention-deficit/hyperactivity disorder (ADHD), school phobia, separation anxiety, panic disorder, and some sleep disorders (such as night terrors). It comes in brand name Norpramin and generic tablets.

How Can This Medicine Help?

Desipramine can decrease symptoms of ADHD, anxiety (nervousness), panic, and night terrors or sleepwalking. The medicine may take several weeks to work.

How Does This Medicine Work?

Tricyclic antidepressants affect the natural substances (*neurotransmitters*) that are needed for certain parts of the brain to work more normally. They increase the activity of *serotonin* and *norepinephrine* to more normal levels in the parts of the brain that regulate concentration, motivation, and mood.

How Long Does This Medicine Last?

Although in adults and older teenagers a dose lasts for a whole day, in younger children several doses a day may be needed.

How Will the Doctor Monitor This Medicine?

The doctor will review your child's medical history and physical examination, paying special attention to pulse rate, blood pressure, weight, and height, before starting desipramine. These measurements will be taken when the dose is increased and occasionally as long as the medicine is continued. The doctor may order some blood or urine tests to be sure your child does not have a hidden medical condition.

Tricyclic antidepressants can slow the speed at which signals move through the heart. This effect is not dangerous if the heart is normal, which is why an ECG (electrocardiogram or heart rhythm test) is done before starting the medicine. The ECG may be repeated as the dose is increased and occasionally while the medicine is being taken. Changes in the heart from the medicine usually can be seen on the ECG before they become a problem, so your child's doctor will order an ECG every so often. To find possible hidden heart risks, it is especially important to tell the doctor if your child or anyone in the family has a history of fainting, palpitations, or irregular heartbeat or if anyone in the family died suddenly.

Be sure to tell the doctor if your child or anyone in the family has bipolar illness (manic-depressive illness) or has tried to kill himself or herself.

Because tricyclic antidepressants may increase the risk of seizures (fits, convulsions), the doctor will want to know whether your child has ever had a seizure or a head injury and if there is any family history of epilepsy. Your child's doctor may want to order an EEG (electroencephalogram or brain wave test) before starting the medicine.

Experts do not agree on whether blood tests are needed to measure the level of this medicine. Blood levels seem to be most useful when your doctor suspects that the dose of medicine is too high or too low. The most accurate level is obtained by drawing blood first thing in the morning, after at least 5 days on the same dose, approximately 12 hours after the evening dose of medicine and before the morning dose.

After the medicine is started, the doctor will want to have regular appointments with you and your child to see how the medicine is working, to see if a dose change is needed, to watch for side effects, to see if desipramine is still needed, and to see if any other treatment is needed. The doctor or nurse may check your child's height, weight, pulse, and blood pressure or order tests, such as an ECG or blood level.

If desipramine is being used for ADHD, the doctor may ask for your child's teacher to fill out reports on your child's learning and behavior at school. Before using medicine and at times afterward, the doctor may ask your child to fill out a rating scale about anxiety and depression, to help see how your child is doing.

What Side Effects Can This Medicine Have?

Any medicine can have side effects, including an allergy to the medicine. Because each patient is different, the doctor will monitor the youth closely, especially when the medicine is started. The doctor will work with you to increase the positive effects and decrease the negative effects of the medicine. Please tell the doctor if any of the listed side effects appear or if you think that the medicine is causing any other problems. Not all of the rare or unusual side effects are listed.

Side effects are most common after starting the medicine or after a dose increase. Many side effects can be avoided or lessened by starting with a very low dose and increasing it slowly—ask the doctor.

Allergic Reaction

Tell the doctor in a day or two (if possible, before the next dose of medicine):

- Hives
- Itching
- Rash

  Stop the medicine and get *immediate* medical care:

- Trouble breathing or chest tightness
- Swelling of lips, tongue, or throat

Common Side Effects

Tell the doctor within a week or two:

- Dry mouth—Have your child try using sugar-free gum or candy.
- Constipation—Encourage your child to drink more fluids and eat high-fiber foods; if necessary, the doctor may recommend a fiber medicine such as Benefiber or a stool softener such as Colace or mineral oil.
- Daytime sleepiness—Do not allow your child to drive, ride a bicycle or motorcycle, or operate machinery if this happens.
- Dizziness—This side effect is worse when the child stands up quickly, especially when getting out of bed in the morning; try having the child stand up slowly.
- Weight gain
- Loss of appetite and weight loss
- Irritability

Occasional Side Effects

Tell the doctor within a week or two:

- Nightmares
- Stuttering
- Blurred vision
- Increase in breast size, nipple discharge, or both (in girls)
- Increase in breast size (in boys)

Less Common, but More Serious, Side Effects

Call the doctor within a day or two:

- High or low blood pressure
- Nausea
- Trouble urinating
- Motor tics (fast, repeated movements) or muscle twitches (jerking movements)
- Increased activity, rapid speech, feeling "speeded up," decreased need for sleep, being very excited or irritable (cranky)

Rare, but Potentially Serious, Side Effects

Call the doctor *immediately:*

- Seizure (fit, convulsion)—**Go to an emergency room.**
- Very fast or irregular heartbeat—**Go to an emergency room.**
- Fainting
- Hallucinations (hearing voices or seeing things that are not there)
- Inability to urinate
- Confusion
- Severe change in behavior

Some Interactions With Other Medicines or Food

Please note that the following are only the most likely interactions with food or other medicines.

Check with your child's doctor before giving your child decongestants or over-the-counter cold medicine.

Taking another antidepressant or valproate with desipramine may increase the level of desipramine and increase side effects.

Taking carbamazepine (Tegretol) with desipramine may decrease the positive effects of desipramine and increase the side effects of carbamazepine.

It can be *very dangerous* to take desipramine at the same time as or even within a month of taking another type of medicine called a *monoamine oxidase inhibitor* (MAOI), such as Eldepryl (selegiline), Nardil (phenelzine), Parnate (tranylcypromine), or Marplan (isocarboxazid)).

Caffeine may worsen side effects on the heart or symptoms of anxiety. It is best not to drink coffee, tea, or soft drinks with caffeine while taking this medicine.

What Could Happen if This Medicine Is Stopped Suddenly?

Stopping the medicine suddenly or skipping a dose is not dangerous but can be very uncomfortable. Your child may feel like he or she has the flu—with a headache, muscle aches, stomachache, and upset stomach. Behavioral problems, sadness, nervousness, or trouble sleeping also may occur. If these feelings appear every day, the medicine may need to be given more often during each day.

How Long Will This Medicine Be Needed?

There is no way to know how long a person will need to take this medicine. Parents work together with the doctor to determine what is right for each child. The medicine may be needed for a long time. Some people may need to take the medicine even as adults.

What Else Should I Know About This Medicine?

In youth who have bipolar disorder (manic depression) or who are at risk for bipolar disorder, any antidepressant medicine may increase the risk of hypomania or mania (excitement, agitation, increased activity, decreased sleep).

An overdose by accident or on purpose with tricyclic antidepressants is very dangerous! You must closely supervise the medicine. You may have to lock up the medicine if your child or teenager is suicidal or if young children live in or visit your home.

Tricyclic antidepressants may cause dry mouth, which could increase the chance of tooth decay. Regular brushing of teeth and checkups with the dentist are especially important.

This medicine causes increased risk of sunburn. Be sure that your child wears sunscreen or protective clothing or stays out of the sun.

People who take tricyclic antidepressants must not drink alcohol or use tranquilizers. Severe sleepiness, loss of consciousness, or even death may result.

Black Box Antidepressant Warning

In 2004, an advisory committee to the FDA decided that there might be an increased risk of suicidal behavior for some youth taking medicines called *antidepressants*. In the research studies that the committee reviewed, about 3%–4% of youth with depression who took an antidepressant medicine—and 1%–2% of youth with depression who took a placebo (pill without active medicine)—talked about suicidal thoughts (thinking about killing themselves or wishing they were dead) or did something to harm themselves. This means that almost twice as many youth who were taking an antidepressant to treat their depression talked about suicide or had suicidal behavior compared with youth with depression who were taking inactive medicine. There were *no* completed suicides in any of these research studies, which included more than 4,000 children and adolescents. For youth being treated for anxiety, there was no difference in suicidal talking or behavior between those taking antidepressant medication and those taking placebo.

The FDA told drug companies to add a *black box warning* label to all antidepressant medicines. Because of this label, a doctor (or advanced practice nurse) prescribing one of these medicines has to warn youth and their families that there might be more suicidal thoughts and actions in youth taking these medicines.

On the other hand, in places where more youth are taking the newer antidepressant medicines, the number of adolescents who commit suicide has gotten smaller. Also, thinking about or attempting suicide is more common in surveys of teenagers in the community than it is in depressed youth treated in research studies with antidepressant medicine.

If a youth is being treated with this medicine and is doing well, then no changes are needed as a result of this warning. Increased suicidal talk or action is most likely to happen in the first few months of treatment with a medicine. If your child has recently started this medicine or is about to start, then you and your doctor (or advanced practice nurse) should watch for any changes in behavior. People who are depressed often have suicidal thoughts or actions. It is hard to know whether suicidal thoughts or actions in depressed people are caused by the depression itself or by the medicine. Also, as their depression is getting better, some people talk more about the suicidal thoughts that they had before but did not talk about. As young people get better from depression, they might be at higher risk of doing something about suicidal thoughts that they have had for some time, because they have more energy.

What Should a Parent Do?

1. Be honest with your child about possible risks and benefits of medicine.
2. Talk to your child about whether he or she is having any suicidal thoughts, and tell your child to come to you if he or she is having such thoughts.
3. You, your child, and your child's doctor or nurse should develop a safety plan. Pick adults whom your child can tell if he or she is thinking about suicide.
4. Be sure to tell your child's doctor, nurse, or therapist if you suspect that your child is using alcohol or drugs or if something has happened that might make your child feel worse, such as a family separation, breaking up with a boyfriend or girlfriend, someone close dying or attempting suicide, physical or sexual abuse, or failure in school.
5. Be sure that there are no guns in the home and that all medicines (including over-the-counter medicines like Tylenol) are closely supervised by an adult and kept in a safe place.
6. Watch for new or worse thoughts of suicide, self-harm, depression, anxiety (nerves), feeling very agitated or restless, being angry or aggressive, having more trouble sleeping, or anything else that you see for the first time, seems worse, or worries your child or you. If these appear, contact a mental health professional **right away.** Do not just stop or change the dose of the medicine on your own. If the problems are serious, and you cannot reach one of your clinicians, call a 24-hour psychiatry emergency telephone number or take your child to an emergency room.

Youth on antidepressant medicine should be watched carefully by their parent(s), clinician(s) (doctor, nurse, therapist), and other concerned adults for the first weeks of treatment. It is a good idea to have a visit or telephone call with the doctor, nurse, or therapist weekly for the first month, every 2 weeks for the second month, and after that at least once a month to check for feelings of depression or sadness, thoughts of killing or harming himself or herself, and any problems with the medication. If you have questions, be sure to ask the doctor, nurse, or therapist.

For more information, see http://www.parentsmedguide.org/ (in English and Spanish).

Notes

Use this space to take notes or to write down questions you want to ask the doctor.

_____

_____

_____

_____

_____

_____

_____

_____

_____

_____

_____

_____

Medication Information for Youth

Desipramine—Norpramin

What the Medicine Is Called and What It Is For

The name of your medicine may be confusing. Most drugs have two names: 1) a scientific name that we call a *generic name* and 2) a trade or *brand name*. The generic name of this medicine is desipramine. The brand name is Norpramin.

Desipramine is called an *antidepressant*, or *tricyclic*. Desipramine is used to treat depression, trouble paying attention and being too active or acting without thinking, and feeling too anxious (nervous). It can help people who have attention-deficit/hyperactivity disorder (ADHD), fear of going to school or being away from home, panic disorder, or sleep problems such as waking up at night very scared (night terrors) or sleepwalking.

How You Take the Medicine

It is very important to take the medicine exactly as the doctor or nurse tells you. Do not skip doses or take extra medicine without asking an adult. If you miss a dose, you may feel sick, as though you have the flu. It is very important that you take all the pills you are supposed to take each day. Your doctor will probably recommend that you take your medicine at the same time each day, which may be with meals or at bedtime.

It may take several weeks before you notice that the medicine is helping. Waiting for the full effect may take even longer. You may feel discouraged and think the medicine is never going to help. You may want to give up and stop taking the medicine. Talk to your doctor and parent(s) about how you feel, but **do not stop** taking the medicine unless your doctor tells you to. It is also important not to take extra pills, hoping that you will feel better faster. Doing that could make you *very* sick.

Stopping the medicine suddenly or skipping a dose can be very uncomfortable. You may feel like you have the flu—with a headache, muscle aches, stomachache, and upset stomach. If these feelings appear every day, the medicine may need to be given more often during each day.

Caffeine (in coffee, tea, or soft drinks) may make you feel worse.

Do not use any other medicines without talking to your doctor first. Do not use alcohol, marijuana, or street drugs while taking this medicine—**it can be very dangerous**. Skipping your medicine to take drugs does not work because many medicines stay in your body for a long time.

This medicine is prescribed only for you. It should never be shared with anyone else.

You do not have to tell others that you are taking this medicine, but it is not something you should feel ashamed or embarrassed about. Many young people are helped by desipramine. This medicine is not habit-forming, and you cannot become "hooked" on it. You should talk to your doctor or nurse about any questions you have about the medicine. It is important to remember that the medicine *helps* you. It cannot *make* you do anything or change you as a person.

193

How Your Doctor Will Follow Your Progress

Before giving you the medicine, your doctor or nurse will talk with you and your parent(s) and measure your height, weight, heart rate (pulse), and blood pressure. The doctor may order some blood or urine tests to be sure you are in good health. Be sure to tell the doctor if you have had very fast heartbeat, chest pain, dizziness, or fainting.

Be sure to tell your doctor or nurse about any other medicines or supplements you are taking, including vitamins, herbs, or aids to weight loss or bodybuilding. Also be sure to tell the doctor or nurse if you are using alcohol or drugs. Because many medicines may affect babies, it is very important to tell the doctor if you might be pregnant or if you are at risk of becoming pregnant. Be sure to tell the doctor if you have had thoughts of hurting yourself, have tried to hurt yourself, or sometimes wish that you were not alive.

Before starting desipramine, at times of increasing the dose, and every 6 months to a year after that, your doctor will ask for an ECG (electrocardiogram or heart rhythm test) to be done. This test counts your heartbeats through small wires that are taped to your chest. It takes only a few minutes.

Your teachers may be asked to fill out a form about your grades and behavior in school. A psychologist may give you some tests to see how you learn best.

Before starting the medicine and afterward, the doctor may ask you to answer questions on paper about anxiety and depression.

Most doctors have regular appointments with young people who are taking medicine. You should use these visits to share any concerns you may have about your medicine and to talk about if it has helped you. From time to time, your physician or nurse may measure your height, weight, heart rate (pulse), and blood pressure to be sure that you are in good health while you are taking the medicine. You may need to have blood tests to see if you are on the right dose of desipramine. Your doctor also will ask for regular reports from your parents and maybe from your teachers (with your permission) to see how well the medicine is working.

Some medicines are started at the amount you will take for as long as you are taking that medicine. Other medicines need to be increased or adjusted until your doctor decides you are taking the right amount. Starting at a low dose and increasing it slowly may lessen side effects. If the medicine helps you, your doctor will probably want you to take it for a long time, maybe even as an adult.

How the Medicine Might Affect You

In addition to the ways the medicine can help you, it may have other effects called *side effects*. Different medicines have different side effects. It is helpful to know about some of the most common side effects of your medicine so that you will understand what they are if they happen. Some people do not have any side effects. Some side effects are just uncomfortable, but others may mean a more serious problem with the medicine. Side effects are most common after starting the medicine or after a dose increase. They may go away with time, or the medicine can be adjusted or changed—ask the doctor.

You could have an allergy to any medicine, which might show up as a rash on your skin, swelling, itching, or trouble breathing.

Please tell your parent(s) and your doctor or nurse about any changes that you notice after taking the medicine. It is especially important to tell a responsible adult if you are feeling depressed or that you may not want to live; if you have thoughts of hurting yourself; or if you begin to feel more irritable, nervous, or restless. Also be sure to tell your parent(s) or doctor if you begin to feel "speeded up" or have trouble sleeping.

Some medicines make people feel sleepy or less coordinated. If this medicine is making you sleepy, it is very important not to drive a car or ride a bicycle or motorcycle. After starting a new medicine or increasing the dose of a medicine, please be extra careful when driving a car, riding a bike, or using machines until you can tell how the medicine affects your alertness, attention, and coordination.

One of the most common side effects of this medicine is feeling tired or sleepy during the day, even if you have had a full night's sleep. After you have been taking the medicine for a few weeks, your body will adjust, and this side effect may go away. If you have had trouble sleeping at night, the medicine can help you sleep better, especially if the doctor tells you to take a dose of medicine in the evening. Other people may feel more restless and excited. Tell your parent(s) or doctor if this is uncomfortable.

Another common side effect is dry mouth. You may be more thirsty than usual and find that you are drinking more water or other liquids. Sucking on sugar-free hard candy or cough drops usually helps. You also could try chewing sugar-free gum or sucking on ice chips. Do not chew the ice; you could hurt your teeth. Also, using lip balm will keep your lips from cracking. It is important to be especially good about brushing your teeth.

Sometimes people taking desipramine notice that their heart is beating a little faster than normal. Usually this happens within the first few weeks of taking the medicine and gets better or goes away. However, if you notice that your heart is beating very fast for more than a few minutes when you have not been exercising, if you feel light-headed or dizzy when you are sitting or standing still, or if you faint, you should let your parent(s) and doctor know right away. Some people feel dizzy or light-headed when standing up fast. If this happens, try to get up more slowly, especially first thing in the morning, when getting out of bed.

Some people become constipated (have hard bowel movements). Try drinking more water and eating more fruits, vegetables, and whole grains. If that does not help, tell your parent(s) or doctor—you may need a medicine to help with this side effect.

Some other side effects that could happen are headache, blurred vision, not feeling hungry and not wanting to eat much, eating more than usual, having an upset stomach, changes in your bowel movements, or trouble passing urine. You may have a change in your sexual functioning or in your breasts—it is OK to ask the doctor about this. This medicine may make you more likely to get sick if you get overheated, so be sure to drink plenty of liquids and rest in the shade in hot weather.

Please let your parent(s) and doctor know if you notice anything different or unusual about how you feel once you start taking the medicine. This includes good things, such as feeling less sad or less nervous or sleeping better at night.

Notes

Use this space to take notes or to write down questions you want to ask the doctor or nurse.

_____

_____

_____

_____

_____

_____

_____

_____

_____

_____

_____

_____

Medication Information for Parents and Teachers

Desmopressin Acetate—DDAVP, Stimate

General Information About Medication

Each child and adolescent is different. No one has exactly the same combination of medical and psychological problems. It is a good idea to talk with the doctor or nurse about the reasons a medicine is being used. It is very important to keep all appointments and to be in touch by telephone if you have concerns. It is important to communicate with the doctor, nurse, or therapist.

It is very important that the medicine be taken exactly as the doctor instructs. However, once in a while, everyone forgets to give a medicine on time. It is a good idea to ask the doctor or nurse what to do if this happens. Do not stop or change a medicine without asking the doctor or nurse first.

If the medicine seems to stop working, it may be because it is not being taken regularly. The youth may be "cheeking" or hiding the medicine or forgetting to take it (especially at school). The doses may be too far apart, or a different dose may be needed. Something at school, at home, or in the neighborhood may be upsetting the youth, or he or she may need special help for learning disabilities or tutoring. Please discuss your concerns with the doctor. **Do not just increase the dose.**

All medicines should be kept in a safe place, out of the reach of children, and should be supervised by an adult. If someone takes too much of a medicine, call the doctor, the poison control center, or a hospital emergency room.

Each medicine has a "generic" or chemical name. Just like laundry detergents or paper towels, some medicines are sold by more than one company under different brand names. The same medicine may be available under a generic name and several brand names. The generic medications are usually less expensive than the brand name ones. The generic medications have the same chemical formula, but they may or may not be exactly the same strength as the brand-name medications. Also, some brands of pills contain dye that can cause allergic reactions. It is a good idea to talk to the doctor and the pharmacist about whether it is important to use a specific brand of medicine.

All medicines can cause an allergic reaction. Examples are hives, itching, rashes, swelling, and trouble breathing. Even a tiny amount of a medicine can cause a reaction in patients who are allergic to that medicine. Be *sure* to talk to the doctor before restarting a medicine that has caused an allergic reaction.

Taking more than one medicine at the same time may cause more side effects or cause one of the medicines to not work as well. Always ask the doctor, nurse, or pharmacist before adding another medicine, whether prescription or over-the-counter. Be sure that each doctor knows about *all* of the medicines your child is taking. Also tell the doctor about any vitamins, herbal medicines, or supplements your child may be taking (including those used for dieting or bodybuilding). Some of these may have side effects alone or when taken with this medication.

Everyone taking medicine should have a physical examination at least once a year.

If you suspect the youth is using drugs or alcohol, please tell the doctor right away.

Pregnancy requires special care in the use of medicine. Please tell the doctor immediately if you suspect the teenager is pregnant or might become pregnant.

Printed information like this applies to children and adolescents in general. If you have questions about the medicine, or if you notice changes or anything unusual, please ask the doctor or nurse. As scientific research advances, knowledge increases and advice changes. Even experts do not always agree. Many medicines have not been approved by the U.S. Food and Drug Administration (FDA) for use in children. For this reason, use of the medicine for a particular problem or age group often is not listed in the *Physicians' Desk Reference*. This does not necessarily mean that the medicine is dangerous or does not work, only that the company that makes the medicine has not received permission to advertise the medicine for use in children. Companies often do not apply for this permission because it is expensive to do the tests needed to apply for approval for use in children. Once a medication is approved by the FDA for any purpose, a doctor is allowed to prescribe it according to research and clinical experience.

Note to Teachers

It is a good idea to talk with the parent(s) about the reason(s) that a medication is being used. If the parent(s) sign consent to release information, it is often helpful to talk with the doctor. If the parent(s) give permission, the doctor may ask you to fill out rating forms about your experience with the student's behavior, feelings, academic performance, and medication side effects. This information is very useful in selecting and monitoring medication treatment. If you have observations that you think are important, do not hesitate to share these with the student's parent(s) and treating clinicians.

All medicines should be kept in a secure place and should be supervised by an adult. If someone takes too much of a medicine, follow your school procedure for an urgent medical problem.

Taking medicine is a private matter and is best managed discreetly and confidentially. It is important to be sensitive to the student's feelings about taking medicine.

If you suspect that the student is using drugs or alcohol, please tell the parent(s) or a school counselor right away.

Desmopressin (DDAVP, Stimate) may cause increased urination in the daytime. The student may need extra trips to the bathroom.

Please tell the parent(s) or school nurse if you suspect medication side effects.

Modifications of the classroom environment or assignments may be useful in addition to medication. The student may need to be evaluated for additional help or for an Individualized Education Plan for learning or behavior.

Any expression of suicidal thoughts or feelings or self-harm by a child or adolescent is a clear signal of distress and should be taken seriously. These behaviors should not be dismissed as "attention seeking."

What Is Desmopressin (DDAVP, Stimate)?

Desmopressin is a man-made version of a naturally occurring hormone—the antidiuretic hormone *vasopressin*, which is made by the *pituitary gland*. Desmopressin comes in two forms: a nasal (nose) spray (DDAVP, Stimate) and DDAVP tablets.

How Can This Medicine Help?

When given at bedtime, desmopressin can prevent bed-wetting (also called nocturnal enuresis). It may be used every night or only for nights when the youth is sleeping away from home (camp, sleepovers) and would be embarrassed by wetting the bed.

How Does This Medicine Work?

Desmopressin temporarily stops or slows the kidney from making urine. After the medicine wears off, there is an increase in urine the next day.

How Long Does This Medicine Last?

Desmopressin lasts for about 10 hours, only for nights on which it is given (at bedtime). When the medicine is stopped, bed-wetting usually returns. If desmopressin is being used regularly, several times a year it may be stopped to see if the youth has grown out of bed-wetting.

How Will the Doctor Monitor This Medicine?

The doctor will review your child's medical history and physical examination before starting desmopressin. The doctor may order blood or urine tests to be sure your child does not have a hidden medical condition that would make it unsafe to use this medicine. The doctor or nurse may measure your child's pulse and blood pressure before starting desmopressin.

After the medicine is started, the doctor will want to have regular appointments with you and your child to see how the medicine is working, to see if a dose change is needed, to watch for side effects, to see if desmopressin is still needed, and to see if any other treatment is needed. The doctor or nurse may check your child's height, weight, pulse, and blood pressure, or order a blood or urine test to see how much water and salt is in your child's body.

What Side Effects Can This Medicine Have?

Any medicine can have side effects, including an allergy to the medicine. Because each patient is different, the doctor will monitor the youth closely, especially when the medicine is started. The doctor will work with you to increase the positive effects and decrease the negative effects of the medicine. Please tell the doctor if any of the listed side effects appear or if you think that the medicine is causing any other problems. Not all of the rare or unusual side effects are listed.

Side effects are most common after starting the medicine or after a dose increase. Many side effects can be avoided or lessened by starting with a very low dose and increasing it slowly—ask the doctor.

Allergic Reaction

Tell the doctor in a day or two (if possible, before the next dose of medicine):

- Hives
- Itching
- Rash

Stop the medicine and get *immediate* medical care:

- Trouble breathing or chest tightness
- Swelling of lips, tongue, or throat

Common Side Effects

Tell the doctor within a week or two:

- Headaches
- Nausea (upset stomach)
- Sore and/or stuffy nose (from the nasal spray form)
- Dizziness

Very Rare, but Serious, Side Effect

If the youth drinks too much water or takes medicines that increase the action of desmopressin, "water poisoning" and a seizure (convulsion) may result. **Seek medical attention *immediately*.**

Some Interactions With Other Medicines or Food

Please note that the following are only the most likely interactions with food or other medicines.

Taking carbamazepine (Tegretol) with desmopressin may dangerously increase the action of desmopressin.

What Could Happen if This Medicine Is Stopped Suddenly?

There are no known medical withdrawal effects, but the bed-wetting could return.

How Long Will This Medicine Be Needed?

Most young people who wet the bed grow out of it sooner or later. That is why it is a good idea to try stopping the desmopressin every so often to see if the bed-wetting has gone away on its own.

What Else Should I Know About This Medicine?

Because desmopressin blocks the usual way the body corrects for amounts of water, drinking of fluids (especially water) should be limited in the evening and night.

This medicine is very expensive. Many families prefer to try using behavior therapy or the "bell and pad" system to stop bed-wetting. If these methods work, the effects last longer than medicine does.

Store the nasal spray upright. Protect it from heat, high humidity, and bright light. The Stimate brand nasal spray should be kept in the refrigerator.

Notes

Use this space to take notes or to write down questions you want to ask the doctor.

_____

_____

_____

_____

_____

_____

_____

_____

_____

_____

_____

_____

_____

From Dulcan MK (editor): _Helping Parents, Youth, and Teachers Understand Medications for Behavioral and Emotional Problems: A Resource Book of Medication Information Handouts_, Third Edition. Washington, DC, American Psychiatric Publishing, 2007

Medication Information
for Youth

Desmopressin Acetate—DDAVP, Stimate

What the Medicine Is Called and What It Is For

The name of your medicine may be confusing. Most drugs have two names: 1) a scientific name that we call a *generic name* and 2) a trade or *brand name*. The generic name of this medicine is desmopressin. The brand names are DDAVP and Stimate.

Desmopressin is a man-made version of a natural hormone. When used at bedtime, your kidneys will make less urine during the night so that you do not wet the bed. After the medicine wears off, there is an increase in urine during the day.

How You Take the Medicine

Desmopressin comes in both pills and a nose spray. It may be used every night or only for nights when you are sleeping away from home (camp, sleepovers) and would be embarrassed by wetting the bed.

Do not take more than the doctor says—this could be dangerous.

This medicine is prescribed only for you. It should never be shared with anyone else.

You do not have to tell others that you are taking this medicine, but it is not something you should feel ashamed or embarrassed about. Many young people are helped by desmopressin. This medicine is not habit-forming, and you cannot become "hooked" on it. You should talk to your doctor or nurse about any questions you have about the medicine. Also, you can talk to the doctor if you would rather use a behavioral program ("bell and pad," for example) instead of taking this medicine.

How Your Doctor Will Follow Your Progress

Before giving you the medicine, your doctor or nurse will talk with you and your parent(s) and may measure your height, weight, heart rate (pulse), and blood pressure. There may be other tests, such as blood or urine tests, to be sure that you are in good health.

Be sure to tell your doctor or nurse about any other medicines or supplements you are taking, including vitamins, herbs, or aids to weight loss or bodybuilding. Also be sure to tell the doctor or nurse if you are using alcohol or drugs. Be sure to tell the doctor if you might be pregnant or if you are at risk of becoming pregnant.

Most doctors have regular appointments with young people who are taking medicine. You should use these visits to share any concerns you may have about your medicine and to talk about if it has helped you. From time to time, your physician or nurse may measure your height, weight, heart rate (pulse), and blood pressure to be sure that you are in good health while you are taking the medicine. There may be a blood or urine test. Your doctor also will ask for regular reports to see how well the medicine is working.

When the medicine is stopped, bed-wetting usually returns. If desmopressin is being used regularly, several times a year the doctor may tell you to stop it to see if you have grown out of bed-wetting, which most people do.

How the Medicine Might Affect You

In addition to the ways the medicine can help you, it may have other effects called *side effects*. Different medicines have different side effects. It is helpful to know about some of the most common side effects of your medicine so that you will understand what they are if they happen. Some people do not have any side effects. Some side effects are just uncomfortable, but others may mean a more serious problem with the medicine. Side effects are most common after starting the medicine or after a dose increase. They may go away with time, or the medicine can be adjusted or changed—ask the doctor.

You could have an allergy to any medicine, which might show up as a rash on your skin, swelling, itching, or trouble breathing.

Some people taking desmopressin have headaches, upset stomach, dizziness, or a sore or stuffy nose (if using the nose spray). Tell your parent(s) or doctor if this happens.

It is **very important** *not* to drink a lot of fluids (especially water) in the evening and at night, when taking desmopressin. You could get very sick!

Please tell your parent(s) and your doctor or nurse about any changes that you notice after taking the medicine. It is especially important to tell a responsible adult if you are feeling depressed or that you may not want to live; if you have thoughts of hurting yourself; or if you begin to feel more irritable, nervous, or restless.

Notes

Use this space to take notes or to write down questions you want to ask the doctor or nurse.

_____

_____

_____

_____

_____

_____

_____

_____

_____

_____

_____

_____

_____

_____

From Dulcan MK (editor): _Helping Parents, Youth, and Teachers Understand Medications for Behavioral and Emotional Problems: A Resource Book of Medication Information Handouts_, Third Edition. Washington, DC, American Psychiatric Publishing, 2007

Medication Information for Parents and Teachers

Diazepam—Valium

General Information About Medication

Each child and adolescent is different. No one has exactly the same combination of medical and psychological problems. It is a good idea to talk with the doctor or nurse about the reasons a medicine is being used. It is very important to keep all appointments and to be in touch by telephone if you have concerns. It is important to communicate with the doctor, nurse, or therapist.

It is very important that the medicine be taken exactly as the doctor instructs. However, once in a while, everyone forgets to give a medicine on time. It is a good idea to ask the doctor or nurse what to do if this happens. Do not stop or change a medicine without asking the doctor or nurse first.

If the medicine seems to stop working, it may be because it is not being taken regularly. The youth may be "cheeking" or hiding the medicine or forgetting to take it (especially at school). The doses may be too far apart, or a different dose may be needed. Something at school, at home, or in the neighborhood may be upsetting the youth, or he or she may need special help for learning disabilities or tutoring. Please discuss your concerns with the doctor. **Do not just increase the dose.**

All medicines should be kept in a safe place, out of the reach of children, and should be supervised by an adult. If someone takes too much of a medicine, call the doctor, the poison control center, or a hospital emergency room.

Each medicine has a "generic" or chemical name. Just like laundry detergents or paper towels, some medicines are sold by more than one company under different brand names. The same medicine may be available under a generic name and several brand names. The generic medications are usually less expensive than the brand name ones. The generic medications have the same chemical formula, but they may or may not be exactly the same strength as the brand-name medications. Also, some brands of pills contain dye that can cause allergic reactions. It is a good idea to talk to the doctor and the pharmacist about whether it is important to use a specific brand of medicine.

All medicines can cause an allergic reaction. Examples are hives, itching, rashes, swelling, and trouble breathing. Even a tiny amount of a medicine can cause a reaction in patients who are allergic to that medicine. Be *sure* to talk to the doctor before restarting a medicine that has caused an allergic reaction.

Taking more than one medicine at the same time may cause more side effects or cause one of the medicines to not work as well. Always ask the doctor, nurse, or pharmacist before adding another medicine, whether prescription or over-the-counter. Be sure that each doctor knows about *all* of the medicines your child is taking. Also tell the doctor about any vitamins, herbal medicines, or supplements your child may be taking. Some of these may have side effects alone or when taken with this medication.

Everyone taking medicine should have a physical examination at least once a year.

If you suspect the youth is using drugs or alcohol, please tell the doctor right away.

207

Pregnancy requires special care in the use of medicine. Please tell the doctor immediately if you suspect the teenager is pregnant or might become pregnant.

Printed information like this applies to children and adolescents in general. If you have questions about the medicine, or if you notice changes or anything unusual, please ask the doctor or nurse. As scientific research advances, knowledge increases and advice changes. Even experts do not always agree. Many medicines have not been approved by the U.S. Food and Drug Administration (FDA) for use in children. For this reason, use of the medicine for a particular problem or age group often is not listed in the *Physicians' Desk Reference*. This does not necessarily mean that the medicine is dangerous or does not work, only that the company that makes the medicine has not received permission to advertise the medicine for use in children. Companies often do not apply for this permission because it is expensive to do the tests needed to apply for approval for use in children. Once a medication is approved by the FDA for any purpose, a doctor is allowed to prescribe it according to research and clinical experience.

Note to Teachers

It is a good idea to talk with the parent(s) about the reason(s) that a medication is being used. If the parent(s) sign consent to release information, it is often helpful to talk with the doctor. If the parent(s) give permission, the doctor may ask you to fill out rating forms about your experience with the student's behavior, feelings, academic performance, and medication side effects. This information is very useful in selecting and monitoring medication treatment. If you have observations that you think are important, do not hesitate to share these with the student's parent(s) and treating clinicians.

It is very important that the medicine be taken exactly as the doctor instructs. However, everyone forgets to give a medicine on time once in a while. It is a good idea to ask the parent(s) in advance what to do if this happens. Do not stop or change the time you are giving a medicine at school without parental permission. If a medication is to be taken with food, but lunchtime or snack time changes, be sure to notify the parent(s) so appropriate adjustments can be made.

All medicines should be kept in a secure place and should be supervised by an adult. If someone takes too much of a medicine, follow your school procedure for an urgent medical problem.

Taking medicine is a private matter and is best managed discreetly and confidentially. It is important to be sensitive to the student's feelings about taking medicine.

If you suspect that the student is using drugs or alcohol, please tell the parent(s) or a school counselor right away.

Please tell the parent(s) or school nurse if you suspect medication side effects.

Modifications of the classroom environment or assignments may be useful in addition to medication. The student may need to be evaluated for additional help or for an Individualized Education Plan for learning or behavior.

Any expression of suicidal thoughts or feelings or self-harm by a child or adolescent is a clear signal of distress and should be taken seriously. These behaviors should not be dismissed as "attention seeking."

What Is Diazepam (Valium)?

Diazepam is a *benzodiazepine*, or *antianxiety* medicine. It used to be called a *minor tranquilizer*. It is sometimes called an *anxiolytic* or *sedative*. It comes in brand name Valium and generic tablets, liquid, and injection (a shot).

How Can This Medicine Help?

Diazepam can decrease anxiety, nervousness, fears, and excessive worrying. It can help anxious people to be calm enough to learn—with therapy and practice (exposure to feared things or situations)—to understand and tolerate their worries or fears and even to overcome them. People with generalized anxiety disorder, social phobia, posttraumatic stress disorder (PTSD), or panic disorder can be helped by diazepam. Most often, it is used for a short time when symptoms are very uncomfortable or frightening or when they make it hard to do important things such as go to school. Diazepam can decrease the severe physical symptoms (rapid heartbeat, trouble breathing, dizziness, sweating) of panic attacks and phobias.

Diazepam also can be used for sleep problems, such as night terrors (sudden waking up from sleep with great fear) or sleepwalking, when these problems put the youth at risk of an accident or make it impossible for other family members to get enough sleep. Diazepam can help with insomnia (difficulty falling asleep) when used for a short time along with a behavioral program.

Sometimes diazepam is used for a few days to treat agitation in mania or psychosis until other medicines start to work.

How Does This Medicine Work?

Diazepam works by calming the parts of the brain that are too excitable in anxious people. The medicine does this by working on *receptors* (special places on brain cells) in certain parts of the brain to change the action of *GABA*, a *neurotransmitter*—a chemical that the brain makes for brain cells to communicate with each other.

How Long Does This Medicine Last?

Diazepam usually needs to be taken twice a day. For acute symptoms of anxiety or agitation, it can be taken occasionally as needed. When used for sleep, it is taken at bedtime. There may still be some effects in the morning, because it lasts a long time.

How Will the Doctor Monitor This Medicine?

The doctor will review your child's medical history and physical examination before starting diazepam. The doctor may order some blood or urine tests or an ECG (electrocardiogram or heart rhythm test) to be sure your child does not have a hidden medical condition. The doctor or nurse may measure your child's height, weight, pulse, and blood pressure before starting diazepam.

After the medicine is started, the doctor will want to have regular appointments with you and your child to see how the medicine is working, to see if a dose change is needed, to watch for side effects, to see if diazepam is still needed, and to see if any other treatment is needed. The doctor or nurse may check your child's height, weight, pulse, and blood pressure.

What Side Effects Can This Medicine Have?

Any medicine can have side effects, including an allergy to the medicine. Because each patient is different, the doctor will monitor the youth closely, especially when the medicine is started. The doctor will work with you to increase the positive effects and decrease the negative effects of the medicine. Please tell the doctor if any of the listed side effects appear or if you think that the medicine is causing any other problems. Not all of the rare or unusual side effects are listed.

Side effects are most common after starting the medicine or after a dose increase. Many side effects can be avoided or lessened by starting with a very low dose and increasing it slowly—ask the doctor.

Allergic Reaction

Tell the doctor in a day or two (if possible, before the next dose of medicine):

- Hives
- Itching
- Rash

Stop the medicine and get *immediate* medical care:

- Trouble breathing or chest tightness
- Swelling of lips, tongue, or throat

Diazepam is usually very safe when used for short periods as the doctor prescribes. The most common side effect is daytime sleepiness. Diazepam can also cause dizziness, feeling "spacey," or decreased coordination. If the medicine is causing any of these problems it is very important not to drive a car, ride a bicycle or motorcycle, or operate machinery.

Diazepam can cause decreased concentration and memory. These problems, along with daytime sleepiness, may decrease learning and performance in school.

People who take diazepam must not drink alcohol. Severe sleepiness or even loss of consciousness may result.

It is possible to become psychologically and physically dependent on diazepam, but that is not a common problem for patients who see their doctors regularly. Because some people abuse benzodiazepines, it is illegal to give or sell these medicines to someone other than the patient for whom they were prescribed.

Very rarely, diazepam causes excitement, irritability, anger, aggression, trouble sleeping, nightmares, uncontrollable behavior, or memory loss. This is called *disinhibition* or a *paradoxical effect*. Stop the medicine and call the doctor if this happens.

Some Interactions With Other Medicines or Food

Please note that the following are only the most likely interactions with food or other medicines.

Diazepam may be taken with or without food.

It is important not to use other sedatives, tranquilizers, or sleeping pills or antihistamines (such as Benadryl) when taking diazepam because of greatly increased side effects.

Oral contraceptives (birth control pills), cimetidine (Tagamet), antifungal agents (such as ketoconazole), fluoxetine (Prozac), propranolol (Inderal), valproate (Depakote), and other medicines may increase the levels of diazepam and increase side effects.

It is better to limit drinks with caffeine (coffee, tea, soft drinks) because caffeine works in the opposite way from this medicine, and the positive effects might be decreased.

What Could Happen if This Medicine Is Stopped Suddenly?

Many medicines cause problems if stopped suddenly. Diazepam must be decreased slowly (tapered) rather than stopped suddenly. When diazepam is stopped suddenly, there are withdrawal symptoms that are uncomfortable and may even be dangerous, although because diazepam is longer lasting, it causes fewer withdrawal problems than shorter-acting benzodiazepines such as alprazolam (Xanax). Problems are more likely in patients taking high doses of diazepam for 2 months or longer, but even after just a few weeks of taking diazepam it is important to stop it slowly. Withdrawal symptoms may include anxiety, irritability, shaking, sweating, aches and pains, muscle cramps, vomiting, confusion, and trouble sleeping. If large doses taken for a long time are stopped suddenly, seizures (fits, convulsions), hallucinations (hearing voices or seeing things that are not there), or out-of-control behavior may result.

How Long Will This Medicine Be Needed?

Diazepam is usually prescribed for only a few weeks to allow the patient to be calm enough to learn new ways to cope with anxiety and to allow the nervous system to become less excitable. Sometimes antianxiety medicines are used for longer periods to treat panic attacks or anxiety that remains after therapy is completed. Each person is unique, and some people may need these medicines for months or years.

What Else Should I Know About This Medicine?

Because benzodiazepines can be abused (especially by people who abuse alcohol or drugs) and can cause psychological dependence or physical dependence (addiction), they are regulated by special state and federal laws as *controlled substances*. These laws place limitations on telephone prescriptions and refills, and prescriptions expire if they are not filled promptly.

People with sleep apnea (breathing stops while they are asleep) should not take diazepam. Tell the doctor if your child snores very loudly.

Diazepam should be avoided during pregnancy, especially in the first 3 months, because it may cause birth defects in the baby. If taken regularly at the end of pregnancy, diazepam may cause withdrawal symptoms in the baby.

Notes

Use this space to take notes or to write down questions you want to ask the doctor.

_____

_____

_____

_____

_____

_____

_____

_____

_____

_____

_____

_____

From Dulcan MK (editor): _Helping Parents, Youth, and Teachers Understand Medications for Behavioral and Emotional Problems: A Resource Book of Medication Information Handouts_, Third Edition. Washington, DC, American Psychiatric Publishing, 2007

Medication Information for Youth

Diazepam—Valium

What the Medicine Is Called and What It Is For

The name of your medicine may be confusing. Most drugs have two names: 1) a scientific name that we call a *generic name* and 2) a trade or *brand name*. The generic name of this medicine is diazepam. The brand name is Valium.

Diazepam is a *benzodiazepine* or *antianxiety* medicine. It works by calming the parts of the brain that are too excitable in anxious people. It can decrease anxiety, nervousness, fears, and excessive worrying. Diazepam can decrease the physical symptoms (rapid heartbeat, trouble breathing, dizziness, sweating) of panic attacks and phobias. It can help anxious people to be calm enough to learn—with therapy and practice—to understand and tolerate their worries or fears and even to overcome them. Your doctor may have told you that you have a condition such as social phobia, generalized anxiety disorder, separation anxiety disorder, posttraumatic stress disorder (PTSD), or panic disorder. Most often, this medicine is used for a short time when symptoms are very uncomfortable or frightening or when they make it hard to do important things such as go to school.

Diazepam also can be used for sleep problems, such as night terrors (sudden waking up from sleep very scared) or sleepwalking. Diazepam can help with insomnia (difficulty falling asleep) when used for a short time along with routines that help you to relax and fall asleep.

Sometimes diazepam is used for a few days to treat agitation in mania or psychosis until other medicines start to work.

How You Take the Medicine

It is very important to take the medicine exactly as the doctor or nurse tells you. Do not skip doses or take extra medicine without asking an adult. If you forget a dose, ask your parent(s) what to do.

It is better to limit drinks with caffeine (coffee, tea, soft drinks) because caffeine works in the opposite way from this medicine, and the positive effects might be decreased.

This medicine is prescribed only for you. It should never be shared with anyone else.

You do not have to tell others that you are taking this medicine, but it is not something you should feel ashamed or embarrassed about. Many young people are helped by diazepam. You should talk to your doctor or nurse about any questions you have about the medicine. It is important to remember that the medicine *helps* you. It cannot *make* you do anything or change you as a person.

Many medicines cause problems if stopped suddenly. Always ask your doctor before stopping a medicine. Problems are more likely to happen in patients taking high doses of diazepam for 2 months or longer, but it is important to decrease the medicine slowly (taper) even after a few weeks. If you notice anxiety, irritability, shaking, sweating, aches and pains, muscle cramps, vomiting, or trouble sleeping, you may need to decrease the medicine more slowly. If large doses are stopped suddenly, seizures (fits, convulsions), hallucinations (hearing voices or seeing things that are not there), or out-of-control behavior may result.

How Your Doctor Will Follow Your Progress

Before giving you the medicine, your doctor or nurse will talk with you and your parent(s) and may measure your height, weight, heart rate (pulse), and blood pressure.

Be sure to tell your doctor or nurse about any other medicines or supplements you are taking, including vitamins, herbs, or aids to weight loss or bodybuilding. Also be sure to tell the doctor or nurse if you are using alcohol or drugs. Because many medicines may affect babies, it is very important to tell the doctor if you might be pregnant or if you are at risk of becoming pregnant.

Your teachers may be asked to fill out a form about your grades and behavior in school. A psychologist may give you some tests to see how you learn best.

Most doctors have regular appointments with young people who are taking medicine. You should use these visits to share any concerns you may have about your medicine and to talk about if it has helped you. From time to time, your physician or nurse may measure your height, weight, heart rate (pulse), and blood pressure to be sure that you are in good health while you are taking the medicine. Your doctor also will ask for regular reports from your parents and maybe from your teachers (with your permission) to see how well the medicine is working.

Diazepam is usually prescribed for only a few weeks to allow you to be calm enough to learn new ways to cope with anxiety and to allow the nervous system to become less excitable. Sometimes antianxiety medicines are used for longer periods to treat panic attacks or anxiety that remains after therapy is completed. Each person is unique, and some people may need these medicines for months or years.

How the Medicine Might Affect You

In addition to the ways the medicine can help you, it may have other effects called *side effects*. Different medicines have different side effects. It is helpful to know about some of the most common side effects of your medicine so that you will understand what they are if they happen. Some people do not have any side effects. Some side effects are just uncomfortable, but others may mean a more serious problem with the medicine. Side effects are most common after starting the medicine or after a dose increase. They may go away with time, or the medicine can be adjusted or changed—ask the doctor.

You could have an allergy to any medicine, which might show up as a rash on your skin, swelling, itching, or trouble breathing.

Please tell your parent(s) and your doctor or nurse about any changes that you notice after taking the medicine. It is especially important to tell a responsible adult if you are feeling depressed or that you may not want to live; if you have thoughts of hurting yourself; or if you begin to feel more irritable, nervous, or restless.

The most common side effect of diazepam is daytime sleepiness. If this medicine is making you sleepy, it is very important not to drive a car or ride a bicycle or motorcycle. After starting diazepam or increasing the dose, please be extra careful when driving a car, riding a bike, or using machines until you can tell how the medicine affects your alertness, attention, and coordination.

Sometimes antianxiety medicines seem to work in the opposite way, causing excitement, irritability, anger, aggression, and other problems. If this happens, tell your parent(s) or your doctor.

Drinking alcohol while taking this medicine can cause severe drowsiness or even passing out. **Don't do it!** Do not use marijuana or street drugs while taking this medicine. They can cause serious side effects. Skipping your medicine to take drugs does not work because many medicines stay in your body for a long time.

Diazepam can be habit-forming, but that is not a common problem for people who take their medicine as the doctor says.

Notes

Use this space to take notes or to write down questions you want to ask the doctor or nurse.

_____

_____

_____

_____

_____

_____

_____

_____

_____

_____

_____

From Dulcan MK (editor): *Helping Parents, Youth, and Teachers Understand Medications for Behavioral and Emotional Problems: A Resource Book of Medication Information Handouts*, Third Edition. Washington, DC, American Psychiatric Publishing, 2007

Medication Information for Parents and Teachers

Diphenhydramine—Benadryl

General Information About Medication

Each child and adolescent is different. No one has exactly the same combination of medical and psychological problems. It is a good idea to talk with the doctor or nurse about the reasons a medicine is being used. It is very important to keep all appointments and to be in touch by telephone if you have concerns. It is important to communicate with the doctor, nurse, or therapist.

It is very important that the medicine be taken exactly as the doctor instructs. However, once in a while, everyone forgets to give a medicine on time. It is a good idea to ask the doctor or nurse what to do if this happens. Do not stop or change a medicine without asking the doctor or nurse first.

If the medicine seems to stop working, it may be because it is not being taken regularly. The youth may be "cheeking" or hiding the medicine or forgetting to take it (especially at school). The doses may be too far apart, or a different dose may be needed. Something at school at home, or in the neighborhood may be upsetting the youth, or he or she may need special help for learning disabilities or tutoring. Please discuss your concerns with the doctor. **Do not just increase the dose.**

All medicines should be kept in a safe place, out of the reach of children, and should be supervised by an adult. If someone takes too much of a medicine, call the doctor the poison control center, or a hospital emergency room.

Each medicine has a "generic" or chemical name. Just like laundry detergents or paper towels, some medicines are sold by more than one company under different brand names. The same medicine may be available under a generic name and several brand names. The generic medications are usually less expensive than the brand name ones. The generic medications have the same chemical formula, but they may or may not be exactly the same strength as the brand-name medications. Also, some brands of pills contain dye that can cause allergic reactions. It is a good idea to talk to the doctor and the pharmacist about whether it is important to use a specific brand of medicine.

All medicines can cause an allergic reaction. Examples are hives, itching, rashes, swelling, and trouble breathing. Even a tiny amount of a medicine can cause a reaction in patients who are allergic to that medicine. Be *sure* to talk to the doctor before restarting a medicine that has caused an allergic reaction.

Taking more than one medicine at the same time may cause more side effects or cause one of the medicines to not work as well. Always ask the doctor, nurse, or pharmacist before adding another medicine, whether prescription or over-the-counter. Be sure that each doctor knows about *all* of the medicines your child is taking. Also tell the doctor about any vitamins, herbal medicines, or supplements your child may be taking. Some of these may have side effects alone or when taken with this medication.

Everyone taking medicine should have a physical examination at least once a year.

If you suspect the youth is using drugs or alcohol, please tell the doctor right away.

Pregnancy requires special care in the use of medicine. Please tell the doctor immediately if you suspect the teenager is pregnant or might become pregnant.

217

Printed information like this applies to children and adolescents in general. If you have questions about the medicine, or if you notice changes or anything unusual, please ask the doctor or nurse. As scientific research advances, knowledge increases and advice changes. Even experts do not always agree. Many medicines have not been approved by the U.S. Food and Drug Administration (FDA) for use in children. For this reason, use of the medicine for a particular problem or age group often is not listed in the *Physicians' Desk Reference*. This does not necessarily mean that the medicine is dangerous or does not work, only that the company that makes the medicine has not received permission to advertise the medicine for use in children. Companies often do not apply for this permission because it is expensive to do the tests needed to apply for approval for use in children. Once a medication is approved by the FDA for any purpose, a doctor is allowed to prescribe it according to research and clinical experience.

Note to Teachers

It is a good idea to talk with the parent(s) about the reason(s) that a medication is being used. If the parent(s) sign consent to release information, it is often helpful to talk with the doctor. If the parent(s) give permission, the doctor may ask you to fill out rating forms about your experience with the student's behavior, feelings, academic performance, and medication side effects. This information is very useful in selecting and monitoring medication treatment. If you have observations that you think are important, do not hesitate to share these with the student's parent(s) and treating clinicians.

It is very important that the medicine be taken exactly as the doctor instructs. However, everyone forgets to give a medicine on time once in a while. It is a good idea to ask the parent(s) in advance what to do if this happens. Do not stop or change the time you are giving a medicine at school without parental permission. If a medication is to be taken with food, but lunchtime or snack time changes, be sure to notify the parent(s) so appropriate adjustments can be made.

All medicines should be kept in a secure place and should be supervised by an adult. If someone takes too much of a medicine, follow your school procedure for an urgent medical problem.

Taking medicine is a private matter and is best managed discreetly and confidentially. It is important to be sensitive to the student's feelings about taking medicine.

If you suspect that the student is using drugs or alcohol, please tell the parent(s) or a school counselor right away.

Please tell the parent(s) or school nurse if you suspect medication side effects.

Modifications of the classroom environment or assignments may be useful in addition to medication. The student may need to be evaluated for additional help or for an Individualized Education Plan for learning or behavior.

Any expression of suicidal thoughts or feelings or self-harm by a child or adolescent is a clear signal of distress and should be taken seriously. These behaviors should not be dismissed as "attention seeking."

What Is Diphenhydramine (Benadryl)?

Diphenhydramine is called an *antihistamine*. These medicines were developed to treat allergies. It is sometimes used to treat anxiety (nervousness), insomnia (difficulty falling asleep), or the side effects of certain other medicines (such as antipsychotics).

Diphenhydramine comes in many different forms—including tablet, capsule, chewable tablet, orally disintegrating tablet (dissolves in the mouth), suspension (liquid), and as one ingredient in many combination over-the-counter medicines for colds and allergies. The medicine also comes in an injection (shot).

How Can This Medicine Help?

Diphenhydramine may decrease nervousness. When used for anxiety, it works best when used for a short time along with psychotherapy. Diphenhydramine can help with insomnia when used for a short time along with a behavioral program, such as regular soothing routines at bedtime and increased exercise in the daytime. It can reduce some of the movement side effects of the antipsychotic medicines, such as severe restlessness, agitation, and pacing *(akathisia)*; muscle spasms *(dystonia)*; muscle stiffness *(cogwheeling rigidity)*; or trembling. Sometimes these are called *parkinsonian* or *extrapyramidal* symptoms. Diphenhydramine can be given regularly to prevent or treat these problems. If there is a sudden, severe muscle spasm, diphenhydramine may be given as a shot so that it works within 15 minutes.

How Does This Medicine Work?

Diphenhydramine can help decrease anxiety and help falling asleep because of its *sedative* effect—that is, it makes people a little sleepy so that they feel less nervous and also fall asleep more easily.

Diphenhydramine counteracts the effects of the antipsychotic medicines in parts of the brain that control muscle action, but without decreasing the effects of the antipsychotic medicines on thinking and other psychiatric symptoms. It balances the *cholinergic* and *dopamine* systems in the brain.

How Long Does This Medicine Last?

Diphenhydramine lasts for 4–7 hours. When used with an antipsychotic medicine, it is usually taken three or four times a day.

How Will the Doctor Monitor This Medicine?

The doctor will review your child's medical history and physical examination before starting diphenhydramine. Be sure to tell the doctor if your child or anyone in the family has a history of asthma or of heart rhythm problems, palpitations, or fainting. The doctor or nurse may measure your child's height, weight, pulse, and blood pressure before starting the medicine. An examination such as the AIMS (Abnormal Involuntary Movement Scale) test may be used to check your child's tongue, legs, and arms for unusual movements that could be helped by the medicine.

After the medicine is started, the doctor will want to have regular appointments with you and your child to see how the medicine is working, to see if a dose change is needed, to watch for side effects, to see if diphenhydramine is still needed, and to see if any other treatment is needed. The doctor or nurse may check your child's height, weight, pulse, and blood pressure.

What Side Effects Can This Medicine Have?

Any medicine can have side effects, including an allergy to the medicine. Because each patient is different, the doctor will monitor the youth closely, especially when the medicine is started. The doctor will work with you

to increase the positive effects and decrease the negative effects of the medicine. Please tell the doctor if any of the listed side effects appear or if you think that the medicine is causing any other problems. Not all of the rare or unusual side effects are listed.

Side effects are most common after starting the medicine or after a dose increase. Many side effects can be avoided or lessened by starting with a very low dose and increasing it slowly—ask the doctor.

Allergic Reaction

Tell the doctor in a day or two (if possible, before the next dose of medicine):

- Hives
- Itching
- Rash

Stop the medicine and get *immediate* medical care:

- Trouble breathing or chest tightness
- Swelling of lips, tongue, or throat

Common Side Effects

Tell the doctor within a week or two:

- Daytime sleepiness—Do not allow your child to drive, ride a bicycle or motorcycle, or operate machinery if this happens.
- Decreased attention, memory, or learning in school
- Dry mouth—Have your child try using sugar-free gum or candy.
- Headache
- Blurred vision
- Constipation—Encourage your child to drink more fluids and eat high-fiber foods; if necessary, the doctor may recommend a fiber medicine such as Benefiber or a stool softener such as Colace or mineral oil.
- Trouble passing urine
- Dizziness or light-headedness—This side effect is worse when the child stands up quickly, especially when getting out of bed in the morning; try having the child stand up slowly.
- Loss of appetite, nausea, or upset stomach

Less Common Side Effects

Call the doctor within a day or two:

- Poor coordination
- Motor tics (fast, repeated movements)
- Unusual muscle movements
- Irritability, overactivity
- Waking up after sleeping for a short time and being unable to get back to sleep.
- Exposure to sunlight may cause severe sunburn, skin rash, redness, or itching; avoid direct exposure to sunlight or use sunscreen.

Very Rare, but Serious, Side Effects

Call the doctor immediately:

- Worsening of asthma or trouble breathing
- Seizure (fit, convulsion)
- Uncontrollable behavior
- Hallucinations (seeing things that are not really there)
- Severe muscle stiffness
- Irregular heartbeat (pulse), fainting, palpitations

Some Interactions With Other Medicines or Food

Please note that the following are only the most likely interactions with food or other medicines.

If other medicines that can cause sleepiness are taken with diphenhydramine, severe sleepiness can result.

What Could Happen if This Medicine Is Stopped Suddenly?

Stopping these medicines suddenly does not usually cause problems, but diarrhea or feeling sick may result if diphenhydramine has been taken for a long time. The problem being treated may come back. Always ask the doctor whether a medicine can be stopped suddenly or must be decreased slowly (tapered).

How Long Will This Medicine Be Needed?

When used for nervousness or sleep, diphenhydramine is usually prescribed for a very short time to allow the patient to be calm enough to learn new ways to cope. If the person needs treatment for a longer time, another medicine is usually prescribed.

When being used to reduce the motor side effects of an antipsychotic medicine, sometimes the diphenhydramine will be needed as long as the person is on the antipsychotic medicine, but sometimes it can be carefully tapered (decreased) and stopped if the person has gotten used to the antipsychotic medicine and there are no longer motor side effects.

What Else Should I Know About This Medicine?

People who take diphenhydramine must not drink alcohol. Severe sleepiness or even loss of consciousness may result.

Diphenhydramine may be confused with desipramine. Benadryl may be confused with Caladryl. Be sure to check the medicine when you get it from the pharmacist.

Notes

Use this space to take notes or to write down questions you want to ask the doctor.

_____

_____

_____

_____

_____

_____

_____

_____

_____

_____

_____

_____

From Dulcan MK (editor): _Helping Parents, Youth, and Teachers Understand Medications for Behavioral and Emotional Problems: A Resource Book of Medication Information Handouts_, Third Edition. Washington, DC, American Psychiatric Publishing, 2007

Medication Information for Youth

Diphenhydramine—Benadryl

What the Medicine Is Called and What It Is For

The name of your medicine may be confusing. Most drugs have two names: 1) a scientific name that we call a *generic name* and 2) a trade or *brand name*. The generic name of this medicine is diphenhydramine. The brand name is Benadryl.

Diphenhydramine is called an *antihistamine*. These medicines were developed to treat allergies. It is sometimes used to treat anxiety (nervousness) or insomnia (difficulty falling asleep). It can help anxious people to be calm enough to learn—with therapy and practice—to understand and tolerate their worries or fears and even to overcome them. Most often, this medicine is used for a short time when symptoms are very uncomfortable or frightening or when they make it hard to do important things such as go to school. Diphenhydramine can help with insomnia when used for a short time along with calming routines that help to fall asleep. It is sometimes used to help lessen the side effects of other medicines.

How You Take the Medicine

It is very important to take the medicine exactly as the doctor or nurse tells you. Do not skip doses or take extra medicine without asking an adult. If you forget a dose, ask your parent(s) what to do. It is best to take this medicine with milk or with food. Do not use any other medicines without talking to your doctor first.

Caffeine (in coffee, tea, or soft drinks) could make you feel worse.

This medicine is prescribed only for you. It should never be shared with anyone else.

You do not have to tell others that you are taking this medicine, but it is not something you should feel ashamed or embarrassed about. Many young people are helped by diphenhydramine. This medicine is not habit-forming, and you cannot become "hooked" on it. You should talk to your doctor or nurse about any questions you have about the medicine. It is important to remember that the medicine *helps* you. It cannot *make* you do anything or change you as a person.

If you stop the medicine suddenly, it might cause you to feel sick, or the problem being treated may come back. Do not stop the medicine unless the doctor tells you to.

How Your Doctor Will Follow Your Progress

Before giving you the medicine, your doctor or nurse will talk with you and your parent(s) and may measure your height, weight, heart rate (pulse), and blood pressure.

Be sure to tell your doctor or nurse about any other medicines or supplements you are taking, including vitamins, herbs, or aids to weight loss or bodybuilding. Also be sure to tell the doctor or nurse if you are using alcohol or drugs. Because many medicines may affect babies, it is very important to tell the doctor if you might be pregnant or if you are at risk of becoming pregnant.

Most doctors have regular appointments with young people who are taking medicine. You should use these visits to share any concerns you may have about your medicine and to talk about if it has helped you. From time to time, your physician or nurse may measure your height, weight, heart rate (pulse), and blood pressure to be sure that you are in good health while you are taking the medicine. Your doctor also will ask for regular reports from your parents and maybe from your teachers (with your permission) to see how well the medicine is working.

How the Medicine Might Affect You

In addition to the ways the medicine can help you, it may have other effects called *side effects.* Different medicines have different side effects. It is helpful to know about some of the most common side effects of your medicine so that you will understand what they are if they happen. Some people do not have any side effects. Some side effects are just uncomfortable, but others may mean a more serious problem with the medicine. Side effects are most common after starting the medicine or after a dose increase. They may go away with time, or the medicine can be adjusted or changed—ask the doctor.

You could have an allergy to any medicine, which might show up as a rash on your skin, swelling, itching, or trouble breathing.

Please tell your parent(s) and your doctor or nurse about any changes that you notice after taking the medicine. It is especially important to tell a responsible adult if you are feeling depressed or that you may not want to live; if you have thoughts of hurting yourself; or if you begin to feel more irritable, nervous, or restless.

The most common side effect of diphenhydramine is daytime sleepiness. If this medicine is making you sleepy, it is very important not to drive a car or ride a bicycle or motorcycle. After starting diphenhydramine or increasing the dose, please be extra careful when driving a car, riding a bike, or using machines until you can tell how the medicine affects your alertness, attention, and coordination.

Drinking alcohol while taking this medicine can cause severe drowsiness or even passing out. **Don't do it!** Do not use marijuana or street drugs while taking this medicine. They can cause serious side effects. Skipping your medicine to take drugs does not work because many medicines stay in your body for a long time.

Tell your parent(s) or the doctor if you wake up at night after sleeping for a short time and cannot get back to sleep.

Sometimes diphenhydramine seems to work in the opposite way, causing excitement, irritability, anger, aggression, and other problems. If this happens, tell your parent(s) or your doctor.

You might feel dizzy, tired, or even faint when you stand up fast. Try standing up slowly, especially first thing in the morning when getting out of bed.

Another common side effect is dry mouth. You may be more thirsty than usual and find that you are drinking more water or other liquids than usual. Sucking on sugar-free hard candy or cough drops usually helps. You also could try chewing sugar-free gum or sucking on ice chips. Do not chew the ice; you could hurt your teeth. Also, using lip balm will keep your lips from cracking. It is important to be especially good about brushing your teeth.

Some people become constipated (have hard bowel movements) when taking this medicine. Try drinking more water and eating more fruits, vegetables, and whole grains. If that does not help, tell your parent(s) or doctor—you may need a medicine to help with this side effect.

Taking this medicine could make you more likely to get badly sunburned or very sick in hot weather. Be sure to drink plenty of liquids and cover up or use sunscreen when you go outside in hot weather. Be careful to rest in the shade and not get overheated.

Other side effects that some people get from diphenhydramine include having trouble passing urine, blurred vision, stomachache, upset stomach, or headache.

Serious side effects hardly ever happen when taking this medicine. You should tell your parent(s) and doctor if you notice anything different or unusual about how you feel once you start taking the medicine, especially if you are having trouble breathing or your body seems to be moving differently than usual.

Notes

Use this space to take notes or to write down questions you want to ask the doctor or nurse.

_____

_____

_____

_____

_____

_____

_____

_____

_____

_____

_____

From Dulcan MK (editor): *Helping Parents, Youth, and Teachers Understand Medications for Behavioral and Emotional Problems: A Resource Book of Medication Information Handouts,* Third Edition. Washington, DC, American Psychiatric Publishing, 2007

Medication Information for Parents and Teachers

Duloxetine—Cymbalta

General Information About Medication

Each child and adolescent is different. No one has exactly the same combination of medical and psychological problems. It is a good idea to talk with the doctor or nurse about the reasons a medicine is being used. It is very important to keep all appointments and to be in touch by telephone if you have concerns. It is important to communicate with the doctor, nurse, or therapist.

It is very important that the medicine be taken exactly as the doctor instructs. However, once in a while, everyone forgets to give a medicine on time. It is a good idea to ask the doctor or nurse what to do if this happens. Do not stop or change a medicine without asking the doctor or nurse first.

If the medicine seems to stop working, it may be because it is not being taken regularly. The youth may be "cheeking" or hiding the medicine or forgetting to take it (especially at school). The doses may be too far apart, or a different dose may be needed. Something at school, at home, or in the neighborhood may be upsetting the youth, or he or she may need special help for learning disabilities or tutoring. Please discuss your concerns with the doctor. **Do not just increase the dose.**

All medicines should be kept in a safe place, out of the reach of children, and should be supervised by an adult. If someone takes too much of a medicine, call the doctor, the poison control center, or a hospital emergency room.

Each medicine has a "generic" or chemical name. Just like laundry detergents or paper towels, some medicines are sold by more than one company under different brand names. The same medicine may be available under a generic name and several brand names. The generic medications are usually less expensive than the brand name ones. The generic medications have the same chemical formula, but they may or may not be exactly the same strength as the brand-name medications. Also, some brands of pills contain dye that can cause allergic reactions. It is a good idea to talk to the doctor and the pharmacist about whether it is important to use a specific brand of medicine.

All medicines can cause an allergic reaction. Examples are hives, itching, rashes, swelling, and trouble breathing. Even a tiny amount of a medicine can cause a reaction in patients who are allergic to that medicine. Be *sure* to talk to the doctor before restarting a medicine that has caused an allergic reaction.

Taking more than one medicine at the same time may cause more side effects or cause one of the medicines to not work as well. Always ask the doctor, nurse, or pharmacist before adding another medicine, whether prescription or over-the-counter. Be sure that each doctor knows about *all* of the medicines your child is taking. Also tell the doctor about any vitamins, herbal medicines, or supplements your child may be taking. Some of these may have side effects alone or when taken with this medication.

Everyone taking medicine should have a physical examination at least once a year.

If you suspect the youth is using drugs or alcohol, please tell the doctor right away.

227

Pregnancy requires special care in the use of medicine. Please tell the doctor immediately if you suspect the teenager is pregnant or might become pregnant.

Printed information like this applies to children and adolescents in general. If you have questions about the medicine, or if you notice changes or anything unusual, please ask the doctor or nurse. As scientific research advances, knowledge increases and advice changes. Even experts do not always agree. Many medicines have not been approved by the U.S. Food and Drug Administration (FDA) for use in children. For this reason, use of the medicine for a particular problem or age group often is not listed in the *Physicians' Desk Reference*. This does not necessarily mean that the medicine is dangerous or does not work, only that the company that makes the medicine has not received permission to advertise the medicine for use in children. Companies often do not apply for this permission because it is expensive to do the tests needed to apply for approval for use in children. Once a medication is approved by the FDA for any purpose, a doctor is allowed to prescribe it according to research and clinical experience.

Note to Teachers

It is a good idea to talk with the parent(s) about the reason(s) that a medication is being used. If the parent(s) sign consent to release information, it is often helpful to talk with the doctor. If the parent(s) give permission, the doctor may ask you to fill out rating forms about your experience with the student's behavior, feelings, academic performance, and medication side effects. This information is very useful in selecting and monitoring medication treatment. If you have observations that you think are important, do not hesitate to share these with the student's parent(s) and treating clinicians.

It is very important that the medicine be taken exactly as the doctor instructs. However, everyone forgets to give a medicine on time once in a while. It is a good idea to ask the parent(s) in advance what to do if this happens. Do not stop or change the time you are giving a medicine at school without parental permission. If a medication is to be taken with food, but lunchtime or snack time changes, be sure to notify the parent(s) so appropriate adjustments can be made.

All medicines should be kept in a secure place and should be supervised by an adult. If someone takes too much of a medicine, follow your school procedure for an urgent medical problem.

Taking medicine is a private matter and is best managed discreetly and confidentially. It is important to be sensitive to the student's feelings about taking medicine.

If you suspect that the student is using drugs or alcohol, please tell the parent(s) or a school counselor right away.

Please tell the parent(s) or school nurse if you suspect medication side effects.

Modifications of the classroom environment or assignments may be useful in addition to medication. The student may need to be evaluated for additional help or for an Individualized Education Plan for learning or behavior.

Any expression of suicidal thoughts or feelings or self-harm by a child or adolescent is a clear signal of distress and should be taken seriously. These behaviors should not be dismissed as "attention seeking."

What Is Duloxetine (Cymbalta)?

Duloxetine is a new *antidepressant*. It is known as a *serotonin-norepinephrine reuptake inhibitor* (SNRI). It comes in brand name Cymbalta capsules. Compared with the *selective serotonin reuptake inhibitors* (SSRIs), less is known about duloxetine's safety and effectiveness in children and adolescents.

How Can This Medicine Help?

Duloxetine is used to treat depression. Less is known about whether it helps anxiety disorders such as obsessive-compulsive disorder (OCD), posttraumatic stress disorder (PTSD), panic disorder, or separation anxiety disorder. It is also used to treat nerve pain in adults with diabetes.

How Does This Medicine Work?

Duloxetine increases the amount of two neurotransmitters—*serotonin* and *norepinephrine*—in parts of the brain. *Neurotransmitters* are the chemicals used by brain cells to communicate. People with depression and anxiety may have low levels of serotonin and norepinephrine in certain parts of the brain. Duloxetine helps by increasing the action of these neurotransmitters to more normal levels.

How Long Does This Medicine Last?

Duloxetine is taken twice a day.

How Will the Doctor Monitor This Medicine?

The doctor will review your child's medical history and physical examination before starting duloxetine. Be sure to tell the doctor if your child or anyone in the family has had liver problems. The doctor may order some blood or urine tests to be sure your child does not have a hidden medical condition that would make it unsafe to use this medicine. Extra care is needed when using duloxetine in youth with seizures (epilepsy), liver or kidney problems, or diabetes. The doctor or nurse may measure your child's pulse, blood pressure, and weight before starting the medicine.

Be sure to tell the doctor if your child or anyone in the family has bipolar illness (manic-depressive illness) or has tried to kill himself or herself.

After the medicine is started, the doctor will want to have regular appointments with you and your child to see how the medicine is working, to see if a dose change is needed, to watch for side effects, to see if duloxetine is still needed, and to see if any other treatment is needed. The doctor or nurse may check your child's height, weight, pulse, and blood pressure. Duloxetine may cause small increases in blood pressure.

Before using medicine and at times afterward, the doctor may ask your child to fill out a rating scale about depression and anxiety, to help see how your child is doing.

What Side Effects Can This Medicine Have?

Any medicine can have side effects, including an allergy to the medicine. Because each patient is different, the doctor will monitor the youth closely, especially when the medicine is started. The doctor will work with you to increase the positive effects and decrease the negative effects of the medicine. Please tell the doctor if any of the listed side effects appear or if you think that the medicine is causing any other problems. Not all of the rare or unusual side effects are listed.

Side effects are most common after starting the medicine or after a dose increase. Many side effects can be avoided or lessened by starting with a very low dose and increasing it slowly—ask the doctor.

Allergic Reaction

Tell the doctor in a day or two (if possible, before the next dose of medicine):

- Hives
- Itching
- Rash

Stop the medicine and get *immediate* medical care:

- Trouble breathing or chest tightness
- Swelling of lips, tongue, or throat

Common Side Effects

Tell the doctor within a week or two:

- Nausea, upset stomach, vomiting
- Decreased appetite
- Dry mouth—Have your child try using sugar-free gum or candy.
- Constipation—Encourage your child to drink more fluids and eat high-fiber foods; if necessary, the doctor may recommend a fiber medicine such as Benefiber or a stool softener such as Colace or mineral oil.
- Insomnia (trouble sleeping)
- Daytime sleepiness or tiredness—Do not allow your child to drive, ride a bicycle or motorcycle, or operate machinery if this happens.
- Dizziness—This side effect is worse when the child stands up quickly, especially when getting out of bed in the morning; try having the child stand up slowly.
- Excessive sweating

Less Common, but More Serious, Side Effects

Call the doctor within a day or two:

- Significant suicidal thoughts or self-injurious behavior
- Increased activity, rapid speech, feeling "speeded up," decreased need for sleep, being very excited or irritable (cranky)

Serious Side Effects

Call the doctor *immediately* or go to the nearest emergency room:

- Seizure (fit, convulsion)
- Stiffness, high fever, confusion, tremors (shaking)
- Overheating or heatstroke—Prevent by decreasing activity in hot weather, staying out of the sun, and drinking water.

Serotonin Syndrome

A very serious side effect called *serotonin syndrome* can happen when certain kinds of medicines (including some medicines for migraine headaches—triptans) are taken by the same person. *Very* rarely, it can happen at high doses of just one medicine. The early signs are restlessness, confusion, shaking, skin turning red, sweating, and jerking of muscles. If you see these symptoms, stop the medicine and send or take the youth to an emergency room right away.

Some Interactions With Other Medicines or Food

Please note that the following are only the most likely interactions with food or other medicines.

Duloxetine interacts with many other medicines, including some antibiotics and other psychiatric medicines. It is especially important to tell the doctor and pharmacist about all of the medicines your child is taking or has taken in the past few months, including over-the-counter and herbal medicines. Sometimes one medicine can increase or decrease the blood level of another medicine, so that different doses are needed. Cipro and Tagamet both increase the level of duloxetine. When switching from fluvoxamine, paroxetine, or fluoxetine to duloxetine, lower doses of duloxetine are needed, because those other antidepressants increase the levels of duloxetine. The herbal medicine St. John's wort also increases serotonin and can cause serious side effects if taken with duloxetine.

It can be *very dangerous* to take duloxetine at the same time as or even within a month of taking another type of medicine called a *monoamine oxidase inhibitor* (MAOI), such as Eldepryl (selegiline), Nardil (phenelzine), Parnate (tranylcypromine), or Marplan (isocarboxazid).

Duloxetine does not usually cause problems when taken with decongestant cold medicines.

Duloxetine can be taken with or without food.

Caffeine may increase side effects.

What Could Happen if This Medicine Is Stopped Suddenly?

If duloxetine is stopped suddenly, there may be uncomfortable withdrawal feelings, including dizziness, headache, irritability, and nightmares. Do not stop this medicine suddenly, and ask the doctor if these symptoms happen as the medicine is being tapered (dose decreased).

How Long Will This Medicine Be Needed?

Duloxetine may take up to 1–2 months to reach its full effect. If your child has a good response to duloxetine, it is a good idea to continue the medicine for at least 6 months.

What Else Should I Know About This Medicine?

In youth who have bipolar disorder (manic depression) or who are at risk for bipolar disorder, any antidepressant medicine may increase the risk of hypomania or mania (excitement, agitation, increased activity, decreased sleep).

Smoking may lower the levels of duloxetine, making it not work as well.

In hot weather, make sure your child drinks enough water or other liquids and does not get overheated.

Sometimes, after a person has improved while taking duloxetine, he or she loses interest in school or friends or just stops trying. Please tell your child's doctor if this happens—it may be a side effect of the medicine. A lower dose or a different medicine may be needed.

Store the medicine away from sunlight, heat, moisture, and humidity.

Duloxetine capsules should not be crushed, chewed, sprinkled on food, or mixed with juice but should be swallowed whole.

Black Box Antidepressant Warning

In 2004, an advisory committee to the FDA decided that there might be an increased risk of suicidal behavior for some youth taking medicines called *antidepressants*. In the research studies that the committee reviewed, about 3%–4% of youth with depression who took an antidepressant medicine—and 1%–2% of youth with depression who took a placebo (pill without active medicine)—talked about suicidal thoughts (thinking about killing themselves or wishing they were dead) or did something to harm themselves. This means that almost twice as many youth who were taking an antidepressant to treat their depression talked about suicide or had suicidal behavior compared with youth with depression who were taking inactive medicine. There were *no* completed suicides in any of these research studies, which included more than 4,000 children and adolescents. For youth being treated for anxiety, there was no difference in suicidal talking or behavior between those taking antidepressant medication and those taking placebo.

The FDA told drug companies to add a *black box warning* label to all antidepressant medicines. Because of this label, a doctor (or advanced practice nurse) prescribing one of these medicines has to warn youth and their families that there might be more suicidal thoughts and actions in youth taking these medicines.

On the other hand, in places where more youth are taking the newer antidepressant medicines, the number of adolescents who commit suicide has gotten smaller. Also, thinking about or attempting suicide is more common in surveys of teenagers in the community than it is in depressed youth treated in research studies with antidepressant medicine.

If a youth is being treated with this medicine and is doing well, then no changes are needed as a result of this warning. Increased suicidal talk or action is most likely to happen in the first few months of treatment with a medicine. If your child has recently started this medicine or is about to start, then you and your doctor (or advanced practice nurse) should watch for any changes in behavior. People who are depressed often have suicidal thoughts or actions. It is hard to know whether suicidal thoughts or actions in depressed people are caused by the depression itself or by the medicine. Also, as their depression is getting better, some people talk more about the suicidal thoughts that they had before but did not talk about. As young people get better from depression, they might be at higher risk of doing something about suicidal thoughts that they have had for some time, because they have more energy.

What Should A Parent Do?

1. Be honest with your child about possible risks and benefits of medicine.
2. Talk to your child about whether he or she is having any suicidal thoughts, and tell your child to come to you if he or she is having such thoughts.
3. You, your child, and your child's doctor or nurse should develop a safety plan. Pick adults whom your child can tell if he or she is thinking about suicide.
4. Be sure to tell your child's doctor, nurse, or therapist if you suspect that your child is using alcohol or drugs or if something has happened that might make your child feel worse, such as a family separation, breaking up with a boyfriend or girlfriend, someone close dying or attempting suicide, physical or sexual abuse, or failure in school.

5. Be sure that there are no guns in the home and that all medicines (including over-the-counter medicines like Tylenol) are closely supervised by an adult and kept in a safe place.

6. Watch for new or worse thoughts of suicide, self-harm, depression, anxiety (nerves), feeling very agitated or restless, being angry or aggressive, having more trouble sleeping, or anything else that you see for the first time, seems worse, or worries your child or you. If these appear, contact a mental health professional **right away.** Do not just stop or change the dose of the medicine on your own. If the problems are serious, and you cannot reach one of your clinicians, call a 24-hour psychiatry emergency telephone number or take your child to an emergency room.

Youth on antidepressant medicine should be watched carefully by their parent(s), clinician(s) (doctor, nurse, therapist), and other concerned adults for the first weeks of treatment. It is a good idea to have a visit or telephone call with the doctor, nurse, or therapist weekly for the first month, every 2 weeks for the second month, and after that at least once a month to check for feelings of depression or sadness, thoughts of killing or harming himself or herself, and any problems with the medication. If you have questions, be sure to ask the doctor, nurse, or therapist.

For more information, see http://www.parentsmedguide.org/ (in English and Spanish).

Notes

Use this space to take notes or to write down questions you want to ask the doctor.

_____

_____

_____

_____

_____

_____

_____

_____

_____

_____

_____

From Dulcan MK (editor): *Helping Parents, Youth, and Teachers Understand Medications for Behavioral and Emotional Problems: A Resource Book of Medication Information Handouts*, Third Edition. Washington, DC, American Psychiatric Publishing, 2007

Medication Information for Youth

Duloxetine—Cymbalta

What the Medicine Is Called and What It Is For

The name of your medicine may be confusing. Most drugs have two names: 1) a scientific name that we call a *generic name* and 2) a trade or *brand name*. The generic name of this medicine is duloxetine. The brand name is Cymbalta.

Duloxetine is called an *antidepressant*. Duloxetine is used to treat depression. It is also used to treat nerve pain.

How You Take the Medicine

It is very important to take the medicine exactly as the doctor or nurse tells you. Do not skip doses or take extra medicine without asking an adult. If you forget a dose, ask your parent(s) what to do. It is very important that you take all the pills you are supposed to take each day. Your doctor will probably recommend that you take your medicine at the same time each day, which may be with meals or at bedtime.

It may take a month before you notice that the medicine is helping. Waiting for the full effect may take even longer. You may feel discouraged and think the medicine is never going to help. You may want to give up and stop taking the medicine. Talk to your doctor and parent(s) about how you feel, but **do not stop** taking the medicine unless your doctor tells you to. It is also important not to take extra pills, hoping that you will feel better faster. Doing that could make you sick.

Duloxetine capsules should not be crushed or chewed but should be swallowed whole.

Caffeine (in coffee, tea, or soft drinks) may make you feel worse.

Smoking may lower the levels of duloxetine so that it does not work as well.

This medicine is prescribed only for you. It should never be shared with anyone else.

You do not have to tell others that you are taking this medicine, but it is not something you should feel ashamed or embarrassed about. Many young people are helped by duloxetine. This medicine is not habit-forming, and you cannot become "hooked" on it. You should talk to your doctor or nurse about any questions you have about the medicine. It is important to remember that the medicine *helps* you. It cannot *make* you do anything or change you as a person.

How Your Doctor Will Follow Your Progress

Before giving you the medicine, your doctor or nurse will talk with you and your parent(s) and may measure your height, weight, heart rate (pulse), and blood pressure. The doctor may order some blood or urine tests to be sure you are in good health.

Be sure to tell your doctor or nurse about any other medicines or supplements you are taking, including vitamins, herbs, or aids to weight loss or bodybuilding. Also be sure to tell the doctor or nurse if you are using alcohol or drugs. Because many medicines may affect babies, it is very important to tell the doctor if you might be pregnant or if you are at risk of becoming pregnant. Be sure to tell the doctor if you have had thoughts of hurting yourself, have tried to hurt yourself, or sometimes wish that you were not alive.

Your teachers may be asked to fill out a form about your grades and behavior in school. A psychologist may give you some tests to see how you learn best.

Before starting the medicine and afterward, the doctor may ask you to answer questions on paper about depression and anxiety.

Most doctors have regular appointments with young people who are taking medicine. You should use these visits to share any concerns you may have about your medicine and to talk about if it has helped you. From time to time, your physician or nurse may measure your height, weight, heart rate (pulse), and blood pressure to be sure that you are in good health while you are taking the medicine. Your doctor also will ask for regular reports from your parents and maybe from your teachers (with your permission) to see how well the medicine is working.

Some medicines are started at the amount you will take for as long as you are taking that medicine. Other medicines need to be increased or adjusted until your doctor decides you are taking the right amount. Starting at a low dose and increasing it slowly may lessen side effects. If the medicine helps you, your doctor will probably want you to take it for 6 months to a year.

Stopping the medicine suddenly can cause uncomfortable feelings. Do not stop the medicine unless the doctor tells you to.

How the Medicine Might Affect You

In addition to the ways the medicine can help you, it may have other effects called *side effects*. Different medicines have different side effects. It is helpful to know about some of the most common side effects of your medicine so that you will understand what they are if they happen. Some people do not have any side effects. Some side effects are just uncomfortable, but others may mean a more serious problem with the medicine. Side effects are most common after starting the medicine or after a dose increase. They may go away with time, or the medicine can be adjusted or changed—ask the doctor.

You could have an allergy to any medicine, which might show up as a rash on your skin, swelling, itching, or trouble breathing.

Please tell your parent(s) and your doctor or nurse about any changes that you notice after taking the medicine. It is especially important to tell a responsible adult if you are feeling depressed or that you may not want to live; if you have thoughts of hurting yourself; or if you begin to feel more irritable, nervous, or restless. Also be sure to tell your parent(s) or doctor if you begin to feel "speeded up" or have trouble sleeping.

Some medicines make people feel sleepy or less coordinated. If this medicine is making you sleepy, it is very important not to drive a car or ride a bicycle or motorcycle. After starting a new medicine or increasing the dose of a medicine, please be extra careful when driving a car, riding a bike, or using machines until you can tell how the medicine affects your alertness, attention, and coordination.

One of the most common side effects of this medicine is feeling tired or sleepy during the day, even if you have had a full night's sleep. After you have been taking the medicine for a few weeks, your body will adjust, and this side effect may go away. If you have had trouble sleeping at night, the medicine can help you sleep better, especially if your doctor tells you to take a dose of medicine at bedtime. Other people may feel more restless and excited. Tell your parent(s) or doctor if this is uncomfortable.

This medicine may make your mouth dry. You may be more thirsty than usual and find that you are drinking more water or other liquids. Sucking on sugar-free hard candy or cough drops usually helps. You also could try chewing sugar-free gum or sucking on ice chips. Do not chew the ice; you could hurt your teeth.

Also, using lip balm will keep your lips from cracking. It is important to be especially good about brushing your teeth.

Some other side effects that could happen are headache, not feeling hungry and not wanting to eat much, eating more than usual, having an upset stomach, or changes in your bowel movements. You may have a change in your sexual functioning—it is OK to ask the doctor about this. This medicine may make you more likely to get sick if you get overheated, so be sure to drink plenty of liquids and rest in the shade in hot weather.

Please let your parent(s) and doctor know if you notice anything different or unusual about how you feel once you start taking the medicine. This includes good things, such as feeling less sad or less nervous or sleeping better at night.

Notes

Use this space to take notes or to write down questions you want to ask the doctor or nurse.

_____

_____

_____

_____

_____

_____

_____

_____

_____

_____

From Dulcan MK (editor): *Helping Parents, Youth, and Teachers Understand Medications for Behavioral and Emotional Problems: A Resource Book of Medication Information Handouts*, Third Edition. Washington, DC, American Psychiatric Publishing, 2007

Escitalopram—Lexapro

General Information About Medication

Each child and adolescent is different. No one has exactly the same combination of medical and psychological problems. It is a good idea to talk with the doctor or nurse about the reasons a medicine is being used. It is very important to keep all appointments and to be in touch by telephone if you have concerns. It is important to communicate with the doctor, nurse, or therapist.

It is very important that the medicine be taken exactly as the doctor instructs. However, once in a while, everyone forgets to give a medicine on time. It is a good idea to ask the doctor or nurse what to do if this happens. Do not stop or change a medicine without asking the doctor or nurse first.

If the medicine seems to stop working, it may be because it is not being taken regularly. The youth may be "cheeking" or hiding the medicine or forgetting to take it (especially at school). The doses may be too far apart, or a different dose may be needed. Something at school at home, or in the neighborhood may be upsetting the youth, or he or she may need special help for learning disabilities or tutoring. Please discuss your concerns with the doctor. **Do not just increase the dose.**

All medicines should be kept in a safe place, out of the reach of children, and should be supervised by an adult. If someone takes too much of a medicine, call the doctor, the poison control center, or a hospital emergency room.

Each medicine has a "generic" or chemical name. Just like laundry detergents or paper towels, some medicines are sold by more than one company under different brand names. The same medicine may be available under a generic name and several brand names. The generic medications are usually less expensive than the brand name ones. The generic medications have the same chemical formula, but they may or may not be exactly the same strength as the brand-name medications. Also, some brands of pills contain dye that can cause allergic reactions. It is a good idea to talk to the doctor and the pharmacist about whether it is important to use a specific brand of medicine.

All medicines can cause an allergic reaction. Examples are hives, itching, rashes, swelling, and trouble breathing. Even a tiny amount of a medicine can cause a reaction in patients who are allergic to that medicine. Be *sure* to talk to the doctor before restarting a medicine that has caused an allergic reaction.

Taking more than one medicine at the same time may cause more side effects or cause one of the medicines to not work as well. Always ask the doctor, nurse, or pharmacist before adding another medicine, whether prescription or over-the-counter. Be sure that each doctor knows about *all* of the medicines your child is taking. Also tell the doctor about any vitamins, herbal medicines, or supplements your child may be taking. Some of these may have side effects alone or when taken with this medication.

Everyone taking medicine should have a physical examination at least once a year.

If you suspect the youth is using drugs or alcohol, please tell the doctor right away.

Pregnancy requires special care in the use of medicine. Please tell the doctor immediately if you suspect the teenager is pregnant or might become pregnant.

Printed information like this applies to children and adolescents in general. If you have questions about the medicine, or if you notice changes or anything unusual, please ask the doctor or nurse. As scientific research advances, knowledge increases and advice changes. Even experts do not always agree. Many medicines have not been approved by the U.S. Food and Drug Administration (FDA) for use in children. For this reason, use of the medicine for a particular problem or age group often is not listed in the *Physicians' Desk Reference*. This does not necessarily mean that the medicine is dangerous or does not work, only that the company that makes the medicine has not received permission to advertise the medicine for use in children. Companies often do not apply for this permission because it is expensive to do the tests needed to apply for approval for use in children. Once a medication is approved by the FDA for any purpose, a doctor is allowed to prescribe it according to research and clinical experience.

Note to Teachers

It is a good idea to talk with the parent(s) about the reason(s) that a medication is being used. If the parent(s) sign consent to release information, it is often helpful to talk with the doctor. If the parent(s) give permission, the doctor may ask you to fill out rating forms about your experience with the student's behavior, feelings, academic performance, and medication side effects. This information is very useful in selecting and monitoring medication treatment. If you have observations that you think are important, do not hesitate to share these with the student's parent(s) and treating clinicians.

It is very important that the medicine be taken exactly as the doctor instructs. However, everyone forgets to give a medicine on time once in a while. It is a good idea to ask the parent(s) in advance what to do if this happens. Do not stop or change the time you are giving a medicine at school without parental permission. If a medication is to be taken with food, but lunchtime or snack time changes, be sure to notify the parent(s) so appropriate adjustments can be made.

All medicines should be kept in a secure place and should be supervised by an adult. If someone takes too much of a medicine, follow your school procedure for an urgent medical problem.

Taking medicine is a private matter and is best managed discreetly and confidentially. It is important to be sensitive to the student's feelings about taking medicine.

If you suspect that the student is using drugs or alcohol, please tell the parent(s) or a school counselor right away.

Please tell the parent(s) or school nurse if you suspect medication side effects.

Modifications of the classroom environment or assignments may be useful in addition to medication. The student may need to be evaluated for additional help or for an Individualized Education Plan for learning or behavior.

Any expression of suicidal thoughts or feelings or self-harm by a child or adolescent is a clear signal of distress and should be taken seriously. These behaviors should not be dismissed as "attention seeking."

What Is Escitalopram (Lexapro)?

Escitalopram is an antidepressant known as a *selective serotonin reuptake inhibitor* (SSRI). Lexapro is a purified form of citalopram, including only one of the two forms, called *isomers*. Lexapro comes in tablets and in liquid.

How Can This Medicine Help?

Escitalopram is used to treat depression and anxiety disorders such as obsessive-compulsive disorder (OCD), posttraumatic stress disorder (PTSD), panic disorder, and separation anxiety disorder. Lexapro may have more positive action with fewer side effects than citalopram.

How Does This Medicine Work?

Escitalopram increases the amount of a *neurotransmitter* called *serotonin* in certain parts of the brain. People with emotional and behavioral problems, such as depression and anxiety, may have low levels of serotonin in certain parts of the brain. SSRIs such as escitalopram help by increasing the action of brain serotonin to more normal levels.

How Long Does This Medicine Last?

Escitalopram can be taken only once a day.

How Will the Doctor Monitor This Medicine?

The doctor will review your child's medical history and physical examination before starting escitalopram. The doctor may order some blood or urine tests to be sure your child does not have a hidden medical condition that would make it unsafe to use this medicine. Extra care is needed when using SSRIs in youth with seizures (epilepsy), liver or kidney problems, or diabetes. The doctor or nurse may measure your child's pulse, blood pressure, and weight before starting the medicine.

Be sure to tell the doctor if your child or anyone in the family has bipolar illness (manic-depressive illness) or has tried to kill himself or herself.

After the medicine is started, the doctor will want to have regular appointments with you and your child to see how the medicine is working, to see if a dose change is needed, to watch for side effects, to see if escitalopram is still needed, and to see if any other treatment is needed. The doctor or nurse may check your child's height, weight, pulse, and blood pressure.

Before using medicine and at times afterward, the doctor may ask your child to fill out a rating scale about depression, to help see how your child is doing.

What Side Effects Can This Medicine Have?

Any medicine can have side effects, including an allergy to the medicine. Because each patient is different, the doctor will monitor the youth closely, especially when the medicine is started. The doctor will work with you to increase the positive effects and decrease the negative effects of the medicine. Please tell the doctor if any of the listed side effects appear or if you think that the medicine is causing any other problems. Not all of the rare or unusual side effects are listed.

Side effects are most common after starting the medicine or after a dose increase. Many side effects can be avoided or lessened by starting with a very low dose and increasing it slowly—ask the doctor.

241

Allergic Reaction

Tell the doctor in a day or two (if possible, before the next dose of medicine):

- Hives
- Itching
- Rash

  Stop the medicine and get *immediate* medical care:

- Trouble breathing or chest tightness
- Swelling of lips, tongue, or throat

Common Side Effects

Tell the doctor within a week or two:

- Nausea, upset stomach, vomiting
- Diarrhea
- Dry mouth—Have your child try using sugar-free gum or candy.
- Constipation—Encourage your child to drink more fluids and eat high-fiber foods; if necessary, the doctor may recommend a fiber medicine such as Benefiber or a stool softener such as Colace or mineral oil.
- Headache
- Anxiety or nervousness
- Insomnia (trouble sleeping)
- Restlessness, increased activity level
- Daytime sleepiness or tiredness—Do not allow your child to drive, ride a bicycle or motorcycle, or operate machinery if this side effect is present.
- Dizziness—This side effect is worse when the child stands up quickly, especially when getting out of bed in the morning; try having the child stand up slowly.
- Tremor (shakiness)
- Excessive sweating
- Apathy, lack of interest in school or friends—This may happen after a initial good response to treatment.
- Decreased sexual interest, trouble with sexual functioning
- Weight gain
- Weight loss

Less Common, but More Serious, Side Effects

Call the doctor within a day or two:

- Significant suicidal thoughts or self-injurious behavior
- Increased activity, rapid speech, feeling "speeded up," decreased need for sleep, being very excited or irritable (cranky)

Serious Side Effects

Call the doctor *immediately* or go to the nearest emergency room:

- Seizure (fit, convulsion)
- Stiffness, high fever, confusion, tremors (shaking)
- Overheating or heatstroke—Prevent by decreasing activity in hot weather, staying out of the sun, and drinking water.

Serotonin Syndrome

A very serious side effect called *serotonin syndrome* can happen when certain kinds of medicines (including some medicines for migraine headaches—triptans) are taken by the same person. *Very* rarely, it can happen at high doses of just one medicine. The early signs are restlessness, confusion, shaking, skin turning red, sweating, and jerking of muscles. If you see these symptoms, stop the medicine and send or take the youth to an emergency room right away.

Some Interactions With Other Medicines or Food

Please note that the following are only the most likely interactions with food or other medicines.

Escitalopram interacts with many other medicines, including some antibiotics and other psychiatric medicines. It is especially important to tell the doctor and pharmacist about all of the medicines your child is taking or has taken in the past few months, including over-the-counter and herbal medicines. Sometimes one medicine can increase or decrease the blood level of another medicine so that different doses are needed. Generally, escitalopram has fewer interactions with other medicines than does fluoxetine, paroxetine, or sertraline. Erythromycin and similar antibiotics may increase levels of escitalopram and increase side effects. Escitalopram may increase the heart side effects of pimozide (Orap), so those two medicines should not be taken by the same person. The herbal medicine St. John's wort also increases serotonin and can cause serious side effects if taken with escitalopram.

It can be *very dangerous* to take an SSRI at the same time as or even within a month of taking another type of medicine called a *monoamine oxidase inhibitor* (MAOI), such as Eldepryl (selegiline), Nardil (phenelzine), Parnate (tranylcypromine), or Marplan (isocarboxazid).

Escitalopram does not usually cause problems when taken with decongestant cold medicines.

Escitalopram can be taken with or without food.

Caffeine may increase side effects.

What Could Happen if This Medicine Is Stopped Suddenly?

No known serious medical effects occur if escitalopram is stopped suddenly, but there may be uncomfortable feelings, which should be avoided if possible. Your child might have trouble sleeping, nervousness, irritability, dizziness, and flu-like symptoms. Ask the doctor before stopping escitalopram or if these symptoms happen while the dose is being decreased.

How Long Will This Medicine Be Needed?

Escitalopram may take up to 1–2 months to reach its full effect. If your child has a good response to escitalopram, it is a good idea to continue the medicine for at least 6 months.

What Else Should I Know About This Medicine?

In youth who have bipolar disorder (manic depression) or who are at risk for bipolar disorder, any antidepressant medicine may increase the risk of hypomania or mania (excitement, agitation, increased activity, decreased sleep).

In hot weather, make sure your child drinks enough water or other liquids and does not get overheated.

Sometimes, after a person has improved while taking escitalopram, he or she loses interest in school or friends or just stops trying. Please tell your child's doctor if this happens—it may be a side effect of the medicine. A lower dose or a different medicine may be needed.

Store the medicine away from sunlight, heat, moisture, and humidity.

Black Box Antidepressant Warning

In 2004, an advisory committee to the FDA decided that there might be an increased risk of suicidal behavior for some youth taking medicines called *antidepressants*. In the research studies that the committee reviewed, about 3%–4% of youth with depression who took an antidepressant medicine—and 1%–2% of youth with depression who took a placebo (pill without active medicine)—talked about suicidal thoughts (thinking about killing themselves or wishing they were dead) or did something to harm themselves. This means that almost twice as many youth who were taking an antidepressant to treat their depression talked about suicide or had suicidal behavior compared with youth with depression who were taking inactive medicine. There were *no* completed suicides in any of these research studies, which included more than 4,000 children and adolescents. For youth being treated for anxiety, there was no difference in suicidal talking or behavior between those taking antidepressant medication and those taking placebo.

The FDA told drug companies to add a *black box warning* label to all antidepressant medicines. Because of this label, a doctor (or advanced practice nurse) prescribing one of these medicines has to warn youth and their families that there might be more suicidal thoughts and actions in youth taking these medicines.

On the other hand, in places where more youth are taking the newer antidepressant medicines, the number of adolescents who commit suicide has gotten smaller. Also, thinking about or attempting suicide is more common in surveys of teenagers in the community than it is in depressed youth treated in research studies with antidepressant medicine.

If a youth is being treated with this medicine and is doing well, then no changes are needed as a result of this warning. Increased suicidal talk or action is most likely to happen in the first few months of treatment with a medicine. If your child has recently started this medicine or is about to start, then you and your doctor (or advanced practice nurse) should watch for any changes in behavior. People who are depressed often have suicidal thoughts or actions. It is hard to know whether suicidal thoughts or actions in depressed people are caused by the depression itself or by the medicine. Also, as their depression is getting better, some people talk more about the suicidal thoughts that they had before but did not talk about. As young people get better from depression, they might be at higher risk of doing something about suicidal thoughts that they have had for some time, because they have more energy.

What Should a Parent Do?

1. Be honest with your child about possible risks and benefits of medicine.
2. Talk to your child about whether he or she is having any suicidal thoughts, and tell your child to come to you if he or she is having such thoughts.
3. You, your child, and your child's doctor or nurse should develop a safety plan. Pick adults whom your child can tell if he or she is thinking about suicide.
4. Be sure to tell your child's doctor, nurse, or therapist if you suspect that your child is using alcohol or drugs or if something has happened that might make your child feel worse, such as a family separation, breaking up with a boyfriend or girlfriend, someone close dying or attempting suicide, physical or sexual abuse, or failure in school.
5. Be sure that there are no guns in the home and that all medicines (including over-the-counter medicines like Tylenol) are closely supervised by an adult and kept in a safe place.
6. Watch for new or worse thoughts of suicide, self-harm, depression, anxiety (nerves), feeling very agitated or restless, being angry or aggressive, having more trouble sleeping, or anything else that you see for the first time, seems worse, or worries your child or you. If these appear, contact a mental health professional **right away.** Do not just stop or change the dose of the medicine on your own. If the problems are serious, and you cannot reach one of your clinicians, call a 24-hour psychiatry emergency telephone number or take your child to an emergency room.

Youth on antidepressant medicine should be watched carefully by parent(s), clinician(s) (doctor, nurse, therapist), and other concerned adults for the first weeks of treatment. It is a good idea to have a visit or telephone call with the doctor, nurse, or therapist weekly for the first month, every 2 weeks for the second month, and after that at least once a month to check for feelings of depression or sadness, thoughts of killing or harming himself or herself, and any problems with the medication. If you have questions, be sure to ask the doctor, nurse, or therapist.

For more information, see http://www.parentsmedguide.org/ (in English and Spanish).

Notes

Use this space to take notes or to write down questions you want to ask the doctor.

_____

_____

_____

_____

_____

_____

_____

_____

_____

_____

_____

_____

Medication Information for Youth

Escitalopram—Lexapro

What the Medicine Is Called and What It Is For

The name of your medicine may be confusing. Most drugs have two names: 1) a scientific name that we call a *generic name* and 2) a trade or *brand name*. The generic name of this medicine is escitalopram. The brand name is Lexapro.

Escitalopram is called an *antidepressant,* or *selective serotonin reuptake inhibitor* (SSRI). Lexapro is a form of citalopram that may have fewer side effects. Escitalopram is used to treat depression and anxiety disorders such as obsessive-compulsive disorder (OCD), posttraumatic stress disorder (PTSD), panic disorder, and separation anxiety disorder. It helps people who feel very sad or depressed, anxious (nervous), or afraid, or who have obsessions (uncomfortable thoughts that will not go away) or compulsions (habits that get in the way of daily life).

How You Take the Medicine

It is very important to take the medicine exactly as the doctor or nurse tells you. Do not skip doses or take extra medicine without asking an adult. If you forget a dose, ask your parent(s) what to do. It is very important that you take all the pills you are supposed to take each day. Your doctor will probably recommend that you take your medicine at the same time each day, which may be with meals or at bedtime.

It may take several weeks before you notice that the medicine is helping. Waiting for the full effect may take even longer. You may feel discouraged and think the medicine is never going to help. You may want to give up and stop taking the medicine. Talk to your doctor and parent(s) about how you feel, but **do not stop** taking the medicine unless your doctor tells you to. It is also important not to take extra pills, hoping that you will feel better faster. Doing that could make you very sick.

Caffeine (in coffee, tea, or soft drinks) may make you feel worse.

This medicine is prescribed only for you. It should never be shared with anyone else.

You do not have to tell others that you are taking this medicine, but it is not something you should feel ashamed or embarrassed about. Many young people are helped by escitalopram. This medicine is not habit-forming, and you cannot become "hooked" on it. You should talk to your doctor or nurse about any questions you have about the medicine. It is important to remember that the medicine *helps* you. It cannot *make* you do anything or change you as a person.

247

How Your Doctor Will Follow Your Progress

Before giving you the medicine, your doctor or nurse will talk with you and your parent(s) and may measure your height, weight, heart rate (pulse), and blood pressure. The doctor may order some blood or urine tests to be sure you are in good health.

Be sure to tell your doctor or nurse about any other medicines or supplements you are taking, including vitamins, herbs, or aids to weight loss or bodybuilding. Also be sure to tell the doctor or nurse if you are using alcohol or drugs. Because many medicines may affect babies, it is very important to tell the doctor if you might be pregnant or if you are at risk of becoming pregnant. Be sure to tell the doctor if you have had thoughts of hurting yourself, have tried to hurt yourself, or sometimes wish that you were not alive.

Your teachers may be asked to fill out a form about your grades and behavior in school. A psychologist may give you some tests to see how you learn best.

Before starting the medicine and afterward, the doctor may ask you to answer questions on paper about depression and anxiety.

Most doctors have regular appointments with young people who are taking medicine. You should use these visits to share any concerns you may have about your medicine and to talk about if it has helped you. From time to time, your physician or nurse may measure your height, weight, heart rate (pulse), and blood pressure to be sure that you are in good health while you are taking the medicine. Your doctor also will ask for regular reports from your parents and maybe from your teachers (with your permission) to see how well the medicine is working.

Some medicines are started at the amount you will take for as long as you are taking that medicine. Other medicines need to be increased or adjusted until your doctor decides you are taking the right amount. Starting at a low dose and increasing it slowly may lessen side effects. If the medicine helps you, your doctor will probably want you to take it for 6 months to a year if you are taking it to treat depression. If you are taking it for another problem, your doctor will decide how long you will need to take the medicine as he or she watches your progress.

It is not dangerous to stop escitalopram suddenly, but there might be uncomfortable feelings, such as trouble sleeping, nervousness, irritability, or feeling sick. It is better to decrease it slowly. Do not stop taking a medicine unless the doctor tells you to. If you have any problems after stopping or decreasing this medicine, tell your parent(s) or doctor.

How the Medicine Might Affect You

In addition to the ways the medicine can help you, it may have other effects called *side effects*. Different medicines have different side effects. It is helpful to know about some of the most common side effects of your medicine so that you will understand what they are if they happen. Some people do not have any side effects. Some side effects are just uncomfortable, but others may mean a more serious problem with the medicine. Side effects are most common after starting the medicine or after a dose increase. They may go away with time, or the medicine can be adjusted or changed—ask the doctor.

You could have an allergy to any medicine, which might show up as a rash on your skin, swelling, itching, or trouble breathing.

Please tell your parent(s) and your doctor or nurse about any changes that you notice after taking the medicine. It is especially important to tell a responsible adult if you are feeling depressed or that you may not want to live; if you have thoughts of hurting yourself; or if you begin to feel more irritable, nervous, or restless. Also be sure to tell your parent(s) or doctor if you begin to feel "speeded up" or have trouble sleeping.

Some medicines make people feel sleepy or less coordinated. If this medicine is making you sleepy, it is very important not to drive a car or ride a bicycle or motorcycle. After starting a new medicine or increasing the dose of a medicine, please be extra careful when driving a car, riding a bike, or using machines until you can tell how the medicine affects your alertness, attention, and coordination.

One of the most common side effects of this medicine is feeling tired or sleepy during the day, even if you have had a full night's sleep. After you have been taking the medicine for a few weeks, your body will adjust, and this side effect may go away. If you have had trouble sleeping at night, the medicine can help you sleep better, especially if the doctor tells you to take a dose of medicine in the evening. Other people may feel more restless and excited. Tell your parent(s) or doctor if this is uncomfortable. Sometimes after being on the medicine for a while, people do not care as much about school or friends. Changing the dose or the type of medicine can help this.

This medicine may make your mouth dry. You may be more thirsty than usual and find that you are drinking more water or other liquids. Sucking on sugar-free hard candy or cough drops usually helps. You also could try chewing sugar-free gum or sucking on ice chips. Do not chew the ice; you could hurt your teeth. Also, using lip balm will keep your lips from cracking. It is important to be especially good about brushing your teeth.

Some other side effects that could happen are headache, not feeling hungry and not wanting to eat much, eating more than usual, having an upset stomach, or changes in your bowel movements. You may have a change in your sexual functioning—it is OK to ask the doctor about this. This medicine may make you more likely to get sick if you get overheated, so be sure to drink plenty of liquids and rest in the shade in hot weather.

Please let your parent(s) and doctor know if you notice anything different or unusual about how you feel once you start taking the medicine. This includes good things, such as feeling less sad or less nervous or sleeping better at night.

Notes

Use this space to take notes or to write down questions you want to ask the doctor or nurse.

_____

_____

_____

_____

_____

_____

_____

_____

_____

_____

_____

_____

Estazolam—ProSom

General Information About Medication

Each child and adolescent is different. No one has exactly the same combination of medical and psychological problems. It is a good idea to talk with the doctor or nurse about the reasons a medicine is being used. It is very important to keep all appointments and to be in touch by telephone if you have concerns. It is important to communicate with the doctor, nurse, or therapist.

It is very important that the medicine be taken exactly as the doctor instructs. However, once in a while, everyone forgets to give a medicine on time. It is a good idea to ask the doctor or nurse what to do if this happens. Do not stop or change a medicine without asking the doctor or nurse first.

If the medicine seems to stop working, it may be because it is not being taken regularly. The youth may be "cheeking" or hiding the medicine or forgetting to take it (especially at school). The doses may be too far apart, or a different dose may be needed. Something at school, at home, or in the neighborhood may be upsetting the youth, or he or she may need special help for learning disabilities or tutoring. Please discuss your concerns with the doctor. **Do not just increase the dose.**

All medicines should be kept in a safe place, out of the reach of children, and should be supervised by an adult. If someone takes too much of a medicine, call the doctor, the poison control center, or a hospital emergency room.

Each medicine has a "generic" or chemical name. Just like laundry detergents or paper towels, some medicines are sold by more than one company under different brand names. The same medicine may be available under a generic name and several brand names. The generic medications are usually less expensive than the brand name ones. The generic medications have the same chemical formula, but they may or may not be exactly the same strength as the brand-name medications. Also, some brands of pills contain dye that can cause allergic reactions. It is a good idea to talk to the doctor and the pharmacist about whether it is important to use a specific brand of medicine.

All medicines can cause an allergic reaction. Examples are hives, itching, rashes, swelling, and trouble breathing. Even a tiny amount of a medicine can cause a reaction in patients who are allergic to that medicine. Be *sure* to talk to the doctor before restarting a medicine that has caused an allergic reaction.

Taking more than one medicine at the same time may cause more side effects or cause one of the medicines to not work as well. Always ask the doctor, nurse, or pharmacist before adding another medicine, whether prescription or over-the-counter. Be sure that each doctor knows about *all* of the medicines your child is taking. Also tell the doctor about any vitamins, herbal medicines, or supplements your child may be taking. Some of these may have side effects alone or when taken with this medication.

Everyone taking medicine should have a physical examination at least once a year.

If you suspect the youth is using drugs or alcohol, please tell the doctor right away.

Pregnancy requires special care in the use of medicine. Please tell the doctor immediately if you suspect the teenager is pregnant or might become pregnant.

Printed information like this applies to children and adolescents in general. If you have questions about the medicine, or if you notice changes or anything unusual, please ask the doctor or nurse. As scientific research advances, knowledge increases and advice changes. Even experts do not always agree. Many medicines have not been approved by the U.S. Food and Drug Administration (FDA) for use in children. For this reason, use of the medicine for a particular problem or age group often is not listed in the *Physicians' Desk Reference*. This does not necessarily mean that the medicine is dangerous or does not work, only that the company that makes the medicine has not received permission to advertise the medicine for use in children. Companies often do not apply for this permission because it is expensive to do the tests needed to apply for approval for use in children. Once a medication is approved by the FDA for any purpose, a doctor is allowed to prescribe it according to research and clinical experience.

Note to Teachers

It is a good idea to talk with the parent(s) about the reason(s) that a medication is being used. If the parent(s) sign consent to release information, it is often helpful to talk with the doctor. If the parent(s) give permission, the doctor may ask you to fill out rating forms about your experience with the student's behavior, feelings, academic performance, and medication side effects. This information is very useful in selecting and monitoring medication treatment. If you have observations that you think are important, do not hesitate to share these with the student's parent(s) and treating clinicians.

It is very important that the medicine be taken exactly as the doctor instructs. However, everyone forgets to give a medicine on time once in a while. It is a good idea to ask the parent(s) in advance what to do if this happens. Do not stop or change the time you are giving a medicine at school without parental permission. If a medication is to be taken with food, but lunchtime or snack time changes, be sure to notify the parent(s) so appropriate adjustments can be made.

All medicines should be kept in a secure place and should be supervised by an adult. If someone takes too much of a medicine, follow your school procedure for an urgent medical problem.

Taking medicine is a private matter and is best managed discreetly and confidentially. It is important to be sensitive to the student's feelings about taking medicine.

If you suspect that the student is using drugs or alcohol, please tell the parent(s) or a school counselor right away.

Please tell the parent(s) or school nurse if you suspect medication side effects.

Modifications of the classroom environment or assignments may be useful in addition to medication. The student may need to be evaluated for additional help or for an Individualized Education Plan for learning or behavior.

Any expression of suicidal thoughts or feelings or self-harm by a child or adolescent is a clear signal of distress and should be taken seriously. These behaviors should not be dismissed as "attention seeking."

What Is Estazolam (ProSom)?

Estazolam is a *benzodiazepine* medicine. It is called a *hypnotic* or *sedative-hypnotic*. It comes in brand name ProSom and generic tablets.

How Can This Medicine Help?

Estazolam is used to treat insomnia—problems falling asleep—when used for a short time along with a behavioral program. It can also be used for problem sleep behaviors, called *parasomnias*, such as night terrors (sudden waking up from sleep with great fear), sleepwalking, or sleeptalking, when these put the youth at risk of an accident or make it impossible for other family members to get enough sleep.

How Does This Medicine Work?

Estazolam works on *receptors* (special places on brain cells) in certain parts of the brain to change the action of *GABA*—a *neurotransmitter*—a chemical that the brain makes for brain cells to communicate with each other.

How Long Does This Medicine Last?

Estazolam is taken before bedtime and starts working within 15–30 minutes. There may still be some effects in the morning.

How Will the Doctor Monitor This Medicine?

The doctor will review your child's medical history and physical examination before starting estazolam.

After the medicine is started, the doctor will want to have regular appointments with you and your child to see how the medicine is working, to see if a dose change is needed, to watch for side effects, to see if estazolam is still needed, and to see if any other treatment is needed.

What Side Effects Can This Medicine Have?

Any medicine can have side effects, including an allergy to the medicine. Because each patient is different, the doctor will monitor the youth closely, especially when the medicine is started. The doctor will work with you to increase the positive effects and decrease the negative effects of the medicine. Please tell the doctor if any of the listed side effects appear or if you think that the medicine is causing any other problems. Not all of the rare or unusual side effects are listed.

Side effects are most common after starting the medicine or after a dose increase. Many side effects can be avoided or lessened by starting with a very low dose and increasing it slowly—ask the doctor.

Allergic Reaction

Tell the doctor in a day or two (if possible, before the next dose of medicine):

* Hives
* Itching
* Rash

Stop the medicine and get *immediate* medical care:

* Trouble breathing or chest tightness
* Swelling of lips, tongue, or throat

Estazolam is usually very safe when used for short periods as the doctor prescribes.

The most common side effect is daytime sleepiness. Estazolam can also cause dizziness, feeling "spacey," or decreased coordination. If the medicine is causing any of these problems it is very important not to drive a car, ride a bicycle or motorcycle, or operate machinery.

Estazolam can cause decreased concentration and memory. These problems, along with daytime sleepiness, may decrease learning and performance in school.

People who take estazolam must not drink alcohol. Severe sleepiness or even loss of consciousness may result.

It is possible to become psychologically and physically dependent on estazolam, but that is not a common problem for patients who see their doctors regularly. Because some people abuse benzodiazepines, it is illegal to give or sell these medicines to someone other than the patient for whom they were prescribed.

Very rarely, estazolam causes excitement, irritability, anger, aggression, agitation, trouble sleeping, nightmares, uncontrollable behavior, or memory loss. This is called *disinhibition* or a *paradoxical effect*. This may be more common in younger children. Stop the medicine and call the doctor if this happens.

Some Interactions With Other Medicines or Food

Please note that the following are only the most likely interactions with food or other medicines.

Caffeine may cause trouble sleeping and make estazolam less effective. If caffeine is eliminated, less estazolam may be needed, or estazolam may not be needed at all.

Oral contraceptives (birth control pills), cimetidine (Tagamet), antifungal agents (such as ketoconazole), fluoxetine (Prozac), fluvoxamine (Luvox), antibiotics (such as ciprofloxacin [Cipro]), and other medicines may increase the levels of estazolam and increase side effects.

It is important not to use other sedatives, tranquilizers, or sleeping pills or antihistamines (such as Benadryl) when taking estazolam because of greatly increased side effects.

What Could Happen if This Medicine Is Stopped Suddenly?

Many medicines cause problems if stopped suddenly. Estazolam must be decreased slowly (tapered) rather than stopped suddenly. When estazolam is stopped suddenly, there are withdrawal symptoms that are uncomfortable and may even be dangerous. Problems are more likely in patients taking high doses of estazolam for 2 months or longer, but even after just a few weeks of taking estazolam it is important to stop it slowly. Withdrawal symptoms may include anxiety, irritability, shaking, sweating, aches and pains, muscle cramps, vomiting, confusion, and trouble sleeping. If large doses taken for a long time are stopped suddenly, seizures (fits, convulsions), hallucinations (hearing voices or seeing things that are not there), or out-of-control behavior may result.

How Long Will This Medicine Be Needed?

The length of time depends on why estazolam is being used. When used for sleep, it is usually prescribed for only a week or so. A behavioral program, such as regular soothing routines at bedtime and increased exercise in the daytime, should be used along with the medicine to improve sleep. This program can be continued after the medicine is tapered or when the medicine is used only occasionally.

When used for night terrors or other parasomnias, the medicine may be needed for months or years.

What Else Should I Know About This Medicine?

Because benzodiazepines can be abused (especially by people who abuse alcohol or drugs) and can cause psychological dependence or physical dependence (addiction), they are regulated by special state and federal laws as *controlled substances*. These laws place limitations on telephone prescriptions and refills, and prescriptions expire if they are not filled promptly.

People with sleep apnea (breathing stops while they are asleep) should not take estazolam. Tell the doctor if your child snores very loudly.

Estazolam should be avoided during pregnancy, especially in the first 3 months, because it may cause birth defects in the baby. If taken regularly at the end of pregnancy, estazolam may cause withdrawal symptoms in the baby.

Notes

Use this space to take notes or to write down questions you want to ask the doctor.

_____

_____

_____

_____

_____

_____

_____

_____

From Dulcan MK (editor): *Helping Parents, Youth, and Teachers Understand Medications for Behavioral and Emotional Problems: A Resource Book of Medication Information Handouts*, Third Edition. Washington, DC, American Psychiatric Publishing, 2007

Medication Information for Youth

Estazolam—ProSom

What the Medicine Is Called and What It Is For

The name of your medicine may be confusing. Most drugs have two names: 1) a scientific name that we call a *generic name* and 2) a trade or *brand name*. The generic name of this medicine is estazolam. The brand name is ProSom.

Estazolam is a *benzodiazepine* medicine. It works by calming the parts of the brain that are too excitable. Estazolam can help with insomnia (difficulty falling asleep) when used for a short time along with routines that help you to relax and fall asleep. Estazolam also can be used for sleep problems such as night terrors (sudden waking up from sleep very scared) or sleepwalking.

How You Take the Medicine

It is very important to take the medicine exactly as the doctor or nurse tells you. Do not skip doses or take extra medicine without asking an adult. If you forget a dose, ask your parent(s) what to do.

It is better to limit drinks with caffeine (coffee, tea, soft drinks) because caffeine works in the opposite way from this medicine, and the positive effects might be decreased.

This medicine is prescribed only for you. It should never be shared with anyone else.

You do not have to tell others that you are taking this medicine, but it is not something you should feel ashamed or embarrassed about. Many young people are helped by estazolam. You should talk to your doctor or nurse about any questions you have about the medicine. It is important to remember that the medicine *helps* you. It cannot *make* you do anything or change you as a person.

Many medicines cause problems if stopped suddenly. Always ask your doctor before stopping a medicine. Problems are more likely to happen in patients taking high doses of estazolam for 2 months or longer, but it is important to decrease the medicine slowly (taper) even after a few weeks. If you notice anxiety, irritability, shaking, sweating, aches and pains, muscle cramps, vomiting, or trouble sleeping, you may need to decrease the medicine more slowly. If large doses are stopped suddenly, seizures (fits, convulsions), hallucinations (hearing voices or seeing things that are not there), or out-of-control behavior may result.

How Your Doctor Will Follow Your Progress

Before giving you the medicine, your doctor or nurse will talk with you and your parent(s) and may measure your height, weight, heart rate (pulse), and blood pressure.

Be sure to tell your doctor or nurse about any other medicines or supplements you are taking, including vitamins, herbs, or aids to weight loss or bodybuilding. Also be sure to tell the doctor or nurse if you are using alcohol or drugs. Because many medicines may affect babies, it is very important to tell the doctor if you might be pregnant or if you are at risk of becoming pregnant.

Most doctors have regular appointments with young people who are taking medicine. You should use these visits to share any concerns you may have about your medicine and to talk about if it has helped you. From time to time, your physician or nurse may measure your height, weight, heart rate (pulse), and blood pressure to be sure that you are in good health while you are taking the medicine. Your doctor also will ask for regular reports from your parents to see how well the medicine is working.

Estazolam is usually prescribed for only a week or so to allow you to develop better sleep habits. Regular exercise in the daytime usually helps with sleep at night.

Each person is unique, and some people may need this medicine for months or years.

How the Medicine Might Affect You

In addition to the ways the medicine can help you, it may have other effects called *side effects*. Different medicines have different side effects. It is helpful to know about some of the most common side effects of your medicine so that you will understand what they are if they happen. Some people do not have any side effects. Some side effects are just uncomfortable, but others may mean a more serious problem with the medicine. Side effects are most common after starting the medicine or after a dose increase. They may go away with time, or the medicine can be adjusted or changed—ask the doctor.

You could have an allergy to any medicine, which might show up as a rash on your skin, swelling, itching, or trouble breathing.

Please tell your parent(s) and your doctor or nurse about any changes that you notice after taking the medicine. It is especially important to tell a responsible adult if you are feeling depressed or that you may not want to live; if you have thoughts of hurting yourself; or if you begin to feel more irritable, nervous, or restless.

The most common side effect of estazolam is daytime sleepiness. If this medicine is making you sleepy, it is very important not to drive a car or ride a bicycle or motorcycle. After starting estazolam or increasing the dose, please be extra careful when driving a car, riding a bike, or using machines until you can tell how the medicine affects your alertness, attention, and coordination.

Sometimes sleep medicines seem to work in the opposite way, causing excitement, irritability, anger, aggression, and other problems. If this happens, tell your parent(s) or your doctor.

Drinking alcohol while taking this medicine is dangerous and can cause severe drowsiness or even passing out. **Don't do it!** Do not use marijuana or street drugs while taking this medicine. They can cause serious side effects. Skipping your medicine to take drugs does not work because many medicines stay in your body for a long time.

Estazolam can be habit-forming, but that is not a common problem for people who take their medicine as the doctor says.

Notes

Use this space to take notes or to write down questions you want to ask the doctor or nurse.

_____

_____

_____

_____

_____

_____

_____

_____

_____

_____

_____

_____

_____

_____

From Dulcan MK (editor): _Helping Parents, Youth, and Teachers Understand Medications for Behavioral and Emotional Problems: A Resource Book of Medication Information Handouts_, Third Edition. Washington, DC, American Psychiatric Publishing, 2007

Medication Information for Parents and Teachers

Eszopiclone—Lunesta

General Information About Medication

Each child and adolescent is different. No one has exactly the same combination of medical and psychological problems. It is a good idea to talk with the doctor or nurse about the reasons a medicine is being used. It is very important to keep all appointments and to be in touch by telephone if you have concerns. It is important to communicate with the doctor, nurse, or therapist.

It is very important that the medicine be taken exactly as the doctor instructs. However, once in a while, everyone forgets to give a medicine on time. It is a good idea to ask the doctor or nurse what to do if this happens. Do not stop or change a medicine without asking the doctor or nurse first.

If the medicine seems to stop working, it may be because it is not being taken regularly. The youth may be "cheeking" or hiding the medicine or forgetting to take it. A different dose may be needed. Something at school, at home, or in the neighborhood may be upsetting the youth, or he or she may need special help for learning disabilities or tutoring. Please discuss your concerns with the doctor. **Do not just increase the dose.**

All medicines should be kept in a safe place, out of the reach of children, and should be supervised by an adult. If someone takes too much of a medicine, call the doctor, the poison control center, or a hospital emergency room.

Each medicine has a "generic" or chemical name. Just like laundry detergents or paper towels, some medicines are sold by more than one company under different brand names. The same medicine may be available under a generic name and several brand names. The generic medications are usually less expensive than the brand name ones. The generic medications have the same chemical formula, but they may or may not be exactly the same strength as the brand-name medications. Also, some brands of pills contain dye that can cause allergic reactions. It is a good idea to talk to the doctor and the pharmacist about whether it is important to use a specific brand of medicine.

All medicines can cause an allergic reaction. Examples are hives, itching, rashes, swelling, and trouble breathing. Even a tiny amount of a medicine can cause a reaction in patients who are allergic to that medicine. Be *sure* to talk to the doctor before restarting a medicine that has caused an allergic reaction.

Taking more than one medicine at the same time may cause more side effects or cause one of the medicines to not work as well. Always ask the doctor, nurse, or pharmacist before adding another medicine, whether prescription or over-the-counter. Be sure that each doctor knows about *all* of the medicines your child is taking. Also tell the doctor about any vitamins, herbal medicines, or supplements your child may be taking. Some of these may have side effects alone or when taken with this medication.

Everyone taking medicine should have a physical examination at least once a year.

If you suspect the youth is using drugs or alcohol, please tell the doctor right away.

Pregnancy requires special care in the use of medicine. Please tell the doctor immediately if you suspect the teenager is pregnant or might become pregnant.

261

Printed information like this applies to children and adolescents in general. If you have questions about the medicine, or if you notice changes or anything unusual, please ask the doctor or nurse. As scientific research advances, knowledge increases and advice changes. Even experts do not always agree. Many medicines have not been approved by the U.S. Food and Drug Administration (FDA) for use in children. For this reason, use of the medicine for a particular problem or age group often is not listed in the *Physicians' Desk Reference*. This does not necessarily mean that the medicine is dangerous or does not work, only that the company that makes the medicine has not received permission to advertise the medicine for use in children. Companies often do not apply for this permission because it is expensive to do the tests needed to apply for approval for use in children. Once a medication is approved by the FDA for any purpose, a doctor is allowed to prescribe it according to research and clinical experience.

Note to Teachers

It is a good idea to talk with the parent(s) about the reason(s) that a medication is being used. If the parent(s) sign consent to release information, it is often helpful to talk with the doctor. If the parent(s) give permission, the doctor may ask you to fill out rating forms about your experience with the student's behavior, feelings, academic performance, and medication side effects. This information is very useful in selecting and monitoring medication treatment. If you have observations that you think are important, do not hesitate to share these with the student's parent(s) and treating clinicians.

All medicines should be kept in a secure place and should be supervised by an adult. If someone takes too much of a medicine, follow your school procedure for an urgent medical problem.

Taking medicine is a private matter and is best managed discreetly and confidentially. It is important to be sensitive to the student's feelings about taking medicine.

If you suspect that the student is using drugs or alcohol, please tell the parent(s) or a school counselor right away.

Please tell the parent(s) or school nurse if you suspect medication side effects.

Any expression of suicidal thoughts or feelings or self-harm by a child or adolescent is a clear signal of distress and should be taken seriously. These behaviors should not be dismissed as "attention seeking."

What Is Eszopiclone (Lunesta)?

Eszopiclone is a *hypnotic* medicine or *sedative-hypnotic*. It is *not* a *benzodiazepine*. It comes in brand name Lunesta tablets.

How Can This Medicine Help?

Eszopiclone is used to treat insomnia—problems falling asleep or staying asleep—when used for a short time along with a behavioral program.

How Does This Medicine Work?

Eszopiclone works to change the activity of *GABA*, one of the *neurotransmitters* that the brain makes for nerve cells to communicate with each other.

How Long Does This Medicine Last?

Eszopiclone is taken before bedtime and starts working within 1 hour. It lasts about 8 hours.

How Will the Doctor Monitor This Medicine?

The doctor will review your child's medical history and physical examination before starting eszopiclone. Be sure to tell the doctor if your child has liver disease.

After the medicine is started, the doctor will want to have regular appointments with you and your child to see how the medicine is working, to see if a dose change is needed, to watch for side effects, to see if eszopiclone is still needed, and to see if any other treatment is needed.

What Side Effects Can This Medicine Have?

Any medicine can have side effects, including an allergy to the medicine. Because each patient is different, the doctor will monitor the youth closely, especially when the medicine is started. The doctor will work with you to increase the positive effects and decrease the negative effects of the medicine. Please tell the doctor if any of the listed side effects appear or if you think that the medicine is causing any other problems. Not all of the rare or unusual side effects are listed.

Side effects are most common after starting the medicine or after a dose increase. Many side effects can be avoided or lessened by starting with a very low dose and increasing it slowly—ask the doctor.

Allergic Reaction

Tell the doctor in a day or two (if possible, before the next dose of medicine):

- Hives
- Itching
- Rash

  Stop the medicine and get *immediate* medical care:

- Trouble breathing or chest tightness
- Swelling of lips, tongue, or throat

Common Side Effects

Tell the doctor in a week or two:

- Daytime sleepiness—Do not allow your child to drive a car, ride a bicycle or motorcycle, or operate machinery if this happens.
- Dizziness, feeling "spacey," or decreased coordination
- Low energy or tiredness
- Headache
- Bad taste in the mouth

263

Less Common Side Effects

Tell the doctor within a week or two:

- More trouble sleeping
- Nausea
- Vomiting
- Diarrhea
- Memory loss
- Nervousness (anxiety)
- Dry mouth
- Nightmares

Rare, but Serious, Side Effects

Tell the doctor right away:

- Depression
- Thoughts of suicide or self-harm
- Hallucinations (seeing or hearing things that are not really there)
- Agitation
- Loss of coordination
- Signs of infection—Fever, chills, sore throat

Some Interactions With Other Medicines or Food

Please note that the following are only the most likely interactions with food or other medicines.

Caffeine may cause trouble sleeping and make eszopiclone less effective. If caffeine is eliminated, less eszopiclone may be needed, or eszopiclone may not be needed at all.

Taking this medicine with or right after a high-fat or large meal may delay or reduce its effect. For faster results, take this medicine several hours after a meal.

It is important not to use other sedatives, tranquilizers, or sleeping pills or antihistamines (such as Benadryl) when taking eszopiclone because of increased daytime sleepiness.

Eszopiclone interacts with many other medicines. Be sure to tell the doctor everything your child is taking.

What Could Happen if This Medicine Is Stopped Suddenly?

When eszopiclone is stopped, there may be more trouble sleeping *(rebound insomnia)* for a few nights.

If eszopiclone has been used regularly for more than a week or in high doses and it is stopped suddenly, withdrawal symptoms may occur. This may include anxiety (nervousness), stomach cramps, vomiting, sweating, or shakiness. Report any such reactions to the doctor right away. It is important to taper the medicine (decrease and stop it slowly).

How Long Will This Medicine Be Needed?

Eszopiclone is usually prescribed for a short time, but some people may need to take it for longer. A behavioral program, such as regular soothing routines at bedtime and increased exercise in the daytime, should be used along with the medicine to improve sleep. Finding developmentally appropriate bed- and wake-times and sticking to them is very important. These strategies should be continued after the medicine is stopped or when the medicine is used only occasionally.

What Else Should I Know About This Medicine?

The tablet should be swallowed whole. Do not break, crush, or allow your child to chew the tablets.

It is possible to become psychologically and physically dependent on eszopiclone, but that is not a common problem for patients who see their doctors regularly and take the medicine as prescribed. It is against the law to give or sell this medicine to someone other than the patient for whom it was prescribed.

People who take eszopiclone must not drink alcohol. Severe sleepiness or even loss of consciousness may result.

People with *sleep apnea* (breathing stops while they are asleep) should not take eszopiclone. Tell the doctor if your child snores very loudly.

Notes

Use this space to take notes or to write down questions you want to ask the doctor.

_____

_____

_____

_____

_____

_____

_____

_____

_____

_____

_____

_____

_____

_____

From Dulcan MK (editor): _Helping Parents, Youth, and Teachers Understand Medications for Behavioral and Emotional Problems: A Resource Book of Medication Information Handouts_, Third Edition. Washington, DC, American Psychiatric Publishing, 2007

Medication Information for Youth

Eszopiclone—Lunesta

What the Medicine Is Called and What It Is For

The name of your medicine may be confusing. Most drugs have two names: 1) a scientific name that we call a *generic name* and 2) a trade or *brand name*. The generic name of this medicine is eszopiclone. The brand name is Lunesta.

Eszopiclone works by calming the parts of the brain that are too excitable. Eszopiclone can help with insomnia (difficulty falling asleep or staying asleep) when used for a short time along with routines that help you to relax and fall asleep.

How You Take the Medicine

It is very important to take the medicine exactly as the doctor or nurse tells you. Do not skip doses or take extra medicine without asking an adult. If you forget a dose, ask your parent(s) what to do.

Swallow the tablet whole. Do not break, crush, or chew the tablets.

Eszopiclone works best if combined with a regular bedtime, calming routines before bedtime, and physical exercise during the day. Getting up on time is also important in keeping a regular sleep schedule.

It is better to limit drinks with caffeine (coffee, tea, soft drinks) because caffeine works in the opposite way from eszopiclone, and the positive effects might be decreased.

Taking this medicine with or right after a big meal may make it not work as well. It works best when taken several hours after eating.

This medicine is prescribed only for you. It should never be shared with anyone else.

You do not have to tell others that you are taking this medicine, but it is not something you should feel ashamed or embarrassed about. Many young people are helped by eszopiclone. You should talk to your doctor or nurse about any questions you have about the medicine. It is important to remember that the medicine *helps* you. It cannot *make* you do anything or change you as a person.

Many medicines cause problems if stopped suddenly. Always ask your doctor before stopping a medicine. Problems are more likely to happen in patients taking high doses of eszopiclone for 2 months or longer, but it is important to decrease the medicine slowly (taper) even after a few weeks. If you notice anxiety, irritability, shaking, sweating, aches and pains, muscle cramps, vomiting, or trouble sleeping, you may need to decrease the medicine more slowly.

How Your Doctor Will Follow Your Progress

Before giving you the medicine, your doctor or nurse will talk with you and your parent(s) and may measure your height, weight, heart rate (pulse), and blood pressure.

Be sure to tell your doctor or nurse about any other medicines or supplements you are taking, including vitamins, herbs, or aids to weight loss or bodybuilding. Also be sure to tell the doctor or nurse if you are using alcohol or drugs. Because many medicines may affect babies, it is very important to tell the doctor if you might be pregnant or if you are at risk of becoming pregnant.

Most doctors have regular appointments with young people who are taking medicine. You should use these visits to share any concerns you may have about your medicine and to talk about if it has helped you. From time to time, your physician or nurse may measure your height, weight, heart rate (pulse), and blood pressure to be sure that you are in good health while you are taking the medicine. Your doctor also will ask for regular reports from your parents to see how well the medicine is working.

Eszopiclone is usually prescribed for only a week or so to allow you to develop better sleep habits. Regular exercise in the daytime usually helps with sleep at night.

Each person is unique, and some people may need this medicine for months or years.

How the Medicine Might Affect You

In addition to the ways the medicine can help you, it may have other effects called *side effects*. Different medicines have different side effects. It is helpful to know about some of the most common side effects of your medicine so that you will understand what they are if they happen. Some people do not have any side effects. Some side effects are just uncomfortable, but others may mean a more serious problem with the medicine. Side effects are most common after starting the medicine or after a dose increase. They may go away with time, or the medicine can be adjusted or changed—ask the doctor.

You could have an allergy to any medicine, which might show up as a rash on your skin, swelling, itching, or trouble breathing.

Please tell your parent(s) and your doctor or nurse about any changes that you notice after taking the medicine. It is especially important to tell a responsible adult if you are feeling depressed or that you may not want to live; if you have thoughts of hurting yourself; or if you begin to feel more irritable, nervous, or restless.

The most common side effect of eszopiclone is daytime sleepiness. If this medicine is making you sleepy, it is very important not to drive a car or ride a bicycle or motorcycle. After starting eszopiclone or increasing the dose, please be extra careful when driving a car, riding a bike, or using machines until you can tell how the medicine affects your alertness, attention, and coordination.

Sometimes sleep medicines seem to work in the opposite way, causing more trouble sleeping, nightmares, excitement, irritability, anger, aggression, or other problems. If this happens, tell your parent(s) or your doctor.

Some people have dry mouth or a bad taste in the mouth when taking this medicine or headache, stomach upset, changes in their bowel movements, or more trouble remembering things. Be sure to tell your parent(s) or doctor if any of these happen.

Drinking alcohol while taking this medicine can cause severe drowsiness or even passing out. **Don't do it!** Do not use marijuana or street drugs while taking this medicine. They can cause serious side effects. Skipping your medicine to take drugs does not work because many medicines stay in your body for a long time.

Eszopiclone can be habit-forming, but that is not a common problem for people who take their medicine as the doctor says.

Notes

Use this space to take notes or to write down questions you want to ask the doctor or nurse.

_____

_____

_____

_____

_____

_____

_____

_____

_____

_____

_____

_____

_____

From Dulcan MK (editor): _Helping Parents, Youth, and Teachers Understand Medications for Behavioral and Emotional Problems: A Resource Book of Medication Information Handouts,_ Third Edition. Washington, DC, American Psychiatric Publishing, 2007

Medication Information for Parents and Teachers

Fluoxetine—Prozac

General Information About Medication

Each child and adolescent is different. No one has exactly the same combination of medical and psychological problems. It is a good idea to talk with the doctor or nurse about the reasons a medicine is being used. It is very important to keep all appointments and to be in touch by telephone if you have concerns. It is important to communicate with the doctor, nurse, or therapist.

It is very important that the medicine be taken exactly as the doctor instructs. However, once in a while, everyone forgets to give a medicine on time. It is a good idea to ask the doctor or nurse what to do if this happens. Do not stop or change a medicine without asking the doctor or nurse first.

If the medicine seems to stop working, it may be because it is not being taken regularly. The youth may be "cheeking" or hiding the medicine or forgetting to take it (especially at school). The doses may be too far apart, or a different dose may be needed. Something at school at home, or in the neighborhood may be upsetting the youth, or he or she may need special help for learning disabilities or tutoring. Please discuss your concerns with the doctor. **Do not just increase the dose.**

All medicines should be kept in a safe place, out of the reach of children, and should be supervised by an adult. If someone takes too much of a medicine, call the doctor the poison control center, or a hospital emergency room.

Each medicine has a "generic" or chemical name. Just like laundry detergents or paper towels, some medicines are sold by more than one company under different brand names. The same medicine may be available under a generic name and several brand names. The generic medications are usually less expensive than the brand name ones. The generic medications have the same chemical formula, but they may or may not be exactly the same strength as the brand-name medications. Also, some brands of pills contain dye that can cause allergic reactions. It is a good idea to talk to the doctor and the pharmacist about whether it is important to use a specific brand of medicine.

All medicines can cause an allergic reaction. Examples are hives, itching, rashes, swelling, and trouble breathing. Even a tiny amount of a medicine can cause a reaction in patients who are allergic to that medicine. Be *sure* to talk to the doctor before restarting a medicine that has caused an allergic reaction.

Taking more than one medicine at the same time may cause more side effects or cause one of the medicines to not work as well. Always ask the doctor, nurse, or pharmacist before adding another medicine, whether prescription or over-the-counter. Be sure that each doctor knows about *all* of the medicines your child is taking. Also tell the doctor about any vitamins, herbal medicines, or supplements your child may be taking. Some of these may have side effects alone or when taken with this medication.

Everyone taking medicine should have a physical examination at least once a year.

If you suspect the youth is using drugs or alcohol, please tell the doctor right away.

271

Pregnancy requires special care in the use of medicine. Please tell the doctor immediately if you suspect the teenager is pregnant or might become pregnant.

Printed information like this applies to children and adolescents in general. If you have questions about the medicine, or if you notice changes or anything unusual, please ask the doctor or nurse. As scientific research advances, knowledge increases and advice changes. Even experts do not always agree. Many medicines have not been approved by the U.S. Food and Drug Administration (FDA) for use in children. For this reason, use of the medicine for a particular problem or age group often is not listed in the *Physicians' Desk Reference*. This does not necessarily mean that the medicine is dangerous or does not work, only that the company that makes the medicine has not received permission to advertise the medicine for use in children. Companies often do not apply for this permission because it is expensive to do the tests needed to apply for approval for use in children. Once a medication is approved by the FDA for any purpose, a doctor is allowed to prescribe it according to research and clinical experience.

Note to Teachers

It is a good idea to talk with the parent(s) about the reason(s) that a medication is being used. If the parent(s) sign consent to release information, it is often helpful to talk with the doctor. If the parent(s) give permission, the doctor may ask you to fill out rating forms about your experience with the student's behavior, feelings, academic performance, and medication side effects. This information is very useful in selecting and monitoring medication treatment. If you have observations that you think are important, do not hesitate to share these with the student's parent(s) and treating clinicians.

It is very important that the medicine be taken exactly as the doctor instructs. However, everyone forgets to give a medicine on time once in a while. It is a good idea to ask the parent(s) in advance what to do if this happens. Do not stop or change the time you are giving a medicine at school without parental permission. If a medication is to be taken with food, but lunchtime or snack time changes, be sure to notify the parent(s) so appropriate adjustments can be made.

All medicines should be kept in a secure place and should be supervised by an adult. If someone takes too much of a medicine, follow your school procedure for an urgent medical problem.

Taking medicine is a private matter and is best managed discreetly and confidentially. It is important to be sensitive to the student's feelings about taking medicine.

If you suspect that the student is using drugs or alcohol, please tell the parent(s) or a school counselor right away.

Please tell the parent(s) or school nurse if you suspect medication side effects.

Modifications of the classroom environment or assignments may be useful in addition to medication. The student may need to be evaluated for additional help or for an Individualized Education Plan for learning or behavior.

Any expression of suicidal thoughts or feelings or self-harm by a child or adolescent is a clear signal of distress and should be taken seriously. These behaviors should not be dismissed as "attention seeking."

What Is Fluoxetine (Prozac)?

Fluoxetine is an *antidepressant* known as a *selective serotonin reuptake inhibitor* (SSRI). It is sold in both brand name Prozac and generic forms. It comes in tablets, capsules, a once-weekly extended-release capsule, and in liquid form. For very small doses or for children who cannot swallow pills, the pill form can be dissolved in cranberry or orange juice and kept in the refrigerator. Fluoxetine is also sold under the brand name of Sarafem for premenstrual syndrome.

How Can This Medicine Help?

Fluoxetine is used to treat depression and anxiety disorders such as obsessive-compulsive disorder (OCD), posttraumatic stress disorder (PTSD), panic disorder, and separation anxiety disorder.

How Does This Medicine Work?

Fluoxetine increases the amount of a *neurotransmitter* called *serotonin* in certain parts of the brain. People with emotional and behavioral problems, such as depression and anxiety, may have low levels of serotonin in certain parts of the brain. SSRIs such as fluoxetine help by increasing the action of brain serotonin to more normal levels.

How Long Does This Medicine Last?

Fluoxetine lasts a very long time. It has some action in the body for as long as 4 weeks after it is stopped.

How Will the Doctor Monitor This Medicine?

The doctor will review your child's medical history and physical examination before starting fluoxetine. The doctor may order some blood or urine tests to be sure your child does not have a hidden medical condition that would make it unsafe to use this medicine. Extra care is needed when using SSRIs in youth with seizures (epilepsy), liver or kidney problems, or diabetes. The doctor or nurse may measure your child's pulse, blood pressure, and weight before starting the medicine.

Be sure to tell the doctor if your child or anyone in the family has bipolar illness (manic-depressive illness) or has tried to kill himself or herself.

After the medicine is started, the doctor will want to have regular appointments with you and your child to see how the medicine is working, to see if a dose change is needed, to watch for side effects, to see if fluoxetine is still needed, and to see if any other treatment is needed. The doctor or nurse may check your child's height, weight, pulse, and blood pressure.

Before using medicine and at times afterward, the doctor may ask your child to fill out a rating scale about depression, to help see how your child is doing.

What Side Effects Can This Medicine Have?

Any medicine can have side effects, including an allergy to the medicine. Because each patient is different, the doctor will monitor the youth closely, especially when the medicine is started. The doctor will work with you to increase the positive effects and decrease the negative effects of the medicine. Please tell the doctor if any of the listed side effects appear or if you think that the medicine is causing any other problems. Not all of the rare or unusual side effects are listed.

Fluoxetine stays in the body for a long time, so side effects may last for days after the medicine is stopped.

Side effects are most common after starting the medicine or after a dose increase. Many side effects can be avoided or lessened by starting with a very low dose and increasing it slowly—ask the doctor.

Allergic Reaction

Tell the doctor in a day or two (if possible, before the next dose of medicine):

- Hives
- Itching
- Rash

Stop the medicine and get *immediate* medical care:

- Trouble breathing or chest tightness
- Swelling of lips, tongue, or throat

Common Side Effects

Tell the doctor within a week or two:

- Nausea, upset stomach, vomiting
- Diarrhea
- Dry mouth—Have your child try using sugar-free gum or candy.
- Constipation—Encourage your child to drink more fluids and eat high-fiber foods; if necessary, the doctor may recommend a fiber medicine such as Benefiber or a stool softener such as Colace or mineral oil.
- Headache
- Anxiety or nervousness
- Insomnia (trouble sleeping)
- Restlessness, increased activity level
- Daytime sleepiness or tiredness—Do not allow your child to drive, ride a bicycle or motorcycle, or operate machinery if this side effect is present.
- Dizziness—This side effect is worse when the child stands up quickly, especially when getting out of bed in the morning; try having the child stand up slowly.
- Tremor (shakiness)
- Excessive sweating
- Apathy, lack of interest in school or friends—This may happen after a initial good response to treatment.
- Decreased sexual interest, trouble with sexual functioning
- Weight gain
- Weight loss

Less Common, but More Serious, Side Effects

Call the doctor within a day or two:

- Significant suicidal thoughts or self-injurious behavior
- Increased activity, rapid speech, feeling "speeded up," decreased need for sleep, being very excited or irritable (cranky)

Serious Side Effects

Call the doctor *immediately* or go to the nearest emergency room:

- Seizure (fit, convulsion)
- Stiffness, high fever, confusion, tremors (shaking)
- Overheating or heatstroke—Prevent by decreasing activity in hot weather, staying out of the sun, and drinking water.

Serotonin Syndrome

A very serious side effect called *serotonin syndrome* can happen when certain kinds of medicines (including some medicines for migraine headaches—triptans) are taken by the same person. *Very* rarely, it can happen at high doses of just one medicine. The early signs are restlessness, confusion, shaking, skin turning red, sweating, and jerking of muscles. If you see these symptoms, stop the medicine and send or take the youth to an emergency room right away.

Some Interactions With Other Medicines or Food

Please note that the following are only the most likely interactions with food or other medicines.

Fluoxetine interacts with many other medicines, including some antibiotics and other psychiatric medicines. It is especially important to tell the doctor and pharmacist about all of the medicines your child is taking or has taken in the past few months, including over-the-counter and herbal medicines. Sometimes one medicine can increase or decrease the blood level of another medicine, so that different doses are needed. Fluoxetine may increase levels of Dilantin (phenytoin), Tegretol (carbamazepine), and Depakote (divalproex sodium), increasing side effects. The herbal medicine St. John's wort also increases serotonin and can cause serious side effects if taken with fluoxetine.

It can be *very dangerous* to take an SSRI at the same time as or even within a month of taking another type of medicine called a *monoamine oxidase inhibitor* (MAOI), such as Eldepryl (selegiline), Nardil (phenelzine), Parnate (tranylcypromine), or Marplan (isocarboxazid).

Fluoxetine does not usually cause problems when taken with decongestant cold medicines.

Fluoxetine can be taken with or without food.

Caffeine may increase side effects.

What Could Happen if This Medicine Is Stopped Suddenly?

No known serious medical effects occur if fluoxetine is stopped suddenly, but there may be uncomfortable feelings, which should be avoided if possible. Fluoxetine stays in the body for a long time and decreases slowly, so withdrawal effects are rare. If your child has trouble sleeping, nervousness, irritability, dizziness, or flu-like symptoms after stopping fluoxetine, consult with your child's doctor.

How Long Will This Medicine Be Needed?

Fluoxetine may take up to 1–2 months to reach its full effect. If your child has a good response to fluoxetine, it is a good idea to continue the medicine for at least 6 months.

What Else Should I Know About This Medicine?

In youth who have bipolar disorder (manic depression) or who are at risk for bipolar disorder, any antidepressant medicine may increase the risk of hypomania or mania (excitement, agitation, increased activity, decreased sleep).

In hot weather, make sure your child drinks enough water or other liquids and does not get overheated.

Sometimes, after a person has improved while taking fluoxetine, he or she loses interest in school or friends or just stops trying. Please tell your child's doctor if this happens—it may be a side effect of the medicine. A lower dose or a different medicine may be needed.

Store the medicine away from sunlight, heat, moisture, and humidity.

Fluoxetine (Prozac) and fluvoxamine (Luvox) are sometimes confused. Be sure to check the prescription.

Black Box Antidepressant Warning

In 2004, an advisory committee to the FDA decided that there might be an increased risk of suicidal behavior for some youth taking medicines called *antidepressants*. In the research studies that the committee reviewed, about 3%–4% of youth with depression who took an antidepressant medicine—and 1%–2% of youth with depression who took a placebo (pill without active medicine)—talked about suicidal thoughts (thinking about killing themselves or wishing they were dead) or did something to harm themselves. This means that almost twice as many youth who were taking an antidepressant to treat their depression talked about suicide or had suicidal behavior compared with youth with depression who were taking inactive medicine. There were *no* completed suicides in any of these research studies, which included more than 4,000 children and adolescents. For youth being treated for anxiety, there was no difference in suicidal talking or behavior between those taking antidepressant medication and those taking placebo.

The FDA told drug companies to add a *black box warning* label to all antidepressant medicines. Because of this label, a doctor (or advanced practice nurse) prescribing one of these medicines has to warn youth and their families that there might be more suicidal thoughts and actions in youth taking these medicines.

On the other hand, in places where more youth are taking the newer antidepressant medicines, the number of adolescents who commit suicide has gotten smaller. Also, thinking about or attempting suicide is more common in surveys of teenagers in the community than it is in depressed youth treated in research studies with antidepressant medicine.

If a youth is being treated with this medicine and is doing well, then no changes are needed as a result of this warning. Increased suicidal talk or action is most likely to happen in the first few months of treatment with a medicine. If your child has recently started this medicine or is about to start, then you and your doctor (or advanced practice nurse) should watch for any changes in behavior. People who are depressed often have suicidal thoughts or actions. It is hard to know whether suicidal thoughts or actions in depressed people are caused by the depression itself or by the medicine. Also, as their depression is getting better, some people talk more about the suicidal thoughts that they had before but did not talk about. As young people get better from depression, they might be at higher risk of doing something about suicidal thoughts that they have had for some time, because they have more energy.

What Should a Parent Do?

1. Be honest with your child about possible risks and benefits of medicine.
2. Talk to your child about whether he or she is having any suicidal thoughts, and tell your child to come to you if he or she is having such thoughts.
3. You, your child, and your child's doctor or nurse should develop a safety plan. Pick adults whom your child can tell if he or she is thinking about suicide.

4. Be sure to tell your child's doctor, nurse, or therapist if you suspect that your child is using alcohol or drugs or if something has happened that might make your child feel worse, such as a family separation, breaking up with a boyfriend or girlfriend, someone close dying or attempting suicide, physical or sexual abuse, or failure in school.

5. Be sure that there are no guns in the home and that all medicines (including over-the-counter medicines like Tylenol) are closely supervised by an adult and kept in a safe place.

6. Watch for new or worse thoughts of suicide, self-harm, depression, anxiety (nerves), feeling very agitated or restless, being angry or aggressive, having more trouble sleeping, or anything else that you see for the first time, seems worse, or worries your child or you. If these appear, contact a mental health professional **right away.** Do not just stop or change the dose of the medicine on your own. If the problems are serious, and you cannot reach one of your clinicians, call a 24-hour psychiatry emergency telephone number or take your child to an emergency room.

Youth on antidepressant medicine should be watched carefully by their parent(s), clinician(s) (doctor, nurse, therapist), and other concerned adults for the first weeks of treatment. It is a good idea to have a visit or telephone call with the doctor, nurse, or therapist weekly for the first month, every 2 weeks for the second month, and after that at least once a month to check for feelings of depression or sadness, thoughts of killing or harming him- or herself, and any problems with the medication. If you have questions, be sure to ask the doctor, nurse, or therapist.

For more information, see http://www.parentsmedguide.org/ (in English and Spanish).

Notes

Use this space to take notes or to write down questions you want to ask the doctor.

_____

_____

_____

_____

_____

_____

_____

_____

_____

_____

_____

_____

Medication Information
for Youth

Fluoxetine—Prozac

What the Medicine Is Called and What It Is For

The name of your medicine may be confusing. Most drugs have two names: 1) a scientific name that we call a *generic name* and 2) a trade or *brand name*. The generic name of this medicine is fluoxetine. The brand name is Prozac.

Fluoxetine is called an *antidepressant*, or *selective serotonin reuptake inhibitor* (SSRI). Fluoxetine is used to treat depression and anxiety disorders such as obsessive-compulsive disorder (OCD), posttraumatic stress disorder (PTSD), panic disorder, and separation anxiety disorder. It helps people who feel very sad or depressed, anxious (nervous), or afraid, or who have *obsessions* (uncomfortable thoughts that will not go away) or *compulsions* (habits that get in the way of daily life).

How You Take the Medicine

It is very important to take the medicine exactly as the doctor or nurse tells you. Do not skip doses or take extra medicine without asking an adult. If you forget a dose, ask your parent(s) what to do. It is very important that you take all the pills you are supposed to take each day. Your doctor will probably recommend that you take your medicine at the same time each day, which may be with meals or at bedtime.

It may take several weeks before you notice that the medicine is helping. Waiting for the full effect may take even longer. You may feel discouraged and think the medicine is never going to help. You may want to give up and stop taking the medicine. Talk to your doctor and parent(s) about how you feel, but **do not stop** taking the medicine unless your doctor tells you to. It is also important not to take extra pills, hoping that you will feel better faster. Doing that could make you very sick.

Caffeine (in coffee, tea, or soft drinks) may make you feel worse.

This medicine is prescribed only for you. It should never be shared with anyone else.

You do not have to tell others that you are taking this medicine, but it is not something you should feel ashamed or embarrassed about. Many young people are helped by fluoxetine. This medicine is not habit-forming, and you cannot become "hooked" on it. You should talk to your doctor or nurse about any questions you have about the medicine. It is important to remember that the medicine *helps* you. It cannot *make* you do anything or change you as a person.

How Your Doctor Will Follow Your Progress

Before giving you the medicine, your doctor or nurse will talk with you and your parent(s) and may measure your height, weight, heart rate (pulse), and blood pressure. The doctor may order some blood or urine tests to be sure you are in good health.

Be sure to tell your doctor or nurse about any other medicines or supplements you are taking, including vitamins, herbs, or aids to weight loss or bodybuilding. Also be sure to tell the doctor or nurse if you are using alcohol or drugs. Because many medicines may affect babies, it is very important to tell the doctor if you might be pregnant or if you are at risk of becoming pregnant. Be sure to tell the doctor if you have had thoughts of hurting yourself, have tried to hurt yourself, or sometimes wish that you were not alive.

Your teachers may be asked to fill out a form about your grades and behavior in school. A psychologist may give you some tests to see how you learn best.

Before starting the medicine and afterward, the doctor may ask you to answer questions on paper about depression and anxiety.

Most doctors have regular appointments with young people who are taking medicine. You should use these visits to share any concerns you may have about your medicine and to talk about if it has helped you. From time to time, your physician or nurse may measure your height, weight, heart rate (pulse), and blood pressure to be sure that you are in good health while you are taking the medicine. Your doctor also will ask for regular reports from your parents and maybe from your teachers (with your permission) to see how well the medicine is working.

Some medicines are started at the amount you will take for as long as you are taking that medicine. Other medicines need to be increased or adjusted until your doctor decides you are taking the right amount. Starting at a low dose and increasing it slowly may lessen side effects. If the medicine helps you, your doctor will probably want you to take it for 6 months to a year if you are taking it to treat depression. If you are taking it for another problem, your doctor will decide how long you will need to take the medicine as he or she watches your progress.

It is not dangerous to stop fluoxetine suddenly, but there might be uncomfortable feelings, such as trouble sleeping, nervousness, irritability, or feeling sick. It is better to decrease it slowly. Do not stop taking a medicine unless the doctor tells you to. If you have any problems after stopping or decreasing this medicine, tell your parent(s) or doctor.

How the Medicine Might Affect You

In addition to the ways the medicine can help you, it may have other effects called *side effects*. Different medicines have different side effects. It is helpful to know about some of the most common side effects of your medicine so that you will understand what they are if they happen. Some people do not have any side effects. Some side effects are just uncomfortable, but others may mean a more serious problem with the medicine. Side effects are most common after starting the medicine or after a dose increase. They may go away with time, or the medicine can be adjusted or changed—ask the doctor.

You could have an allergy to any medicine, which might show up as a rash on your skin, swelling, itching, or trouble breathing.

Please tell your parent(s) and your doctor or nurse about any changes that you notice after taking the medicine. It is especially important to tell a responsible adult if you are feeling depressed or that you may not want to live; if you have thoughts of hurting yourself; or if you begin to feel more irritable, nervous, or restless. Also be sure to tell your parent(s) or doctor if you begin to feel "speeded up" or have trouble sleeping.

Some medicines make people feel sleepy or less coordinated. If this medicine is making you sleepy, it is very important not to drive a car or ride a bicycle or motorcycle. After starting a new medicine or increasing the dose of a medicine, please be extra careful when driving a car, riding a bike, or using machines until you can tell how the medicine affects your alertness, attention, and coordination.

One of the most common side effects of this medicine is feeling tired or sleepy during the day, even if you have had a full night's sleep. After you have been taking the medicine for a few weeks, your body will adjust, and this side effect may go away. If you have had trouble sleeping at night, fluoxetine may improve your sleep when other symptoms improve. Fluoxetine may make you feel more restless and excited. Tell your parent(s) or doctor if this side effect is uncomfortable. Sometimes after being on the medicine for a while, people do not care as much about school or friends. Changing the dose or the type of medicine can help this—ask the doctor.

This medicine may make your mouth dry. You may be more thirsty than usual and find that you are drinking more water or other liquids. Sucking on sugar-free hard candy or cough drops usually helps. You also could try chewing sugar-free gum or sucking on ice chips. Do not chew the ice; you could hurt your teeth. Also, using lip balm will keep your lips from cracking. It is important to be especially good about brushing your teeth.

Some other side effects that could happen are headache, not feeling hungry and not wanting to eat much, eating more than usual, having an upset stomach, or changes in your bowel movements. You may have a change in your sexual functioning—it is OK to ask the doctor about this. This medicine may make you more likely to get sick if you get overheated, so be sure to drink plenty of liquids and rest in the shade in hot weather.

Please let your parent(s) and doctor know if you notice anything different or unusual about how you feel once you start taking the medicine. This includes good things, such as feeling less sad or less nervous or sleeping better at night.

Notes

Use this space to take notes or to write down questions you want to ask the doctor or nurse.

_____

_____

_____

_____

_____

_____

_____

_____

_____

_____

From Dulcan MK (editor): *Helping Parents, Youth, and Teachers Understand Medications for Behavioral and Emotional Problems: A Resource Book of Medication Information Handouts,* Third Edition. Washington, DC, American Psychiatric Publishing, 2007

Medication Information for Parents and Teachers

Fluphenazine—Prolixin

General Information About Medication

Each child and adolescent is different. No one has exactly the same combination of medical and psychological problems. It is a good idea to talk with the doctor or nurse about the reasons a medicine is being used. It is very important to keep all appointments and to be in touch by telephone if you have concerns. It is important to communicate with the doctor, nurse, or therapist.

It is very important that the medicine be taken exactly as the doctor instructs. However, once in a while, everyone forgets to give a medicine on time. It is a good idea to ask the doctor or nurse what to do if this happens. Do not stop or change a medicine without asking the doctor or nurse first.

If the medicine seems to stop working, it may be because it is not being taken regularly. The youth may be "cheeking" or hiding the medicine or forgetting to take it (especially at school). The doses may be too far apart, or a different dose may be needed. Something at school, at home, or in the neighborhood may be upsetting the youth, or he or she may need special help for learning disabilities or tutoring. Please discuss your concerns with the doctor. **Do not just increase the dose.**

All medicines should be kept in a safe place, out of the reach of children, and should be supervised by an adult. If someone takes too much of a medicine, call the doctor, the poison control center, or a hospital emergency room.

Each medicine has a "generic" or chemical name. Just like laundry detergents or paper towels, some medicines are sold by more than one company under different brand names. The same medicine may be available under a generic name and several brand names. The generic medications are usually less expensive than the brand name ones. The generic medications have the same chemical formula, but they may or may not be exactly the same strength as the brand-name medications. Also, some brands of pills contain dye that can cause allergic reactions. It is a good idea to talk to the doctor and the pharmacist about whether it is important to use a specific brand of medicine.

All medicines can cause an allergic reaction. Examples are hives, itching, rashes, swelling, and trouble breathing. Even a tiny amount of a medicine can cause a reaction in patients who are allergic to that medicine. Be *sure* to talk to the doctor before restarting a medicine that has caused an allergic reaction.

Taking more than one medicine at the same time may cause more side effects or cause one of the medicines to not work as well. Always ask the doctor, nurse, or pharmacist before adding another medicine, whether prescription or over-the-counter. Be sure that each doctor knows about *all* of the medicines your child is taking. Also tell the doctor about any vitamins, herbal medicines, or supplements your child may be taking. Some of these may have side effects alone or when taken with this medication.

Everyone taking medicine should have a physical examination at least once a year.

If you suspect the youth is using drugs or alcohol, please tell the doctor right away.

283

Pregnancy requires special care in the use of medicine. Please tell the doctor immediately if you suspect the teenager is pregnant or might become pregnant.

Printed information like this applies to children and adolescents in general. If you have questions about the medicine, or if you notice changes or anything unusual, please ask the doctor or nurse. As scientific research advances, knowledge increases and advice changes. Even experts do not always agree. Many medicines have not been approved by the U.S. Food and Drug Administration (FDA) for use in children. For this reason, use of the medicine for a particular problem or age group often is not listed in the *Physicians' Desk Reference*. This does not necessarily mean that the medicine is dangerous or does not work, only that the company that makes the medicine has not received permission to advertise the medicine for use in children. Companies often do not apply for this permission because it is expensive to do the tests needed to apply for approval for use in children. Once a medication is approved by the FDA for any purpose, a doctor is allowed to prescribe it according to research and clinical experience.

Note to Teachers

It is a good idea to talk with the parent(s) about the reason(s) that a medication is being used. If the parent(s) sign consent to release information, it is often helpful to talk with the doctor. If the parent(s) give permission, the doctor may ask you to fill out rating forms about your experience with the student's behavior, feelings, academic performance, and medication side effects. This information is very useful in selecting and monitoring medication treatment. If you have observations that you think are important, do not hesitate to share these with the student's parent(s) and treating clinicians.

It is very important that the medicine be taken exactly as the doctor instructs. However, everyone forgets to give a medicine on time once in a while. It is a good idea to ask the parent(s) in advance what to do if this happens. Do not stop or change the time you are giving a medicine at school without parental permission. If a medication is to be taken with food, but lunchtime or snack time changes, be sure to notify the parent(s) so appropriate adjustments can be made.

All medicines should be kept in a secure place and should be supervised by an adult. If someone takes too much of a medicine, follow your school procedure for an urgent medical problem.

Taking medicine is a private matter and is best managed discreetly and confidentially. It is important to be sensitive to the student's feelings about taking medicine.

If you suspect that the student is using drugs or alcohol, please tell the parent(s) or a school counselor right away.

Please tell the parent(s) or school nurse if you suspect medication side effects.

Modifications of the classroom environment or assignments may be useful in addition to medication. The student may need to be evaluated for additional help or for an Individualized Education Plan for learning or behavior.

Any expression of suicidal thoughts or feelings or self-harm by a child or adolescent is a clear signal of distress and should be taken seriously. These behaviors should not be dismissed as "attention seeking."

What Is Fluphenazine (Prolixin)?

Fluphenazine is sometimes called a *typical, conventional,* or *first-generation antipsychotic* medicine. It is also called a *neuroleptic* or *phenothiazine.* It used to be called a *major tranquilizer.* It comes in brand name Prolixin and generic tablets, liquid, and two kinds of shots (injections)—immediate-acting and very long-acting (fluphenazine decanoate).

How Can This Medicine Help?

Fluphenazine is used to treat psychosis, such as in schizophrenia, mania, or very severe depression. It can reduce hallucinations (hearing voices or seeing things that are not there) and delusions (troubling beliefs that other people do not share). It can help the patient be less upset and agitated. It can improve the patient's ability to think clearly.

Sometimes fluphenazine is used to decrease severe aggression or very serious behavioral problems in young people with conduct disorder, mental retardation, or autism.

This medicine is very powerful and should be used to treat very serious problems or symptoms that other medicines do not help. Be patient; the positive effects of this medicine may not appear for 2–3 weeks.

How Does This Medicine Work?

Cells in the brain (neurons) communicate using chemicals called *neurotransmitters*. Too much or too little of these substances in certain parts of the brain can cause problems. Fluphenazine reduces the activity of one of these neurotransmitters, *dopamine*. Blocking the effect of dopamine in certain parts of the brain reduces what have been called *positive symptoms* of psychosis: delusions; hallucinations; disorganized and unusual thinking, speaking, and behavior; excessive activity (agitation); and lack of activity (catatonia). Blocking dopamine can also reduce tics. Reducing dopamine action in other parts of the brain may lead to the side effects of this medicine.

How Long Does This Medicine Last?

Fluphenazine usually may be taken only once a day, unless divided doses are used to lessen side effects. An injection of fluphenazine decanoate lasts for 2–3 weeks.

How Will the Doctor Monitor This Medicine?

The doctor will review your child's medical history and physical examination before starting fluphenazine. The doctor may order some blood or urine tests to be sure your child does not have a hidden medical condition. The doctor or nurse may measure your child's pulse and blood pressure before starting fluphenazine.

Before your child starts taking fluphenazine and every so often afterward, a test such as the AIMS (Abnormal Involuntary Movement Scale) may be used to check your child's tongue, legs, and arms for unusual movements that could be caused by the medicine.

After the medicine is started, the doctor will want to have regular appointments with you and your child to see how the medicine is working, to see if a dose change is needed, to watch for side effects, to see if fluphenazine is still needed, and to see if any other treatment is needed. The doctor or nurse may check your child's height, weight, pulse, and blood pressure, and watch for abnormal movements.

What Side Effects Can This Medicine Have?

Any medicine can have side effects, including an allergy to the medicine. Because each patient is different, the doctor will monitor the youth closely, especially when the medicine is started. The doctor will work with you

to increase the positive effects and decrease the negative effects of the medicine. Please tell the doctor if any of the listed side effects appear or if you think that the medicine is causing any other problems. Not all of the rare or unusual side effects are listed.

Side effects are most common after starting the medicine or after a dose increase. Many side effects can be avoided or lessened by starting with a very low dose and increasing it slowly—ask the doctor.

Allergic Reaction

Tell the doctor in a day or two (if possible, before the next dose of medicine):

- Hives
- Itching
- Rash

Stop the medicine and get *immediate* medical care:

- Trouble breathing or chest tightness
- Swelling of lips, tongue, or throat

Common, but Not Usually Serious, Side Effects

Discuss the following side effects with your child's doctor within a week or two. They often can be helped by lowering the dose of medicine, changing the times medicine is taken, or adding another medicine.

- Dry mouth—Have your child try using sugar-free gum or candy.
- Constipation—Encourage your child to drink more fluids and eat high-fiber foods; if necessary, a fiber medicine such as Benefiber or a stool softener such as Colace or mineral oil may be used.
- Mild trouble urinating
- Blurred vision
- Weight gain—Seek nutritional counseling; provide your child with low-calorie snacks and encourage regular exercise.
- Sadness, irritability, nervousness, clinginess, not wanting to go to school
- Restlessness or inability to sit still
- Shaking of hands and fingers

Less Common, but Not Usually Serious, Side Effects

Discuss the following side effects with your child's doctor within a week or two. They often can be helped by lowering the dose of medicine, changing the times medicine is taken, or adding another medicine.

- Daytime sleepiness or tiredness—Do not allow your child to drive, ride a bicycle or motorcycle, or operate machinery if this happens. This problem may be lessened by taking the medicine at bedtime.
- Dizziness—This side effect is worse when the child stands up quickly, especially when getting out of bed in the morning; try having the child stand up slowly.
- Decreased or slowed movement and decreased facial expressions
- Drooling
- Decreased sexual interest or ability

- Changes in menstrual cycle
- Increase in breast size or discharge from the breasts (in both boys and girls)—This may go away with time.

Less Common, but Potentially Serious, Side Effects

Call the doctor or go to an emergency room *right away:*

- Stiffness of the tongue, jaw, neck, back, or legs
- Overheating or heatstroke—Prevent by decreasing activity in hot weather, staying out of the sun, and drinking water.
- Seizure (fit, convulsion)—This is more likely in people with a history of seizures or head injury.
- Severe confusion

Serious, but Rare, Side Effects

- Extreme stiffness or lack of movement, very high fever, mental confusion, irregular pulse rate, or eye pain—**This is a medical emergency. Go to an emergency room *right away.***
- Sudden stiffness and inability to breathe or swallow—**Go to an emergency room or call 911.** Tell the paramedics, nurses, and doctors that the patient is taking fluphenazine. Other medicines can be used to treat this problem fast.
- Increased thirst, frequent urination, lethargy, tiredness, dizziness—These could be signs of diabetes (especially if your child is overweight or there is a family history of diabetes). **Talk to a doctor within a day.**

What Else Should I Know About Side Effects?

Most side effects lessen over time. If they are troublesome, talk with your child's doctor. Some side effects can be decreased by taking a smaller dose of medicine, by stopping the medicine, by changing to another medicine, or by adding another medicine (see table below).

One side effect that may not go away is *tardive dyskinesia* (or TD). Patients with tardive dyskinesia have involuntary movements of the body, especially the mouth and tongue. The patient may look as though he or she is making faces over and over again. Jerky movements of the arms, legs, or body may occur. There may be fine, wormlike, or sudden repeated movements of the tongue, or the person may appear to be chewing something or smacking or puckering his or her lips. The fingers may look as though they are rolling something. If you notice any unusual movements, be sure to tell the doctor. The doctor may use the AIMS test to look for these movements.

The medicine may increase the level of *prolactin*, a natural hormone made in the part of the brain called the *pituitary*. This may cause side effects such as breast tenderness or swelling or production of milk, in both boys and girls. It also may interfere with sexual functioning in teenage boys and with regular menstrual cycles (periods) in teenage girls. A blood test can measure the level of prolactin. If these side effects do not go away and are troublesome, talk with your child's doctor about substituting another medicine for fluphenazine.

Heart problems are more common if other medicines are being taken also. Be sure to tell your child's doctors and your pharmacist about all medications your child is taking.

Neuroleptic malignant syndrome is a very rare side effect that can lead to death. The symptoms are severe muscle stiffness, high fever, increased heart rate and blood pressure, irregular heartbeat (pulse), and sweating. It may lead to unconsciousness. If you suspect this, **call 911 or go to an emergency room right away.**

What Medicines Are Used to Treat the Side Effects of Fluphenazine?

The following medicines may be used to treat the movement side effects of fluphenazine. These medicines may have their own side effects as well; ask the doctor if you suspect a problem.

Brand name	Generic name
Akineton	Biperiden
Artane	Trihexyphenidyl
Ativan	Lorazepam*
Benadryl	Diphenhydramine*
Catapres	Clonidine*
Cogentin	Benztropine mesylate*
Inderal	Propranolol*
Klonopin	Clonazepam*
Symmetrel	Amantadine

*This medicine has its own information sheet in this book.

Some Interactions With Other Medicines or Food

Please note that the following are only the most likely interactions with food or other medicines.

Fluphenazine may be taken with or without food. If the medicine causes stomach upset, taking it with food may help.

Fluoxetine (Prozac) or paroxetine (Paxil) may increase the levels of fluphenazine, increasing the risk of side effects.

It is better to limit drinks with caffeine (coffee, tea, soft drinks) because caffeine works in the opposite way from this medicine, and the positive effects might be decreased.

What Could Happen if This Medicine Is Stopped Suddenly?

Involuntary movements, or *withdrawal dyskinesias*, may appear within 1–4 weeks of lowering the dose or stopping the medicine. Usually these go away, but they can last for days to months. If fluphenazine is stopped suddenly, emotional problems such as irritability, nervousness, or moodiness; behavior problems; or physical problems such as stomachache, loss of appetite, nausea, vomiting, diarrhea, sweating, indigestion, trouble sleeping, trembling, or shaking may appear. These problems usually last only a few days to a few weeks. If they happen, tell your child's doctor. The medicine dose may need to be lowered more slowly (tapered). Always check with the doctor before stopping a medicine!

How Long Will This Medicine Be Needed?

How long your child will need to be on fluphenazine depends partly on the reason that it was prescribed. Some problems last for only a few months, whereas others last much longer. Sometimes fluphenazine is used for only a short time until other medicines or behavioral treatments start to work. Some people need to take fluphenazine for years. It is especially important with medicines as powerful as this one to ask the doctor whether it is still needed. Every few months, you should discuss with your child's doctor the reasons for using fluphenazine and whether it is time for a trial of lowering the dose.

What Else Should I Know About This Medicine?

There are many older and newer medicines that are used for the same kinds of problems. If your child is having bad side effects or the medicine does not seem to be working, ask the doctor if another medicine in this group might work as well or better and have fewer side effects for your child.

Be sure to tell the doctor if there is anyone in your family who died suddenly or had a heart problem.

Notes

Use this space to take notes or to write down questions you want to ask the doctor.

_____

_____

_____

_____

_____

_____

_____

_____

From Dulcan MK (editor): _Helping Parents, Youth, and Teachers Understand Medications for Behavioral and Emotional Problems: A Resource Book of Medication Information Handouts,_ Third Edition. Washington, DC, American Psychiatric Publishing, 2007

Fluphenazine—Prolixin

What the Medicine Is Called and What It Is For

The name of your medicine may be confusing. Most drugs have two names: 1) a scientific name that we call a *generic name* and 2) a trade or *brand name*. The generic name of this medicine is fluphenazine. The brand name is Prolixin.

Fluphenazine can help people who feel very confused and have severe problems thinking clearly. It can lessen *hallucinations* (seeing or hearing things that are not really there) and *delusions* (troubling beliefs that other people do not share). This medicine also is sometimes used to help young people who have mania or very severe depression or who get very angry and hit people or break things.

How You Take the Medicine

It is very important to take the medicine exactly as the doctor or nurse tells you. Do not skip doses or take extra medicine without asking an adult. If you forget a dose, ask your parent(s) what to do.

It is better to limit drinks with caffeine (coffee, tea, soft drinks) because caffeine works in the opposite way from this medicine, and the positive effects might be decreased.

If your stomach is upset, taking the medicine with food may help.

This medicine is prescribed only for you. It should never be shared with anyone else.

You do not have to tell others that you are taking this medicine, but it is not something you should feel ashamed or embarrassed about. Many young people are helped by fluphenazine. This medicine is not habit-forming, and you cannot become "hooked" on it. You should talk to your doctor or nurse about any questions you have about the medicine. It is important to remember that the medicine *helps* you. It cannot *make* you do anything or change you as a person.

How Your Doctor Will Follow Your Progress

Before giving you the medicine, your doctor or nurse will talk with you and your parent(s) and may measure your height, weight, heart rate (pulse), and blood pressure. There may be other tests, such as blood tests for sugar and cholesterol. Before you start taking the medicine and every so often afterward, the doctor or nurse will look at your tongue, arms, and legs to check for unusual movements. This is called the AIMS (Abnormal Involuntary Movement Scale) test.

Be sure to tell your doctor or nurse about any other medicines or supplements you are taking, including vitamins, herbs, or aids to weight loss or bodybuilding. Also be sure to tell the doctor or nurse if you are using alcohol or drugs. Because many medicines may affect babies, it is very important to tell the doctor if you might be pregnant or if you are at risk of becoming pregnant.

Your teachers may be asked to fill out a form about your grades and behavior in school. A psychologist may give you some tests to see how you learn best.

Most doctors have regular appointments with young people who are taking medicine. You should use these visits to share any concerns you may have about your medicine and to talk about if it has helped you. From time to time, your physician or nurse may measure your height, weight, heart rate (pulse), and blood pressure to be sure that you are in good health while you are taking the medicine. There may be blood tests to watch for diabetes or high cholesterol. Your doctor also will ask for regular reports from your parents and maybe from your teachers (with your permission) to see how well the medicine is working.

If the medicine helps you, your doctor will probably want you to take it for several months to a year. Your doctor will decide how long you will need to take the medicine as he or she watches your progress.

How the Medicine Might Affect You

In addition to the ways the medicine can help you, it may have other effects called *side effects*. Different medicines have different side effects. It is helpful to know about some of the most common side effects of your medicine so that you will understand what they are if they happen. Some people do not have any side effects. Some side effects are just uncomfortable, but others may mean a more serious problem with the medicine. Side effects are most common after starting the medicine or after a dose increase. They may go away with time, or the medicine can be adjusted or changed—ask the doctor.

You could have an allergy to any medicine, which might show up as a rash on your skin, swelling, itching, or trouble breathing.

Please tell your parent(s) and your doctor or nurse about any changes that you notice after taking the medicine. It is especially important to tell a responsible adult if you are feeling depressed or that you may not want to live; if you have thoughts of hurting yourself; or if you begin to feel more irritable, nervous, or restless.

One of the most common side effects of this medicine is feeling tired or sleepy during the day, even if you have had a full night's sleep. If this medicine is making you sleepy, it is very important not to drive a car or ride a bicycle or motorcycle. After starting the medicine or increasing the dose of medicine, please be extra careful when driving a car, riding a bike, or using machines until you can tell how the medicine affects your alertness, attention, and coordination. After you have been taking the medicine for a few weeks, your body will adjust, and this side effect will likely go away. If you had trouble sleeping at night before taking the medicine, it can help you sleep better, especially if the doctor tells you to take a dose of medicine in the evening.

You might feel dizzy or light-headed if you stand up fast. Try standing up slowly, especially when getting out of bed in the morning.

Another common side effect is dry mouth. You may be more thirsty than usual and find that you are drinking more water or other liquids than usual. Sucking on sugar-free hard candy or cough drops usually helps. You also could try chewing sugar-free gum or sucking on ice chips. Do not chew the ice; you could hurt your teeth. Also, using lip balm will keep your lips from cracking. It is important to be especially good about brushing your teeth.

Taking this medicine could make you more likely to get badly sunburned or very sick in hot weather. Be sure to drink plenty of liquids and cover up or use sunscreen when you go outside in hot weather. Be careful to rest in the shade and not get overheated.

Sometimes teenagers who take fluphenazine gain weight. The weight gain may be from increased appetite and also from ways that the medicine changes how the body processes food. It is much easier to prevent weight gain than to lose weight later. It is a good idea to eat a well-balanced diet without "junk food" and with healthy snacks like fruits and vegetables, not sweets or fried foods. It is better to drink water or skim milk, not pop, sodas, soft drinks, or sugary juices. Regular exercise is important for maintaining a healthy weight (and may also help with sleep).

Some people become constipated (have hard bowel movements) when taking this medicine. Try drinking more water and eating more fruits, vegetables, and whole grains. If that does not help, tell your parent(s) or doctor—you may need a medicine to help with this side effect. Sometimes people have trouble passing urine. Tell your parent(s) or the doctor if this happens.

This is a very powerful medicine. Some side effects include feeling nervous, restless, or shaky or having stiff muscles. Talk with your doctor about these side effects. They can be helped by adding another medicine, adjusting the dose, or switching to another medicine.

Another, more serious, side effect can be longer lasting and more difficult to treat. This very rare side effect is called *tardive dyskinesia* (or TD). A person taking fluphenazine may develop movements of the mouth, tongue, face, arms, legs, or body that are not being made on purpose. This side effect can go away when the medicine is stopped, but in some people it does not go away. Your doctor will explain this effect to you and your parent(s) and how he or she will watch for any signs that you are developing this problem. Be sure to ask your doctor any questions that you may have about this, but do not worry too much about it. It hardly ever happens to teenagers.

You may notice changes in your sexual functioning or in your breasts—it is OK to ask the doctor about this.

You should tell your parent(s) and doctor if you notice anything different or unusual about how you feel once you start taking the medicine. This includes good things, such as feeling less confused, feeling less sad or angry, not hearing voices anymore, or sleeping better at night.

You cannot become addicted to this medicine, but you should not stop it suddenly. Never stop a medicine without talking to the doctor. If fluphenazine is stopped or decreased suddenly you may notice more moodiness or irritability, stomachaches or upset stomach, trouble sleeping, or trembling or shaking. Let your parent(s) or doctor know if this happens—the medicine may need to be decreased more slowly.

Notes

Use this space to take notes or to write down questions you want to ask the doctor or nurse.

_____

_____

_____

Copyright © 2007 American Psychiatric Publishing, Inc. The purchaser of this book is licensed to distribute copies of these forms in limited amounts. Please see copyright page for further information. The authors have worked to ensure that all information in this book concerning drug dosages, schedules, routes of administration, and side effects is accurate as of the time of publication and consistent with standards set by the U.S. Food and Drug Administration and the general medical community and accepted child psychiatric practice. The information on this medication sheet does not cover all the possible uses, precautions, side effects, or interactions of this drug. For a complete listing of side effects, see the manufacturer's package insert, which can be obtained from your physician or pharmacist. As medical research and practice advance, therapeutic standards may change. For this reason and because human and mechanical errors sometimes occur, we recommend that readers follow the advice of a physician who is directly involved in their care or the care of a member of their family.

From Dulcan MK (editor): _Helping Parents, Youth, and Teachers Understand Medications for Behavioral and Emotional Problems: A Resource Book of Medication Information Handouts_, Third Edition. Washington, DC, American Psychiatric Publishing, 2007

Medication Information for Parents and Teachers

Flurazepam—Dalmane

General Information About Medication

Each child and adolescent is different. No one has exactly the same combination of medical and psychological problems. It is a good idea to talk with the doctor or nurse about the reasons a medicine is being used. It is very important to keep all appointments and to be in touch by telephone if you have concerns. It is important to communicate with the doctor, nurse, or therapist.

It is very important that the medicine be taken exactly as the doctor instructs. However, once in a while, everyone forgets to give a medicine on time. It is a good idea to ask the doctor or nurse what to do if this happens. Do not stop or change a medicine without asking the doctor or nurse first.

If the medicine seems to stop working, it may be because it is not being taken regularly. The youth may be "cheeking" or hiding the medicine or forgetting to take it (especially at school). The doses may be too far apart, or a different dose may be needed. Something at school, at home, or in the neighborhood may be upsetting the youth, or he or she may need special help for learning disabilities or tutoring. Please discuss your concerns with the doctor. **Do not just increase the dose.**

All medicines should be kept in a safe place, out of the reach of children, and should be supervised by an adult. If someone takes too much of a medicine, call the doctor, the poison control center, or a hospital emergency room.

Each medicine has a "generic" or chemical name. Just like laundry detergents or paper towels, some medicines are sold by more than one company under different brand names. The same medicine may be available under a generic name and several brand names. The generic medications are usually less expensive than the brand name ones. The generic medications have the same chemical formula, but they may or may not be exactly the same strength as the brand-name medications. Also, some brands of pills contain dye that can cause allergic reactions. It is a good idea to talk to the doctor and the pharmacist about whether it is important to use a specific brand of medicine.

All medicines can cause an allergic reaction. Examples are hives, itching, rashes, swelling, and trouble breathing. Even a tiny amount of a medicine can cause a reaction in patients who are allergic to that medicine. Be *sure* to talk to the doctor before restarting a medicine that has caused an allergic reaction.

Taking more than one medicine at the same time may cause more side effects or cause one of the medicines to not work as well. Always ask the doctor, nurse, or pharmacist before adding another medicine, whether prescription or over-the-counter. Be sure that each doctor knows about *all* of the medicines your child is taking. Also tell the doctor about any vitamins, herbal medicines, or supplements your child may be taking. Some of these may have side effects alone or when taken with this medication.

Everyone taking medicine should have a physical examination at least once a year.

If you suspect the youth is using drugs or alcohol, please tell the doctor right away.

Pregnancy requires special care in the use of medicine. Please tell the doctor immediately if you suspect the teenager is pregnant or might become pregnant.

295

Printed information like this applies to children and adolescents in general. If you have questions about the medicine, or if you notice changes or anything unusual, please ask the doctor or nurse. As scientific research advances, knowledge increases and advice changes. Even experts do not always agree. Many medicines have not been approved by the U.S. Food and Drug Administration (FDA) for use in children. For this reason, use of the medicine for a particular problem or age group often is not listed in the *Physicians' Desk Reference*. This does not necessarily mean that the medicine is dangerous or does not work, only that the company that makes the medicine has not received permission to advertise the medicine for use in children. Companies often do not apply for this permission because it is expensive to do the tests needed to apply for approval for use in children. Once a medication is approved by the FDA for any purpose, a doctor is allowed to prescribe it according to research and clinical experience.

Note to Teachers

It is a good idea to talk with the parent(s) about the reason(s) that a medication is being used. If the parent(s) sign consent to release information, it is often helpful to talk with the doctor. If the parent(s) give permission, the doctor may ask you to fill out rating forms about your experience with the student's behavior, feelings, academic performance, and medication side effects. This information is very useful in selecting and monitoring medication treatment. If you have observations that you think are important, do not hesitate to share these with the student's parent(s) and treating clinicians.

It is very important that the medicine be taken exactly as the doctor instructs. However, everyone forgets to give a medicine on time once in a while. It is a good idea to ask the parent(s) in advance what to do if this happens. Do not stop or change the time you are giving a medicine at school without parental permission. If a medication is to be taken with food, but lunchtime or snack time changes, be sure to notify the parent(s) so appropriate adjustments can be made.

All medicines should be kept in a secure place and should be supervised by an adult. If someone takes too much of a medicine, follow your school procedure for an urgent medical problem.

Taking medicine is a private matter and is best managed discreetly and confidentially. It is important to be sensitive to the student's feelings about taking medicine.

If you suspect that the student is using drugs or alcohol, please tell the parent(s) or a school counselor right away.

Please tell the parent(s) or school nurse if you suspect medication side effects.

Modifications of the classroom environment or assignments may be useful in addition to medication. The student may need to be evaluated for additional help or for an Individualized Education Plan for learning or behavior.

Any expression of suicidal thoughts or feelings or self-harm by a child or adolescent is a clear signal of distress and should be taken seriously. These behaviors should not be dismissed as "attention seeking."

What Is Flurazepam (Dalmane)?

Flurazepam is a *benzodiazepine* medicine. It is called a *hypnotic* or *sedative-hypnotic*. It comes in Dalmane brand name and generic capsules.

How Can This Medicine Help?

Flurazepam is used to treat insomnia—problems falling asleep or staying asleep—when used for a short time along with a behavioral program. It can also be used for problem sleep behaviors, called *parasomnias*, such as

296

night terrors (sudden waking up from sleep with great fear), sleepwalking, or sleeptalking, when these put the youth at risk of an accident or make it impossible for other family members to get enough sleep.

How Does This Medicine Work?

Flurazepam works on *receptors* (special places on brain cells) in certain parts of the brain to change the action of *GABA*—a *neurotransmitter*—a chemical that the brain makes for brain cells to communicate with each other.

How Long Does This Medicine Last?

Flurazepam is taken before bedtime and starts working within an hour. There may still be some effects in the morning. Benzodiazepine hypnotics differ in how long they last. Flurazepam is a long-acting benzodiazepine, so it is more likely to cause sleepiness and memory problems the next day. The medicine builds up in the body if taken every day, which can make daytime drowsiness worse

How Will the Doctor Monitor This Medicine?

The doctor will review your child's medical history and physical examination before starting flurazepam.

After the medicine is started, the doctor will want to have regular appointments with you and your child to see how the medicine is working, to see if a dose change is needed, to watch for side effects, to see if flurazepam is still needed, and to see if any other treatment is needed.

What Side Effects Can This Medicine Have?

Any medicine can have side effects, including an allergy to the medicine. Because each patient is different, the doctor will monitor the youth closely, especially when the medicine is started. The doctor will work with you to increase the positive effects and decrease the negative effects of the medicine. Please tell the doctor if any of the listed side effects appear or if you think that the medicine is causing any other problems. Not all of the rare or unusual side effects are listed.

Side effects are most common after starting the medicine or after a dose increase. Many side effects can be avoided or lessened by starting with a very low dose and increasing it slowly—ask the doctor.

Allergic Reaction

Tell the doctor in a day or two (if possible, before the next dose of medicine):

- Hives
- Itching
- Rash

Stop the medicine and get *immediate* medical care:

- Trouble breathing or chest tightness
- Swelling of lips, tongue, or throat

Flurazepam is usually very safe when used for short periods as the doctor prescribes.

The most common side effect is daytime sleepiness. Flurazepam can also cause dizziness, feeling "spacey," or decreased coordination. If the medicine is causing any of these problems it is very important not to drive a car, ride a bicycle or motorcycle, or operate machinery.

Flurazepam can cause decreased concentration and memory. These problems, along with daytime sleepiness, may decrease learning and performance in school.

People who take flurazepam must not drink alcohol. Severe sleepiness or even loss of consciousness may result.

It is possible to become psychologically and physically dependent on flurazepam, but that is not a common problem for patients who see their doctors regularly. Because some people abuse benzodiazepines, it is illegal to give or sell these medicines to someone other than the patient for whom they were prescribed.

Very rarely, flurazepam causes excitement, irritability, anger, aggression, agitation, trouble sleeping, nightmares, uncontrollable behavior, or memory loss. This is called *disinhibition* or a *paradoxical effect*. This may be more common in younger children. Stop the medicine and call the doctor if this happens.

Some Interactions With Other Medicines or Food

Please note that the following are only the most likely interactions with food or other medicines.

Caffeine (in soft drinks, coffee, tea) may cause trouble sleeping and make flurazepam less effective. If caffeine is eliminated, less flurazepam may be needed, or flurazepam may not be needed at all.

Oral contraceptives (birth control pills), antifungal agents (such as ketoconazole), fluoxetine (Prozac), fluvoxamine (Luvox), cimetidine (Tagamet), and other medicines may increase the levels of flurazepam and increase side effects.

It is important not to use other sedatives, tranquilizers, or sleeping pills or antihistamines (such as Benadryl) when taking flurazepam because of greatly increased side effects.

What Could Happen if This Medicine Is Stopped Suddenly?

Many medicines cause problems if stopped suddenly. Flurazepam must be decreased slowly (tapered) rather than stopped suddenly. When flurazepam is stopped suddenly, there are withdrawal symptoms that are uncomfortable and may even be dangerous. Problems are more likely in patients taking high doses of flurazepam for 2 months or longer, but even after just a few weeks of taking flurazepam it is important to stop it slowly. Withdrawal symptoms may include anxiety, irritability, shaking, sweating, aches and pains, muscle cramps, vomiting, confusion, and trouble sleeping. If large doses taken for a long time are stopped suddenly, seizures (fits, convulsions), hallucinations (hearing voices or seeing things that are not there), or out-of-control behavior may result.

How Long Will This Medicine Be Needed?

The length of time depends on why flurazepam is being used. When used for sleep, it is usually prescribed for only a week or so. A behavioral program, such as regular soothing routines at bedtime and increased exercise in the daytime, should be used along with the medicine to improve sleep. This program can be continued after the medicine is tapered (stopped slowly) or when the medicine is used only occasionally.

When used for night terrors or other parasomnias, the medicine may be needed for months or years.

What Else Should I Know About This Medicine?

Because benzodiazepines can be abused (especially by people who abuse alcohol or drugs) and can cause psychological dependence or physical dependence (addiction), they are regulated by special state and federal laws as *controlled substances*. These laws place limitations on telephone prescriptions and refills.

People with sleep apnea (breathing stops while they are asleep) should not take flurazepam. Tell the doctor if your child snores very loudly.

Flurazepam should be avoided during pregnancy, especially in the first 3 months, because it may cause birth defects in the baby. If taken regularly at the end of pregnancy, flurazepam may cause withdrawal symptoms in the baby.

Notes

Use this space to take notes or to write down questions you want to ask the doctor.

_____

_____

_____

_____

_____

_____

_____

_____

_____

_____

_____

_____

_____

From Dulcan MK (editor): *Helping Parents, Youth, and Teachers Understand Medications for Behavioral and Emotional Problems: A Resource Book of Medication Information Handouts,* Third Edition. Washington, DC, American Psychiatric Publishing, 2007

Medication Information for Youth

Flurazepam—Dalmane

What the Medicine Is Called and What It Is For

The name of your medicine may be confusing. Most drugs have two names: 1) a scientific name that we call a *generic name* and 2) a trade or *brand name*. The generic name of this medicine is flurazepam. The brand name is Dalmane.

Flurazepam is a *benzodiazepine* medicine. It works by calming the parts of the brain that are too excitable. Flurazepam can help with insomnia (difficulty falling asleep or staying asleep) when used for a short time along with routines that help you to relax and fall asleep. Flurazepam also can be used for sleep problems such as night terrors (sudden waking up from sleep very scared) or sleepwalking.

How You Take the Medicine

It is very important to take the medicine exactly as the doctor or nurse tells you. Do not skip doses or take extra medicine without asking an adult. If you forget a dose, ask your parent(s) what to do.

It is better to limit drinks with caffeine (coffee, tea, soft drinks) because caffeine works in the opposite way from this medicine, and the positive effects might be decreased.

This medicine is prescribed only for you. It should never be shared with anyone else.

You do not have to tell others that you are taking this medicine, but it is not something you should feel ashamed or embarrassed about. Many young people are helped by flurazepam. You should talk to your doctor or nurse about any questions you have about the medicine. It is important to remember that the medicine *helps* you. It cannot *make* you do anything or change you as a person.

Many medicines cause problems if stopped suddenly. Always ask your doctor before stopping a medicine. Problems are more likely to happen in patients taking high doses of flurazepam for 2 months or longer, but it is important to decrease the medicine slowly (taper) even after a few weeks. If you notice anxiety, irritability, shaking, sweating, aches and pains, muscle cramps, vomiting, or trouble sleeping, you may need to decrease the medicine more slowly. If large doses are stopped suddenly, seizures (fits, convulsions), hallucinations (hearing voices or seeing things that are not there), or out-of-control behavior may result.

How Your Doctor Will Follow Your Progress

Before giving you the medicine, your doctor or nurse will talk with you and your parent(s) and may measure your height, weight, heart rate (pulse), and blood pressure.

Be sure to tell your doctor or nurse about any other medicines or supplements you are taking, including vitamins, herbs, or aids to weight loss or bodybuilding. Also be sure to tell the doctor or nurse if you are using alcohol or drugs. Because many medicines may affect babies, it is very important to tell the doctor if you might be pregnant or if you are at risk of becoming pregnant.

Most doctors have regular appointments with young people who are taking medicine. You should use these visits to share any concerns you may have about your medicine and to talk about if it has helped you. From time to time, your physician or nurse may measure your height, weight, heart rate (pulse), and blood pressure to be sure that you are in good health while you are taking the medicine. Your doctor also will ask for regular reports from your parents to see how well the medicine is working.

Flurazepam is usually prescribed for only a week or so to allow you to develop better sleep habits. Regular exercise in the daytime usually helps with sleep at night.

Each person is unique, and some people may need this medicine for months or years.

How the Medicine Might Affect You

In addition to the ways the medicine can help you, it may have other effects called *side effects*. Different medicines have different side effects. It is helpful to know about some of the most common side effects of your medicine so that you will understand what they are if they happen. Some people do not have any side effects. Some side effects are just uncomfortable, but others may mean a more serious problem with the medicine. Side effects are most common after starting the medicine or after a dose increase. They may go away with time, or the medicine can be adjusted or changed—ask the doctor.

You could have an allergy to any medicine, which might show up as a rash on your skin, swelling, itching, or trouble breathing.

Please tell your parent(s) and your doctor or nurse about any changes that you notice after taking the medicine. It is especially important to tell a responsible adult if you are feeling depressed or that you may not want to live; if you have thoughts of hurting yourself; or if you begin to feel more irritable, nervous, or restless.

The most common side effect of flurazepam is daytime sleepiness. If this medicine is making you sleepy, it is very important not to drive a car or ride a bicycle or motorcycle. After starting flurazepam or increasing the dose, please be extra careful when driving a car, riding a bike, or using machines until you can tell how the medicine affects your alertness, attention, and coordination.

Sometimes sleep medicines seem to work in the opposite way, causing excitement, irritability, anger, aggression, and other problems. If this happens, tell your parent(s) or your doctor.

Drinking alcohol while taking this medicine can cause severe drowsiness or even passing out. **Don't do it!** Do not use marijuana or street drugs while taking this medicine. They can cause serious side effects. Skipping your medicine to take drugs does not work because many of the medicines stay in your body for a long time.

Flurazepam can be habit-forming, but that is not a common problem for people who take their medicine as the doctor says.

Notes

Use this space to take notes or to write down questions you want to ask the doctor or nurse.

_____

_____

_____

_____

_____

_____

_____

_____

_____

_____

_____

_____

_____

From Dulcan MK (editor): _Helping Parents, Youth, and Teachers Understand Medications for Behavioral and Emotional Problems: A Resource Book of Medication Information Handouts,_ Third Edition. Washington, DC, American Psychiatric Publishing, 2007

Medication Information for Parents and Teachers

Fluvoxamine—Luvox

General Information About Medication

Each child and adolescent is different. No one has exactly the same combination of medical and psychological problems. It is a good idea to talk with the doctor or nurse about the reasons a medicine is being used. It is very important to keep all appointments and to be in touch by telephone if you have concerns. It is important to communicate with the doctor, nurse, or therapist.

It is very important that the medicine be taken exactly as the doctor instructs. However, once in a while, everyone forgets to give a medicine on time. It is a good idea to ask the doctor or nurse what to do if this happens. Do not stop or change a medicine without asking the doctor or nurse first.

If the medicine seems to stop working, it may be because it is not being taken regularly. The youth may be "cheeking" or hiding the medicine or forgetting to take it (especially at school). The doses may be too far apart, or a different dose may be needed. Something at school, at home, or in the neighborhood may be upsetting the youth, or he or she may need special help for learning disabilities or tutoring. Please discuss your concerns with the doctor. **Do not just increase the dose.**

All medicines should be kept in a safe place, out of the reach of children, and should be supervised by an adult. If someone takes too much of a medicine, call the doctor, the poison control center, or a hospital emergency room.

Each medicine has a "generic" or chemical name. Just like laundry detergents or paper towels, some medicines are sold by more than one company under different brand names. The same medicine may be available under a generic name and several brand names. The generic medications are usually less expensive than the brand name ones. The generic medications have the same chemical formula, but they may or may not be exactly the same strength as the brand-name medications. Also, some brands of pills contain dye that can cause allergic reactions. It is a good idea to talk to the doctor and the pharmacist about whether it is important to use a specific brand of medicine.

All medicines can cause an allergic reaction. Examples are hives, itching, rashes, swelling, and trouble breathing. Even a tiny amount of a medicine can cause a reaction in patients who are allergic to that medicine. Be *sure* to talk to the doctor before restarting a medicine that has caused an allergic reaction.

Taking more than one medicine at the same time may cause more side effects or cause one of the medicines to not work as well. Always ask the doctor, nurse, or pharmacist before adding another medicine, whether prescription or over-the-counter. Be sure that each doctor knows about *all* of the medicines your child is taking. Also tell the doctor about any vitamins, herbal medicines, or supplements your child may be taking. Some of these may have side effects alone or when taken with this medication.

Everyone taking medicine should have a physical examination at least once a year.

If you suspect the youth is using drugs or alcohol, please tell the doctor right away.

Pregnancy requires special care in the use of medicine. Please tell the doctor immediately if you suspect the teenager is pregnant or might become pregnant.

Printed information like this applies to children and adolescents in general. If you have questions about the medicine, or if you notice changes or anything unusual, please ask the doctor or nurse. As scientific research advances, knowledge increases and advice changes. Even experts do not always agree. Many medicines have not been approved by the U.S. Food and Drug Administration (FDA) for use in children. For this reason, use of the medicine for a particular problem or age group often is not listed in the *Physicians' Desk Reference*. This does not necessarily mean that the medicine is dangerous or does not work, only that the company that makes the medicine has not received permission to advertise the medicine for use in children. Companies often do not apply for this permission because it is expensive to do the tests needed to apply for approval for use in children. Once a medication is approved by the FDA for any purpose, a doctor is allowed to prescribe it according to research and clinical experience.

Note to Teachers

It is a good idea to talk with the parent(s) about the reason(s) that a medication is being used. If the parent(s) sign consent to release information, it is often helpful to talk with the doctor. If the parent(s) give permission, the doctor may ask you to fill out rating forms about your experience with the student's behavior, feelings, academic performance, and medication side effects. This information is very useful in selecting and monitoring medication treatment. If you have observations that you think are important, do not hesitate to share these with the student's parent(s) and treating clinicians.

It is very important that the medicine be taken exactly as the doctor instructs. However, everyone forgets to give a medicine on time once in a while. It is a good idea to ask the parent(s) in advance what to do if this happens. Do not stop or change the time you are giving a medicine at school without parental permission. If a medication is to be taken with food, but lunchtime or snack time changes, be sure to notify the parent(s) so appropriate adjustments can be made.

All medicines should be kept in a secure place and should be supervised by an adult. If someone takes too much of a medicine, follow your school procedure for an urgent medical problem.

Taking medicine is a private matter and is best managed discreetly and confidentially. It is important to be sensitive to the student's feelings about taking medicine.

If you suspect that the student is using drugs or alcohol, please tell the parent(s) or a school counselor right away.

Please tell the parent(s) or school nurse if you suspect medication side effects.

Modifications of the classroom environment or assignments may be useful in addition to medication. The student may need to be evaluated for additional help or for an Individualized Education Plan for learning or behavior.

Any expression of suicidal thoughts or feelings or self-harm by a child or adolescent is a clear signal of distress and should be taken seriously. These behaviors should not be dismissed as "attention seeking."

What Is Fluvoxamine (Luvox)?

Fluvoxamine is an *antidepressant* known as a *selective serotonin reuptake inhibitor* (SSRI). It comes in brand name Luvox and generic tablets.

How Can This Medicine Help?

Fluvoxamine is used to treat depression and anxiety disorders such as obsessive-compulsive disorder (OCD), posttraumatic stress disorder (PTSD), panic disorder, and separation anxiety disorder.

How Does This Medicine Work?

Fluvoxamine increases the amount of a *neurotransmitter* called *serotonin* in certain parts of the brain. People with emotional and behavioral problems, such as depression and anxiety, may have low levels of serotonin in certain parts of the brain. SSRIs such as fluvoxamine help by increasing the action of brain serotonin to more normal levels.

How Long Does This Medicine Last?

Fluvoxamine can be taken only once a day, although at higher doses it should be divided into two daily doses to lessen side effects.

How Will the Doctor Monitor This Medicine?

The doctor will review your child's medical history and physical examination before starting fluvoxamine. The doctor may order some blood or urine tests to be sure your child does not have a hidden medical condition that would make it unsafe to use this medicine. Extra care is needed when using SSRIs in youth with seizures (epilepsy), liver or kidney problems, or diabetes. The doctor or nurse may measure your child's pulse, blood pressure, and weight before starting the medicine.

Be sure to tell the doctor if your child or anyone in the family has bipolar illness (manic-depressive illness) or has tried to kill himself or herself.

After the medicine is started, the doctor will want to have regular appointments with you and your child to see how the medicine is working, to see if a dose change is needed, to watch for side effects, to see if fluvoxamine is still needed, and to see if any other treatment is needed. The doctor or nurse may check your child's height, weight, pulse, and blood pressure.

Before using medicine and at times afterward, the doctor may ask your child to fill out a rating scale about depression, to help see how your child is doing.

What Side Effects Can This Medicine Have?

Any medicine can have side effects, including an allergy to the medicine. Because each patient is different, the doctor will monitor the youth closely, especially when the medicine is started. The doctor will work with you to increase the positive effects and decrease the negative effects of the medicine. Please tell the doctor if any of the listed side effects appear or if you think that the medicine is causing any other problems. Not all of the rare or unusual side effects are listed.

Side effects are most common after starting the medicine or after a dose increase. Many side effects can be avoided or lessened by starting with a very low dose and increasing it slowly—ask the doctor.

Allergic Reaction

Tell the doctor in a day or two (if possible, before the next dose of medicine):

- Hives
- Itching
- Rash

Stop the medicine and get *immediate* medical care:

- Trouble breathing or chest tightness
- Swelling of lips, tongue, or throat

Common Side Effects

Tell the doctor within a week or two:

- Nausea, upset stomach, vomiting
- Diarrhea
- Dry mouth—Have your child try using sugar-free gum or candy.
- Constipation—Encourage your child to drink more fluids and eat high-fiber foods; if necessary, a fiber medicine such as Benefiber or a stool softener such as Colace or mineral oil may be used.
- Headache
- Anxiety or nervousness
- Insomnia (trouble sleeping)
- Restlessness, increased activity level
- Daytime sleepiness or tiredness—Do not allow your child to drive, ride a bicycle or motorcycle, or operate machinery if this happens.
- Dizziness—This side effect is worse when the child stands up quickly, especially when getting out of bed in the morning; try having the child stand up slowly.
- Tremor (shakiness)
- Excessive sweating
- Apathy, lack of interest in school or friends—This may happen after a initial good response to treatment.
- Decreased sexual interest, trouble with sexual functioning
- Weight gain
- Weight loss

Less Common, but More Serious, Side Effects

Call the doctor within a day or two:

- Significant suicidal thoughts or self-injurious behavior
- Increased activity, rapid speech, feeling "speeded up," decreased need for sleep, being very excited or irritable (cranky)

Serious Side Effects

Call the doctor *immediately* or go to the nearest emergency room:

- Seizure (fit, convulsion)
- Stiffness, high fever, confusion, tremors (shaking)
- Overheating or heatstroke—Prevent by decreasing activity in hot weather, staying out of the sun, and drinking water.

Serotonin Syndrome

A very serious side effect called *serotonin syndrome* can happen when certain kinds of medicines (including some medicines for migraine headaches—triptans) are taken by the same person. *Very* rarely, it can happen at high doses of just one medicine. The early signs are restlessness, confusion, shaking, skin turning red, sweating, and jerking of muscles. If you see these symptoms, stop the medicine and send or take the youth to an emergency room right away.

Some Interactions With Other Medicines or Food

Please note that the following are only the most likely interactions with food or other medicines.

Fluvoxamine interacts with many other medicines, including some antibiotics and other psychiatric medicines. It is especially important to tell the doctor and pharmacist about all of the medicines your child is taking or has taken in the past few months, including over-the-counter and herbal medicines. Sometimes one medicine can increase or decrease the blood level of another medicine so that different doses are needed. Fluvoxamine may increase levels of theophylline (used for asthma) and carbamazepine (Tegretol), increasing the risk of side effects. The herbal medicine St. John's wort also increases serotonin and can cause serious side effects if taken with fluvoxamine.

It can be *very dangerous* to take an SSRI at the same time as or even within a month of taking another type of medicine called a *monoamine oxidase inhibitor* (MAOI), such as Eldepryl (selegiline), Nardil (phenelzine), Parnate (tranylcypromine), or Marplan (isocarboxazid).

Fluvoxamine does not usually cause problems when taken with decongestant cold medicines.

Fluvoxamine can be taken with or without food.

Caffeine may increase side effects.

What Could Happen if This Medicine Is Stopped Suddenly?

No known serious medical effects occur if fluvoxamine is stopped suddenly, but there may be uncomfortable feelings, which should be avoided if possible. Your child might have trouble sleeping, nervousness, irritability, dizziness, and flu-like symptoms. Ask the doctor before stopping fluvoxamine or if these symptoms happen while the dose is being decreased.

How Long Will This Medicine Be Needed?

Fluvoxamine may take up to 1–2 months to reach its full effect. If your child has a good response to fluvoxamine, it is a good idea to continue the medicine for at least 6 months.

What Else Should I Know About This Medicine?

In youth who have bipolar disorder (manic depression) or who are at risk for bipolar disorder, any antidepressant medicine may increase the risk of hypomania or mania (excitement, agitation, increased activity, decreased sleep).

In hot weather, make sure your child drinks enough water or other liquids and does not get overheated.

Sometimes, after a person has improved while taking fluvoxamine, he or she loses interest in school or friends or just stops trying. Please tell your child's doctor if this happens—it may be a side effect of the medicine. A lower dose or a different medicine may be needed.

Store the medicine away from sunlight, heat, moisture, and humidity.

Fluoxetine (Prozac) and fluvoxamine (Luvox) are sometimes confused. Be sure to check the prescription.

Black Box Antidepressant Warning

In 2004, an advisory committee to the FDA decided that there might be an increased risk of suicidal behavior for some youth taking medicines called *antidepressants*. In the research studies that the committee reviewed, about 3%–4% of youth with depression who took an antidepressant medicine—and 1%–2% of youth with depression who took a placebo (pill without active medicine)—talked about suicidal thoughts (thinking about killing themselves or wishing they were dead) or did something to harm themselves. This means that almost twice as many youth who were taking an antidepressant to treat their depression talked about suicide or had suicidal behavior compared with youth with depression who were taking inactive medicine. There were *no* completed suicides in any of these research studies, which included more than 4,000 children and adolescents. For youth being treated for anxiety, there was no difference in suicidal talking or behavior between those taking antidepressant medication and those taking placebo.

The FDA told drug companies to add a *black box warning* label to all antidepressant medicines. Because of this label, a doctor (or advanced practice nurse) prescribing one of these medicines has to warn youth and their families that there might be more suicidal thoughts and actions in youth taking these medicines.

On the other hand, in places where more youth are taking the newer antidepressant medicines, the number of adolescents who commit suicide has gotten smaller. Also, thinking about or attempting suicide is more common in surveys of teenagers in the community than it is in depressed youth treated in research studies with antidepressant medicine.

If a youth is being treated with this medicine and is doing well, then no changes are needed as a result of this warning. Increased suicidal talk or action is most likely to happen in the first few months of treatment with a medicine. If your child has recently started this medicine or is about to start, then you and your doctor (or advanced practice nurse) should watch for any changes in behavior. People who are depressed often have suicidal thoughts or actions. It is hard to know whether suicidal thoughts or actions in depressed people are caused by the depression itself or by the medicine. Also, as their depression is getting better, some people talk more about the suicidal thoughts that they had before but did not talk about. As young people get better from depression, they might be at higher risk of doing something about suicidal thoughts that they have had for some time, because they have more energy.

What Should a Parent Do?

1. Be honest with your child about possible risks and benefits of medicine.
2. Talk to your child about whether he or she is having any suicidal thoughts, and tell your child to come to you if he or she is having such thoughts.
3. You, your child, and your child's doctor or nurse should develop a safety plan. Pick adults whom your child can tell if he or she is thinking about suicide.

4. Be sure to tell your child's doctor, nurse, or therapist if you suspect that your child is using alcohol or drugs or if something has happened that might make your child feel worse, such as a family separation, breaking up with a boyfriend or girlfriend, someone close dying or attempting suicide, physical or sexual abuse, or failure in school.

5. Be sure that there are no guns in the home and that all medicines (including over-the-counter medicines like Tylenol) are closely supervised by an adult and kept in a safe place.

6. Watch for new or worse thoughts of suicide, self-harm, depression, anxiety (nerves), feeling very agitated or restless, being angry or aggressive, having more trouble sleeping, or anything else that you see for the first time, seems worse, or worries your child or you. If these appear, contact a mental health professional **right away.** Do not just stop or change the dose of the medicine on your own. If the problems are serious, and you cannot reach one of your clinicians, call a 24-hour psychiatry emergency telephone number or take your child to an emergency room.

Youth on antidepressant medicine should be watched carefully by their parent(s), clinician(s) (doctor, nurse, therapist), and other concerned adults for the first weeks of treatment. It is a good idea to have a visit or telephone call with the doctor, nurse, or therapist weekly for the first month, every 2 weeks for the second month, and after that at least once a month to check for feelings of depression or sadness, thoughts of killing or harming himself or herself, and any problems with the medication. If you have questions, be sure to ask the doctor, nurse, or therapist.

For more information, see http://www.parentsmedguide.org/ (in English and Spanish).

Notes

Use this space to take notes or to write down questions you want to ask the doctor.

_____

_____

_____

_____

_____

_____

_____

_____

_____

_____

_____

_____

_____

From Dulcan MK (editor): *Helping Parents, Youth, and Teachers Understand Medications for Behavioral and Emotional Problems: A Resource Book of Medication Information Handouts,* Third Edition. Washington, DC, American Psychiatric Publishing, 2007

Medication Information
for Youth

Fluvoxamine—Luvox

What the Medicine Is Called and What It Is For

The name of your medicine may be confusing. Most drugs have two names: 1) a scientific name that we call a *generic name* and 2) a trade or *brand name*. The generic name of this medicine is fluvoxamine. The brand name is Luvox.

Fluvoxamine is called an *antidepressant*, or *selective serotonin reuptake inhibitor* (SSRI). Fluvoxamine is used to treat depression and anxiety disorders such as obsessive-compulsive disorder (OCD), posttraumatic stress disorder (PTSD), panic disorder, and separation anxiety disorder. It helps people who feel very sad or depressed, anxious (nervous), or afraid, or who have *obsessions* (uncomfortable thoughts that will not go away) or *compulsions* (habits that get in the way of daily life).

How You Take the Medicine

It is very important to take the medicine exactly as the doctor or nurse tells you. Do not skip doses or take extra medicine without asking an adult. If you forget a dose, ask your parent(s) what to do. It is very important that you take all the pills you are supposed to take each day. Your doctor will probably recommend that you take your medicine at the same time each day, which may be with meals or at bedtime.

It may take several weeks before you notice that the medicine is helping. Waiting for the full effect may take even longer. You may feel discouraged and think the medicine is never going to help. You may want to give up and stop taking the medicine. Talk to your doctor and parent(s) about how you feel, but **do not stop** taking the medicine unless your doctor tells you to. It is also important not to take extra pills, hoping that you will feel better faster. Doing that could make you very sick.

Caffeine (in coffee, tea, or soft drinks) may make you feel worse.

This medicine is prescribed only for you. It should never be shared with anyone else.

You do not have to tell others that you are taking this medicine, but it is not something you should feel ashamed or embarrassed about. Many young people are helped by fluvoxamine. This medicine is not habit-forming, and you cannot become "hooked" on it. You should talk to your doctor or nurse about any questions you have about the medicine. It is important to remember that the medicine *helps* you. It cannot *make* you do anything or change you as a person.

How Your Doctor Will Follow Your Progress

Before giving you the medicine, your doctor or nurse will talk with you and your parent(s) and may measure your height, weight, heart rate (pulse), and blood pressure. The doctor may order some blood or urine tests to be sure you are in good health.

Be sure to tell your doctor or nurse about any other medicines or supplements you are taking, including vitamins, herbs, or aids to weight loss or bodybuilding. Also be sure to tell the doctor or nurse if you are using alcohol or drugs. Because many medicines may affect babies, it is very important to tell the doctor if you might be pregnant or if you are at risk of becoming pregnant. Be sure to tell the doctor if you have had thoughts of hurting yourself, have tried to hurt yourself, or sometimes wish that you were not alive.

Your teachers may be asked to fill out a form about your grades and behavior in school. A psychologist may give you some tests to see how you learn best.

Before starting the medicine and afterward, the doctor may ask you to answer questions on paper about depression and anxiety.

Most doctors have regular appointments with young people who are taking medicine. You should use these visits to share any concerns you may have about your medicine and to talk about if it has helped you. From time to time, your physician or nurse may measure your height, weight, heart rate (pulse), and blood pressure to be sure that you are in good health while you are taking the medicine. Your doctor also will ask for regular reports from your parents and maybe from your teachers (with your permission) to see how well the medicine is working.

Some medicines are started at the amount you will take for as long as you are taking that medicine. Other medicines need to be increased or adjusted until your doctor decides you are taking the right amount. Starting at a low dose and increasing it slowly may lessen side effects. If the medicine helps you, your doctor will probably want you to take it for 6 months to a year if you are taking it to treat depression. If you are taking it for another problem, your doctor will decide how long you will need to take the medicine as he or she watches your progress.

It is not dangerous to stop fluvoxamine suddenly, but there might be uncomfortable feelings, such as trouble sleeping, nervousness, irritability, or feeling sick. It is better to decrease it slowly. Do not stop taking a medicine unless the doctor tells you to. If you have any problems after stopping or decreasing this medicine, tell your parent(s) or doctor.

How the Medicine Might Affect You

In addition to the ways the medicine can help you, it may have other effects called *side effects*. Different medicines have different side effects. It is helpful to know about some of the most common side effects of your medicine so that you will understand what they are if they happen. Some people do not have any side effects. Some side effects are just uncomfortable, but others may mean a more serious problem with the medicine. Side effects are most common after starting the medicine or after a dose increase. They may go away with time, or the medicine can be adjusted or changed—ask the doctor.

You could have an allergy to any medicine, which might show up as a rash on your skin, swelling, itching, or trouble breathing.

Please tell your parent(s) and your doctor or nurse about any changes that you notice after taking the medicine. It is especially important to tell a responsible adult if you are feeling depressed or that you may not want to live; if you have thoughts of hurting yourself; or if you begin to feel more irritable, nervous, or restless. Also be sure to tell your parent(s) or doctor if you begin to feel "speeded up" or have trouble sleeping.

Some medicines make people feel sleepy or less coordinated. If this medicine is making you sleepy, it is very important not to drive a car or ride a bicycle or motorcycle. After starting a new medicine or increasing the dose of a medicine, please be extra careful when driving a car, riding a bike, or using machines until you can tell how the medicine affects your alertness, attention, and coordination.

One of the most common side effects of this medicine is feeling tired or sleepy during the day, even if you have had a full night's sleep. After you have been taking the medicine for a few weeks, your body will adjust, and this side effect may go away. If you have had trouble sleeping at night, the medicine can help you sleep better, especially if the doctor tells you to take a dose of medicine in the evening. Other people may feel more restless and excited. Tell your parent(s) or doctor if this is uncomfortable. Sometimes after being on the medicine for a while, people do not care as much about school or friends. Changing the dose or the type of medicine can help this.

This medicine may make your mouth dry. You may be more thirsty than usual and find that you are drinking more water or other liquids. Sucking on sugar-free hard candy or cough drops usually helps. You also could try chewing sugar-free gum or sucking on ice chips. Do not chew the ice; you could hurt your teeth. Also, using lip balm will keep your lips from cracking. It is important to be especially good about brushing your teeth.

Some other side effects that could happen are headache, not feeling hungry and not wanting to eat much, eating more than usual, having an upset stomach, or changes in your bowel movements. You may have a change in your sexual functioning—it is OK to ask the doctor about this. This medicine may make you more likely to get sick if you get overheated, so be sure to drink plenty of liquids and rest in the shade in hot weather.

Please let your parent(s) and doctor know if you notice anything different or unusual about how you feel once you start taking the medicine. This includes good things, such as feeling less sad or less nervous or sleeping better at night.

Notes

Use this space to take notes or to write down questions you want to ask the doctor or nurse.

_____

_____

_____

_____

_____

_____

_____

From Dulcan MK (editor): _Helping Parents, Youth, and Teachers Understand Medications for Behavioral and Emotional Problems: A Resource Book of Medication Information Handouts_, Third Edition. Washington, DC, American Psychiatric Publishing, 2007

Medication Information for Parents and Teachers

Gabapentin—Neurontin

General Information About Medication

Each child and adolescent is different. No one has exactly the same combination of medical and psychological problems. It is a good idea to talk with the doctor or nurse about the reasons a medicine is being used. It is very important to keep all appointments and to be in touch by telephone if you have concerns. It is important to communicate with the doctor, nurse, or therapist.

It is very important that the medicine be taken exactly as the doctor instructs. However, once in a while, everyone forgets to give a medicine on time. It is a good idea to ask the doctor or nurse what to do if this happens. Do not stop or change a medicine without asking the doctor or nurse first.

If the medicine seems to stop working, it may be because it is not being taken regularly. The youth may be "cheeking" or hiding the medicine or forgetting to take it (especially at school). The doses may be too far apart, or a different dose may be needed. Something at school, at home, or in the neighborhood may be upsetting the youth, or he or she may need special help for learning disabilities or tutoring. Please discuss your concerns with the doctor. **Do not just increase the dose.**

All medicines should be kept in a safe place, out of the reach of children, and should be supervised by an adult. If someone takes too much of a medicine, call the doctor, the poison control center, or a hospital emergency room.

Each medicine has a "generic" or chemical name. Just like laundry detergents or paper towels, some medicines are sold by more than one company under different brand names. The same medicine may be available under a generic name and several brand names. The generic medications are usually less expensive than the brand name ones. The generic medications have the same chemical formula, but they may or may not be exactly the same strength as the brand-name medications. Also, some brands of pills contain dye that can cause allergic reactions. It is a good idea to talk to the doctor and the pharmacist about whether it is important to use a specific brand of medicine.

All medicines can cause an allergic reaction. Examples are hives, itching, rashes, swelling, and trouble breathing. Even a tiny amount of a medicine can cause a reaction in patients who are allergic to that medicine. Be *sure* to talk to the doctor before restarting a medicine that has caused an allergic reaction.

Taking more than one medicine at the same time may cause more side effects or cause one of the medicines to not work as well. Always ask the doctor, nurse, or pharmacist before adding another medicine, whether prescription or over-the-counter. Be sure that each doctor knows about *all* of the medicines your child is taking. Also tell the doctor about any vitamins, herbal medicines, or supplements your child may be taking. Some of these may have side effects alone or when taken with this medication.

Everyone taking medicine should have a physical examination at least once a year.

If you suspect the youth is using drugs or alcohol, please tell the doctor right away.

Pregnancy requires special care in the use of medicine. Please tell the doctor immediately if you suspect the teenager is pregnant or might become pregnant.

Printed information like this applies to children and adolescents in general. If you have questions about the medicine, or if you notice changes or anything unusual, please ask the doctor or nurse. As scientific research advances, knowledge increases and advice changes. Even experts do not always agree. Many medicines have not been approved by the U.S. Food and Drug Administration (FDA) for use in children. For this reason, use of the medicine for a particular problem or age group often is not listed in the *Physicians' Desk Reference*. This does not necessarily mean that the medicine is dangerous or does not work, only that the company that makes the medicine has not received permission to advertise the medicine for use in children. Companies often do not apply for this permission because it is expensive to do the tests needed to apply for approval for use in children. Once a medication is approved by the FDA for any purpose, a doctor is allowed to prescribe it according to research and clinical experience.

Note to Teachers

It is a good idea to talk with the parent(s) about the reason(s) that a medication is being used. If the parent(s) sign consent to release information, it is often helpful to talk with the doctor. If the parent(s) give permission, the doctor may ask you to fill out rating forms about your experience with the student's behavior, feelings, academic performance, and medication side effects. This information is very useful in selecting and monitoring medication treatment. If you have observations that you think are important, do not hesitate to share these with the student's parent(s) and treating clinicians.

It is very important that the medicine be taken exactly as the doctor instructs. However, everyone forgets to give a medicine on time once in a while. It is a good idea to ask the parent(s) in advance what to do if this happens. Do not stop or change the time you are giving a medicine at school without parental permission. If a medication is to be taken with food, but lunchtime or snack time changes, be sure to notify the parent(s) so appropriate adjustments can be made.

All medicines should be kept in a secure place and should be supervised by an adult. If someone takes too much of a medicine, follow your school procedure for an urgent medical problem.

Taking medicine is a private matter and is best managed discreetly and confidentially. It is important to be sensitive to the student's feelings about taking medicine.

If you suspect that the student is using drugs or alcohol, please tell the parent(s) or a school counselor right away.

Please tell the parent(s) or school nurse if you suspect medication side effects.

Modifications of the classroom environment or assignments may be useful in addition to medication. The student may need to be evaluated for additional help or for an Individualized Education Plan for learning or behavior.

Any expression of suicidal thoughts or feelings or self-harm by a child or adolescent is a clear signal of distress and should be taken seriously. These behaviors should not be dismissed as "attention seeking."

What Is Gabapentin (Neurontin)?

Gabapentin was first used to treat seizures (fits, convulsions), so it is sometimes called an *anticonvulsant*. Now it is also used for behavioral problems or bipolar disorder (manic-depressive disorder) whether or not the patient has seizures. It also may be used when the patient has a history of severe mood changes, sometimes called *mood swings*. When used in psychiatry, this medicine is more commonly called a *mood stabilizer*.

It comes in brand name Neurontin tablets, capsules, and liquid as well as in generic tablets and capsules.

How Can This Medicine Help?

Gabapentin can reduce aggression, anger, and severe mood swings.

How Does This Medicine Work?

Gabapentin is thought to work by stabilizing a part of the brain cell (the cell membrane or envelope) and by changing the concentrations of certain *neurotransmitters* (chemicals in the brain) such as *GABA* and *serotonin*.

How Long Does This Medicine Last?

Gabapentin needs to be taken two or three times a day.

How Will the Doctor Monitor This Medicine?

The doctor will review your child's medical history and physical examination before starting gabapentin. The doctor may order some blood tests to be sure your child does not have a hidden kidney condition that would make it unsafe to use this medicine. The doctor or nurse may measure your child's pulse and blood pressure before starting gabapentin.

After the medicine is started, the doctor will want to have regular appointments with you and your child to see how the medicine is working, to see if a dose change is needed, to watch for side effects, to see if gabapentin is still needed, and to see if any other treatment is needed. The doctor or nurse may check your child's height, weight, pulse, and blood pressure.

What Side Effects Can This Medicine Have?

Any medicine can have side effects, including an allergy to the medicine. Because each patient is different, the doctor will monitor the youth closely, especially when the medicine is started. The doctor will work with you to increase the positive effects and decrease the negative effects of the medicine. Please tell the doctor if any of the listed side effects appear or if you think that the medicine is causing any other problems. Not all of the rare or unusual side effects are listed.

Side effects are most common after starting the medicine or after a dose increase. Many side effects can be avoided or lessened by starting with a very low dose and increasing it slowly—ask the doctor.

Allergic Reaction

Tell the doctor in a day or two (if possible, before the next dose of medicine):

- Hives
- Itching
- Rash

319

Stop the medicine and get *immediate* medical care:

- Trouble breathing or chest tightness
- Swelling of lips, tongue, or throat

General Side Effects

These side effects are more common when first starting the medicine. Tell the doctor within a week or two:

- Daytime sleepiness or tiredness—Do not allow your child to drive, ride a bicycle or motorcycle, or operate machinery if this happens.
- Dizziness
- Unsteadiness
- Rapid, involuntary movements of the eyes
- Tremor
- Double vision
- Fatigue
- Muscle pain

Side Effects on Thinking, Behavior, and Emotions

Tell the doctor within a week:

- Worsening of behavioral problems
- Temper tantrums, increased anger and/or aggression
- Irritability
- Problems with concentration or doing schoolwork

Some Interactions With Other Medicines or Food

Please note that the following are only the most likely interactions with food or other medicines.

Caffeine may increase side effects.

Taking gabapentin with another medicine may cause more side effects. Be sure that each doctor knows about *all* of the medicines being taken.

Gabapentin does not interact with other anticonvulsants.

Antacids decrease the levels of gabapentin so that it does not work as well. Do not give antacids within 2 hours before or after gabapentin.

What Could Happen if This Medicine Is Stopped Suddenly?

Stopping gabapentin suddenly could lead to an increase in seizures or convulsions if your child is being treated for epilepsy (seizures).

How Long Will This Medicine Be Needed?

The length of time a person needs to take gabapentin depends on what problem is being treated. For example, someone with an impulse control disorder usually takes the medicine only until behavioral therapy begins to work. Someone with bipolar disorder may need to take the medicine for many years. Please ask the doctor about the length of treatment needed.

What Else Should I Know About This Medicine?

Taking gabapentin with food may decrease stomach upset.

Keep the medicine in a safe place under close supervision. Keep the pill container tightly closed and in a dry place, away from bathrooms, showers, and humidifiers.

Notes

Use this space to take notes or to write down questions you want to ask the doctor.

_____

_____

_____

_____

_____

_____

_____

_____

From Dulcan MK (editor): _Helping Parents, Youth, and Teachers Understand Medications for Behavioral and Emotional Problems: A Resource Book of Medication Information Handouts_, Third Edition. Washington, DC, American Psychiatric Publishing, 2007

Medication Information for Youth

Gabapentin—Neurontin

What the Medicine Is Called and What It Is For

The name of your medicine may be confusing. Most drugs have two names: 1) a scientific name that we call a *generic name* and 2) a trade or *brand name*. The generic name of this medicine is gabapentin. The brand name is Neurontin.

Gabapentin was first used to help people with epilepsy (seizures, fits, convulsions), so it is sometimes called an *anticonvulsant*. It is now also called a *mood stabilizer*, because it is used to help people who have severe mood changes, sometimes called *mood swings*, especially in children and adolescents with bipolar disorder (manic-depressive disorder), depression, or trouble controlling anger. Gabapentin can reduce aggression, anger, and severe mood swings. It is thought to work by making brain cells less excitable.

How You Take the Medicine

It is very important to take the medicine exactly as the doctor or nurse tells you. Do not skip doses or take extra medicine without asking an adult. If you forget a dose, ask your parent(s) what to do.

This medicine is prescribed only for you. It should never be shared with anyone else.

You do not have to tell others that you are taking this medicine, but it is not something you should feel ashamed or embarrassed about. Many young people are helped by gabapentin. This medicine is not habit-forming, and you cannot become "hooked" on it. You should talk to your doctor or nurse about any questions you have about the medicine. It is important to remember that the medicine *helps* you. It cannot *make* you do anything or change you as a person.

If your stomach is upset, taking the medicine with food may help.

Caffeine (in coffee, tea, or soft drinks) may make you feel worse.

It is very important not to stop this medicine suddenly—it could be uncomfortable or even dangerous.

How Your Doctor Will Follow Your Progress

Before giving you the medicine, your doctor or nurse will talk with you and your parent(s) and may measure your height, weight, heart rate (pulse), and blood pressure. The doctor may order blood tests to be sure that you are in good health.

323

Be sure to tell your doctor or nurse about any other medicines or supplements you are taking, including vitamins, herbs, or aids to weight loss or bodybuilding. Also be sure to tell the doctor or nurse if you are using alcohol or drugs. Because many medicines may affect babies, it is very important to tell the doctor if you might be pregnant or if you are at risk of becoming pregnant.

Your teachers may be asked to fill out a form about your grades and behavior in school. A psychologist may give you some tests to see how you learn best.

Most doctors have regular appointments with young people who are taking medicine. You should use these visits to share any concerns you may have about your medicine and to talk about if it has helped you. From time to time, your physician or nurse may measure your height, weight, heart rate (pulse), and blood pressure to be sure that you are in good health while you are taking the medicine and that your kidneys are working well. Your doctor also will ask for regular reports from your parents and maybe from your teachers (with your permission) to see how well the medicine is working.

How the Medicine Might Affect You

In addition to the ways the medicine can help you, it may have other effects called *side effects*. Different medicines have different side effects. It is helpful to know about some of the most common side effects of your medicine so that you will understand what they are if they happen. Some people do not have any side effects. Some side effects are just uncomfortable, but others may mean a more serious problem with the medicine. Side effects are most common after starting the medicine or after a dose increase. They may go away with time, or the medicine can be adjusted or changed—ask the doctor.

You could have an allergy to any medicine, which might show up as a rash on your skin, swelling, itching, or trouble breathing.

Please tell your parent(s) and your doctor or nurse about any changes that you notice after taking the medicine. It is especially important to tell a responsible adult if you are feeling depressed or that you may not want to live; if you have thoughts of hurting yourself; or if you begin to feel more irritable, nervous, or restless.

Some medicines make people feel sleepy or less coordinated. If this medicine is making you sleepy, it is very important not to drive a car or ride a bicycle or motorcycle. After starting a new medicine or increasing the dose of a medicine, please be extra careful when driving a car, riding a bike, or using machines until you can tell how the medicine affects your alertness, attention, and coordination.

The most common side effects of gabapentin are dizziness, daytime sleepiness, and feeling tired. Less common side effects are problems with paying attention, feeling irritable or angry, clumsiness, muscle pain, shaking, and double or blurred vision. These sometimes go away after you have been taking the medicine for a while or if the doctor lowers the dose of medicine you are taking. Tell your parent(s) or the doctor if you are having trouble with any of these side effects.

Notes

Use this space to take notes or to write down questions you want to ask the doctor or nurse.

_____

_____

_____

_____

_____

_____

_____

_____

_____

_____

_____

From Dulcan MK (editor): _Helping Parents, Youth, and Teachers Understand Medications for Behavioral and Emotional Problems: A Resource Book of Medication Information Handouts,_ Third Edition. Washington, DC, American Psychiatric Publishing, 2007

Medication Information for Parents and Teachers

Guanfacine—Tenex

General Information About Medication

Each child and adolescent is different. No one has exactly the same combination of medical and psychological problems. It is a good idea to talk with the doctor or nurse about the reasons a medicine is being used. It is very important to keep all appointments and to be in touch by telephone if you have concerns. It is important to communicate with the doctor, nurse, or therapist.

It is very important that the medicine be taken exactly as the doctor instructs. However, once in a while, everyone forgets to give a medicine on time. It is a good idea to ask the doctor or nurse what to do if this happens. Do not stop or change a medicine without asking the doctor or nurse first.

If the medicine seems to stop working, it may be because it is not being taken regularly. The youth may be "cheeking" or hiding the medicine or forgetting to take it (especially at school). The doses may be too far apart, or a different dose may be needed. Something at school, at home, or in the neighborhood may be upsetting the youth, or he or she may need special help for learning disabilities or tutoring. Please discuss your concerns with the doctor. **Do not just increase the dose.**

All medicines should be kept in a safe place, out of the reach of children, and should be supervised by an adult. If someone takes too much of a medicine, call the doctor, the poison control center, or a hospital emergency room.

Each medicine has a "generic" or chemical name. Just like laundry detergents or paper towels, some medicines are sold by more than one company under different brand names. The same medicine may be available under a generic name and several brand names. The generic medications are usually less expensive than the brand name ones. The generic medications have the same chemical formula, but they may or may not be exactly the same strength as the brand-name medications. Also, some brands of pills contain dye that can cause allergic reactions. It is a good idea to talk to the doctor and the pharmacist about whether it is important to use a specific brand of medicine.

All medicines can cause an allergic reaction. Examples are hives, itching, rashes, swelling, and trouble breathing. Even a tiny amount of a medicine can cause a reaction in patients who are allergic to that medicine. Be *sure* to talk to the doctor before restarting a medicine that has caused an allergic reaction.

Taking more than one medicine at the same time may cause more side effects or cause one of the medicines to not work as well. Always ask the doctor, nurse, or pharmacist before adding another medicine, whether prescription or over-the-counter. Be sure that each doctor knows about *all* of the medicines your child is taking. Also tell the doctor about any vitamins, herbal medicines, or supplements your child may be taking. Some of these may have side effects alone or when taken with this medication.

Everyone taking medicine should have a physical examination at least once a year.

If you suspect the youth is using drugs or alcohol, please tell the doctor right away.

327

Pregnancy requires special care in the use of medicine. Please tell the doctor immediately if you suspect the teenager is pregnant or might become pregnant.

Printed information like this applies to children and adolescents in general. If you have questions about the medicine, or if you notice changes or anything unusual, please ask the doctor or nurse. As scientific research advances, knowledge increases and advice changes. Even experts do not always agree. Many medicines have not been approved by the U.S. Food and Drug Administration (FDA) for use in children. For this reason, use of the medicine for a particular problem or age group often is not listed in the *Physicians' Desk Reference*. This does not necessarily mean that the medicine is dangerous or does not work, only that the company that makes the medicine has not received permission to advertise the medicine for use in children. Companies often do not apply for this permission because it is expensive to do the tests needed to apply for approval for use in children. Once a medication is approved by the FDA for any purpose, a doctor is allowed to prescribe it according to research and clinical experience.

Note to Teachers

It is a good idea to talk with the parent(s) about the reason(s) that a medication is being used. If the parent(s) sign consent to release information, it is often helpful to talk with the doctor. If the parent(s) give permission, the doctor may ask you to fill out rating forms about your experience with the student's behavior, feelings, academic performance, and medication side effects. This information is very useful in selecting and monitoring medication treatment. If you have observations that you think are important, do not hesitate to share these with the student's parent(s) and treating clinicians.

It is very important that the medicine be taken exactly as the doctor instructs. However, everyone forgets to give a medicine on time once in a while. It is a good idea to ask the parent(s) in advance what to do if this happens. Do not stop or change the time you are giving a medicine at school without parental permission. If a medication is to be taken with food, but lunchtime or snack time changes, be sure to notify the parent(s) so appropriate adjustments can be made.

All medicines should be kept in a secure place and should be supervised by an adult. If someone takes too much of a medicine, follow your school procedure for an urgent medical problem.

Taking medicine is a private matter and is best managed discreetly and confidentially. It is important to be sensitive to the student's feelings about taking medicine.

If you suspect that the student is using drugs or alcohol, please tell the parent(s) or a school counselor right away.

Please tell the parent(s) or school nurse if you suspect medication side effects.

Modifications of the classroom environment or assignments may be useful in addition to medication. The student may need to be evaluated for additional help or for an Individualized Education Plan for learning or behavior.

Any expression of suicidal thoughts or feelings or self-harm by a child or adolescent is a clear signal of distress and should be taken seriously. These behaviors should not be dismissed as "attention seeking."

What Is Guanfacine (Tenex)?

Guanfacine was first used to treat high blood pressure, so it is sometimes called an *antihypertensive*. Now it is also used to treat symptoms of Tourette's disorder, chronic tics (fast, repeated movements), attention-deficit/hyperactivity disorder (ADHD), and aggression. It comes in brand name Tenex and generic tablets.

How Can This Medicine Help?

Guanfacine can decrease symptoms of hyperactivity, impulsivity, anxiety, irritability, temper tantrums, explosive anger, and tics. It can increase patience and frustration tolerance as well as improve self-control and cooperation with adults. Guanfacine is sometimes used together with a stimulant medication (methylphenidate or amphetamine) for ADHD or with an atypical or pimozide (Orap) for Tourette's disorder. The positive effects usually do not start for 2 weeks after a stable dose is reached. The full benefit may not be seen for 2–4 months.

How Does This Medicine Work?

Guanfacine works by decreasing the level of excitement in parts of the brain. It is sometimes called an *alpha-adrenergic agonist*. It affects the levels of *norepinephrine*, one of the *neurotransmitters*—a chemical that the brain makes for nerve cells to communicate with each other. This effect helps people with tic disorders to stop moving or making noises when they do not want to and helps people with ADHD to slow down and think before doing something. It calms parts of the brain that are too excited in people with severe anxiety. This medicine is chemically different from sedatives or tranquilizers, even though it may make your child sleepy when he or she first starts taking it.

How Long Does This Medicine Last?

Although guanfacine lasts 24 hours in the body after a dose, when children take it for problems with emotions or behavior it must be taken two or three times a day.

How Will the Doctor Monitor This Medicine?

The doctor will review your child's medical history and physical examination before starting guanfacine. The doctor may order some blood or urine tests to be sure your child does not have a hidden medical condition. Be sure to tell the doctor if your child or anyone in the family has high blood pressure, heart disease, or diabetes. The doctor also may want to obtain an ECG (electrocardiogram or heart rhythm test) before starting the medicine. The doctor or nurse will measure your child's height, weight, pulse, and blood pressure before starting guanfacine.

After the medicine is started, the doctor will want to have regular appointments with you and your child to see how the medicine is working, to see if a dose change is needed, to watch for side effects, to see if guanfacine is still needed, and to see if any other treatment is needed. The doctor or nurse will check your child's height, weight, pulse, and blood pressure.

What Side Effects Can This Medicine Have?

Any medicine can have side effects, including an allergy to the medicine. Because each patient is different, the doctor will monitor the youth closely, especially when the medicine is started. The doctor will work with you to increase the positive effects and decrease the negative effects of the medicine. Please tell the doctor if any of the listed side effects appear or if you think that the medicine is causing any other problems. Not all of the rare or unusual side effects are listed.

Side effects are most common after starting the medicine or after a dose increase. Many side effects can be avoided or lessened by starting with a very low dose and increasing it slowly—ask the doctor.

Allergic Reaction

Tell the doctor in a day or two (if possible, before the next dose of medicine):

- Hives
- Itching
- Rash

Stop the medicine and get *immediate* medical care:

- Trouble breathing or chest tightness
- Swelling of lips, tongue, or throat

Common, but Usually Mild, Side Effects

The following side effects are more common at first or as the dose is increased. If they do not go away after a week or two, ask the doctor about lowering the dose.

- Daytime sleepiness, especially when bored or not doing anything (usually worst in the first 2–4 weeks)—Do not allow your child to drive, ride a bicycle or motorcycle, or operate machinery if this happens.
- Fatigue or tiredness
- Low blood pressure (rarely a serious problem)
- Dizziness or light-headedness—This side effect is worse when the child stands up quickly, especially when getting out of bed in the morning; try having the child stand up slowly.
- Headache
- Stomachache

If one of the following side effects appears, call the doctor within a day or two:

- Slow pulse rate (heartbeat)
- Temporary worsening of tics in Tourette's disorder
- Insomnia (trouble sleeping)—This may be caused by the medicine wearing off.
- Ringing in the ears

Less Common Side Effects

Call the doctor within a day or two:

- Depression or increased irritability
- Confusion
- Bed-wetting
- Muscle cramps
- Itching
- Runny nose

330

Less Common, but Serious, Side Effects

Call the doctor *immediately:*

- Severe or increased dizziness or light-headedness
- Fainting

Very Rare, but Serious, Side Effects

Call the doctor *immediately:*

- Irregular heartbeat
- Trouble breathing
- Decreased frequency of urination; rapid, puffy swelling of the body (especially the legs and feet); sudden headaches with nausea and vomiting—These could be signs of kidney failure.

Side Effects Reported in Adults but Rare in Children

Tell the doctor within a week:

- Dry mouth—Have your child try using sugar-free gum or candy.
- Constipation—Encourage your child to drink more fluids and eat high-fiber foods; if necessary, the doctor may recommend a fiber medicine such as Benefiber or a stool softener such as Colace or mineral oil.
- Low blood pressure
- Weakness
- Nightmares
- Increased blood sugar (mainly in persons with diabetes)
- Sensation of cold or pain in fingers or toes
- Weight gain

Some Interactions With Other Medicines or Food

Please note that the following are only the most likely interactions with food or other medicines.

Increased sleepiness will occur in combination with medications for anxiety (sedatives or tranquilizers), sleep (hypnotics), allergy or colds (antihistamines), psychosis, or seizures (anticonvulsants).

What Could Happen if This Medicine Is Stopped Suddenly?

Withdrawal effects are rare, but the following could happen:

- Very high blood pressure, even if blood pressure was normal before starting the medicine *(rebound hypertension):* This occurs 2–4 days after withdrawal.
- Temporary worsening of behavioral problems or tics
- Nervousness or anxiety

- Rapid or irregular heartbeat
- Chest pain
- Headache
- Stomach cramps, nausea, vomiting
- Trouble sleeping

Because of these effects, it is important not to stop guanfacine suddenly but to decrease it slowly (taper) as directed by the doctor. It is also important not to miss a dose of guanfacine, because withdrawal symptoms such as heart or blood pressure problems may occur. **Be sure not to let the prescription run out!**

How Long Will This Medicine Be Needed?

There is no way to know how long a person will need to take guanfacine. The parent(s), the doctor, and the school will work together to determine what is right for each patient. Some people need the medicine for a few years; some people may need it longer.

What Else Should I Know About This Medicine?

If a child is sleepy from the guanfacine, something active or interesting to do will help the child to stay awake. Sleeping extra hours will not help. Sleepiness usually decreases as the child gets used to the medicine. If the youth is still sleepy in the daytime after 4 weeks on the same dose, a lower dose or a different medicine may be needed.

Tenex may be confused with Xanax. Be sure to check the prescription when you get it from the pharmacy.

Notes

Use this space to take notes or to write down questions you want to ask the doctor.

_____

_____

_____

_____

_____

_____

_____

_____

_____

_____

_____

_____

_____

Medication Information for Youth

Guanfacine—Tenex

What the Medicine Is Called and What It Is For

The name of your medicine may be confusing. Most drugs have two names: 1) a scientific name that we call a *generic name* and 2) a trade or *brand name*. The generic name of this medicine is guanfacine. The brand name is Tenex.

Guanfacine was first used to treat high blood pressure, so it is sometimes called an *antihypertensive*. Now it is also used to help children and teenagers who have trouble sitting still, are too active ("hyperactive") or impulsive, have a bad temper, are hitting people or breaking things, or have tics (fast, repeated movements or repeated sounds that are hard to control). Your doctor may have told you that you have attention-deficit/hyperactivity disorder (ADHD) or Tourette's disorder.

How You Take the Medicine

It is very important to take the medicine exactly as the doctor or nurse tells you. Do not skip doses or take extra medicine without asking an adult. If you forget a dose, ask your parent(s) what to do.

It is *very important* that you take *all* the pills you are supposed to take each day. Your doctor will probably recommend that you take your medicine at the same time each day, which may be with meals and at bedtime. You may notice some help from the medicine within the first few weeks. However, guanfacine does not take full effect until as long as 2–4 months after you start taking it. You may feel discouraged and think it is not really helping you. You may want to give up and stop taking the medicine. Talk to your doctor and parent(s) about how you feel, but **do not stop** taking your medicine unless your doctor tells you to. **It can be very dangerous to stop this medicine suddenly.**

Do not use any other medicines without talking to your doctor first. Some people with ADHD or Tourette's disorder will take guanfacine together with another medicine because the doctor tells them to.

Do not use alcohol, marijuana, or street drugs while taking guanfacine. They can cause serious side effects. Skipping your medicine to take drugs does not work because many medicines stay in your body for a long time.

This medicine is prescribed only for you. It should never be shared with anyone else.

You do not have to tell others that you are taking this medicine, but it is not something you should feel ashamed or embarrassed about. Many young people are helped by guanfacine. This medicine is not habit-forming, and you cannot become "hooked" on it. You should talk to your doctor or nurse about any questions you have about the medicine. It is important to remember that the medicine *helps* you. It cannot *make* you do anything or change you as a person.

How Your Doctor Will Follow Your Progress

Before giving you the medicine, your doctor or nurse will talk with you and your parent(s) and may measure your height, weight, heart rate (pulse), and blood pressure. You also may need to take a test called an ECG (electrocardiogram or heart rhythm test). This simple test counts your heartbeats through small wires that are taped to your chest. It takes only a few minutes. This test may need to be repeated at some time while you are taking the medicine. It is important to tell the doctor if you have ever had a very fast heartbeat, chest pain, dizziness, or fainting.

Be sure to tell your doctor or nurse about any other medicines or supplements you are taking, including vitamins, herbs, or aids to weight loss or bodybuilding. Also be sure to tell the doctor or nurse if you are using alcohol or drugs. Because many medicines may affect babies, it is very important to tell the doctor if you might be pregnant or if you are at risk of becoming pregnant.

Your teachers may be asked to fill out a form about your grades and behavior in school. A psychologist may give you some tests to see how you learn best.

You will probably start by taking one pill or part of a pill each day. Your doctor will tell you if and when you should start taking more medicine. He or she will watch your progress and decide when you are taking the right amount and how long you need to take the medicine.

Most doctors have regular appointments with young people who are taking medicine. You should use these visits to share any concerns you may have about your medicine and to talk about if it has helped you. From time to time, your physician or nurse may measure your height, weight, heart rate (pulse), and blood pressure to be sure that you are in good health while you are taking the medicine. Your doctor also will ask for regular reports from your parents and maybe from your teachers (with your permission) to see how well the medicine is working.

How the Medicine Might Affect You

In addition to the ways the medicine can help you, it may have other effects called *side effects*. Different medicines have different side effects. It is helpful to know about some of the most common side effects of your medicine so that you will understand what they are if they happen. Some people do not have any side effects. Some side effects are just uncomfortable, but others may mean a more serious problem with the medicine. Side effects are most common after starting the medicine or after a dose increase. They may go away with time, or the medicine can be adjusted or changed—ask the doctor.

You could have an allergy to any medicine, which might show up as a rash on your skin, swelling, itching, or trouble breathing.

Please tell your parent(s) and your doctor or nurse about any changes that you notice after taking the medicine. It is especially important to tell a responsible adult if you are feeling depressed or that you may not want to live; if you have thoughts of hurting yourself; or if you begin to feel more irritable, nervous, or restless.

Some medicines make people feel sleepy or less coordinated. If this medicine is making you sleepy, it is very important not to drive a car or ride a bicycle or motorcycle. After starting a new medicine or increasing the dose of a medicine, please be extra careful when driving a car, riding a bike, or using machines until you can tell how the medicine affects your alertness, attention, and coordination.

One of the most common side effects of guanfacine is feeling tired or sleepy during the day, especially if things are boring. After you have been taking the medicine for a few weeks, your body will adjust, and you should not feel as sleepy during the day. If you do not stop feeling sleepy during the day or if you start to feel more sleepy than you did before, let your parent(s) and your doctor know. If you have had trouble sleeping at night or have had problems with nightmares, the medicine can help you sleep better. If you wake up in the middle of the night and have trouble going back to sleep or have nightmares, be sure to tell the doctor.

If you become very sad while taking guanfacine, let your doctor know how you are feeling. Your medicine may need to be changed.

Because guanfacine can lower blood pressure, you may have problems if your blood pressure gets too low. If you become dizzy or light-headed or if you faint, let your parent(s) and doctor know right away. It will help if you get up slowly in the morning instead of jumping right out of bed.

Remember that even if you are bothered by some side effect, you should not just stop taking the pills. Doing that could cause you to feel very nervous and anxious and also could cause your blood pressure to go very high. If you have any side effects that make you so uncomfortable that you want to stop taking the medicine, talk to your doctor. **Do not just stop taking it!**

Other side effects that people sometimes have from guanfacine are headache or stomachache.

You should tell your parent(s) and doctor if you notice anything different or unusual about how you feel once you start taking the medicine.

Notes

Use this space to take notes or to write down questions you want to ask the doctor or nurse.

_____

_____

_____

_____

_____

_____

_____

_____

_____

_____

_____

_____

_____

From Dulcan MK (editor): *Helping Parents, Youth, and Teachers Understand Medications for Behavioral and Emotional Problems: A Resource Book of Medication Information Handouts*, Third Edition. Washington, DC, American Psychiatric Publishing, 2007

Medication Information for Parents and Teachers

Haloperidol—Haldol

General Information About Medication

Each child and adolescent is different. No one has exactly the same combination of medical and psychological problems. It is a good idea to talk with the doctor or nurse about the reasons a medicine is being used. It is very important to keep all appointments and to be in touch by telephone if you have concerns. It is important to communicate with the doctor, nurse, or therapist.

It is very important that the medicine be taken exactly as the doctor instructs. However, once in a while, everyone forgets to give a medicine on time. It is a good idea to ask the doctor or nurse what to do if this happens. Do not stop or change a medicine without asking the doctor or nurse first.

If the medicine seems to stop working, it may be because it is not being taken regularly. The youth may be "cheeking" or hiding the medicine or forgetting to take it (especially at school). The doses may be too far apart, or a different dose may be needed. Something at school, at home, or in the neighborhood may be upsetting the youth, or he or she may need special help for learning disabilities or tutoring. Please discuss your concerns with the doctor. **Do not just increase the dose.**

All medicines should be kept in a safe place, out of the reach of children, and should be supervised by an adult. If someone takes too much of a medicine, call the doctor, the poison control center, or a hospital emergency room.

Each medicine has a "generic" or chemical name. Just like laundry detergents or paper towels, some medicines are sold by more than one company under different brand names. The same medicine may be available under a generic name and several brand names. The generic medications are usually less expensive than the brand name ones. The generic medications have the same chemical formula, but they may or may not be exactly the same strength as the brand-name medications. Also, some brands of pills contain dye that can cause allergic reactions. It is a good idea to talk to the doctor and the pharmacist about whether it is important to use a specific brand of medicine.

All medicines can cause an allergic reaction. Examples are hives, itching, rashes, swelling, and trouble breathing. Even a tiny amount of a medicine can cause a reaction in patients who are allergic to that medicine. Be *sure* to talk to the doctor before restarting a medicine that has caused an allergic reaction.

Taking more than one medicine at the same time may cause more side effects or cause one of the medicines to not work as well. Always ask the doctor, nurse, or pharmacist before adding another medicine, whether prescription or over-the-counter. Be sure that each doctor knows about *all* of the medicines your child is taking. Also tell the doctor about any vitamins, herbal medicines, or supplements your child may be taking. Some of these may have side effects alone or when taken with this medication.

Everyone taking medicine should have a physical examination at least once a year.

If you suspect the youth is using drugs or alcohol, please tell the doctor right away.

Pregnancy requires special care in the use of medicine. Please tell the doctor immediately if you suspect the teenager is pregnant or might become pregnant.

Printed information like this applies to children and adolescents in general. If you have questions about the medicine, or if you notice changes or anything unusual, please ask the doctor or nurse. As scientific research advances, knowledge increases and advice changes. Even experts do not always agree. Many medicines have not been approved by the U.S. Food and Drug Administration (FDA) for use in children. For this reason, use of the medicine for a particular problem or age group often is not listed in the *Physicians' Desk Reference*. This does not necessarily mean that the medicine is dangerous or does not work, only that the company that makes the medicine has not received permission to advertise the medicine for use in children. Companies often do not apply for this permission because it is expensive to do the tests needed to apply for approval for use in children. Once a medication is approved by the FDA for any purpose, a doctor is allowed to prescribe it according to research and clinical experience.

Note to Teachers

It is a good idea to talk with the parent(s) about the reason(s) that a medication is being used. If the parent(s) sign consent to release information, it is often helpful to talk with the doctor. If the parent(s) give permission, the doctor may ask you to fill out rating forms about your experience with the student's behavior, feelings, academic performance, and medication side effects. This information is very useful in selecting and monitoring medication treatment. If you have observations that you think are important, do not hesitate to share these with the student's parent(s) and treating clinicians.

It is very important that the medicine be taken exactly as the doctor instructs. However, everyone forgets to give a medicine on time once in a while. It is a good idea to ask the parent(s) in advance what to do if this happens. Do not stop or change the time you are giving a medicine at school without parental permission. If a medication is to be taken with food, but lunchtime or snack time changes, be sure to notify the parent(s) so appropriate adjustments can be made.

All medicines should be kept in a secure place and should be supervised by an adult. If someone takes too much of a medicine, follow your school procedure for an urgent medical problem.

Taking medicine is a private matter and is best managed discreetly and confidentially. It is important to be sensitive to the student's feelings about taking medicine.

If you suspect that the student is using drugs or alcohol, please tell the parent(s) or a school counselor right away.

Please tell the parent(s) or school nurse if you suspect medication side effects.

Modifications of the classroom environment or assignments may be useful in addition to medication. The student may need to be evaluated for additional help or for an Individualized Education Plan for learning or behavior.

Any expression of suicidal thoughts or feelings or self-harm by a child or adolescent is a clear signal of distress and should be taken seriously. These behaviors should not be dismissed as "attention seeking."

What Is Haloperidol (Haldol)?

Haloperidol is sometimes called a *typical, conventional,* or *first-generation antipsychotic* medicine. It is also called a *neuroleptic.* It used to be called a *major tranquilizer.* It comes in brand name Haldol and generic tablets, liquid, and two kinds of shots (injections): immediate acting and very long-acting (haloperidol decanoate).

How Can This Medicine Help?

Haloperidol is used to treat psychosis, such as in schizophrenia, mania, or very severe depression. It can reduce hallucinations (hearing voices or seeing things that are not there) and delusions (troubling beliefs that other people do not share). It can help the patient be less upset and agitated. It can improve the patient's ability to think clearly.

Sometimes haloperidol is used to decrease severe aggression or very serious behavioral problems in young people with conduct disorder, mental retardation, or autism.

Haloperidol is also used to reduce motor and vocal tics (fast, repeated movements or sounds) and behavioral problems in people with Tourette's disorder.

This medicine is very powerful and should be used to treat very serious problems or symptoms that other medicines do not help. Be patient; the positive effects of this medicine may not appear for 2–3 weeks.

How Does This Medicine Work?

Cells in the brain (neurons) communicate using chemicals called *neurotransmitters*. Too much or too little of these substances in certain parts of the brain can cause problems. Haloperidol reduces the activity of one of these neurotransmitters, *dopamine*. Blocking the effect of dopamine in certain parts of the brain reduces what have been called *positive symptoms* of psychosis: delusions; hallucinations; disorganized and unusual thinking, speaking, and behavior; excessive activity (agitation); and lack of activity (catatonia). Blocking dopamine can also reduce tics. Reducing dopamine action in other parts of the brain may lead to the side effects of this medicine.

How Long Does This Medicine Last?

Haloperidol usually may be taken only once a day, unless divided doses are used to lessen side effects. An injection of haloperidol decanoate lasts for 3–4 weeks.

How Will the Doctor Monitor This Medicine?

The doctor will review your child's medical history and physical examination before starting haloperidol. The doctor may order some blood or urine tests to be sure your child does not have a hidden medical condition. The doctor or nurse may measure your child's pulse and blood pressure before starting haloperidol.

Be sure to tell the doctor if anyone in the family is hearing impaired or has had heart problems or died suddenly.

Before your child starts taking haloperidol and every so often afterward, a test such as the AIMS (Abnormal Involuntary Movement Scale) may be used to check your child's tongue, legs, and arms for unusual movements that could be caused by the medicine.

After the medicine is started, the doctor will want to have regular appointments with you and your child to see how the medicine is working, to see if a dose change is needed, to watch for side effects, to see if haloperidol is still needed, and to see if any other treatment is needed. The doctor or nurse may check your child's height, weight, pulse, and blood pressure, and watch for abnormal movements.

341

What Side Effects Can This Medicine Have?

Any medicine can have side effects, including an allergy to the medicine. Because each patient is different, the doctor will monitor the youth closely, especially when the medicine is started. The doctor will work with you to increase the positive effects and decrease the negative effects of the medicine. Please tell the doctor if any of the listed side effects appear or if you think that the medicine is causing any other problems. Not all of the rare or unusual side effects are listed.

Side effects are most common after starting the medicine or after a dose increase. Many side effects can be avoided or lessened by starting with a very low dose and increasing it slowly—ask the doctor.

Allergic Reaction

Tell the doctor in a day or two (if possible, before the next dose of medicine):

- Hives
- Itching
- Rash

    Stop the medicine and get *immediate* medical care:

- Trouble breathing or chest tightness
- Swelling of lips, tongue, or throat

Common, but Not Usually Serious, Side Effects

Discuss the following side effects with your child's doctor within a week or two. They often can be helped by lowering the dose of medicine, changing the times medicine is taken, or adding another medicine.

- Dry mouth—Have your child try using sugar-free gum or candy.
- Constipation—Encourage your child to drink more fluids and eat high-fiber foods; if necessary, the doctor may recommend a fiber medicine such as Benefiber or a stool softener such as Colace or mineral oil.
- Mild trouble urinating
- Blurred vision
- Weight gain—Seek nutritional counseling; provide your child with low-calorie snacks and encourage regular exercise.
- Sadness, irritability, nervousness, clinginess, not wanting to go to school
- Restlessness or inability to sit still
- Shaking of hands and fingers

Less Common, but Not Usually Serious, Side Effects

Discuss the following side effects with your child's doctor within a week or two. They often can be helped by lowering the dose of medicine, changing the times medicine is taken, or adding another medicine.

- Daytime sleepiness or tiredness—Do not allow your child to drive, ride a bicycle or motorcycle, or operate machinery if this happens. This problem may be lessened by taking the medicine at bedtime.

- Dizziness—This side effect is worse when the child stands up quickly, especially when getting out of bed in the morning; try having the child stand up slowly.
- Decreased or slowed movement and decreased facial expressions
- Drooling
- Decreased sexual interest or ability
- Changes in menstrual cycle
- Increase in breast size or discharge from the breasts (in both boys and girls)—This may go away with time.

Less Common, but Potentially Serious, Side Effects

Call the doctor or go to an emergency room *right away*:

- Stiffness of the tongue, jaw, neck, back, or legs
- Overheating or heatstroke—Prevent by decreasing activity in hot weather, staying out of the sun, and drinking water.
- Seizure (fit, convulsion)—This is more likely in people with a history of seizures or head injury.
- Severe confusion

Rare, but Serious, Side Effects

- Extreme stiffness or lack of movement, very high fever, mental confusion, irregular pulse rate, or eye pain—**This is a medical emergency. Go to an emergency room *right away.***
- Sudden stiffness and inability to breathe or swallow—**Go to an emergency room or call 911.** Tell the paramedics, nurses, and doctors that the patient is taking haloperidol. Other medicines can be used to treat this problem fast.
- Increased thirst, frequent urination, lethargy, tiredness, dizziness—These could be signs of diabetes (especially if your child is overweight or there is a family history of diabetes). **Talk to a doctor within a day.**

What Else Should I Know About Side Effects?

Most side effects lessen over time. If they are troublesome, talk with your child's doctor. Some side effects can be decreased by taking a smaller dose of medicine, by stopping the medicine, by changing to another medicine, or by adding another medicine (see the table).

One side effect that may not go away is *tardive dyskinesia* (or TD). Patients with tardive dyskinesia have involuntary movements of the body, especially the mouth and tongue. The patient may look as though he or she is making faces over and over again. Jerky movements of the arms, legs, or body may occur. There may be fine, wormlike, or sudden repeated movements of the tongue, or the person may appear to be chewing something or smacking or puckering his or her lips. The fingers may look as though they are rolling something. If you notice any unusual movements, be sure to tell the doctor. The doctor may use the AIMS test to look for these movements.

The medicine may increase the level of *prolactin*, a natural hormone made in the part of the brain called the *pituitary*. This may cause side effects such as breast tenderness or swelling or production of milk, in both boys and girls. It also may interfere with sexual functioning in teenage boys and with regular menstrual cycles (periods) in teenage girls. A blood test can measure the level of prolactin. If these side effects do not go away and are troublesome, talk with your child's doctor about substituting another medicine for haloperidol.

Heart problems are more common if other medicines are being taken as well. Be sure to tell all your child's doctors and your pharmacist about all medications your child is taking.

Neuroleptic malignant syndrome is a very rare side effect that can lead to death. The symptoms are severe muscle stiffness, high fever, increased heart rate and blood pressure, irregular heartbeat (pulse), and sweating. It may lead to unconsciousness. If you suspect this, **call 911 or go to an emergency room right away.**

What Medicines Are Used to Treat the Side Effects of Haloperidol?

The following medicines may be used to treat the movement side effects of haloperidol. All of these medicines may have their own side effects as well; ask the doctor if you suspect a problem.

Brand name	Generic name
Akineton	Biperiden
Artane	Trihexyphenidyl
Ativan	Lorazepam*
Benadryl	Diphenhydramine*
Catapres	Clonidine*
Cogentin	Benztropine mesylate*
Inderal	Propranolol*
Klonopin	Clonazepam*
Symmetrel	Amantadine

*This medicine has its own information sheet in this book.

Some Interactions With Other Medicines or Food

Please note that the following are only the most likely interactions with food or other medicines.

Haloperidol may be taken with or without food. If the medicine causes stomach upset, taking it with food may help.

Carbamazepine (Tegretol) may decrease levels of haloperidol so that it does not work as well.

Fluoxetine (Prozac) may increase the levels of haloperidol, increasing the risk of side effects.

It is better to limit drinks with caffeine (coffee, tea, soft drinks) because caffeine works in the opposite way from this medicine, and the positive effects might be decreased.

What Could Happen if This Medicine Is Stopped Suddenly?

Involuntary movements, or *withdrawal dyskinesias*, may appear within 1–4 weeks of lowering the dose or stopping the medicine. Usually these go away, but they can last for days to months. If haloperidol is stopped suddenly, emotional problems such as irritability, nervousness, or moodiness; behavior problems; or physical problems such as stomachache, loss of appetite, nausea, vomiting, diarrhea, sweating, indigestion, trouble sleeping, trembling, or shaking may appear. These problems usually last only a few days to a few weeks. If they happen, tell your child's doctor. The medicine dose may need to be lowered more slowly (tapered). Always check with the doctor before stopping a medicine!

How Long Will This Medicine Be Needed?

How long your child will need to be on haloperidol depends partly on the reason that it was prescribed. Some problems last for only a few months, whereas others last much longer. Sometimes haloperidol is used for only a short time until other medicines or behavioral treatments start to work. Some people need to take haloperidol for years. It is especially important with medicines as powerful as this one to ask the doctor whether it is still needed. Every few months, you should discuss with your child's doctor the reasons for using haloperidol and whether it is time for a trial of lowering the dose.

What Else Should I Know About This Medicine?

There are many older and newer medicines that are used for the same kinds of problems. If your child is having bad side effects or the medicine does not seem to be working, ask the doctor if another medicine in this group might work as well or better and have fewer side effects for your child.

Be sure to tell the doctor if there is anyone in your family who died suddenly or had a heart problem.

Notes

Use this space to take notes or to write down questions you want to ask the doctor.

_____

_____

_____

_____

_____

_____

_____

_____

_____

_____

Medication Information for Youth

Haloperidol—Haldol

What the Medicine Is Called and What It Is For

The name of your medicine may be confusing. Most drugs have two names: 1) a scientific name that we call a *generic name* and 2) a trade or *brand name*. The generic name of this medicine is haloperidol. The brand name is Haldol.

Haloperidol can help people who feel very confused and have severe problems thinking clearly. It can lessen *hallucinations* (seeing or hearing things that are not really there) and *delusions* (troubling beliefs that other people do not share). This medicine also is sometimes used to help young people who have mania or very severe depression or who get very angry and hit people or break things. It is also used to reduce motor and vocal tics (fast, repeated movements or sounds) in people with Tourette's disorder.

How You Take the Medicine

It is very important to take the medicine exactly as the doctor or nurse tells you. Do not skip doses or take extra medicine without asking an adult. If you forget a dose, ask your parent(s) what to do.

It is better to limit drinks with caffeine (coffee, tea, soft drinks) because caffeine works in the opposite way from this medicine, and the positive effects might be decreased.

If your stomach is upset, taking the medicine with food may help.

This medicine is prescribed only for you. It should never be shared with anyone else.

You do not have to tell others that you are taking this medicine, but it is not something you should feel ashamed or embarrassed about. Many young people are helped by haloperidol. This medicine is not habit-forming, and you cannot become "hooked" on it. You should talk to your doctor or nurse about any questions you have about the medicine. It is important to remember that the medicine *helps* you. It cannot *make* you do anything or change you as a person.

How Your Doctor Will Follow Your Progress

Before giving you the medicine, your doctor or nurse will talk with you and your parent(s) and may measure your height, weight, heart rate (pulse), and blood pressure. There may be other tests, such as blood tests for sugar and cholesterol. Before you start taking the medicine and every so often afterward, the doctor or nurse will look at your tongue, arms, and legs to check for unusual movements. This is called the AIMS (Abnormal Involuntary Movement Scale) test.

Be sure to tell your doctor or nurse about any other medicines or supplements you are taking, including vitamins, herbs, or aids to weight loss or bodybuilding. Also be sure to tell the doctor or nurse if you are using alcohol or drugs. Because many medicines may affect babies, it is very important to tell the doctor if you might be pregnant or if you are at risk of becoming pregnant.

Your teachers may be asked to fill out a form about your grades and behavior in school. A psychologist may give you some tests to see how you learn best.

Most doctors have regular appointments with young people who are taking medicine. You should use these visits to share any concerns you may have about your medicine and to talk about if it has helped you. From time to time, your physician or nurse may measure your height, weight, heart rate (pulse), and blood pressure to be sure that you are in good health while you are taking the medicine. Your doctor also will ask for regular reports from your parents and maybe from your teachers (with your permission) to see how well the medicine is working.

If the medicine helps you, your doctor will probably want you to take it for several months to a year. Your doctor will decide how long you will need to take the medicine as he or she watches your progress.

How the Medicine Might Affect You

In addition to the ways the medicine can help you, it may have other effects called *side effects*. Different medicines have different side effects. It is helpful to know about some of the most common side effects of your medicine so that you will understand what they are if they happen. Some people do not have any side effects. Some side effects are just uncomfortable, but others may mean a more serious problem with the medicine. Side effects are most common after starting the medicine or after a dose increase. They may go away with time, or the medicine can be adjusted or changed—ask the doctor.

You could have an allergy to any medicine, which might show up as a rash on your skin, swelling, itching, or trouble breathing.

Please tell your parent(s) and your doctor or nurse about any changes that you notice after taking the medicine. It is especially important to tell a responsible adult if you are feeling depressed or that you may not want to live; if you have thoughts of hurting yourself; or if you begin to feel more irritable, nervous, or restless.

One of the most common side effects of this medicine is feeling tired or sleepy during the day, even if you have had a full night's sleep. If this medicine is making you sleepy, it is very important not to drive a car or ride a bicycle or motorcycle. After starting the medicine or increasing the dose of medicine, please be extra careful when driving a car, riding a bike, or using machines until you can tell how the medicine affects your alertness, attention, and coordination. After you have been taking the medicine for a few weeks, your body will adjust, and this side effect will likely go away. If you had trouble sleeping at night before taking the medicine, it can help you sleep better, especially if the doctor tells you to take a dose of medicine in the evening.

You might feel dizzy or light-headed if you stand up fast. Try standing up slowly, especially when getting out of bed in the morning.

Another common side effect is dry mouth. You may be more thirsty than usual and find that you are drinking more water or other liquids than usual. Sucking on sugar-free hard candy or cough drops usually helps. You also could try chewing sugar-free gum or sucking on ice chips. Do not chew the ice; you could hurt your teeth. Also, using lip balm will keep your lips from cracking. It is important to be especially good about brushing your teeth.

Taking this medicine could make you more likely to get badly sunburned or very sick in hot weather. Be sure to drink plenty of liquids and cover up or use sunscreen when you go outside in hot weather. Be careful to rest in the shade and not get overheated.

Sometimes teenagers who take haloperidol gain weight. The weight gain may be from increased appetite and also from ways that the medicine changes how the body processes food. It is much easier to prevent weight gain than to lose weight later. It is a good idea to eat a well-balanced diet without "junk food" and with healthy snacks like fruits and vegetables, not sweets or fried foods. It is better to drink water or skim milk, not pop, sodas, soft drinks, or sugary juices. Regular exercise is important for maintaining a healthy weight (and may also help with sleep).

Some people become constipated (have hard bowel movements) when taking this medicine. Try drinking more water and eating more fruits, vegetables, and whole grains. If that does not help, tell your parent(s) or doctor—you may need a medicine to help with this side effect. Sometimes people have trouble passing urine. Tell your parent(s) or the doctor if this happens.

This is a very powerful medicine. Some side effects include feeling nervous, restless, or shaky or having stiff muscles. Talk with your doctor about these side effects. They can be helped by adding another medicine, adjusting the dose, or switching to another medicine.

Another, more serious, side effect can be longer lasting and more difficult to treat. This very rare side effect is called *tardive dyskinesia* (or TD). A person taking haloperidol may develop movements of the mouth, tongue, face, arms, legs, or body that are not being made on purpose. This side effect can go away when the medicine is stopped, but in some people it does not go away. Your doctor will explain this effect to you and your parent(s) and how he or she will watch for any signs that you are developing this problem. Be sure to ask your doctor any questions that you may have about this, but do not worry too much about it. It hardly ever happens to teenagers.

You may notice changes in your sexual functioning or in your breasts—it is OK to ask the doctor about this.

You should tell your parent(s) and doctor if you notice anything different or unusual about how you feel once you start taking the medicine. This includes good things, such as feeling less confused, feeling less sad or angry, not hearing voices anymore, or sleeping better at night.

You cannot become addicted to this medicine, but you should not stop it suddenly. Never stop a medicine without talking to the doctor. If haloperidol is stopped or decreased suddenly you may notice more moodiness or irritability, stomachaches or upset stomach, trouble sleeping, or trembling or shaking. Let your parent(s) or doctor know if this happens—the medicine may need to be decreased more slowly.

Notes

Use this space to take notes or to write down questions you want to ask the doctor or nurse.

_____

_____

_____

_____

_____

_____

_____

_____

_____

_____

_____

_____

_____

From Dulcan MK (editor): *Helping Parents, Youth, and Teachers Understand Medications for Behavioral and Emotional Problems: A Resource Book of Medication Information Handouts,* Third Edition. Washington, DC, American Psychiatric Publishing, 2007

Medication Information for Parents and Teachers

Hydroxyzine—Atarax, Vistaril

General Information About Medication

Each child and adolescent is different. No one has exactly the same combination of medical and psychological problems. It is a good idea to talk with the doctor or nurse about the reasons a medicine is being used. It is very important to keep all appointments and to be in touch by telephone if you have concerns. It is important to communicate with the doctor, nurse, or therapist.

It is very important that the medicine be taken exactly as the doctor instructs. However, once in a while, everyone forgets to give a medicine on time. It is a good idea to ask the doctor or nurse what to do if this happens. Do not stop or change a medicine without asking the doctor or nurse first.

If the medicine seems to stop working, it may be because it is not being taken regularly. The youth may be "cheeking" or hiding the medicine or forgetting to take it (especially at school). The doses may be too far apart, or a different dose may be needed. Something at school, at home, or in the neighborhood may be upsetting the youth, or he or she may need special help for learning disabilities or tutoring. Please discuss your concerns with the doctor. **Do not just increase the dose.**

All medicines should be kept in a safe place, out of the reach of children, and should be supervised by an adult. If someone takes too much of a medicine, call the doctor, the poison control center, or a hospital emergency room.

Each medicine has a "generic" or chemical name. Just like laundry detergents or paper towels, some medicines are sold by more than one company under different brand names. The same medicine may be available under a generic name and several brand names. The generic medications are usually less expensive than the brand name ones. The generic medications have the same chemical formula, but they may or may not be exactly the same strength as the brand-name medications. Also, some brands of pills contain dye that can cause allergic reactions. It is a good idea to talk to the doctor and the pharmacist about whether it is important to use a specific brand of medicine.

All medicines can cause an allergic reaction. Examples are hives, itching, rashes, swelling, and trouble breathing. Even a tiny amount of a medicine can cause a reaction in patients who are allergic to that medicine. Be *sure* to talk to the doctor before restarting a medicine that has caused an allergic reaction.

Taking more than one medicine at the same time may cause more side effects or cause one of the medicines to not work as well. Always ask the doctor, nurse, or pharmacist before adding another medicine, whether prescription or over-the-counter. Be sure that each doctor knows about *all* of the medicines your child is taking. Also tell the doctor about any vitamins, herbal medicines, or supplements your child may be taking. Some of these may have side effects alone or when taken with this medication.

Everyone taking medicine should have a physical examination at least once a year.

If you suspect the youth is using drugs or alcohol, please tell the doctor right away.

351

Pregnancy requires special care in the use of medicine. Please tell the doctor immediately if you suspect the teenager is pregnant or might become pregnant.

Printed information like this applies to children and adolescents in general. If you have questions about the medicine, or if you notice changes or anything unusual, please ask the doctor or nurse. As scientific research advances, knowledge increases and advice changes. Even experts do not always agree. Many medicines have not been approved by the U.S. Food and Drug Administration (FDA) for use in children. For this reason, use of the medicine for a particular problem or age group often is not listed in the *Physicians' Desk Reference*. This does not necessarily mean that the medicine is dangerous or does not work, only that the company that makes the medicine has not received permission to advertise the medicine for use in children. Companies often do not apply for this permission because it is expensive to do the tests needed to apply for approval for use in children. Once a medication is approved by the FDA for any purpose, a doctor is allowed to prescribe it according to research and clinical experience.

Note to Teachers

It is a good idea to talk with the parent(s) about the reason(s) that a medication is being used. If the parent(s) sign consent to release information, it is often helpful to talk with the doctor. If the parent(s) give permission, the doctor may ask you to fill out rating forms about your experience with the student's behavior, feelings, academic performance, and medication side effects. This information is very useful in selecting and monitoring medication treatment. If you have observations that you think are important, do not hesitate to share these with the student's parent(s) and treating clinicians.

It is very important that the medicine be taken exactly as the doctor instructs. However, everyone forgets to give a medicine on time once in a while. It is a good idea to ask the parent(s) in advance what to do if this happens. Do not stop or change the time you are giving a medicine at school without parental permission. If a medication is to be taken with food, but lunchtime or snack time changes, be sure to notify the parent(s) so appropriate adjustments can be made.

All medicines should be kept in a secure place and should be supervised by an adult. If someone takes too much of a medicine, follow your school procedure for an urgent medical problem.

Taking medicine is a private matter and is best managed discreetly and confidentially. It is important to be sensitive to the student's feelings about taking medicine.

If you suspect that the student is using drugs or alcohol, please tell the parent(s) or a school counselor right away.

Please tell the parent(s) or school nurse if you suspect medication side effects.

Modifications of the classroom environment or assignments may be useful in addition to medication. The student may need to be evaluated for additional help or for an Individualized Education Plan for learning or behavior.

Any expression of suicidal thoughts or feelings or self-harm by a child or adolescent is a clear signal of distress and should be taken seriously. These behaviors should not be dismissed as "attention seeking."

What Is Hydroxyzine (Atarax, Vistaril)?

Hydroxyzine is called an *antihistamine*. Antihistamines were developed to treat allergies. Hydroxyzine is sometimes used to treat anxiety (nervousness) or insomnia (difficulty falling asleep). It comes in generic or brand name Vistaril capsules and liquid and generic or brand name Atarax tablets. It also comes in an injection (shot).

How Can This Medicine Help?

Hydroxyzine may decrease nervousness. When used for anxiety, it works best when used for a short time along with psychotherapy. Hydroxyzine can help with insomnia when used for a short time along with a behavioral program, such as regular soothing routines at bedtime and increased exercise in the daytime.

How Does This Medicine Work?

Hydroxyzine can help decrease anxiety and help falling asleep because of its *sedative* effect. That is, it makes people a little sleepy so that they feel less nervous and also fall asleep more easily.

How Long Does This Medicine Last?

Hydroxyzine lasts for 4–6 hours.

How Will the Doctor Monitor This Medicine?

The doctor will review your child's medical history and physical examination before starting hydroxyzine. Be sure to tell the doctor if your child or anyone in the family has a history of asthma or of heart rhythm problems, palpitations, or fainting. The doctor or nurse may measure your child's height, weight, pulse, and blood pressure before starting the medicine.

After the medicine is started, the doctor will want to have regular appointments with you and your child to see how the medicine is working, to see if a dose change is needed, to watch for side effects, to see if hydroxyzine is still needed, and to see if any other treatment is needed. The doctor or nurse may check your child's height, weight, pulse, and blood pressure.

What Side Effects Can This Medicine Have?

Any medicine can have side effects, including an allergy to the medicine. Because each patient is different, the doctor will monitor the youth closely, especially when the medicine is started. The doctor will work with you to increase the positive effects and decrease the negative effects of the medicine. Please tell the doctor if any of the listed side effects appear or if you think that the medicine is causing any other problems. Not all of the rare or unusual side effects are listed.

Side effects are most common after starting the medicine or after a dose increase. Many side effects can be avoided or lessened by starting with a very low dose and increasing it slowly—ask the doctor.

Allergic Reaction

Tell the doctor in a day or two (if possible, before the next dose of medicine):

- Hives
- Itching
- Rash

Stop the medicine and get *immediate* medical care:

- Trouble breathing or chest tightness
- Swelling of lips, tongue, or throat

Common Side Effects

Tell the doctor within a week or two:

- Daytime sleepiness—Do not allow your child to drive, ride a bicycle or motorcycle, or operate machinery if this happens.
- Decreased attention, memory, or learning in school
- Dry mouth—Have your child try using sugar-free gum or candy.
- Headache
- Blurred vision
- Constipation—Encourage your child to drink more fluids and eat high-fiber foods; if necessary, the doctor may recommend a fiber medicine such as Benefiber or a stool softener such as Colace or mineral oil.
- Dizziness or light-headedness—This side effect is worse when the child stands up quickly, especially when getting out of bed in the morning; try having the child stand up slowly.
- Loss of appetite, nausea, or upset stomach

Less Common Side Effects

Call the doctor within a day or two:

- Poor coordination
- Motor tics (fast, repeated movements)
- Unusual muscle movements
- Irritability, overactivity
- Waking up after sleeping for a short time and being unable to get back to sleep
- Exposure to sunlight may cause severe sunburn, skin rash, redness, or itching; avoid direct exposure to sunlight or use sunscreen.
- Trouble passing urine

Very Rare, but Serious, Side Effects

Call the doctor *immediately*:

- Worsening of asthma or trouble breathing
- Seizure (fit, convulsion)
- Uncontrollable behavior
- Hallucinations (seeing things that are not really there)
- Severe muscle stiffness
- Irregular heartbeat (pulse), fainting, palpitations

Some Interactions With Other Medicines or Food

Please note that the following are only the most likely interactions with food or other medicines.
If other medicines that can cause sleepiness are taken with hydroxyzine, severe sleepiness can result.

What Could Happen if This Medicine Is Stopped Suddenly?

Stopping these medicines suddenly does not usually cause problems, but diarrhea or feeling sick may result if it has been taken for a long time. The problem being treated may come back. Always ask the doctor whether a medicine can be stopped suddenly or must be decreased slowly (tapered).

How Long Will This Medicine Be Needed?

When used for nervousness or sleep, hydroxyzine is usually prescribed for a very short time to allow the patient to be calm enough to learn new ways to cope. If the person needs treatment for a longer time, another medicine is usually prescribed.

What Else Should I Know About This Medicine?

People who take hydroxyzine must not drink alcohol. Severe sleepiness or even loss of consciousness may result.

Notes

Use this space to take notes or to write down questions you want to ask the doctor.

_____

_____

_____

_____

_____

_____

_____

_____

_____

_____

_____

_____

_____

Medication Information for Youth

Hydroxyzine—Atarax, Vistaril

What the Medicine Is Called and What It Is For

The name of your medicine may be confusing. Most drugs have two names: 1) a scientific name that we call a *generic name* and 2) a trade or *brand name*. The generic name of this medicine is hydroxyzine. The brand names are Atarax or Vistaril.

Hydroxyzine is called an *antihistamine*. These medicines were developed to treat allergies. Hydroxyzine is sometimes used to treat anxiety (nervousness) or insomnia (difficulty falling asleep). It can help anxious people to be calm enough to learn—with therapy and practice—to understand and tolerate their worries or fears and even to overcome them. Most often, this medicine is used for a short time when symptoms are very uncomfortable or frightening or when they make it hard to do important things such as go to school. Hydroxyzine can help with insomnia when used for a short time along with calming routines that help to fall asleep. It is sometimes used to help lessen the side effects of other medicines.

How You Take the Medicine

It is very important to take the medicine exactly as the doctor or nurse tells you. Do not skip doses or take extra medicine without asking an adult. If you forget a dose, ask your parent(s) what to do. It is best to take this medicine with milk or with food.

Do not use any other medicines without talking to your doctor first. Do not use alcohol, marijuana, or street drugs while taking this medicine. They can cause serious side effects. Skipping your medicine to take drugs does not work because many medicines stay in your body for a long time.

Caffeine (in coffee, tea, or soft drinks) could make you feel worse.

This medicine is prescribed only for you. It should never be shared with anyone else.

You do not have to tell others that you are taking this medicine, but it is not something you should feel ashamed or embarrassed about. Many young people are helped by hydroxyzine. This medicine is not habit-forming, and you cannot become "hooked" on it. You should talk to your doctor or nurse about any questions you have about the medicine. It is important to remember that the medicine *helps* you. It cannot *make* you do anything or change you as a person.

If you stop the medicine suddenly, it might cause you to feel sick, or the problem being treated may come back. Do not stop the medicine unless the doctor tells you to.

357

How Your Doctor Will Follow Your Progress

Before giving you the medicine, your doctor or nurse will talk with you and your parent(s) and may measure your height, weight, heart rate (pulse), and blood pressure.

Be sure to tell your doctor or nurse about any other medicines or supplements you are taking, including vitamins, herbs, or aids to weight loss or bodybuilding. Also be sure to tell the doctor or nurse if you are using alcohol or drugs. Because many medicines may affect babies, it is very important to tell the doctor if you might be pregnant or if you are at risk of becoming pregnant.

Most doctors have regular appointments with young people who are taking medicine. You should use these visits to share any concerns you may have about your medicine and to talk about if it has helped you. From time to time, your physician or nurse may measure your height, weight, heart rate (pulse), and blood pressure to be sure that you are in good health while you are taking the medicine. Your doctor also will ask for regular reports from your parents and maybe from your teachers (with your permission) to see how well the medicine is working.

How the Medicine Might Affect You

In addition to the ways the medicine can help you, it may have other effects called *side effects*. Different medicines have different side effects. It is helpful to know about some of the most common side effects of your medicine so that you will understand what they are if they happen. Some people do not have any side effects. Some side effects are just uncomfortable, but others may mean a more serious problem with the medicine. Side effects are most common after starting the medicine or after a dose increase. They may go away with time, or the medicine can be adjusted or changed—ask the doctor.

You could have an allergy to any medicine, which might show up as a rash on your skin, swelling, itching, or trouble breathing.

Please tell your parent(s) and your doctor or nurse about any changes that you notice after taking the medicine. It is especially important to tell a responsible adult if you are feeling depressed or that you may not want to live; if you have thoughts of hurting yourself; or if you begin to feel more irritable, nervous, or restless.

The most common side effect of hydroxyzine is daytime sleepiness. If this medicine is making you sleepy, it is very important not to drive a car or ride a bicycle or motorcycle. After starting a new medicine or increasing the dose of a medicine, please be extra careful when driving a car, riding a bike, or using machines until you can tell how the medicine affects your alertness, attention, and coordination.

Drinking alcohol while taking this medicine can cause severe drowsiness or even passing out. **Don't do it!**

Tell your parent(s) or the doctor if you wake up at night after sleeping for a short time and cannot get back to sleep.

Sometimes hydroxyzine seems to work in the opposite way, causing excitement, irritability, anger, aggression, and other problems. If this happens, tell your parent(s) or your doctor.

You might feel dizzy, tired, or even faint when you stand up fast. Try standing up slowly, especially first thing in the morning when getting out of bed.

Another common side effect is dry mouth. You may be more thirsty than usual and find that you are drinking more water or other liquids than usual. Sucking on sugar-free hard candy or cough drops usually helps. You also could try chewing sugar-free gum or sucking on ice chips. Do not chew the ice; you could hurt your teeth. Also, using lip balm will keep your lips from cracking. It is important to be especially good about brushing your teeth.

Some people become constipated (have hard bowel movements) when taking this medicine. Try drinking more water and eating more fruits, vegetables, and whole grains. If that does not help, tell your parent(s) or doctor—you may need a medicine to help with this side effect.

Taking this medicine could make you more likely to get badly sunburned or very sick in hot weather. Be sure to drink plenty of liquids and cover up or use sunscreen when you go outside in hot weather. Be careful to rest in the shade and not get overheated.

Other side effects that some people get from hydroxyzine include having trouble passing urine, blurred vision, stomachache, upset stomach, or headache.

Serious side effects hardly ever happen when taking this medicine. You should tell your parent(s) and doctor if you notice anything different or unusual about how you feel once you start taking the medicine, especially if you are having trouble breathing or your body seems to be moving differently than usual.

Notes

Use this space to take notes or to write down questions you want to ask the doctor or nurse.

_____

_____

_____

_____

_____

_____

_____

_____

_____

_____

From Dulcan MK (editor): *Helping Parents, Youth, and Teachers Understand Medications for Behavioral and Emotional Problems: A Resource Book of Medication Information Handouts*, Third Edition. Washington, DC, American Psychiatric Publishing, 2007

Medication Information
for Parents and Teachers

Imipramine—Tofranil

General Information About Medication

Each child and adolescent is different. No one has exactly the same combination of medical and psychological problems. It is a good idea to talk with the doctor or nurse about the reasons a medicine is being used. It is very important to keep all appointments and to be in touch by telephone if you have concerns. It is important to communicate with the doctor, nurse, or therapist.

It is very important that the medicine be taken exactly as the doctor instructs. However, once in a while, everyone forgets to give a medicine on time. It is a good idea to ask the doctor or nurse what to do if this happens. Do not stop or change a medicine without asking the doctor or nurse first.

If the medicine seems to stop working, it may be because it is not being taken regularly. The youth may be "cheeking" or hiding the medicine or forgetting to take it (especially at school). The doses may be too far apart, or a different dose may be needed. Something at school, at home, or in the neighborhood may be upsetting the youth, or he or she may need special help for learning disabilities or tutoring. Please discuss your concerns with the doctor. **Do not just increase the dose.**

All medicines should be kept in a safe place, out of the reach of children, and should be supervised by an adult. If someone takes too much of a medicine, call the doctor, the poison control center, or a hospital emergency room.

Each medicine has a "generic" or chemical name. Just like laundry detergents or paper towels, some medicines are sold by more than one company under different brand names. The same medicine may be available under a generic name and several brand names. The generic medications are usually less expensive than the brand name ones. The generic medications have the same chemical formula, but they may or may not be exactly the same strength as the brand-name medications. Also, some brands of pills contain dye that can cause allergic reactions. It is a good idea to talk to the doctor and the pharmacist about whether it is important to use a specific brand of medicine.

All medicines can cause an allergic reaction. Examples are hives, itching, rashes, swelling, and trouble breathing. Even a tiny amount of a medicine can cause a reaction in patients who are allergic to that medicine. Be *sure* to talk to the doctor before restarting a medicine that has caused an allergic reaction.

Taking more than one medicine at the same time may cause more side effects or cause one of the medicines to not work as well. Always ask the doctor, nurse, or pharmacist before adding another medicine, whether prescription or over-the-counter. Be sure that each doctor knows about *all* of the medicines your child is taking. Also tell the doctor about any vitamins, herbal medicines, or supplements your child may be taking. Some of these may have side effects alone or when taken with this medication.

Everyone taking medicine should have a physical examination at least once a year.

If you suspect the youth is using drugs or alcohol, please tell the doctor right away.

Pregnancy requires special care in the use of medicine. Please tell the doctor immediately if you suspect the teenager is pregnant or might become pregnant.

Printed information like this applies to children and adolescents in general. If you have questions about the medicine, or if you notice changes or anything unusual, please ask the doctor or nurse. As scientific research advances, knowledge increases and advice changes. Even experts do not always agree. Many medicines have not been approved by the U.S. Food and Drug Administration (FDA) for use in children. For this reason, use of the medicine for a particular problem or age group often is not listed in the *Physicians' Desk Reference*. This does not necessarily mean that the medicine is dangerous or does not work, only that the company that makes the medicine has not received permission to advertise the medicine for use in children. Companies often do not apply for this permission because it is expensive to do the tests needed to apply for approval for use in children. Once a medication is approved by the FDA for any purpose, a doctor is allowed to prescribe it according to research and clinical experience.

Note to Teachers

It is a good idea to talk with the parent(s) about the reason(s) that a medication is being used. If the parent(s) sign consent to release information, it is often helpful to talk with the doctor. If the parent(s) give permission, the doctor may ask you to fill out rating forms about your experience with the student's behavior, feelings, academic performance, and medication side effects. This information is very useful in selecting and monitoring medication treatment. If you have observations that you think are important, do not hesitate to share these with the student's parent(s) and treating clinicians.

It is very important that the medicine be taken exactly as the doctor instructs. However, everyone forgets to give a medicine on time once in a while. It is a good idea to ask the parent(s) in advance what to do if this happens. Do not stop or change the time you are giving a medicine at school without parental permission. If a medication is to be taken with food, but lunchtime or snack time changes, be sure to notify the parent(s) so appropriate adjustments can be made.

All medicines should be kept in a secure place and should be supervised by an adult. If someone takes too much of a medicine, follow your school procedure for an urgent medical problem.

Taking medicine is a private matter and is best managed discreetly and confidentially. It is important to be sensitive to the student's feelings about taking medicine.

If you suspect that the student is using drugs or alcohol, please tell the parent(s) or a school counselor right away.

Please tell the parent(s) or school nurse if you suspect medication side effects.

Modifications of the classroom environment or assignments may be useful in addition to medication. The student may need to be evaluated for additional help or for an Individualized Education Plan for learning or behavior.

Any expression of suicidal thoughts or feelings or self-harm by a child or adolescent is a clear signal of distress and should be taken seriously. These behaviors should not be dismissed as "attention seeking."

You may notice the following side effects at school:

Common Side Effects

- Dry mouth—Allow the student to chew sugar-free gum or to make extra trips to the water fountain.
- Constipation—Allow the student to drink more fluids or to use the bathroom more often.
- Daytime sleepiness—The student should not drive, ride a bicycle or motorcycle, or operate machinery.
- Dizziness (especially when standing up quickly)—This may happen in the classroom or during physical education). Suggest that the student stand up more slowly.
- Irritability

Occasional Side Effects

- Stuttering
- Increased risk of sunburn (this may be a problem if recess or physical education is outdoors in warm weather)—The student should wear sunscreen or protective clothing or stay out of the sun.

Less Common Side Effects

- Nausea—The student may need to take the medicine after a meal or snack.
- Trouble urinating—The student may need more time in the bathroom.
- Blurred vision—The student may have trouble seeing the blackboard.
- Motor tics (fast, repeated movements) or muscle twitches (jerking movements) of parts of the body
- Increased activity, rapid speech, feeling "speeded up," being very excited or irritable (cranky)
- Skin rash

Rare, but Potentially Serious, Side Effects

Call the parents(s) or follow your school's emergency procedures *immediately*:

- Seizure (fit, convulsion) **(This is a medical emergency.)**
- Very fast or irregular heartbeat **(This is a medical emergency.)**
- Fainting
- Hallucinations (hearing voices or seeing things that are not there)
- Inability to urinate
- Confusion
- Severe change in behavior

What Is Imipramine (Tofranil)?

Imipramine is called a *tricyclic antidepressant*. It was first used to treat depression but is now used to treat enuresis (bed-wetting), attention-deficit/hyperactivity disorder (ADHD), school phobia, separation anxiety, panic disorder, and some sleep disorders (such as night terrors). It comes in brand name Tofranil and generic tablets and Tofranil-PM sustained-release (long-acting) capsules.

How Can This Medicine Help?

Imipramine can decrease symptoms of ADHD, anxiety (nervousness), panic, and night terrors or sleepwalking. The medicine may take several weeks to work. Imipramine can also help control urination and decrease bed-wetting (nocturnal enuresis). When treating enuresis, the medicine works right away.

How Does This Medicine Work?

Tricyclic antidepressants affect *neurotransmitters*—the natural substances that are needed for certain parts of the brain to work normally. They increase the activity of *serotonin* and *norepinephrine* to more normal levels in the parts of the brain that regulate concentration, motivation, and mood. Science does not yet know how imipramine helps stop bed-wetting.

How Long Does This Medicine Last?

Although a dose lasts for a whole day in adults and older teenagers, in younger children several doses a day may be needed.

How Will the Doctor Monitor This Medicine?

The doctor will review your child's medical history and physical examination, paying special attention to pulse rate, blood pressure, weight, and height, before starting imipramine. These measurements will be taken when the dose is increased and occasionally as long as the medicine is continued. The doctor may order some blood or urine tests to be sure your child does not have a hidden medical condition that would make it unsafe to use this medicine.

Tricyclic antidepressants can slow the speed at which signals move through the heart. This effect is not dangerous if the heart is normal, which is why an ECG (electrocardiogram or heart rhythm test) is done before starting the medicine. The ECG may be repeated as the dose is increased and occasionally while the medicine is being taken. Changes in the heart from the medicine usually can be seen on the ECG before they become a problem, so your child's doctor will order an ECG every so often. When imipramine is used only at night in very low doses to treat bed-wetting, an ECG may not be needed.

To find possible hidden heart risks, it is especially important to tell the doctor if your child or anyone in the family has a history of fainting, palpitations, or irregular heartbeat or if anyone in the family died suddenly.

Be sure to tell the doctor if your child or anyone in the family has bipolar illness (manic-depressive illness) or has tried to kill himself or herself.

Because tricyclic antidepressants may increase the risk of seizures (fits, convulsions), the doctor will want to know whether your child has ever had a seizure or a head injury and if there is any family history of epilepsy. Your child's doctor may want to order an EEG (electroencephalogram or brain wave test) before starting the medicine.

Experts do not agree on whether blood tests are needed to measure the level of this medicine. Blood levels seem to be most useful when your doctor suspects that the dose of medicine is too high or too low. The most accurate level is obtained by drawing blood first thing in the morning after at least 5 days on the same dose, approximately 12 hours after the evening dose of medicine and before the morning dose.

After the medicine is started, the doctor will want to have regular appointments with you and your child to see how the medicine is working, to see if a dose change is needed, to watch for side effects, to see if imipramine is still needed, and to see if any other treatment is needed. The doctor or nurse may check your child's height, weight, pulse, and blood pressure or order tests, such as an ECG or blood level.

Before using medicine and at times afterward, the doctor may ask your child to fill out a rating scale about anxiety, to help see how your child is doing.

What Side Effects Can This Medicine Have?

Any medicine can have side effects, including an allergy to the medicine. Because each patient is different, the doctor will monitor the youth closely, especially when the medicine is started. The doctor will work with you to increase the positive effects and decrease the negative effects of the medicine. Please tell the doctor if any of the listed side effects appear or if you think that the medicine is causing any other problems. Not all of the rare or unusual side effects are listed.

Side effects are most common after starting the medicine or after a dose increase. Many side effects can be avoided or lessened by starting with a very low dose and increasing it slowly—ask the doctor.

Allergic Reaction

Tell the doctor in a day or two (if possible, before the next dose of medicine):

- Hives
- Itching
- Rash (may be caused by an allergy to the medicine or to a dye in the specific brand of pill)

Stop the medicine and get *immediate* medical care:

- Trouble breathing or chest tightness
- Swelling of lips, tongue, or throat

Common Side Effects

Tell the doctor within a week or two:

- Dry mouth—Have your child try using sugar-free gum or candy.
- Constipation—Encourage your child to drink more fluids and eat high-fiber foods; if necessary, the doctor may recommend a fiber medicine such as Benefiber or a stool softener such as Colace or mineral oil.
- Daytime sleepiness—Do not allow your child to drive, ride a bicycle or motorcycle, or operate machinery if this happens.
- Dizziness—This side effect is worse when the child stands up quickly, especially when getting out of bed in the morning; try having the child stand up slowly.
- Weight gain
- Loss of appetite and weight loss
- Irritability
- Acne

Occasional Side Effects

Tell the doctor within a week or two:

- Nightmares
- Stuttering
- Blurred vision

365

- Increase in breast size, nipple discharge, or both (in girls)
- Increase in breast size (in boys)

Less Common, but More Serious, Side Effects

Call the doctor within a day or two:

- High or low blood pressure
- Nausea
- Trouble urinating
- Motor tics (fast, repeated movements) or muscle twitches (jerking movements)
- Increased activity, rapid speech, feeling "speeded up," decreased need for sleep, being very excited or irritable (cranky)

Rare, but Potentially Serious, Side Effects

Call the doctor *immediately*:

- Seizure (fit, convulsion)—**Go to an emergency room.**
- Very fast or irregular heartbeat—**Go to an emergency room.**
- Fainting
- Hallucinations (hearing voices or seeing things that are not there)
- Inability to urinate
- Confusion
- Severe change in behavior

Some Interactions With Other Medicines or Food

Please note that the following are only the most likely interactions with food or other medicines.

Check with your child's doctor before giving your child decongestants or over-the-counter cold medicine.

Taking another antidepressant or Depakote with imipramine may increase the level of imipramine and increase side effects.

Taking carbamazepine (Tegretol) with imipramine may decrease the positive effects of imipramine and increase the side effects of carbamazepine.

It can be *very dangerous* to take imipramine at the same time as or even within a month of taking another type of medicine called a *monoamine oxidase inhibitor* (MAOI), such as Eldepryl (selegiline), Nardil (phenelzine), Parnate (tranylcypromine), or Marplan (isocarboxazid).

Caffeine may worsen side effects on the heart or symptoms of anxiety. It is best not to drink coffee, tea, or soft drinks with caffeine while taking this medicine.

What Could Happen if This Medicine Is Stopped Suddenly?

Stopping the medicine suddenly or skipping a dose is not dangerous but can be very uncomfortable. Your child may feel like he or she has the flu—with a headache, muscle aches, stomachache, and upset stomach. Behavioral problems, sadness, nervousness, or trouble sleeping also may occur. If these feelings appear every day, the medicine may need to be given more often during each day.

How Long Will This Medicine Be Needed?

There is no way to know how long a person will need to take this medicine. Parents work together with the doctor to determine what is right for each child. For bed-wetting, the medicine may be used for 6–12 months and may be stopped if the child grows out of bed-wetting. When treating ADHD, the medicine may be needed for a longer time. Some people may need to take the medicine even as adults.

What Else Should I Know About This Medicine?

In youth who have bipolar disorder (manic depression) or who are at risk for bipolar disorder, any antidepressant medicine may increase the risk of hypomania or mania (excitement, agitation, increased activity, decreased sleep).

An overdose by accident or on purpose with tricyclic antidepressants is very dangerous! You must closely supervise the medicine. You may have to lock up the medicine if your child or teenager is suicidal or if young children live in or visit your home.

Tricyclic antidepressants may cause dry mouth, which could increase the chance of tooth decay. Regular brushing of teeth and checkups with the dentist are especially important.

This medicine causes increased risk of sunburn. Be sure that your child wears sunscreen or protective clothing or stays out of the sun.

People who take tricyclic antidepressants must not drink alcohol or use tranquilizers. Severe sleepiness, loss of consciousness, or even death may result.

Black Box Antidepressant Warning

In 2004, an advisory committee to the FDA decided that there might be an increased risk of suicidal behavior for some youth taking medicines called *antidepressants*. In the research studies that the committee reviewed, about 3%–4% of youth with depression who took an antidepressant medicine—and 1%–2% of youth with depression who took a placebo (pill without active medicine)—talked about suicidal thoughts (thinking about killing themselves or wishing they were dead) or did something to harm themselves. This means that almost twice as many youth who were taking an antidepressant to treat their depression talked about suicide or had suicidal behavior compared with youth with depression who were taking inactive medicine. There were *no* completed suicides in any of these research studies, which included more than 4,000 children and adolescents. For youth being treated for anxiety, there was no difference in suicidal talking or behavior between those taking antidepressant medication and those taking placebo.

The FDA told drug companies to add a *black box warning* label to all antidepressant medicines. Because of this label, a doctor (or advanced practice nurse) prescribing one of these medicines has to warn youth and their families that there might be more suicidal thoughts and actions in youth taking these medicines.

On the other hand, in places where more youth are taking the newer antidepressant medicines, the number of adolescents who commit suicide has gotten smaller. Also, thinking about or attempting suicide is more common in surveys of teenagers in the community than it is in depressed youth treated in research studies with antidepressant medicine.

If a youth is being treated with this medicine and is doing well, then no changes are needed as a result of this warning. Increased suicidal talk or action is most likely to happen in the first few months of treatment with a medicine. If your child has recently started this medicine or is about to start, then you and your doctor (or advanced practice nurse) should watch for any changes in behavior. People who are depressed often have suicidal thoughts or actions. It is hard to know whether suicidal thoughts or actions in depressed people are caused by the depression itself or by the medicine. Also, as their depression is getting better, some people talk more about the suicidal thoughts that they had before but did not talk about. As young people get better from depression, they might be at higher risk of doing something about suicidal thoughts that they have had for some time, because they have more energy.

What Should a Parent Do?

1. Be honest with your child about possible risks and benefits of medicine.
2. Talk to your child about whether he or she is having any suicidal thoughts, and tell your child to come to you if he or she is having such thoughts.
3. You, your child, and your child's doctor or nurse should develop a safety plan. Pick adults whom your child can tell if he or she is thinking about suicide.
4. Be sure to tell your child's doctor, nurse, or therapist if you suspect that your child is using alcohol or drugs or if something has happened that might make your child feel worse, such as a family separation, breaking up with a boyfriend or girlfriend, someone close dying or attempting suicide, physical or sexual abuse, or failure in school.
5. Be sure that there are no guns in the home and that all medicines (including over-the-counter medicines like Tylenol) are closely supervised by an adult and kept in a safe place.
6. Watch for new or worse thoughts of suicide, self-harm, depression, anxiety (nerves), feeling very agitated or restless, being angry or aggressive, having more trouble sleeping, or anything else that you see for the first time, seems worse, or worries your child or you. If these appear, contact a mental health professional **right away.** Do not just stop or change the dose of the medicine on your own. If the problems are serious, and you cannot reach one of your clinicians, call a 24-hour psychiatry emergency telephone number or take your child to an emergency room.

Youth on antidepressant medicine should be watched carefully by their parent(s), clinician(s) (doctor, nurse, therapist), and other concerned adults for the first weeks of treatment. It is a good idea to have a visit or telephone call with the doctor, nurse, or therapist weekly for the first month, every 2 weeks for the second month, and after that at least once a month to check for feelings of depression or sadness, thoughts of killing or harming himself or herself, and any problems with the medication. If you have questions, be sure to ask the doctor, nurse, or therapist.

For more information, see http://www.parentsmedguide.org/ (in English and Spanish).

Notes

Use this space to take notes or to write down questions you want to ask the doctor.

_____

_____

_____

_____

_____

_____

_____

_____

_____

_____

_____

_____

_____

Imipramine—Tofranil

What the Medicine Is Called and What It Is For

The name of your medicine may be confusing. Most drugs have two names: 1) a scientific name that we call a *generic name* and 2) a trade or *brand name*. The generic name of this medicine is imipramine. The brand name is Tofranil.

Imipramine is called an *antidepressant*, or *tricyclic*. Imipramine is used to treat depression, trouble paying attention, being too active or acting without thinking, and feeling too anxious (nervous). It can help people who have attention-deficit/hyperactivity disorder (ADHD), fear of going to school or being away from home, panic disorder, or sleep problems such as waking up at night very scared (night terrors) or sleepwalking. Sometimes imipramine is used to help people who wet the bed to stay dry at night.

How You Take the Medicine

It is very important to take the medicine exactly as the doctor or nurse tells you. Do not skip doses or take extra medicine without asking an adult. If you miss a dose, you may feel sick, as though you have the flu. It is very important that you take all the pills you are supposed to take each day. Your doctor will probably recommend that you take your medicine at the same time each day, which may be with meals or at bedtime.

It may take several weeks before you notice that the medicine is helping. Waiting for the full effect may take even longer. You may feel discouraged and think the medicine is never going to help. You may want to give up and stop taking the medicine. Talk to your doctor and parent(s) about how you feel, but **do not stop** taking the medicine unless your doctor tells you to. It is also important not to take extra pills, hoping that you will feel better faster. Doing that could make you *very* sick.

If you are taking imipramine to stop wetting the bed, it may be used every night or only for nights when you are sleeping away from home (camp, sleepovers) and would be embarrassed.

If you are taking imipramine regularly, stopping it suddenly or skipping a dose can be very uncomfortable. You may feel like you have the flu—with a headache, muscle aches, stomachache, and upset stomach. If these feelings appear every day, the medicine may need to be given more often during each day.

Caffeine (in coffee, tea, or soft drinks) may make you feel worse.

Do not use any other medicines without talking to your doctor first. Do not use alcohol, marijuana, or street drugs while taking this medicine—**it can be very dangerous.** Skipping your medicine to take drugs does not work because many medicines stay in your body for a long time.

This medicine is prescribed only for you. It should never be shared with anyone else.

You do not have to tell others that you are taking this medicine, but it is not something you should feel ashamed or embarrassed about. Many young people are helped by imipramine. This medicine is not habit-forming, and you cannot become "hooked" on it. You should talk to your doctor or nurse about any questions you have about the medicine. It is important to remember that the medicine *helps* you. It cannot *make* you do anything or change you as a person.

How Your Doctor Will Follow Your Progress

Before giving you the medicine, your doctor or nurse will talk with you and your parent(s) and measure your height, weight, heart rate (pulse), and blood pressure. The doctor may order some blood or urine tests to be sure you are in good health. Be sure to tell the doctor if you have had very fast heartbeat, chest pain, dizziness, or fainting.

Be sure to tell your doctor or nurse about any other medicines or supplements you are taking, including vitamins, herbs, or aids to weight loss or bodybuilding. Also be sure to tell the doctor or nurse if you are using alcohol or drugs. Because many medicines may affect babies, it is very important to tell the doctor if you might be pregnant or if you are at risk of becoming pregnant. Be sure to tell the doctor if you have had thoughts of hurting yourself, have tried to hurt yourself, or sometimes wish that you were not alive.

Before starting imipramine, at times of increasing the dose, and every 6 months to a year after that, your doctor will ask for an ECG (electrocardiogram or heart rhythm test) to be done. This test counts your heartbeats through small wires that are taped to your chest. It takes only a few minutes.

Your teachers may be asked to fill out a form about your grades and behavior in school. A psychologist may give you some tests to see how you learn best.

Before starting the medicine and afterward, the doctor may ask you to answer questions on paper about anxiety and depression.

Most doctors have regular appointments with young people who are taking medicine. You should use these visits to share any concerns you may have about your medicine and to talk about if it has helped you. From time to time, your physician or nurse may measure your height, weight, heart rate (pulse), and blood pressure to be sure that you are in good health while you are taking the medicine. You may need to have blood tests to see if you are on the right dose of imipramine. Your doctor also will ask for regular reports from your parents and maybe from your teachers (with your permission) to see how well the medicine is working.

Some medicines are started at the amount you will take for as long as you are taking that medicine. Other medicines need to be increased or adjusted until your doctor decides you are taking the right amount. Starting at a low dose and increasing it slowly may lessen side effects. If the medicine helps you, your doctor will probably want you to take it for a long time, maybe even as an adult.

If you are taking imipramine for bed-wetting, you can talk to the doctor if you would rather try a behavioral program ("bell and pad") instead of taking this medicine. When the medicine is stopped, bed-wetting usually returns. If imipramine is being used regularly, several times a year the doctor may tell you to stop it to see if you have grown out of bed-wetting, which most people do.

How the Medicine Might Affect You

In addition to the ways the medicine can help you, it may have other effects called *side effects*. Different medicines have different side effects. It is helpful to know about some of the most common side effects of your medicine so that you will understand what they are if they happen. Some people do not have any side effects. Some side effects are just uncomfortable, but others may mean a more serious problem with the medicine. Side effects are most common after starting the medicine or after a dose increase. They may go away with time, or the medicine can be adjusted or changed—ask the doctor.

You could have an allergy to any medicine, which might show up as a rash on your skin, swelling, itching, or trouble breathing.

Please tell your parent(s) and your doctor or nurse about any changes that you notice after taking the medicine. It is especially important to tell a responsible adult if you are feeling depressed or that you may not want to live; if you have thoughts of hurting yourself; or if you begin to feel more irritable, nervous, or restless. Also be sure to tell if you begin to feel "speeded up" or have trouble sleeping.

Some medicines make people feel sleepy or less coordinated. If this medicine is making you sleepy, it is very important not to drive a car or ride a bicycle or motorcycle. After starting a new medicine or increasing the dose of a medicine, please be extra careful when driving a car, riding a bike, or using machines until you can tell how the medicine affects your alertness, attention, and coordination.

One of the most common side effects of this medicine is feeling tired or sleepy during the day, even if you have had a full night's sleep. After you have been taking the medicine for a few weeks, your body will adjust, and this side effect may go away. If you have had trouble sleeping at night, the medicine can help you sleep better, especially if the doctor tells you to take a dose of medicine in the evening. Other people may feel more restless and excited. Tell your parent(s) or doctor if this is uncomfortable.

Another common side effect is dry mouth. You may be more thirsty than usual and find that you are drinking more water or other liquids. Sucking on sugar-free hard candy or cough drops usually helps. You also could try chewing sugar-free gum or sucking on ice chips. Do not chew the ice; you could hurt your teeth. Also, using lip balm will keep your lips from cracking. It is important to be especially good about brushing your teeth.

Sometimes people taking imipramine notice that their heart is beating a little faster than normal. Usually this happens within the first few weeks of taking the medicine and gets better or goes away. However, if you notice that your heart is beating very fast for more than a few minutes when you have not been exercising, if you feel light-headed or dizzy when you are sitting or standing still, or if you faint, you should let your parent(s) and doctor know right away. Some people feel dizzy or light-headed when standing up fast. If this happens, try to get up more slowly, especially first thing in the morning when getting out of bed.

Some people become constipated (have hard bowel movements). Try drinking more water and eating more fruits, vegetables, and whole grains. If that does not help, tell your parent(s) or doctor—you may need a medicine to help with this side effect.

Other side effects that could happen are acne, headache, blurred vision, not feeling hungry and not wanting to eat much, eating more than usual, having an upset stomach, changes in your bowel movements, or trouble passing urine. You may have a change in your sexual functioning or in your breasts—it is OK to ask the doctor about this. This medicine may make you more likely to get sick if you get overheated, so be sure to drink plenty of liquids and rest in the shade in hot weather.

Please let your parent(s) and doctor know if you notice anything different or unusual about how you feel once you start taking the medicine. This includes good things, such as feeling less sad or nervous or sleeping better at night.

Notes

Use this space to take notes or to write down questions you want to ask the doctor or nurse.

_____

_____

_____

_____

_____

_____

_____

_____

_____

_____

_____

_____

_____

_____

From Dulcan MK (editor): *Helping Parents, Youth, and Teachers Understand Medications for Behavioral and Emotional Problems: A Resource Book of Medication Information Handouts*, Third Edition. Washington, DC, American Psychiatric Publishing, 2007

Medication Information
for Parents and Teachers

Lamotrigine—Lamictal

General Information About Medication

Each child and adolescent is different. No one has exactly the same combination of medical and psychological problems. It is a good idea to talk with the doctor or nurse about the reasons a medicine is being used. It is very important to keep all appointments and to be in touch by telephone if you have concerns. It is important to communicate with the doctor, nurse, or therapist.

It is very important that the medicine be taken exactly as the doctor instructs. However, once in a while, everyone forgets to give a medicine on time. It is a good idea to ask the doctor or nurse what to do if this happens. Do not stop or change a medicine without asking the doctor or nurse first.

If the medicine seems to stop working, it may be because it is not being taken regularly. The youth may be "cheeking" or hiding the medicine or forgetting to take it (especially at school). The doses may be too far apart, or a different dose may be needed. Something at school, at home, or in the neighborhood may be upsetting the youth, or he or she may need special help for learning disabilities or tutoring. Please discuss your concerns with the doctor. **Do not just increase the dose.**

All medicines should be kept in a safe place, out of the reach of children, and should be supervised by an adult. If someone takes too much of a medicine, call the doctor, the poison control center, or a hospital emergency room.

Each medicine has a "generic" or chemical name. Just like laundry detergents or paper towels, some medicines are sold by more than one company under different brand names. The same medicine may be available under a generic name and several brand names. The generic medications are usually less expensive than the brand name ones. The generic medications have the same chemical formula, but they may or may not be exactly the same strength as the brand-name medications. Also, some brands of pills contain dye that can cause allergic reactions. It is a good idea to talk to the doctor and the pharmacist about whether it is important to use a specific brand of medicine.

All medicines can cause an allergic reaction. Examples are hives, itching, rashes, swelling, and trouble breathing. Even a tiny amount of a medicine can cause a reaction in patients who are allergic to that medicine. Be *sure* to talk to the doctor before restarting a medicine that has caused an allergic reaction.

Taking more than one medicine at the same time may cause more side effects or cause one of the medicines to not work as well. Always ask the doctor, nurse, or pharmacist before adding another medicine, whether prescription or over-the-counter. Be sure that each doctor knows about *all* of the medicines your child is taking. Also tell the doctor about any vitamins, herbal medicines, or supplements your child may be taking. Some of these may have side effects alone or when taken with this medication.

Everyone taking medicine should have a physical examination at least once a year.

If you suspect the youth is using drugs or alcohol, please tell the doctor right away.

Pregnancy requires special care in the use of medicine. Please tell the doctor immediately if you suspect the teenager is pregnant or might become pregnant.

Printed information like this applies to children and adolescents in general. If you have questions about the medicine, or if you notice changes or anything unusual, please ask the doctor or nurse. As scientific research advances, knowledge increases and advice changes. Even experts do not always agree. Many medicines have not been approved by the U.S. Food and Drug Administration (FDA) for use in children. For this reason, use of the medicine for a particular problem or age group often is not listed in the *Physicians' Desk Reference*. This does not necessarily mean that the medicine is dangerous or does not work, only that the company that makes the medicine has not received permission to advertise the medicine for use in children. Companies often do not apply for this permission because it is expensive to do the tests needed to apply for approval for use in children. Once a medication is approved by the FDA for any purpose, a doctor is allowed to prescribe it according to research and clinical experience.

Note to Teachers

It is a good idea to talk with the parent(s) about the reason(s) that a medication is being used. If the parent(s) sign consent to release information, it is often helpful to talk with the doctor. If the parent(s) give permission, the doctor may ask you to fill out rating forms about your experience with the student's behavior, feelings, academic performance, and medication side effects. This information is very useful in selecting and monitoring medication treatment. If you have observations that you think are important, do not hesitate to share these with the student's parent(s) and treating clinicians.

It is very important that the medicine be taken exactly as the doctor instructs. However, everyone forgets to give a medicine on time once in a while. It is a good idea to ask the parent(s) in advance what to do if this happens. Do not stop or change the time you are giving a medicine at school without parental permission. If a medication is to be taken with food, but lunchtime or snack time changes, be sure to notify the parent(s) so appropriate adjustments can be made.

All medicines should be kept in a secure place and should be supervised by an adult. If someone takes too much of a medicine, follow your school procedure for an urgent medical problem.

Taking medicine is a private matter and is best managed discreetly and confidentially. It is important to be sensitive to the student's feelings about taking medicine.

If you suspect that the student is using drugs or alcohol, please tell the parent(s) or a school counselor right away.

Please tell the parent(s) or school nurse if you suspect medication side effects.

Modifications of the classroom environment or assignments may be useful in addition to medication. The student may need to be evaluated for additional help or for an Individualized Education Plan for learning or behavior.

Any expression of suicidal thoughts or feelings or self-harm by a child or adolescent is a clear signal of distress and should be taken seriously. These behaviors should not be dismissed as "attention seeking."

What Is Lamotrigine (Lamictal)?

Lamotrigine was first used to treat seizures (fits, convulsions), so it is sometimes called an *anticonvulsant*. Now it is also used for behavioral problems or bipolar disorder (manic-depressive disorder), whether or not the patient has seizures. It also may be used when the patient has a history of severe mood changes, sometimes called *mood swings*. When used in psychiatry, this medicine is more commonly called a *mood stabilizer*.

Lamotrigine comes in brand name Lamictal tablets and chewable tablets.

376

How Can This Medicine Help?

Lamotrigine can reduce aggression, anger, and severe mood swings. It can treat mania or prevent bipolar depression.

How Does This Medicine Work?

Lamotrigine is thought to work by stabilizing a part of the brain cell (the cell membrane or envelope) and by changing the concentration of a *neurotransmitter* (brain chemical) called *glutamate*.

How Long Does This Medicine Last?

Lamotrigine needs to be taken twice a day.

How Will the Doctor Monitor This Medicine?

The doctor will review your child's medical history and physical examination before starting lamotrigine. The doctor may order some blood tests to be sure your child does not have a hidden medical condition that would make it unsafe to use this medicine. The doctor or nurse may measure your child's pulse and blood pressure before starting lamotrigine.

After the medicine is started, the doctor will want to have regular appointments with you and your child to see how the medicine is working, to see if a dose change is needed, to watch for side effects, to see if lamotrigine is still needed, and to see if any other treatment is needed. The doctor or nurse may check your child's height, weight, pulse, and blood pressure. Blood tests are not usually needed during treatment with lamotrigine.

What Side Effects Can This Medicine Have?

Any medicine can have side effects, including an allergy to the medicine. Because each patient is different, the doctor will monitor the youth closely, especially when the medicine is started. The doctor will work with you to increase the positive effects and decrease the negative effects of the medicine. Please tell the doctor if any of the listed side effects appear or if you think that the medicine is causing any other problems. Not all of the rare or unusual side effects are listed.

Side effects are most common after starting the medicine or after a dose increase. Many side effects can be avoided or lessened by starting with a very low dose and increasing it slowly—ask the doctor.

Allergic Reaction

Tell the doctor in a day or two (if possible, before the next dose of medicine):

- Hives
- Itching

  Stop the medicine and get *immediate* medical care:

- Rash
- Trouble breathing or chest tightness
- Swelling of lips, tongue, or throat

General Side Effects

These side effects are more common when first starting the medicine. Tell the doctor within a week or two:

- Daytime sleepiness—Do not allow your child to drive, ride a bicycle or motorcycle, or operate machinery if this happens.
- Dizziness
- Headache
- Blurred vision
- Double vision
- Unsteadiness
- Nausea, vomiting
- Stomach cramps

Behavioral and Emotional Side Effects

Call the doctor within a day or two:

- Anxiety or nervousness
- Agitation or mania
- Tics (motor movements or sounds), thinking unwanted words of phrases over and over

Possibly Dangerous Side Effects

Stop lamotrigine and go to an emergency room *immediately*:

- Vomiting
- Rash, especially when the rash is in the nose or mouth or there is also sore throat, fever, and/or generally feeling sick

Some Interactions With Other Medicines or Food

Please note that the following are only the most likely interactions with food or other medicines.

Caffeine may increase side effects.

Lamotrigine interacts with many other medicines. Taking it with another medicine may make one or both not work as well or may cause more side effects. Be sure that each doctor knows about *all* of the medicines your child is taking.

Valproate (Depakote, Depakene) increases the level of lamotrigine, which increases the risk of very serious skin reaction.

When lamotrigine and birth control pills are taken together, neither one works very well. This could increase the risk of pregnancy.

What Could Happen if This Medicine Is Stopped Suddenly?

Stopping lamotrigine suddenly may cause seizures or convulsions if your child is being treated for epilepsy (seizures).

How Long Will This Medicine Be Needed?

The length of time a person needs to take lamotrigine depends on what problem is being treated. For example, someone with an impulse control disorder usually takes the medicine only until behavioral therapy begins to work. Someone with bipolar disorder may need to take the medicine for many years. Please ask the doctor about the length of treatment needed.

What Else Should I Know About This Medicine?

Taking lamotrigine with food may decrease stomach upset.

The FDA has required a *black box warning* on lamotrigine because of the risk of an extreme skin reaction called *Stevens-Johnson syndrome*, a serious and potentially life-threatening condition. The risk is higher in children than in adults. This very serious blistering of skin and mucous membranes is more likely when lamotrigine is combined with valproate (Depakene or Depakote). Most rashes go away if the lamotrigine is stopped, but all rashes should be seen by a doctor. Some ways that the risk of serious reaction might be decreased include

- Increasing the dose of lamotrigine very slowly
- Avoiding other new medicines in the first 2 months of treatment with lamotrigine
- Avoiding new foods, cosmetics, deodorants, or clothes detergents or fabric softeners in the first 2 months of taking lamotrigine
- Not starting lamotrigine within 2 weeks of a rash, viral illness, or vaccination
- Avoiding sunburn
- Avoiding exposure to poison ivy or poison oak

Keep the medicine in a safe place under close supervision. Keep the pill container tightly closed and in a dry place, away from bathrooms, showers, and humidifiers.

Notes

Use this space to take notes or to write down questions you want to ask the doctor.

_____

_____

_____

_____

_____

_____

_____

_____

_____

_____

_____

_____

From Dulcan MK (editor): _Helping Parents, Youth, and Teachers Understand Medications for Behavioral and Emotional Problems: A Resource Book of Medication Information Handouts,_ Third Edition. Washington, DC, American Psychiatric Publishing, 2007

Medication Information for Youth

Lamotrigine—Lamictal

What the Medicine Is Called and What It Is For

The name of your medicine may be confusing. Most drugs have two names: 1) a scientific name that we call a *generic name* and 2) a trade or *brand name*. The generic name of this medicine is lamotrigine. The brand name is Lamictal.

Lamotrigine was first used to help people with epilepsy (seizures, fits, convulsions), so it is sometimes called an *anticonvulsant*. It is now also called a *mood stabilizer*, because it is used to help people who have severe mood changes, sometimes called *mood swings*, especially in children and adolescents with bipolar disorder (manic-depressive disorder), depression, or trouble controlling anger. Lamotrigine can reduce aggression, anger, and severe mood swings. It can treat mania or prevent relapse (mania coming back). It is thought to work by making brain cells less excitable.

How You Take the Medicine

It is very important to take the medicine exactly as the doctor or nurse tells you. Do not skip doses or take extra medicine without asking an adult. If you forget a dose, ask your parent(s) what to do.

This medicine is prescribed only for you. It should never be shared with anyone else.

You do not have to tell others that you are taking this medicine, but it is not something you should feel ashamed or embarrassed about. Many young people are helped by lamotrigine. This medicine is not habit-forming, and you cannot become "hooked" on it. You should talk to your doctor or nurse about any questions you have about the medicine. It is important to remember that the medicine *helps* you. It cannot *make* you do anything or change you as a person.

If your stomach is upset, taking the medicine with food may help.

Caffeine (in coffee, tea, or soft drinks) may make you feel worse.

It is very important not to stop this medicine suddenly—it could be uncomfortable or even dangerous.

When lamotrigine and birth control pills are taken together, neither one works very well. This could increase the risk of pregnancy.

Until you get used to the medicine, it is best to avoid new foods, skin products, or deodorants and to stay out of the sun.

How Your Doctor Will Follow Your Progress

Before starting lamotrigine, your doctor or nurse will talk with you and your parent(s) and may measure your height, weight, heart rate (pulse), and blood pressure. The doctor may order blood tests to be sure you are healthy before taking the medicine.

Be sure to tell your doctor or nurse about any other medicines or supplements you are taking, including vitamins, herbs, or aids to weight loss or bodybuilding. Also be sure to tell the doctor or nurse if you are using alcohol or drugs. Because many medicines may affect babies, it is very important to tell the doctor if you might be pregnant or if you are at risk of becoming pregnant.

Your teachers may be asked to fill out a form about your grades and behavior in school. A psychologist may give you some tests to see how you learn best.

Most doctors have regular appointments with young people who are taking medicine. You should use these visits to share any concerns you may have about your medicine and to talk about if it has helped you. From time to time, your physician or nurse may measure your height, weight, heart rate (pulse), and blood pressure to be sure that you are in good health while you are taking the medicine. Your doctor also will ask for regular reports from your parents and maybe from your teachers (with your permission) to see how well the medicine is working.

How the Medicine Might Affect You

In addition to the ways the medicine can help you, it may have other effects called *side effects*. Different medicines have different side effects. It is helpful to know about some of the most common side effects of your medicine so that you will understand what they are if they happen. Some people do not have any side effects. Some side effects are just uncomfortable, but others may mean a more serious problem with the medicine. Side effects are most common after starting the medicine or after a dose increase. They may go away with time, or the medicine can be adjusted or changed—ask the doctor.

You could have an allergy to any medicine, which might show up as a rash on your skin, swelling, itching, or trouble breathing.

Please tell your parent(s) and your doctor or nurse about any changes that you notice after taking the medicine. It is especially important to tell a responsible adult if you are feeling depressed or that you may not want to live; if you have thoughts of hurting yourself; or if you begin to feel more irritable, nervous, or restless. Also be sure to tell if you begin to feel more "speeded up" or have trouble sleeping.

Some medicines make people feel sleepy or less coordinated. If this medicine is making you sleepy, it is very important not to drive a car or ride a bicycle or motorcycle. After starting a new medicine or increasing the dose of a medicine, please be extra careful when driving a car, riding a bike, or using machines until you can tell how the medicine affects your alertness, attention, and coordination.

The most common side effects of lamotrigine are dizziness, daytime sleepiness, and feeling tired. Less common side effects are problems with paying attention, feeling irritable or angry, clumsiness, headache, stomachache, nausea, and double or blurred vision. These sometimes go away after you have been taking the medicine for a while or if the doctor lowers the dose of medicine you are taking. Tell your parent(s) or the doctor if you are having trouble with any of these side effects.

It is very important to tell your parent(s) or doctor **right away** if you notice a rash in your nose or mouth, a sore throat, or fever or if you feel sick or throw up.

Rarely, people taking lamotrigine have repeated muscle movements, make sounds, or have repeated unwanted thoughts. Tell your parent(s) and doctor if this happens.

Notes

Use this space to take notes or to write down questions you want to ask the doctor or nurse.

_____

_____

_____

_____

_____

_____

_____

_____

_____

_____

_____

_____

Medication Information for Parents and Teachers

Lithium—Eskalith, Lithobid

General Information About Medication

Each child and adolescent is different. No one has exactly the same combination of medical and psychological problems. It is a good idea to talk with the doctor or nurse about the reasons a medicine is being used. It is very important to keep all appointments and to be in touch by telephone if you have concerns. It is important to communicate with the doctor, nurse, or therapist.

It is very important that the medicine be taken exactly as the doctor instructs. However, once in a while, everyone forgets to give a medicine on time. It is a good idea to ask the doctor or nurse what to do if this happens. Do not stop or change a medicine without asking the doctor or nurse first.

If the medicine seems to stop working, it may be because it is not being taken regularly. The youth may be "cheeking" or hiding the medicine or forgetting to take it (especially at school). The doses may be too far apart, or a different dose may be needed. Something at school, at home, or in the neighborhood may be upsetting the youth, or he or she may need special help for learning disabilities or tutoring. Please discuss your concerns with the doctor. **Do not just increase the dose.**

All medicines should be kept in a safe place, out of the reach of children, and should be supervised by an adult. If someone takes too much of a medicine, call the doctor, the poison control center, or a hospital emergency room.

Each medicine has a "generic" or chemical name. Just like laundry detergents or paper towels, some medicines are sold by more than one company under different brand names. The same medicine may be available under a generic name and several brand names. The generic medications are usually less expensive than the brand name ones. The generic medications have the same chemical formula, but they may or may not be exactly the same strength as the brand-name medications. Also, some brands of pills contain dye that can cause allergic reactions. It is a good idea to talk to the doctor and the pharmacist about whether it is important to use a specific brand of medicine.

All medicines can cause an allergic reaction. Examples are hives, itching, rashes, swelling, and trouble breathing. Even a tiny amount of a medicine can cause a reaction in patients who are allergic to that medicine. Be *sure* to talk to the doctor before restarting a medicine that has caused an allergic reaction.

Taking more than one medicine at the same time may cause more side effects or cause one of the medicines to not work as well. Always ask the doctor, nurse, or pharmacist before adding another medicine, whether prescription or over-the-counter. Be sure that each doctor knows about *all* of the medicines your child is taking. Also tell the doctor about any vitamins, herbal medicines, or supplements your child may be taking. Some of these may have side effects alone or when taken with this medication.

Everyone taking medicine should have a physical examination at least once a year.

If you suspect the youth is using drugs or alcohol, please tell the doctor right away.

Pregnancy requires special care in the use of medicine. Please tell the doctor immediately if you suspect the teenager is pregnant or might become pregnant.

385

Printed information like this applies to children and adolescents in general. If you have questions about the medicine, or if you notice changes or anything unusual, please ask the doctor or nurse. As scientific research advances, knowledge increases and advice changes. Even experts do not always agree. Many medicines have not been approved by the U.S. Food and Drug Administration (FDA) for use in children. For this reason, use of the medicine for a particular problem or age group often is not listed in the *Physicians' Desk Reference*. This does not necessarily mean that the medicine is dangerous or does not work, only that the company that makes the medicine has not received permission to advertise the medicine for use in children. Companies often do not apply for this permission because it is expensive to do the tests needed to apply for approval for use in children. Once a medication is approved by the FDA for any purpose, a doctor is allowed to prescribe it according to research and clinical experience.

Note to Teachers

It is a good idea to talk with the parent(s) about the reason(s) that a medication is being used. If the parent(s) sign consent to release information, it is often helpful to talk with the doctor. If the parent(s) give permission, the doctor may ask you to fill out rating forms about your experience with the student's behavior, feelings, academic performance, and medication side effects. This information is very useful in selecting and monitoring medication treatment. If you have observations that you think are important, do not hesitate to share these with the student's parent(s) and treating clinicians.

It is very important that the medicine be taken exactly as the doctor instructs. However, everyone forgets to give a medicine on time once in a while. It is a good idea to ask the parent(s) in advance what to do if this happens. Do not stop or change the time you are giving a medicine at school without parental permission. If a medication is to be taken with food, but lunchtime or snack time changes, be sure to notify the parent(s) so appropriate adjustments can be made.

You may notice the following side effects at school:

Common Side Effects

The following side effects often go away after 2 weeks or so:

- Weight gain
- Stomachache
- Diarrhea
- Nausea, vomiting—The student may need to take the medicine after a meal or snack to decrease nausea.
- Increased thirst—Allow the student to make extra trips to the water fountain or carry a water bottle.
- Increased frequency of urination—The student may need to go to the bathroom more often.
- Shakiness of hands, tremor—You may notice the student's handwriting getting worse.
- Tiredness, weakness
- Headache
- Dizziness (when standing up quickly—This may happen in the classroom or during physical education). Suggest that the student stand up slowly.

Occasional Side Effects

- Low thyroid function or goiter (enlarged thyroid)—You may notice that the student is tired, feels cold, gains weight, has coarsening of hair, or does less well academically.

386

- Acne
- Skin rash
- Hair loss
- Irritability

Signs That the Lithium Level May Be Too High—Early Symptoms of Lithium Toxicity

If the student has any of these signs, tell the parent(s) or school nurse immediately:

- Vomiting or diarrhea
- Trembling that is worse than usual or very severe
- Weakness
- Lack of coordination
- Unsteadiness when standing or walking
- Extreme sleepiness or tiredness
- Severe dizziness
- Trouble speaking or slurred speech
- Confusion

Serious (Toxic) Effects of Too Much Lithium—Dangerous Lithium Toxicity

Use your school procedure for a medical emergency if the student experiences any of the following side effects:

- Irregular heartbeat
- Fainting
- Staggering
- Blurred vision
- Ringing or buzzing sound in the ears
- Inability to urinate
- Muscle twitches
- High fever
- Seizure (fit, convulsion)
- Unconsciousness

Overdosing with lithium may cause death. Be sure the lithium bottle is in a secure place and medication is taken under supervision.

All medicines should be kept in a secure place and should be supervised by an adult. If someone takes too much of a medicine, follow your school procedure for an urgent medical problem.

Taking medicine is a private matter and is best managed discreetly and confidentially. It is important to be sensitive to the student's feelings about taking medicine.

If you suspect that the student is using drugs or alcohol, please tell the parent(s) or a school counselor right away.

Please tell the parent(s) or school nurse if you suspect medication side effects.

Modifications of the classroom environment or assignments may be useful in addition to medication. The student may need to be evaluated for additional help or for an Individualized Education Plan for learning or behavior.

Any expression of suicidal thoughts or feelings or self-harm by a child or adolescent is a clear signal of distress and should be taken seriously. These behaviors should not be dismissed as "attention seeking."

What Is Lithium (Eskalith, Lithobid)?

Lithium is a naturally occurring salt similar to sodium. Lithium is available in the following forms:

Name	Form
Generic	Lithium carbonate tablets and capsules
Eskalith	Lithium carbonate capsules
Generic*	Slow-release lithium carbonate tablets
Lithobid*	Slow-release lithium carbonate tablets
Eskalith CR*	Controlled-release (long-acting) lithium carbonate tablets
Generic liquid	Lithium citrate syrup

*Do not cut or crush; must be swallowed whole.

How Can This Medicine Help?

Lithium can decrease mood swings. It can reduce fighting or destroying of property. Lithium may be prescribed for bipolar disorder (also known as manic depression), certain types of depression, severe mood swings, or very serious aggression.

How Does This Medicine Work?

Lithium acts by stabilizing nerve cells in the brain. This action works in different ways depending on the problem that is being treated. For children with bipolar disorder, it works by reducing mood swings. In adults with bipolar disorder (manic-depressive disorder), it has been shown to help prevent mania relapse and to reduce depression.

For children and adolescents with depression whose symptoms have not responded to treatment with an antidepressant used alone, lithium can help the antidepressant work better.

For children with explosive aggression caused by rage, lithium works by "turning down" the rage and decreasing the impulsivity. The youth then has time to figure out more constructive ways to deal with his or her rage.

How Long Does This Medicine Last?

Lithium must be taken three or four times a day, except the slow-release forms, which may be taken once or twice a day.

How Will the Doctor Monitor This Medicine?

The doctor will review your child's medical history and physical examination before starting lithium. The doctor may order some blood or urine tests to be sure your child does not have a hidden medical condition that would make it unsafe to use this medicine. Be sure to tell the doctor if your child or anyone in the family has a history of kidney or thyroid problems or diabetes. The doctor or nurse may measure your child's height, weight, pulse, and blood pressure before starting the medicine. The doctor may order other tests, such as an ECG (electrocardiogram or heart rhythm test) and an EEG (electroencephalogram or brain wave test).

After lithium is started, the doctor will want to have regular appointments with you and your child to see how the medicine is working, to see if a dose change is needed, to watch for side effects, to see if lithium is still needed, and to see if any other treatment is needed. The doctor will need to do blood tests (to check lithium levels) regularly to make sure that the medicine is at the right dose. These tests may be done once or twice a week at first and then once every month or two after the dose is set. Blood should be drawn first thing in the morning, 10–12 hours after the evening dose and before the morning dose. The doctor also will perform blood and urine tests regularly to check for kidney or thyroid side effects. The doctor or nurse may check your child's height, weight, pulse, and blood pressure.

What Side Effects Can This Medicine Have?

Any medicine can have side effects, including an allergy to the medicine. Because each patient is different, the doctor will monitor the youth closely, especially when the medicine is started. The doctor will work with you to increase the positive effects and decrease the negative effects of the medicine. Please tell the doctor if any of the listed side effects appear or if you think that the medicine is causing any other problems. Not all of the rare or unusual side effects are listed.

Side effects are most common after starting the medicine or after a dose increase. Many side effects can be avoided or lessened by starting with a very low dose and increasing it slowly—ask the doctor.

Allergic Reaction

Tell the doctor in a day or two (if possible, before the next dose of medicine):

- Hives
- Itching
- Rash

  Stop the medicine and get *immediate* medical care:

- Trouble breathing or chest tightness
- Swelling of lips, tongue, or throat

Lithium should be taken with food to decrease side effects. Make sure that your child drinks plenty of water when taking lithium to prevent dehydration and lithium toxicity. If side effects appear, give your child one or two glasses of water.

Common Side Effects

The following side effects often go away after 2 weeks or so. If they are troublesome, ask the doctor about lowering the dose.

- Weight gain
- Stomachache
- Diarrhea
- Nausea, vomiting
- Increased thirst
- Increased frequency of urination
- Shakiness of hands (tremor)—Another medication, such as Inderal, may be added.
- Tiredness, weakness
- Headache
- Dizziness

Occasional Side Effects

Tell the doctor within a week or two:

- Tiredness, feeling cold, weight gain, dry skin, coarser hair, or decreased school performance—These could be signs of low thyroid function.
- A lump on the front of the neck—This could be a sign of enlarged thyroid gland (goiter).
- New or worse acne or psoriasis
- Hair loss
- Bed-wetting
- Metallic taste in the mouth
- Irritability

Signs That the Lithium Level May Be Too High— Early Symptoms of Lithium Toxicity

Call the doctor *immediately* and do not give lithium for at least 24 hours:

- Vomiting or diarrhea more than once
- Trembling that is worse than usual or very severe
- Weakness
- Lack of coordination
- Unsteadiness when standing or walking
- Extreme sleepiness or tiredness
- Severe dizziness
- Trouble speaking or slurred speech
- Confusion

Serious (Toxic) Effects of Too Much Lithium—Dangerous Lithium Toxicity

If your child has any of the following, go to the doctor's office or to an emergency room *immediately!*

- Irregular heartbeat
- Fainting
- Staggering
- Blurred vision
- Ringing or buzzing sound in the ears
- Inability to urinate
- Muscle twitches
- High fever
- Seizure (fit, convulsion)
- Unconsciousness

Overdosing with lithium may cause death. You must closely supervise the medicine. You should lock up the medicine if your child or teenager is suicidal or if a young child lives in or visits your home.

Some Interactions With Other Medicines or Food

Please note that the following are only the most likely interactions with food or other medicines.

Soft drinks with caffeine may make side effects worse.

Some anti-inflammatory medicines can increase lithium levels and make side effects worse. Examples are listed in the table below.

Brand name	Generic name
Advil, Motrin	Ibuprofen
Indocin	Indomethacin
Aleve, Anaprox, Naprosyn	Naproxen

Taking lithium with theophylline may decrease lithium levels so that it does not work as well. Certain diuretics such as hydrochlorothiazide can increase lithium levels.

What Could Happen if This Medicine Is Stopped Suddenly?

There are no medical withdrawal effects if lithium is stopped suddenly. However, the problem being treated is likely to come back. If lithium is stopped suddenly, some patients with bipolar disorder may become manic more often and may be more difficult to treat. If your child has been taking lithium for 6–8 weeks or longer, the dose should be decreased gradually (tapered) over 8–16 weeks before stopping it to prevent this effect. Always check with your child's doctor before stopping a medicine.

How Long Will This Medicine Be Needed?

How long your child will need to take lithium depends on the reason that it was prescribed. For children and adolescents with bipolar disorder, lithium is often prescribed for 2 years or longer. Depending on how many times your child has had depression or mania, he or she may need to take the medicine for many years. Some patients require lithium for their entire lives to function normally.

For children and adolescents with severe depression who need lithium plus an antidepressant, lithium is usually needed for at least 5–6 months after the child's mood returns to normal. This is necessary to prevent the depression from coming back.

For rage, lithium must be continued for several months to years until the patient, his or her family, and the doctor can find different ways to control the rage. The rage usually becomes more controllable as the child grows, becomes more mature, and develops more effective problem-solving and coping skills. Another medicine also may help.

What Else Should I Know About This Medicine?

Store the medicine at room temperature, away from moisture.

Make sure your child drinks plenty of water, especially in hot weather and when exercising. Avoid extremes of salt intake; large amounts of salty foods or a salt-free diet can make the lithium level too low or too high.

Tell the doctor if the pharmacy changes the brand of lithium—extra blood tests of the lithium level may be needed.

When lithium causes increased thirst, young people may drink large amounts of soft drinks. Drinking soft drinks is not a good idea because it can lead to weight gain (from sugar) or nervousness (from caffeine). Drinking water, fruit juice mixed with water, or salt-free seltzer is fine. Your child may need a note to permit frequent trips to the water fountain and bathroom at school.

Stop the lithium and call the doctor if your child develops an illness with vomiting, diarrhea, fever, or loss of appetite. Talk with the doctor if your child wants to diet to lose weight.

Lithium levels may change with the menstrual cycle. If you suspect that this is happening, keep a log or diary and discuss it with the doctor.

Lithium should not be taken during pregnancy because it can cause birth defects. If there is any chance of your teenager becoming pregnant, please talk with the doctor about this concern.

Notes

Use this space to take notes or to write down questions you want to ask the doctor.

_____

_____

_____

_____

_____

_____

_____

_____

_____

_____

_____

_____

_____

From Dulcan MK (editor): _Helping Parents, Youth, and Teachers Understand Medications for Behavioral and Emotional Problems: A Resource Book of Medication Information Handouts,_ Third Edition. Washington, DC, American Psychiatric Publishing, 2007

Medication Information for Youth

Lithium—Eskalith, Lithobid

What the Medicine Is Called and What It Is For

The name of your medicine may be confusing. Most drugs have two names: 1) a scientific name that we call a *generic name* and 2) a trade or *brand name*. The generic name of this medicine is lithium. The brand names are Eskalith and Lithobid.

Lithium is most often used for people who have bipolar disorder (also called *manic-depressive disorder* or *mood swings*). Lithium is a natural salt that can help steady a person's mood—that is, help the person have fewer big ups and downs. When used alone or with another medicine, lithium can treat mania and depression and may help keep mood steady. It also can help children and teenagers who have problems controlling their anger or impulsive behavior (acting before thinking).

How You Take the Medicine

It is very important that you take all the pills that you are supposed to take each day. Do not skip doses or take extra medicine without asking an adult. Your doctor will probably recommend that you take your medicine at the same time(s) each day, which may be with meals or at bedtime. If you forget a dose, ask your parent(s) what to do.

It usually takes some time for the positive effects of lithium to be noticed. The medicine may not take full effect until several weeks after you start taking it. You may feel discouraged and think the medicine is never going to help. You may want to give up and stop taking the medicine. Talk to your doctor and parent(s) about how you feel, but **do not stop** taking your medicine unless your doctor tells you to. It is also important not to take extra pills hoping that you will feel better faster. Doing that could make you very sick.

Do not chew or crush the long-acting forms of lithium—swallow them whole.

Caffeine (in coffee, tea, or soft drinks) may make you feel worse.

Do not use any other medicines without talking to your doctor first. Even over-the-counter pain medicine like Advil or Aleve can make the side effects of lithium worse.

Do not use alcohol, marijuana, or street drugs while taking these pills. They can cause serious side effects. Skipping your medicine to take drugs does not work because many medicines stay in your body for a long time.

This medicine is prescribed only for you. It should never be shared with anyone else.

You do not have to tell others that you are taking this medicine, but it is not something you should feel ashamed or embarrassed about. Many young people are helped by lithium. This medicine is not habit-forming, and you cannot become "hooked" on it. You should talk to your doctor or nurse about any questions you have about the medicine. It is important to remember that the medicine *helps* you. It cannot *make* you do anything or change you as a person.

How Your Doctor Will Follow Your Progress

Before giving you the medicine, your doctor or nurse will talk with you and your parent(s) and will measure your height, weight, heart rate (pulse), and blood pressure.

Be sure to tell your doctor or nurse about any other medicines or supplements you are taking, including vitamins, herbs, or aids to weight loss or bodybuilding. Also be sure to tell the doctor or nurse if you are using alcohol or drugs. Because lithium can cause birth defects in babies, it is very important to tell the doctor if you might be pregnant or if you are at risk of becoming pregnant.

Blood and urine tests are needed before starting this medicine so the doctor can be sure you are in good health. Do not be surprised when the nurse or lab technician asks you to urinate (pee) in a plastic cup. You may also need to have a test called an ECG (electrocardiogram or heart rhythm test). This test counts your heartbeats through small wires that are taped to your chest. It takes only about 15 minutes. You also may need to take a test called an EEG (electroencephalogram or brain wave test). This test uses wires taped to your head to chart your brain waves. It does not tell anything about what you are thinking or feeling. It takes about an hour. Neither test hurts.

Your teachers may be asked to fill out a form about your grades and behavior in school. A psychologist may give you some tests to see how you learn best.

You will probably begin your medicine by taking only one pill once or twice a day. Your medicine will need to be increased until your doctor decides that you are taking the right amount. How much lithium is in your body must be measured to help your doctor determine how many pills you need to take each day and to make sure you have the right amount of medicine in your body. This is called getting a *lithium level*. You will need to have blood tests regularly while you are taking this medicine, usually first thing in the morning before your morning dose of medicine.

If the medicine helps you, your doctor will decide how long you will need to take it as he or she follows your progress.

Most doctors have regular appointments with young people who are taking medicine. You should use these visits to share any concerns you may have about your medicine and to talk about if it has helped you. From time to time, your physician or nurse will measure your height, weight, heart rate (pulse), and blood pressure to be sure that you are in good health while you are taking the medicine. There will be other blood and urine tests to check your lithium level and to be sure that you stay in good health. Your doctor also will ask for regular reports from your parents and maybe from your teachers (with your permission) to see how well the medicine is working.

How the Medicine Might Affect You

In addition to the ways the medicine can help you, it may have other effects called *side effects*. Different medicines have different side effects. It is helpful to know about some of the most common side effects of your medicine so that you will understand what they are if they happen. Some people do not have any side effects. Some side effects are just uncomfortable, but others may mean a more serious problem with the medicine. Side effects are most common after starting the medicine or after a dose increase. They may go away with time, or the medicine can be adjusted or changed—ask the doctor.

You could have an allergy to any medicine, which might show up as a rash on your skin, swelling, itching, or trouble breathing.

Please tell your parent(s) and your doctor or nurse about any changes that you notice after taking the medicine. It is especially important to tell a responsible adult if you are feeling depressed or that you may not want to live; if you have thoughts of hurting yourself; or if you begin to feel more irritable, nervous, or restless. Also be sure to tell your parent(s) or doctor if you begin to feel more "speeded up" or have more trouble sleeping.

Some medicines make people feel sleepy or less coordinated. If this medicine is making you sleepy, it is very important not to drive a car or ride a bicycle or motorcycle. After starting a new medicine or increasing the dose of a medicine, please be extra careful when driving a car, riding a bike, or using machines until you can tell how the medicine affects your alertness, attention, and coordination.

Many people notice a slight shaking of their hands after they start taking lithium. This shaking is called a *tremor*. Often, the tremor goes away in a few weeks, but sometimes it continues. For some students, their handwriting becomes hard to read. Your parent(s) or doctor can explain this to your teacher. Your doctor may lower the dose of your medicine, change your medicine, or add another medicine (such as Inderal) if this side effect is a big problem for you.

Another common side effect of lithium that can be bothersome is increased thirst and urination. This can be a problem in school if teachers do not like students to leave the classroom to get a drink of water or to go to the bathroom. Talk this over with your parent(s) and doctor so that they can work with your teacher if this becomes a problem. When you get thirsty, drink water or diluted fruit juice. Too many soft drinks can make you gain weight or make the tremor worse. Stay away from very salty foods because they can change your lithium level. It is important to drink plenty of water each day, especially in hot weather.

Some people taking lithium get an upset stomach and diarrhea. Taking the medicine with food or milk can help avoid this problem. Some people gain weight. A skin rash or acne may develop or get worse. Tell your doctor if any of these problems happen so that he or she can talk with you about them and possibly make changes in your medicine that will lessen or stop the problem

Some people get headaches or a bad taste in the mouth while taking lithium.

Too much medicine in your system (toxicity) can make you feel very sick. You may become confused, feel shaky, and have an upset stomach. Toxicity can happen if you take too much medicine or if you do not have enough fluid in your body, which can come from not drinking enough water, sweating a lot, or being sick with vomiting and diarrhea. It is very important to tell your parents and doctor **right away** if this happens to you.

Tell your parent(s) or doctor if you feel much more tired than usual, if you feel cold more than other people do, or if you notice changes in your skin or hair or a lump on the front of your neck.

You should tell your parent(s) and doctor if you notice anything different or unusual about how you feel once you start taking the medicine. This includes good things, such as feeling less confused, less sad, less "hyper," and less angry or sleeping better at night.

Notes

Use this space to take notes or to write down questions you want to ask the doctor or nurse.

_____

_____

_____

_____

_____

_____

_____

_____

_____

_____

_____

_____

_____

From Dulcan MK (editor): _Helping Parents, Youth, and Teachers Understand Medications for Behavioral and Emotional Problems: A Resource Book of Medication Information Handouts,_ Third Edition. Washington, DC, American Psychiatric Publishing, 2007

Medication Information for Parents and Teachers

Lorazepam—Ativan

General Information About Medication

Each child and adolescent is different. No one has exactly the same combination of medical and psychological problems. It is a good idea to talk with the doctor or nurse about the reasons a medicine is being used. It is very important to keep all appointments and to be in touch by telephone if you have concerns. It is important to communicate with the doctor, nurse, or therapist.

It is very important that the medicine be taken exactly as the doctor instructs. However, once in a while, everyone forgets to give a medicine on time. It is a good idea to ask the doctor or nurse what to do if this happens. Do not stop or change a medicine without asking the doctor or nurse first.

If the medicine seems to stop working, it may be because it is not being taken regularly. The youth may be "cheeking" or hiding the medicine or forgetting to take it (especially at school). The doses may be too far apart, or a different dose may be needed. Something at school, at home, or in the neighborhood may be upsetting the youth, or he or she may need special help for learning disabilities or tutoring. Please discuss your concerns with the doctor. **Do not just increase the dose.**

All medicines should be kept in a safe place, out of the reach of children, and should be supervised by an adult. If someone takes too much of a medicine, call the doctor, the poison control center, or a hospital emergency room.

Each medicine has a "generic" or chemical name. Just like laundry detergents or paper towels, some medicines are sold by more than one company under different brand names. The same medicine may be available under a generic name and several brand names. The generic medications are usually less expensive than the brand name ones. The generic medications have the same chemical formula, but they may or may not be exactly the same strength as the brand-name medications. Also, some brands of pills contain dye that can cause allergic reactions. It is a good idea to talk to the doctor and the pharmacist about whether it is important to use a specific brand of medicine.

All medicines can cause an allergic reaction. Examples are hives, itching, rashes, swelling, and trouble breathing. Even a tiny amount of a medicine can cause a reaction in patients who are allergic to that medicine. Be *sure* to talk to the doctor before restarting a medicine that has caused an allergic reaction.

Taking more than one medicine at the same time may cause more side effects or cause one of the medicines to not work as well. Always ask the doctor, nurse, or pharmacist before adding another medicine, whether prescription or over-the-counter. Be sure that each doctor knows about *all* of the medicines your child is taking. Also tell the doctor about any vitamins, herbal medicines, or supplements your child may be taking. Some of these may have side effects alone or when taken with this medication.

Everyone taking medicine should have a physical examination at least once a year.

If you suspect the youth is using drugs or alcohol, please tell the doctor right away.

399

Pregnancy requires special care in the use of medicine. Please tell the doctor immediately if you suspect the teenager is pregnant or might become pregnant.

Printed information like this applies to children and adolescents in general. If you have questions about the medicine, or if you notice changes or anything unusual, please ask the doctor or nurse. As scientific research advances, knowledge increases and advice changes. Even experts do not always agree. Many medicines have not been approved by the U.S. Food and Drug Administration (FDA) for use in children. For this reason, use of the medicine for a particular problem or age group often is not listed in the *Physicians' Desk Reference*. This does not necessarily mean that the medicine is dangerous or does not work, only that the company that makes the medicine has not received permission to advertise the medicine for use in children. Companies often do not apply for this permission because it is expensive to do the tests needed to apply for approval for use in children. Once a medication is approved by the FDA for any purpose, a doctor is allowed to prescribe it according to research and clinical experience.

Note to Teachers

It is a good idea to talk with the parent(s) about the reason(s) that a medication is being used. If the parent(s) sign consent to release information, it is often helpful to talk with the doctor. If the parent(s) give permission, the doctor may ask you to fill out rating forms about your experience with the student's behavior, feelings, academic performance, and medication side effects. This information is very useful in selecting and monitoring medication treatment. If you have observations that you think are important, do not hesitate to share these with the student's parent(s) and treating clinicians.

It is very important that the medicine be taken exactly as the doctor instructs. However, everyone forgets to give a medicine on time once in a while. It is a good idea to ask the parent(s) in advance what to do if this happens. Do not stop or change the time you are giving a medicine at school without parental permission. If a medication is to be taken with food, but lunchtime or snack time changes, be sure to notify the parent(s) so appropriate adjustments can be made.

All medicines should be kept in a secure place and should be supervised by an adult. If someone takes too much of a medicine, follow your school procedure for an urgent medical problem.

Taking medicine is a private matter and is best managed discreetly and confidentially. It is important to be sensitive to the student's feelings about taking medicine.

If you suspect that the student is using drugs or alcohol, please tell the parent(s) or a school counselor right away.

Please tell the parent(s) or school nurse if you suspect medication side effects.

Modifications of the classroom environment or assignments may be useful in addition to medication. The student may need to be evaluated for additional help or for an Individualized Education Plan for learning or behavior.

Any expression of suicidal thoughts or feelings or self-harm by a child or adolescent is a clear signal of distress and should be taken seriously. These behaviors should not be dismissed as "attention seeking."

What Is Lorazepam (Ativan)?

Lorazepam is a *benzodiazepine* or *antianxiety* medicine. It used to be called a *minor tranquilizer*. It is sometimes called an *anxiolytic* or *sedative*. It comes in brand name Ativan and generic tablets, liquid, and injection (a shot).

How Can This Medicine Help?

Lorazepam can decrease anxiety, nervousness, fears, and excessive worrying. It can help anxious people to be calm enough to learn—with therapy and practice (exposure to feared things or situations)—to understand and tolerate their worries or fears and even to overcome them. People with generalized anxiety disorder, social phobia, posttraumatic stress disorder (PTSD), or panic disorder can be helped by lorazepam. Most often, it is used for a short time when symptoms are very uncomfortable or frightening or when they make it hard to do important things such as go to school. Lorazepam can decrease the severe physical symptoms (rapid heartbeat, trouble breathing, dizziness, sweating) of panic attacks and phobias.

Lorazepam also can be used for sleep problems, such as night terrors (sudden waking up from sleep with great fear) or sleepwalking, when these problems put the youth at risk of an accident or make it impossible for other family members to get enough sleep. Lorazepam can help with insomnia (difficulty falling asleep) when used for a short time along with a behavioral program, such as regular soothing routines at bedtime and increased exercise in the daytime.

Sometimes lorazepam is used for a few days to treat agitation in mania or psychosis until other medicines start to work.

Lorazepam can be used to treat seizures (epilepsy).

Occasionally the benzodiazepines are used to reduce the side effects of other medicines.

How Does This Medicine Work?

Lorazepam works by calming the parts of the brain that are too excitable in anxious people. The medicine does this by working on *receptors* (special places on brain cells) in certain parts of the brain to change the action of *GABA*, a *neurotransmitter*—a chemical that the brain makes for brain cells to communicate with each other.

How Long Does This Medicine Last?

Lorazepam usually needs to be taken three times a day. For acute symptoms of anxiety or agitation, it can be taken occasionally, as needed. When used for sleep, it is taken at bedtime. There may still be some effects in the morning.

How Will the Doctor Monitor This Medicine?

The doctor will review your child's medical history and physical examination before starting lorazepam. The doctor may order some blood or urine tests or an ECG (electrocardiogram or heart rhythm test) to be sure your child does not have a hidden medical condition. The doctor or nurse may measure your child's height, weight, pulse, and blood pressure before starting lorazepam.

After the medicine is started, the doctor will want to have regular appointments with you and your child to see how the medicine is working, to see if a dose change is needed, to watch for side effects, to see if lorazepam is still needed, and to see if any other treatment is needed. The doctor or nurse may check your child's height, weight, pulse, and blood pressure.

What Side Effects Can This Medicine Have?

Any medicine can have side effects, including an allergy to the medicine. Because each patient is different, the doctor will monitor the youth closely, especially when the medicine is started. The doctor will work with you to increase the positive effects and decrease the negative effects of the medicine. Please tell the doctor if any of the listed side effects appear or if you think that the medicine is causing any other problems. Not all of the rare or unusual side effects are listed.

Side effects are most common after starting the medicine or after a dose increase. Many side effects can be avoided or lessened by starting with a very low dose and increasing it slowly—ask the doctor.

Allergic Reaction

Tell the doctor in a day or two (if possible, before the next dose of medicine):

- Hives
- Itching
- Rash

Stop the medicine and get *immediate* medical care:

- Trouble breathing or chest tightness
- Swelling of lips, tongue, or throat

Lorazepam is usually very safe when used for short periods as the doctor prescribes.

The most common side effect is daytime sleepiness. Lorazepam can also cause dizziness, feeling "spacey," or decreased coordination. If the medicine is causing any of these problems it is very important not to drive a car, ride a bicycle or motorcycle, or operate machinery.

Lorazepam can cause decreased concentration and memory. These problems, along with daytime sleepiness, may decrease learning and performance in school.

People who take lorazepam must not drink alcohol. Severe sleepiness or even loss of consciousness may result.

It is possible to become psychologically and physically dependent on lorazepam, but that is not a common problem for patients who see their doctors regularly. Because some people abuse benzodiazepines, it is illegal to give or sell these medicines to someone other than the patient for whom they were prescribed.

Very rarely, lorazepam causes excitement, irritability, anger, aggression, trouble sleeping, nightmares, uncontrollable behavior, or memory loss. This is called *disinhibition* or a *paradoxical effect*. Stop the medicine and call the doctor if this happens.

Some Interactions With Other Medicines or Food

Please note that the following are only the most likely interactions with food or other medicines.

Lorazepam may be taken with or without food.

It is important not to use other sedatives, tranquilizers, or sleeping pills or antihistamines (such as Benadryl) when taking lorazepam because of greatly increased side effects.

It is better to limit drinks with caffeine (coffee, tea, soft drinks) because caffeine works in the opposite way from this medicine, and the positive effects might be decreased.

What Could Happen if This Medicine Is Stopped Suddenly?

Many medicines cause problems if stopped suddenly. Lorazepam must be decreased slowly (tapered) rather than stopped suddenly. When lorazepam is stopped suddenly, there are withdrawal symptoms that are uncomfortable and may even be dangerous. Problems are more likely in patients taking high doses of lorazepam for 2 months or longer, but even after taking lorazepam for just a few weeks, it is important to stop it slowly. Withdrawal symptoms may include anxiety, irritability, shaking, sweating, aches and pains, muscle cramps, vomiting, confusion, and trouble sleeping. If large doses taken for a long time are stopped suddenly, seizures (fits, convulsions), hallucinations (hearing voices or seeing things that are not there), or out-of-control behavior may result.

How Long Will This Medicine Be Needed?

Lorazepam is usually prescribed for only a few weeks to allow the patient to be calm enough to learn new ways to cope with anxiety and to allow the nervous system to become less excitable. Sometimes antianxiety medicines are used for longer periods to treat panic attacks or anxiety that remain after therapy is completed. Each person is unique, and some people may need these medicines for months or years.

What Else Should I Know About This Medicine?

Because benzodiazepines can be abused (especially by people who abuse alcohol or drugs) and can cause psychological dependence or physical dependence (addiction), they are regulated by special state and federal laws as *controlled substances*. These laws place limitations on telephone prescriptions and refills, and prescriptions expire if they are not filled promptly.

Sometimes alprazolam (Xanax) and lorazepam (Ativan) get mixed up; be sure to check the prescription.

People with sleep apnea (breathing stops while they are asleep) should not take lorazepam. Tell the doctor if your child snores very loudly.

Lorazepam should be avoided during pregnancy, especially in the first 3 months, because it may cause birth defects in the baby. If taken regularly at the end of pregnancy, lorazepam may cause withdrawal symptoms in the baby.

Notes

Use this space to take notes or to write down questions you want to ask the doctor.

_____

_____

_____

_____

_____

_____

_____

_____

_____

_____

_____

_____

_____

_____

Medication Information for Youth

Lorazepam—Ativan

What the Medicine Is Called and What It Is For

The name of your medicine may be confusing. Most drugs have two names: 1) a scientific name that we call a *generic name* and 2) a trade or *brand name*. The generic name of this medicine is lorazepam. The brand name is Ativan.

Lorazepam is a *benzodiazepine* or *antianxiety* medicine. It works by calming the parts of the brain that are too excitable. It can decrease anxiety, nervousness, fears, and excessive worrying. Lorazepam can decrease the physical symptoms (rapid heartbeat, trouble breathing, dizziness, sweating) of panic attacks and phobias. It can help anxious people to be calm enough to learn—with therapy and practice—to understand and tolerate their worries or fears and even to overcome them. Your doctor may have told you that you have a condition such as social phobia, generalized anxiety disorder, separation anxiety disorder, posttraumatic stress disorder (PTSD), or panic disorder. Most often, this medicine is used for a short time when symptoms are very uncomfortable or frightening or when they make it hard to do important things such as go to school.

Lorazepam also can be used for sleep problems, such as night terrors (sudden waking up from sleep with great fear) or sleepwalking. Lorazepam can help with insomnia (difficulty falling asleep) when used for a short time along with routines that help you to relax and fall asleep.

Sometimes lorazepam is used for a few days to treat agitation in mania or psychosis until other medicines start to work.

Occasionally lorazepam is used to reduce the side effects of other medicines.

How You Take the Medicine

It is very important to take the medicine exactly as the doctor or nurse tells you. Do not skip doses or take extra medicine without asking an adult. If you forget a dose, ask your parent(s) what to do.

It is better to limit drinks with caffeine (coffee, tea, soft drinks) because caffeine works in the opposite way from this medicine, and the positive effects might be decreased.

Many medicines cause problems if stopped suddenly. Always ask your doctor before stopping a medicine. Problems are more likely to happen in patients taking high doses of lorazepam for 2 months or longer, but it is important to decrease the medicine slowly (taper) even after a few weeks. If you notice anxiety, irritability, shaking, sweating, aches and pains, muscle cramps, vomiting, or trouble sleeping, you may need to decrease the medicine more slowly. If large doses are stopped suddenly, seizures (fits, convulsions), hallucinations (hearing voices or seeing things that are not there), or out-of-control behavior may result.

This medicine is prescribed only for you. It should never be shared with anyone else.

You do not have to tell others that you are taking this medicine, but it is not something you should feel ashamed or embarrassed about. Many young people are helped by lorazepam. You should talk to your doctor or nurse about any questions you have about the medicine. It is important to remember that the medicine *helps* you. It cannot *make* you do anything or change you as a person.

How Your Doctor Will Follow Your Progress

Before giving you the medicine, your doctor or nurse will talk with you and your parent(s) and may measure your height, weight, heart rate (pulse), and blood pressure. There may be other tests to be sure that you are in good health.

Be sure to tell your doctor or nurse about any other medicines or supplements you are taking, including vitamins, herbs, or aids to weight loss or bodybuilding. Also be sure to tell the doctor or nurse if you are using alcohol or drugs. Because many medicines may affect babies, it is very important to tell the doctor if you might be pregnant or if you are at risk of becoming pregnant.

Your teachers may be asked to fill out a form about your grades and behavior in school. A psychologist may give you some tests to see how you learn best.

Most doctors have regular appointments with young people who are taking medicine. You should use these visits to share any concerns you may have about your medicine and to talk about if it has helped you. From time to time, your physician or nurse may measure your height, weight, heart rate (pulse), and blood pressure to be sure that you are in good health while you are taking the medicine. Your doctor also will ask for regular reports from your parents and maybe from your teachers (with your permission) to see how well the medicine is working.

Lorazepam is usually prescribed for only a few weeks to allow you to be calm enough to learn new ways to cope with anxiety and to allow the nervous system to become less excitable. Sometimes antianxiety medicines are used for longer periods to treat panic attacks or anxiety that remain after therapy is completed. Each person is unique, and some people may need these medicines for months or years.

How the Medicine Might Affect You

In addition to the ways the medicine can help you, it may have other effects called *side effects*. Different medicines have different side effects. It is helpful to know about some of the most common side effects of your medicine so that you will understand what they are if they happen. Some people do not have any side effects. Some side effects are just uncomfortable, but others may mean a more serious problem with the medicine. Side effects are most common after starting the medicine or after a dose increase. They may go away with time, or the medicine can be adjusted or changed—ask the doctor.

You could have an allergy to any medicine, which might show up as a rash on your skin, swelling, itching, or trouble breathing.

Please tell your parent(s) and your doctor or nurse about any changes that you notice after taking the medicine. It is especially important to tell a responsible adult if you are feeling depressed or that you may not want to live; if you have thoughts of hurting yourself; or if you begin to feel more irritable, nervous, or restless.

The most common side effect of lorazepam is daytime sleepiness. If this medicine is making you sleepy, it is very important not to drive a car or ride a bicycle or motorcycle. After starting lorazepam or increasing the dose, please be extra careful when driving a car, riding a bike, or using machines until you can tell how the medicine affects your alertness, attention, and coordination.

Sometimes antianxiety medicines seem to work in the opposite way, causing excitement, irritability, anger, aggression, and other problems. If this happens, tell your parent(s) or your doctor.

Drinking alcohol while taking this medicine can cause severe drowsiness or even passing out. **Don't do it!** Do not use marijuana or street drugs while taking this medicine. They can cause serious side effects. Skipping your medicine to take drugs does not work because many medicines stay in your body for a long time.

Lorazepam can be habit-forming, but that is not a common problem for people who take their medicine as the doctor says.

Notes

Use this space to take notes or to write down questions you want to ask the doctor or nurse.

_____

_____

_____

_____

_____

_____

_____

_____

_____

_____

_____

From Dulcan MK (editor): *Helping Parents, Youth, and Teachers Understand Medications for Behavioral and Emotional Problems: A Resource Book of Medication Information Handouts,* Third Edition. Washington, DC, American Psychiatric Publishing, 2007

Medication Information for Parents and Teachers

Loxapine—Loxitane

General Information About Medication

Each child and adolescent is different. No one has exactly the same combination of medical and psychological problems. It is a good idea to talk with the doctor or nurse about the reasons a medicine is being used. It is very important to keep all appointments and to be in touch by telephone if you have concerns. It is important to communicate with the doctor, nurse, or therapist.

It is very important that the medicine be taken exactly as the doctor instructs. However, once in a while, everyone forgets to give a medicine on time. It is a good idea to ask the doctor or nurse what to do if this happens. Do not stop or change a medicine without asking the doctor or nurse first.

If the medicine seems to stop working, it may be because it is not being taken regularly. The youth may be "cheeking" or hiding the medicine or forgetting to take it (especially at school). The doses may be too far apart, or a different dose may be needed. Something at school, at home, or in the neighborhood may be upsetting the youth, or he or she may need special help for learning disabilities or tutoring. Please discuss your concerns with the doctor. **Do not just increase the dose.**

All medicines should be kept in a safe place, out of the reach of children, and should be supervised by an adult. If someone takes too much of a medicine, call the doctor, the poison control center, or a hospital emergency room.

Each medicine has a "generic" or chemical name. Just like laundry detergents or paper towels, some medicines are sold by more than one company under different brand names. The same medicine may be available under a generic name and several brand names. The generic medications are usually less expensive than the brand name ones. The generic medications have the same chemical formula, but they may or may not be exactly the same strength as the brand-name medications. Also, some brands of pills contain dye that can cause allergic reactions. It is a good idea to talk to the doctor and the pharmacist about whether it is important to use a specific brand of medicine.

All medicines can cause an allergic reaction. Examples are hives, itching, rashes, swelling, and trouble breathing. Even a tiny amount of a medicine can cause a reaction in patients who are allergic to that medicine. Be *sure* to talk to the doctor before restarting a medicine that has caused an allergic reaction.

Taking more than one medicine at the same time may cause more side effects or cause one of the medicines to not work as well. Always ask the doctor, nurse, or pharmacist before adding another medicine, whether prescription or over-the-counter. Be sure that each doctor knows about *all* of the medicines your child is taking. Also tell the doctor about any vitamins, herbal medicines, or supplements your child may be taking. Some of these may have side effects alone or when taken with this medication.

Everyone taking medicine should have a physical examination at least once a year.

If you suspect the youth is using drugs or alcohol, please tell the doctor right away.

Pregnancy requires special care in the use of medicine. Please tell the doctor immediately if you suspect the teenager is pregnant or might become pregnant.

Printed information like this applies to children and adolescents in general. If you have questions about the medicine, or if you notice changes or anything unusual, please ask the doctor or nurse. As scientific research advances, knowledge increases and advice changes. Even experts do not always agree. Many medicines have not been approved by the U.S. Food and Drug Administration (FDA) for use in children. For this reason, use of the medicine for a particular problem or age group often is not listed in the *Physicians' Desk Reference*. This does not necessarily mean that the medicine is dangerous or does not work, only that the company that makes the medicine has not received permission to advertise the medicine for use in children. Companies often do not apply for this permission because it is expensive to do the tests needed to apply for approval for use in children. Once a medication is approved by the FDA for any purpose, a doctor is allowed to prescribe it according to research and clinical experience.

Note to Teachers

It is a good idea to talk with the parent(s) about the reason(s) that a medication is being used. If the parent(s) sign consent to release information, it is often helpful to talk with the doctor. If the parent(s) give permission, the doctor may ask you to fill out rating forms about your experience with the student's behavior, feelings, academic performance, and medication side effects. This information is very useful in selecting and monitoring medication treatment. If you have observations that you think are important, do not hesitate to share these with the student's parent(s) and treating clinicians.

It is very important that the medicine be taken exactly as the doctor instructs. However, everyone forgets to give a medicine on time once in a while. It is a good idea to ask the parent(s) in advance what to do if this happens. Do not stop or change the time you are giving a medicine at school without parental permission. If a medication is to be taken with food, but lunchtime or snack time changes, be sure to notify the parent(s) so appropriate adjustments can be made.

All medicines should be kept in a secure place and should be supervised by an adult. If someone takes too much of a medicine, follow your school procedure for an urgent medical problem.

Taking medicine is a private matter and is best managed discreetly and confidentially. It is important to be sensitive to the student's feelings about taking medicine.

If you suspect that the student is using drugs or alcohol, please tell the parent(s) or a school counselor right away.

Please tell the parent(s) or school nurse if you suspect medication side effects.

Modifications of the classroom environment or assignments may be useful in addition to medication. The student may need to be evaluated for additional help or for an Individualized Education Plan for learning or behavior.

Any expression of suicidal thoughts or feelings or self-harm by a child or adolescent is a clear signal of distress and should be taken seriously. These behaviors should not be dismissed as "attention seeking."

What Is Loxapine (Loxitane)?

Loxapine is sometimes called a *typical, conventional,* or *first-generation antipsychotic* medicine. It is also called a *neuroleptic.* It used to be called a *major tranquilizer.* It comes in brand name Loxitane and generic capsules.

How Can This Medicine Help?

Loxapine is used to treat psychosis, such as in schizophrenia, mania, or very severe depression. It can reduce hallucinations (hearing voices or seeing things that are not there) and delusions (troubling beliefs that other people do not share). It can help the patient be less upset and agitated. It can improve the patient's ability to think clearly.

Sometimes loxapine is used to decrease severe aggression or very serious behavioral problems in young people with conduct disorder, mental retardation, or autism.

This medicine is very powerful and should be used to treat very serious problems or symptoms that other medicines do not help. Be patient; the positive effects of this medicine may not appear for 2–3 weeks.

How Does This Medicine Work?

Cells in the brain (neurons) communicate using chemicals called *neurotransmitters*. Too much or too little of these substances in certain parts of the brain can cause problems. Loxapine reduces the activity of one of these neurotransmitters, *dopamine*. Blocking the effect of dopamine in certain parts of the brain reduces what have been called *positive symptoms* of psychosis: delusions; hallucinations; disorganized and unusual thinking, speaking, and behavior; excessive activity (agitation); and lack of activity (catatonia). Reducing dopamine action in other parts of the brain may lead to the side effects of this medicine.

How Long Does This Medicine Last?

Loxapine is usually taken several times a day.

How Will the Doctor Monitor This Medicine?

The doctor will review your child's medical history and physical examination before starting loxapine. The doctor may order some blood or urine tests to be sure your child does not have a hidden medical condition. The doctor or nurse may measure your child's pulse and blood pressure before starting loxapine.

Before your child starts taking loxapine and every so often afterward, the doctor may perform a test such as the AIMS (Abnormal Involuntary Movement Scale) to check your child's tongue, legs, and arms for unusual movements that could be caused by the medicine.

After the medicine is started, the doctor will want to have regular appointments with you and your child to see how the medicine is working, to see if a dose change is needed, to watch for side effects, to see if loxapine is still needed, and to see if any other treatment is needed. The doctor or nurse may check your child's height, weight, pulse, and blood pressure, and watch for abnormal movements.

What Side Effects Can This Medicine Have?

Any medicine can have side effects, including an allergy to the medicine. Because each patient is different, the doctor will monitor the youth closely, especially when the medicine is started. The doctor will work with you

to increase the positive effects and decrease the negative effects of the medicine. Please tell the doctor if any of the listed side effects appear or if you think that the medicine is causing any other problems. Not all of the rare or unusual side effects are listed.

Side effects are most common after starting the medicine or after a dose increase. Many side effects can be avoided or lessened by starting with a very low dose and increasing it slowly—ask the doctor.

Allergic Reaction

Tell the doctor in a day or two (if possible, before the next dose of medicine):

- Hives
- Itching
- Rash

    Stop the medicine and get *immediate* medical care:

- Trouble breathing or chest tightness
- Swelling of lips, tongue, or throat

Common, but Not Usually Serious, Side Effects

Discuss the following side effects with your child's doctor within a week or two. They often can be helped by lowering the dose of medicine, changing the times medicine is taken, or adding another medicine.

- Dry mouth—Have your child try using sugar-free gum or candy.
- Constipation—Encourage your child to drink more fluids and eat high-fiber foods; if necessary, the doctor may recommend a fiber medicine such as Benefiber or a stool softener such as Colace or mineral oil.
- Increased risk of sunburn—Have your child wear sunscreen or protective clothing or stay out of the sun.
- Mild trouble urinating
- Blurred vision
- Weight gain—Seek nutritional counseling; provide your child with low-calorie snacks and encourage regular exercise.
- Sadness, irritability, nervousness, clinginess, not wanting to go to school
- Restlessness or inability to sit still
- Shaking of hands and fingers

Less Common, but Not Usually Serious, Side Effects

Discuss the following side effects with your child's doctor within a week or two. They often can be helped by lowering the dose of medicine, changing the times medicine is taken, or adding another medicine.

- Daytime sleepiness or tiredness—Do not allow your child to drive, ride a bicycle or motorcycle, or operate machinery if this happens. This problem may be lessened by taking the medicine at bedtime.
- Dizziness—This side effect is worse when the child stands up quickly, especially when getting out of bed in the morning; try having the child stand up slowly.
- Decreased or slowed movement and decreased facial expressions
- Drooling

- Decreased sexual interest or ability
- Changes in menstrual cycle
- Increase in breast size or discharge from the breasts (in both boys and girls)—This may go away with time.

Less Common, but Potentially Serious, Side Effects

Call the doctor or go to an emergency room *right away:*

- Stiffness of the tongue, jaw, neck, back, or legs
- Overheating or heatstroke—Prevent by decreasing activity in hot weather, staying out of the sun, and drinking water.
- Seizure (fit, convulsion)—This is more likely in people with a history of seizures or head injury.
- Severe confusion

Rare, but Serious, Side Effects

- Extreme stiffness or lack of movement, very high fever, mental confusion, irregular pulse rate, or eye pain—**This is a medical emergency. Go to an emergency room** *right away.*
- Sudden stiffness and inability to breathe or swallow—**Go to an emergency room or call 911.** Tell the paramedics, nurses, and doctors that the patient is taking loxapine. Other medicines can be used to treat this problem fast.
- Increased thirst, frequent urination, lethargy, tiredness, dizziness—These could be signs of diabetes (especially if your child is overweight or there is a family history of diabetes). **Talk to a doctor within a day.**

What Else Should I Know About Side Effects?

Most side effects lessen over time. If they are troublesome, talk with your child's doctor. Some side effects can be decreased by taking a smaller dose of medicine, by stopping the medicine, by changing to another medicine, or by adding another medicine (see the table).

One side effect that may not go away is *tardive dyskinesia* (or TD). Patients with tardive dyskinesia have involuntary movements of the body, especially the mouth and tongue. The patient may look as though he or she is making faces over and over again. Jerky movements of the arms, legs, or body may occur. There may be fine, wormlike, or sudden repeated movements of the tongue, or the person may appear to be chewing something or smacking or puckering his or her lips. The fingers may look as though they are rolling something. If you notice any unusual movements, be sure to tell the doctor. The doctor may use the AIMS test to look for these movements.

The medicine may increase the level of *prolactin*, a natural hormone made in the part of the brain called the *pituitary*. This may cause side effects such as breast tenderness or swelling or production of milk, in both boys and girls. It also may interfere with sexual functioning in teenage boys and with regular menstrual cycles (periods) in teenage girls. A blood test can measure the level of prolactin. If these side effects do not go away and are troublesome, talk with your child's doctor about substituting another medicine for loxapine.

Heart problems are more common if other medicines are being taken also. Be sure to tell all your child's doctors and your pharmacist about all medications your child is taking.

Neuroleptic malignant syndrome is a very rare side effect that can lead to death. The symptoms are severe muscle stiffness, high fever, increased heart rate and blood pressure, irregular heartbeat (pulse), and sweating. It may lead to unconsciousness. If you suspect this, **call 911 or go to an emergency room right away.**

What Medicines Are Used to Treat the Side Effects of Loxapine?

The following medicines may be used to treat the movement side effects of loxapine. All of these medicines may have their own side effects as well. Ask the doctor if you suspect a problem.

Brand name	Generic name
Akineton	Biperiden
Artane	Trihexyphenidyl
Ativan	Lorazepam*
Benadryl	Diphenhydramine*
Catapres	Clonidine*
Cogentin	Benztropine mesylate*
Inderal	Propranolol*
Klonopin	Clonazepam*
Symmetrel	Amantadine

*This medicine has its own information sheet in this book.

Some Interactions With Other Medicines or Food

Please note that the following are only the most likely interactions with food or other medicines.

Loxapine may be taken with or without food. If the medicine causes stomach upset, taking it with food may help.

It is better to limit drinks with caffeine (coffee, tea, soft drinks) because caffeine works in the opposite way from this medicine, and the positive effects might be decreased.

What Could Happen if This Medicine Is Stopped Suddenly?

Involuntary movements, or *withdrawal dyskinesias*, may appear within 1–4 weeks of lowering the dose or stopping the medicine. Usually these go away, but they can last for days to months. If loxapine is stopped suddenly, emotional problems such as irritability, nervousness, moodiness; behavior problems; or physical problems such as stomachache, loss of appetite, nausea, vomiting, diarrhea, sweating, indigestion, trouble sleeping, trembling, or shaking may appear. These problems usually last only a few days to a few weeks. If they happen, tell your child's doctor. The medicine dose may need to be lowered more slowly (tapered). Always check with the doctor before stopping a medicine!

How Long Will This Medicine Be Needed?

How long your child will need to be on loxapine depends partly on the reason that it was prescribed. Some problems last for only a few months, whereas others last much longer. Sometimes loxapine is used for only a short time until other medicines or behavioral treatments start to work. Some people need to take loxapine for years. It is especially important with medicines as powerful as this one to ask the doctor whether it is still needed. Every few months, you should discuss with your child's doctor the reasons for using loxapine and whether it is time for a trial of lowering the dose.

What Else Should I Know About This Medicine?

There are many older and newer medicines that are used for the same kinds of problems. If your child is having bad side effects or the medicine does not seem to be working, ask the doctor if another medicine in this group might work as well or better and have fewer side effects for your child.

Be sure to tell the doctor if there is anyone in your family who died suddenly or had a heart problem.

Notes

Use this space to take notes or to write down questions you want to ask the doctor.

_____

_____

_____

_____

_____

_____

_____

_____

_____

_____

From Dulcan MK (editor): _Helping Parents, Youth, and Teachers Understand Medications for Behavioral and Emotional Problems: A Resource Book of Medication Information Handouts,_ Third Edition. Washington, DC, American Psychiatric Publishing, 2007

Medication Information for Youth

Loxapine—Loxitane

What the Medicine Is Called and What It Is For

The name of your medicine may be confusing. Most drugs have two names: 1) a scientific name that we call a *generic name* and 2) a trade or *brand name*. The generic name of this medicine is loxapine. The brand name is Loxitane.

Loxapine can help people who feel very confused and have severe problems thinking clearly. It can lessen *hallucinations* (seeing or hearing things that are not really there) and *delusions* (troubling beliefs that other people do not share). This medicine also is sometimes used to help young people who have mania or very severe depression or who get very angry and hit people or break things.

How You Take the Medicine

It is very important to take the medicine exactly as the doctor or nurse tells you. Do not skip doses or take extra medicine without asking an adult. If you forget a dose, ask your parent(s) what to do.

It is better to limit drinks with caffeine (coffee, tea, soft drinks) because caffeine works in the opposite way from this medicine, and the positive effects might be decreased.

If your stomach is upset, taking the medicine with food may help.

This medicine is prescribed only for you. It should never be shared with anyone else.

You do not have to tell others that you are taking this medicine, but it is not something you should feel ashamed or embarrassed about. Many young people are helped by loxapine. This medicine is not habit-forming, and you cannot become "hooked" on it. You should talk to your doctor or nurse about any questions you have about the medicine. It is important to remember that the medicine *helps* you. It cannot *make* you do anything or change you as a person.

How Your Doctor Will Follow Your Progress

Before giving you the medicine, your doctor or nurse will talk with you and your parent(s) and may measure your height, weight, heart rate (pulse), and blood pressure. There may be other tests, such as blood tests for sugar and cholesterol. Before you start taking the medicine and every so often afterward, the doctor or nurse will look at your tongue, arms, and legs to check for unusual movements. This is called the AIMS (Abnormal Involuntary Movement Scale) test.

Be sure to tell your doctor or nurse about any other medicines or supplements you are taking, including vitamins, herbs, or aids to weight loss or bodybuilding. Also be sure to tell the doctor or nurse if you are using alcohol or drugs. Because many medicines may affect babies, it is very important to tell the doctor if you might be pregnant or if you are at risk of becoming pregnant.

Your teachers may be asked to fill out a form about your grades and behavior in school. A psychologist may give you some tests to see how you learn best.

Most doctors have regular appointments with young people who are taking medicine. You should use these visits to share any concerns you may have about your medicine and to talk about if it has helped you. From time to time, your physician or nurse may measure your height, weight, heart rate (pulse), and blood pressure to be sure that you are in good health while you are taking the medicine. There may be blood tests to watch for diabetes or high cholesterol. Your doctor also will ask for regular reports from your parents and maybe from your teachers (with your permission) to see how well the medicine is working.

If the medicine helps you, your doctor will probably want you to take it for several months to a year. Your doctor will decide how long you will need to take the medicine as he or she watches your progress.

How the Medicine Might Affect You

In addition to the ways the medicine can help you, it may have other effects called *side effects*. Different medicines have different side effects. It is helpful to know about some of the most common side effects of your medicine so that you will understand what they are if they happen. Some people do not have any side effects. Some side effects are just uncomfortable, but others may mean a more serious problem with the medicine. Side effects are most common after starting the medicine or after a dose increase. They may go away with time, or the medicine can be adjusted or changed—ask the doctor.

You could have an allergy to any medicine, which might show up as a rash on your skin, swelling, itching, or trouble breathing.

Please tell your parent(s) and your doctor or nurse about any changes that you notice after taking the medicine. It is especially important to tell a responsible adult if you are feeling depressed or that you may not want to live; if you have thoughts of hurting yourself; or if you begin to feel more irritable, nervous, or restless.

One of the most common side effects of this medicine is feeling tired or sleepy during the day, even if you have had a full night's sleep. If this medicine is making you sleepy, it is very important not to drive a car or ride a bicycle or motorcycle. After starting the medicine or increasing the dose of medicine, please be extra careful when driving a car, riding a bike, or using machines until you can tell how the medicine affects your alertness, attention, and coordination. After you have been taking the medicine for a few weeks, your body will adjust, and this side effect will likely go away. If you had trouble sleeping at night before taking the medicine, it can help you sleep better, especially if the doctor tells you to take a dose of medicine in the evening.

You might feel dizzy or light-headed if you stand up fast. Try standing up slowly, especially when getting out of bed in the morning.

Another common side effect is dry mouth. You may be more thirsty than usual and find that you are drinking more water or other liquids than usual. Sucking on sugar-free hard candy or cough drops usually helps. You also could try chewing sugar-free gum or sucking on ice chips. Do not chew the ice; you could hurt your teeth. Also, using lip balm will keep your lips from cracking. It is important to be especially good about brushing your teeth.

Taking this medicine could make you more likely to get badly sunburned or very sick in hot weather. Be sure to drink plenty of liquids and cover up or use sunscreen when you go outside in hot weather. Be careful to rest in the shade and not get overheated.

Sometimes teenagers who take loxapine gain weight. The weight gain may be from increased appetite and also from ways that the medicine changes how the body processes food. It is much easier to prevent weight gain than to lose weight later. It is a good idea to eat a well-balanced diet without "junk food" and with healthy snacks like fruits and vegetables, not sweets or fried foods. It is better to drink water or skim milk, not pop, sodas, soft drinks, or sugary juices. Regular exercise is important for maintaining a healthy weight (and may also help with sleep).

Some people become constipated (have hard bowel movements) when taking this medicine. Try drinking more water and eating more fruits, vegetables, and whole grains. If that does not help, tell your parent(s) or doctor—you may need a medicine to help with this side effect. Sometimes people have trouble passing urine. Tell your parent(s) or the doctor if this happens.

This is a very powerful medicine. Some side effects include feeling nervous, restless, or shaky or having stiff muscles. Talk with your doctor about these side effects. They can be helped by adding another medicine, adjusting the dose, or switching to another medicine.

Another, more serious, side effect can be longer lasting and more difficult to treat. This very rare side effect is called *tardive dyskinesia* (or TD). A person taking loxapine may develop movements of the mouth, tongue, face, arms, legs, or body that are not being made on purpose. This side effect can go away when the medicine is stopped, but in some people it does not go away. Your doctor will explain this effect to you and your parent(s) and how he or she will watch for any signs that you are developing this problem. Be sure to ask your doctor any questions that you may have about this, but do not worry too much about it. It hardly ever happens to teenagers.

You may notice changes in your sexual functioning or in your breasts—it is OK to ask the doctor about this.

You should tell your parent(s) and doctor if you notice anything different or unusual about how you feel once you start taking the medicine. This includes good things, such as feeling less confused, feeling less sad or angry, not hearing voices anymore, or sleeping better at night.

You cannot become addicted to this medicine, but you should not stop it suddenly. Never stop a medicine without talking to the doctor. If loxapine is stopped or decreased suddenly you may notice more moodiness or irritability, stomachaches or upset stomach, trouble sleeping, or trembling or shaking. Let your parent(s) or doctor know if this happens—the medicine may need to be decreased more slowly.

Notes

Use this space to take notes or to write down questions you want to ask the doctor or nurse.

_____

_____

_____

_____

_____

_____

_____

_____

_____

_____

_____

_____

From Dulcan MK (editor): _Helping Parents, Youth, and Teachers Understand Medications for Behavioral and Emotional Problems: A Resource Book of Medication Information Handouts_, Third Edition. Washington, DC, American Psychiatric Publishing, 2007

Medication Information for Parents and Teachers

Melatonin

General Information About Medication

Each child and adolescent is different. No one has exactly the same combination of medical and psychological problems. It is a good idea to talk with the doctor or nurse about the reasons a medicine is being used. It is very important to keep all appointments and to be in touch by telephone if you have concerns. It is important to communicate with the doctor, nurse, or therapist.

It is very important that the medicine be taken exactly as the doctor instructs. However, once in a while, everyone forgets to give a medicine on time. It is a good idea to ask the doctor or nurse what to do if this happens. Do not stop or change a medicine without asking the doctor or nurse first.

If the medicine seems to stop working, it may be because it is not being taken regularly. The youth may be "cheeking" or hiding the medicine or forgetting to take it (especially at school). The doses may be too far apart, or a different dose may be needed. Something at school, at home, or in the neighborhood may be upsetting the youth, or he or she may need special help for learning disabilities or tutoring. Please discuss your concerns with the doctor. **Do not just increase the dose.**

All medicines should be kept in a safe place, out of the reach of children, and should be supervised by an adult. If someone takes too much of a medicine, call the doctor, the poison control center, or a hospital emergency room.

Each medicine has a "generic" or chemical name. Just like laundry detergents or paper towels, some medicines are sold by more than one company under different brand names. The same medicine may be available under a generic name and several brand names. The generic medications are usually less expensive than the brand name ones. The generic medications have the same chemical formula, but they may or may not be exactly the same strength as the brand-name medications. Also, some brands of pills contain dye that can cause allergic reactions. It is a good idea to talk to the doctor and the pharmacist about whether it is important to use a specific brand of medicine.

All medicines can cause an allergic reaction. Examples are hives, itching, rashes, swelling, and trouble breathing. Even a tiny amount of a medicine can cause a reaction in patients who are allergic to that medicine. Be *sure* to talk to the doctor before restarting a medicine that has caused an allergic reaction.

Taking more than one medicine at the same time may cause more side effects or cause one of the medicines to not work as well. Always ask the doctor, nurse, or pharmacist before adding another medicine, whether prescription or over-the-counter. Be sure that each doctor knows about *all* of the medicines your child is taking. Also tell the doctor about any vitamins, herbal medicines, or supplements your child may be taking. Some of these may have side effects alone or when taken with this medication.

Everyone taking medicine should have a physical examination at least once a year.

If you suspect the youth is using drugs or alcohol, please tell the doctor right away.

Pregnancy requires special care in the use of medicine. Please tell the doctor immediately if you suspect the teenager is pregnant or might become pregnant.

Printed information like this applies to children and adolescents in general. If you have questions about the medicine, or if you notice changes or anything unusual, please ask the doctor or nurse. As scientific research advances, knowledge increases and advice changes. Even experts do not always agree. Many medicines have not been approved by the U.S. Food and Drug Administration (FDA) for use in children. For this reason, use of the medicine for a particular problem or age group often is not listed in the *Physicians' Desk Reference*. This does not necessarily mean that the medicine is dangerous or does not work, only that the company that makes the medicine has not received permission to advertise the medicine for use in children. Companies often do not apply for this permission because it is expensive to do the tests needed to apply for approval for use in children. Once a medication is approved by the FDA for any purpose, a doctor is allowed to prescribe it according to research and clinical experience.

Note to Teachers

It is a good idea to talk with the parent(s) about the reason(s) that a medication is being used. If the parent(s) sign consent to release information, it is often helpful to talk with the doctor. If the parent(s) give permission, the doctor may ask you to fill out rating forms about your experience with the student's behavior, feelings, academic performance, and medication side effects. This information is very useful in selecting and monitoring medication treatment. If you have observations that you think are important, do not hesitate to share these with the student's parent(s) and treating clinicians.

All medicines should be kept in a secure place and should be supervised by an adult. If someone takes too much of a medicine, follow your school procedure for an urgent medical problem.

Taking medicine is a private matter and is best managed discreetly and confidentially. It is important to be sensitive to the student's feelings about taking medicine.

If you suspect that the student is using drugs or alcohol, please tell the parent(s) or a school counselor right away.

Please tell the parent(s) or school nurse if you suspect medication side effects.

Modifications of the classroom environment or assignments may be useful in addition to medication. The student may need to be evaluated for additional help or for an Individualized Education Plan for learning or behavior.

Any expression of suicidal thoughts or feelings or self-harm by a child or adolescent is a clear signal of distress and should be taken seriously. These behaviors should not be dismissed as "attention seeking."

What Is Melatonin?

Melatonin is a natural hormone produced by the body. Melatonin is produced by the *pineal gland*, which is located just above the middle of the brain. During the day, the pineal gland is not active. It starts producing melatonin after sunset, usually around 9:00 P.M. As a result, melatonin levels in the brain rise sharply, and the person begins to feel less alert and more sleepy. Melatonin levels remain high through the night and fall to low daytime levels by the morning hours, usually around 9:00 A.M.

Melatonin is available in the United States without a prescription as a nutritional supplement.

Melatonin is not a sedative, hypnotic, or tranquilizer.

How Can This Medicine Help?

Melatonin can improve sleep by returning a person to a more natural sleep cycle. It can help with falling asleep and with staying asleep for long enough to be rested. It has been shown to work in children without psychiatric problems who have severe sleep problems as well as in children with attention-deficit/hyperactivity disorder (ADHD), developmental delays, or autism who have severe sleep problems.

Melatonin can reset the body's clock and help to regulate the circadian cycle. Many adolescents have delayed sleep phase syndrome, a disorder of the biological clock in which the youth is not sleepy until very late at night and is unable to get up early in the morning. This causes problems with school attendance and performance. Melatonin is helpful in shifting sleep to a more regular time schedule.

How Does This Medicine Work?

Synthetic (man-made) melatonin can improve sleep in both children and adults. The exact way in which this happens is not known, but it is thought that the synthetic melatonin copies the effects of natural melatonin in the brain. It starts working 1–2 hours after taking it. It is usually given 30 minutes to 1 hour before bedtime.

A behavioral program, such as regular soothing routines at bedtime and increased exercise in the daytime, should be used in combination with the medicine to improve sleep. Finding developmentally appropriate bed- and wake-times and sticking to them is very important. These strategies should be continued after the medicine is stopped or when the medicine is used only occasionally.

How Will the Doctor Monitor This Medicine?

The doctor will review your child's medical history and physical examination before starting melatonin. The doctor may order some blood or urine tests to be sure your child does not have a hidden medical condition.

After the medicine is started, the doctor will want to have regular appointments with you and your child to see how the medicine is working, to see if a dose change is needed, to watch for side effects, to see if melatonin is still needed, and to see if any other treatment is needed.

What Side Effects Can This Medicine Have?

Any medicine can have side effects, including an allergy to the medicine. Because each patient is different, the doctor will monitor the youth closely, especially when the medicine is started. The doctor will work with you to increase the positive effects and decrease the negative effects of the medicine. Please tell the doctor if any of the listed side effects appear or if you think that the medicine is causing any other problems. Not all of the rare or unusual side effects are listed.

Side effects are most common after starting the medicine or after a dose increase. Many side effects can be avoided or lessened by starting with a very low dose and increasing it slowly—ask the doctor.

Allergic Reaction

Tell the doctor in a day or two (if possible, before the next dose of medicine):

- Hives
- Itching
- Rash

    Stop the medicine and get *immediate* medical care:

- Trouble breathing or chest tightness
- Swelling of lips, tongue, or throat

Other Possible Side Effects

Melatonin appears to be well tolerated, with no significant side effects reported. There has not been a lot of research on the safety of melatonin in children. Some children may be sleepy in the morning when it is time to get up and go to school or may have a headache or upset stomach.

Some Interactions With Other Medicines or Food

Please note that the following are only the most likely interactions with food or other medicines.

    There are no reported interactions of melatonin with medicines or food.

    Caffeine may interfere with sleep and make it more difficult for the melatonin to work.

What Could Happen if This Medicine Is Stopped Suddenly?

There are no known effects from stopping melatonin suddenly, although the original sleep problem might return.

How Long Will This Medicine Be Needed?

Some people may need melatonin for a long time (years), but others may need it only until the sleep rhythm improves.

What Else Should I Know About This Medicine?

Because melatonin is not regulated by the FDA, the amount of melatonin that is actually in the pill may not be the same as listed on the package.

Notes

Use this space to take notes or to write down questions you want to ask the doctor.

_____

_____

_____

_____

_____

_____

_____

_____

_____

_____

_____

_____

From Dulcan MK (editor): _Helping Parents, Youth, and Teachers Understand Medications for Behavioral and Emotional Problems: A Resource Book of Medication Information Handouts,_ Third Edition. Washington, DC, American Psychiatric Publishing, 2007

Medication Information for Youth

Melatonin

What the Medicine Is Called and What It Is For

Melatonin is a natural hormone made by a gland in the brain. It has a daily rhythm of high levels and low levels. A man-made form of melatonin is sold over-the-counter as a nutritional supplement. It is not a sedative or a tranquilizer. It is not like sleeping pills, but it can improve sleep by helping a person have a more natural sleep cycle. It can help with falling asleep and staying asleep long enough to feel rested. Some teenagers do not get sleepy until later and later at night and have more and more trouble getting up in the morning for school. Melatonin can help shift sleep to a more regular schedule.

How You Take the Medicine

It is very important to take the medicine exactly as the doctor or nurse tells you. Do not skip doses or take extra medicine without asking an adult. If you forget a dose, ask your parent(s) what to do.

Melatonin works best if combined with a regular bedtime, calming routines before bedtime, and physical exercise during the day. Getting up on time is also important in keeping a regular sleep schedule.

Caffeine (in coffee, tea, or soft drinks) may make it harder to fall asleep and make the melatonin not work as well.

This medicine is prescribed only for you. It should never be shared with anyone else.

You do not have to tell others that you are taking this medicine, but it is not something you should feel ashamed or embarrassed about. Many young people are helped by melatonin. This medicine is not habit-forming, and you cannot become "hooked" on it. You should talk to your doctor or nurse about any questions you have about the medicine. It is important to remember that the medicine *helps* you. It cannot *make* you do anything or change you as a person.

How Your Doctor Will Follow Your Progress

Before giving you the medicine, your doctor or nurse will talk with you and your parent(s) and may measure your height, weight, heart rate (pulse), and blood pressure.

Be sure to tell your doctor or nurse about any other medicines or supplements you are taking, including vitamins, herbs, or aids to weight loss or bodybuilding. Also be sure to tell the doctor or nurse if you are using alcohol or drugs. Because many medicines may affect babies, it is very important to tell the doctor if you might be pregnant or if you are at risk of becoming pregnant.

Most doctors have regular appointments with young people who are taking medicine. You should use these visits to share any concerns you may have about your medicine and to talk about if it has helped you. From time to time, your physician or nurse may measure your height, weight, heart rate (pulse), and blood pressure to be sure that you are in good health while you are taking the medicine. Your doctor also will ask for regular reports from your parents to see how well the medicine is working.

How the Medicine Might Affect You

In addition to the ways the medicine can help you, it may have other effects called *side effects*. Different medicines have different side effects. It is helpful to know about some of the most common side effects of your medicine so that you will understand what they are if they happen. Some people do not have any side effects. Some side effects are just uncomfortable, but others may mean a more serious problem with the medicine. Side effects are most common after starting the medicine or after a dose increase. They may go away with time, or the medicine can be adjusted or changed—ask the doctor.

You could have an allergy to any medicine, which might show up as a rash on your skin, swelling, itching, or trouble breathing.

Please tell your parent(s) and your doctor or nurse about any changes that you notice after taking the medicine. It is especially important to tell a responsible adult if you are feeling depressed or that you may not want to live; if you have thoughts of hurting yourself; or if you begin to feel more irritable, nervous, or restless.

Some medicines make people feel sleepy or less coordinated. If this medicine is making you sleepy, it is very important not to drive a car or ride a bicycle or motorcycle. After starting melatonin or increasing the dose, please be extra careful when driving a car, riding a bike, or using machines until you can tell how the medicine affects your alertness, attention, and coordination.

Some people are sleepy in the morning or may have a headache or upset stomach while taking melatonin.

Notes

Use this space to take notes or to write down questions you want to ask the doctor or nurse.

_____

_____

_____

_____

_____

_____

_____

_____

_____

_____

_____

_____

_____

_____

From Dulcan MK (editor): _Helping Parents, Youth, and Teachers Understand Medications for Behavioral and Emotional Problems: A Resource Book of Medication Information Handouts_, Third Edition. Washington, DC, American Psychiatric Publishing, 2007

Medication Information for Parents and Teachers

Methylphenidate—Methylin, Ritalin, Metadate, Concerta, Daytrana, Focalin

General Information About Medication

Each child and adolescent is different. No one has exactly the same combination of medical and psychological problems. It is a good idea to talk with the doctor or nurse about the reasons a medicine is being used. It is very important to keep all appointments and to be in touch by telephone if you have concerns. It is important to communicate with the doctor, nurse, or therapist.

It is very important that the medicine be taken exactly as the doctor instructs. However, once in a while, everyone forgets to give a medicine on time. It is a good idea to ask the doctor or nurse what to do if this happens. Do not stop or change a medicine without asking the doctor or nurse first.

If the medicine seems to stop working, it may be because it is not being taken regularly. The youth may be "cheeking" or hiding the medicine or forgetting to take it (especially at school). The doses may be too far apart, or a different dose may be needed. Something at school, at home, or in the neighborhood may be upsetting the youth, or he or she may need special help for learning disabilities or tutoring. Please discuss your concerns with the doctor. **Do not just increase the dose.**

All medicines should be kept in a safe place, out of the reach of children, and should be supervised by an adult. If someone takes too much of a medicine, call the doctor, the poison control center, or a hospital emergency room.

Each medicine has a "generic" or chemical name. Just like laundry detergents or paper towels, some medicines are sold by more than one company under different brand names. The same medicine may be available under a generic name and several brand names. The generic medications are usually less expensive than the brand name ones. The generic medications have the same chemical formula, but they may or may not be exactly the same strength as the brand-name medications. Also, some brands of pills contain dye that can cause allergic reactions. It is a good idea to talk to the doctor and the pharmacist about whether it is important to use a specific brand of medicine.

All medicines can cause an allergic reaction. Examples are hives, itching, rashes, swelling, and trouble breathing. Even a tiny amount of a medicine can cause a reaction in patients who are allergic to that medicine. Be *sure* to talk to the doctor before restarting a medicine that has caused an allergic reaction.

Taking more than one medicine at the same time may cause more side effects or cause one of the medicines to not work as well. Always ask the doctor, nurse, or pharmacist before adding another medicine, whether prescription or over-the-counter. Be sure that each doctor knows about *all* of the medicines your child is taking. Also tell the doctor about any vitamins, herbal medicines, or supplements your child may be taking. Some of these may have side effects alone or when taken with this medication.

Everyone taking medicine should have a physical examination at least once a year.

If you suspect the youth is using drugs or alcohol, please tell the doctor right away.

Pregnancy requires special care in the use of medicine. Please tell the doctor immediately if you suspect the teenager is pregnant or might become pregnant.

431

Printed information like this applies to children and adolescents in general. If you have questions about the medicine, or if you notice changes or anything unusual, please ask the doctor or nurse. As scientific research advances, knowledge increases and advice changes. Even experts do not always agree. Many medicines have not been approved by the U.S. Food and Drug Administration (FDA) for use in children. For this reason, use of the medicine for a particular problem or age group often is not listed in the *Physicians' Desk Reference*. This does not necessarily mean that the medicine is dangerous or does not work, only that the company that makes the medicine has not received permission to advertise the medicine for use in children. Companies often do not apply for this permission because it is expensive to do the tests needed to apply for approval for use in children. Once a medication is approved by the FDA for any purpose, a doctor is allowed to prescribe it according to research and clinical experience.

Note to Teachers

It is a good idea to talk with the parent(s) about the reason(s) that a medication is being used. If the parent(s) sign consent to release information, it is often helpful to talk with the doctor. If the parent(s) give permission, the doctor may ask you to fill out rating forms about your experience with the student's behavior, feelings, academic performance, and medication side effects. This information is very useful in selecting and monitoring medication treatment. If you have observations that you think are important, do not hesitate to share these with the student's parent(s) and treating clinicians.

It is very important that the medicine be taken exactly as the doctor instructs. However, everyone forgets to give a medicine on time once in a while. It is a good idea to ask the parent(s) in advance what to do if this happens. Do not stop or change the time you are giving a medicine at school without parental permission. If a medication is to be taken with food, but lunchtime or snack time changes, be sure to notify the parent(s) so appropriate adjustments can be made.

All medicines should be kept in a secure place and should be supervised by an adult. If someone takes too much of a medicine, follow your school procedure for an urgent medical problem.

Taking medicine is a private matter and is best managed discreetly and confidentially. It is important to be sensitive to the student's feelings about taking medicine.

If you suspect that the student is using drugs or alcohol, please tell the parent(s) or a school counselor right away.

Please tell the parent(s) or school nurse if you suspect medication side effects.

Modifications of the classroom environment or assignments may be useful in addition to medication. The student may need to be evaluated for additional help or for an Individualized Education Plan for learning or behavior.

Any expression of suicidal thoughts or feelings or self-harm by a child or adolescent is a clear signal of distress and should be taken seriously. These behaviors should not be dismissed as "attention seeking."

What Is Methylphenidate (Methylin, Ritalin, Metadate, Concerta, Daytrana, Focalin)?

Methylphenidate is called a *stimulant*. It is used to treat attention-deficit/hyperactivity disorder (ADHD or ADD), whether the person has hyperactivity (increased moving around) or not. It comes in a generic form and several brand name formulations (see table below). Although all of these medicines have methylphenidate as the active ingredient, they are made differently, so that there are many different ways to take methylphenidate. This helps the doctor to find just the right form of the medicine for each person.

Generic and brand name formulations
Short-acting or immediate-release methylphenidate (3–4 hours)
Generic methylphenidate
Methylin tablets
Methylin CT chewable tablets
Methylin oral solution (grape flavored)
Ritalin
Long-acting methylphenidate
Methylin ER (extended-release; 6–8 hours) (wax matrix)
Ritalin SR (sustained-release; 6–8 hours) (wax matrix)
Metadate ER (extended-release; 6–8 hours) (wax matrix)
Metadate CD (controlled-delivery; 8 hours) (capsule Diffucap with beads; may be sprinkled on food)
Very long-acting methylphenidate
Ritalin LA (long-acting; 8–10 hours) (capsule with beads; may be sprinkled on food)
Concerta (Oros osmotic controlled-release tablet; 10–12 hours)
Daytrana Transdermal System (skin patch; worn for 9 hours; lasts 12 hours)

Dexmethylphenidate is a form of methylphenidate that has only one of the two chemical shapes (called a *dextroisomer*) of methylphenidate. Dexmethylphenidate is given at half the dose of methylphenidate and may have fewer side effects. Dexmethylphenidate comes in brand name Focalin (immediate-release, short-acting tablets; 3–4 hours) and Focalin XR (extended-release, very long-acting capsules that contain beads of medicine; 8–10 hours; may be sprinkled on food).

How Can This Medicine Help?

Methylphenidate can increase attention and the ability to follow instructions. It can improve attention span, decrease distractibility, increase the ability to finish things, decrease hyperactivity, and improve the ability to think before acting (decrease impulsivity). Handwriting and completion of schoolwork and homework can improve. Methylphenidate can improve willingness to follow directions and decrease stubbornness in youngsters with both ADHD and oppositional defiant disorder.

Many people with Tourette's disorder (chronic motor and vocal tics) also have symptoms of ADHD. Methylphenidate may be used cautiously to reduce the symptoms of hyperactivity, impulsivity, and trouble paying attention and usually does not make the tics worse. If the tics get worse, talk with your child's doctor. Lowering the dose or stopping the methylphenidate will usually lead to the tics decreasing again. Tics also increase and decrease for a lot of reasons that are not related to medicine.

Medicine may not remove all symptoms in children with ADHD. These youth may also need special help in school and behavior modification at home and at school. Some youngsters and families are helped by family therapy or group social skills therapy.

Stimulant medicines last for different amounts of time. ADHD symptoms may come back when the medicine wears off. This does not mean the medicine is not working but that longer coverage may be needed.

Methylphenidate is also used to help people with narcolepsy (sudden and uncontrollable episodes of deep sleep) to stay awake.

How Does This Medicine Work?

In people who have ADHD or ADD, parts of the brain are not working as well as they should. An example would be the part that controls impulsive actions ("the brakes"). Methylphenidate helps these parts of the brain work better by acting as a *stimulant*, increasing the activity of neurotransmitters—mostly *dopamine* but also *norepinephrine*. *Neurotransmitters* are the chemicals that the brain makes for the nerve cells to communicate with each other.

Methylphenidate is not a tranquilizer or sedative. It works in the same way in children and adults and in people with or without ADHD.

Methylphenidate and amphetamine are both stimulant medicines, but they work in different ways on the neurotransmitters. A person with ADHD might be helped by one stimulant but not the other, so if one is not working, the doctor may try the other one.

How Long Does This Medicine Last?

All pill types of methylphenidate start working within 30–60 minutes after taking them.

Different forms of methylphenidate last for different lengths of time. The immediate-release or short-acting forms last for 3–4 hours. The long-acting forms last for 6–8 hours. Ritalin LA and Focalin XR last for 8–10 hours, and Concerta lasts for 10–12 hours. The length of time is different for different people, and the medicine may work longer for some symptoms than for others. An advantage of the longer-acting forms is that they do not have to be given during the school day.

Daytrana (the skin patch) may take longer to start working (1–2 hours after being put on the skin). It is designed to be worn for 9 hours. The effects of the medicine last as long as 3 hours after the skin patch is taken off. If there are too many side effects in the evening, the patch can be taken off earlier in the day.

How Will the Doctor Monitor This Medicine?

The doctor will review your child's medical history and physical examination before starting methylphenidate. The doctor may order some blood or urine tests to be sure your child does not have a hidden medical condition. Be sure to tell the doctor if your child or anyone in the family has had heart problems, very fast or irregular heartbeat, high blood pressure (hypertension), dizziness, fainting, shortness of breath, or severe tiredness. Tell the doctor if anyone in the family has died suddenly. Also tell the doctor if your child or anyone in the family has had motor or vocal tics (hard-to-control repeated movements or sounds) or Tourette's disorder (also called Tourette's syndrome). The doctor or nurse will measure your child's height, weight, pulse, and blood pressure before starting the medicine. The doctor will usually ask parents and teachers to fill out behavior rating scales (checklists).

After the medicine is started, the doctor will want to have regular appointments with you and your child to see how the medicine is working, to see if a dose change is needed, to watch for side effects, to see if methylphenidate is still needed, and to see if any other treatment is needed. The doctor or nurse may check your child's height, weight, pulse, and blood pressure. With parental permission, the doctor will usually ask for reports (rating scale, checklist, testing results, comments) from the teacher(s) to keep track of progress in learning and behavior. Some young people take the medicine three or four times a day, every day. Others need to take it only once or twice a day, or only on school days. You and your child's doctor will work out the dose, timing, and type of methylphenidate that is best for your child and his or her symptoms and schedule.

What Side Effects Can This Medicine Have?

Any medicine can have side effects, including an allergy to the medicine. Because each patient is different, the doctor will monitor the youth closely, especially when the medicine is started. The doctor will work with you to increase the positive effects and decrease the negative effects of the medicine. Please tell the doctor if any of the listed side effects appear or if you think that the medicine is causing any other problems. Not all of the rare or unusual side effects are listed.

Side effects are most common after starting the medicine or after a dose increase. Many side effects can be avoided or lessened by starting with a very low dose and increasing it slowly—ask the doctor.

Allergic Reaction

Tell the doctor in a day or two (if possible, before the next dose of medicine):

- Hives
- Itching
- Rash

A rash under the patch may be a problem with the skin patch, and there may also be bumps, blisters, or swelling. After using the skin patch, a new allergy to methylphenidate pills may develop.

Stop the medicine and get *immediate* medical care:

- Trouble breathing or chest tightness
- Swelling of lips, tongue, or throat

Common Side Effects

If the following side effects do not go away after about 2 weeks, ask the doctor about lowering your child's dose.

- Lack of appetite and weight loss—Encourage your child to eat a good breakfast and afternoon and evening snacks; give medicine during or after meals.
- Insomnia (trouble falling asleep)—This may be the ADHD coming back and not a side effect. Talk with your child's doctor. Changing the time or dose of medicine, starting a bedtime routine, or adding another medicine may help.
- Headaches
- Stomachaches
- Irritability, crankiness, crying, emotional sensitivity
- Loss of interest in friends
- Staring into space
- Rapid pulse rate (heartbeat) or increased blood pressure

Preschool-age children are more likely than older children to have irritability, emotional sensitivity, lack of appetite, and/or insomnia.

Less Common Side Effects

Tell the doctor within a week or two:

- Rebound—As the medicine is wearing off, hyperactivity or bad mood may get worse than before the medicine was taken. The doctor can make adjustments to help this problem.
- Slowing of growth—This is why your child's height and weight are checked regularly; if this is a problem, growth usually catches up if the medicine is stopped or the dose is decreased.
- Nervous habits—Examples are picking at skin or biting nails (although these habits are also common in children with ADHD who do not take medicine).
- Stuttering

Rare, but Serious, Side Effects

Call the doctor within a day or two:

- Motor or vocal tics (fast, repeated movements or sounds) or muscle twitches (jerking movements) of parts of the body
- Sadness that lasts more than a few days
- Auditory, visual, or tactile hallucinations (hearing, seeing, or feeling things that are not there)
- Any behavior that is very unusual for your child

Some Interactions With Other Medicines or Food

Please note that the following are only the most likely interactions with food or other medicines.

Caffeine may increase side effects.

Methylphenidate may be taken with or without food.

The combination of methylphenidate with medicines such as imipramine (Tofranil) or nortriptyline (Pamelor) may cause irritability and confusion or severe emotional and behavioral problems (such as hallucinations and fighting). However, methylphenidate with either of these two medicines rarely may be used together, *very carefully.*

It is not a good idea to combine stimulants with nasal decongestants or cough and cold medicines that contain ingredients such as pseudoephedrine or phenylephrine because rapid pulse rate (heartbeat) or high blood pressure may develop. If a stuffy nose is really troublesome, it is better to use a nasal spray. Check with the pharmacist before giving an over-the-counter medicine. Also, many children with ADHD become cranky or more hyperactive while taking antihistamines (such as Benadryl). If medicine for allergies is needed, ask your child's doctor.

Methylphenidate may increase the levels of selective serotonin reuptake inhibitor (SSRI) antidepressants (such as Prozac, Paxil, Zoloft, and Celexa).

Methylphenidate should not be taken at the same time as or even within a month of taking another type of medicine called a *monoamine oxidase inhibitor* (MAOI), such as Eldepryl (selegiline), Nardil (phenelzine), Parnate (tranylcypromine), or Marplan (isocarboxazid). The combination could cause severe high blood pressure.

What Could Happen if This Medicine Is Stopped Suddenly?

No medical withdrawal effects occur if methylphenidate is stopped suddenly. The ADHD will come back as soon as the medicine wears off. Some people may have irritability, trouble sleeping, or increased hyperactivity for a day or two if they have been taking the medicine every day for a long time, especially at high doses. It may be better to decrease the medicine slowly (taper) over a week or so.

How Long Will This Medicine Be Needed?

There is no way to know how long a person will need to take methylphenidate. The parent(s), the doctor, and the school will work together to determine what is right for each patient. Sometimes the medicine is needed for a few years, but many people need to take medicine for ADHD even as adults.

What Else Should I Know About This Medicine?

Many people have incorrect information about stimulants. If you hear anything that worries you, please check with your doctor.

Although the FDA has not approved methylphenidate for use in children younger than 6 years, this is not because it is dangerous or does not work. It is because there was not enough research on young children at the time that methylphenidate was approved by the FDA. Now there is research that shows that methylphenidate can be used safely and effectively in preschool children with ADHD. Amphetamines are FDA approved for children younger than 6 years, but this is a historical accident that happened as rules changed for approval of medicines. There is actually less research on amphetamines for ADHD in young children than there is for methylphenidate.

Stimulants do not *cause* drug use or addiction. However, because the patient or other people (especially if they have a history of drug abuse) may abuse these medicines, adult supervision is especially important. Some teenagers may try to sell or share their medicine, so it should be kept in a secure place and given by an adult. Methylphenidate will not help people who do not have ADHD to get better grades or do better on tests, but some people think that it will, so they try to take someone else's medicine.

The government considers methylphenidate to be a *controlled substance*. There are special rules for how much of this medicine may be prescribed at one time and how soon prescriptions must be filled after they are written. Prescriptions may not have refills and may not be telephoned to the pharmacy. The doctor must write a new prescription for stimulants each time, and prescriptions may not be written with a date in the future. Prescriptions may be mailed or picked up at the doctor's office.

It is important for the child *not* to chew or crush any of the long-acting tablets or capsules because doing so releases too much medicine all at once. Empty Concerta shells will pass through the digestive system and may be seen in bowel movements. This is harmless. If the patient has trouble swallowing, Concerta may be difficult to swallow or may even get stuck.

For children who cannot swallow pills, a variety of options is available. The capsule long-acting forms may be opened and the tiny beads inside sprinkled onto a spoonful of applesauce. The mixture of applesauce and medicine should be swallowed without chewing. However, the medicine should not be mixed into food and stored, and the beads should not be mixed in liquid. The skin patch may be useful for children who need a long-acting form but who cannot or will not swallow pills. Short-acting methylphenidate in chewable and liquid forms is also available.

437

When using Daytrana (the patch), a new patch is applied to the skin each day. Put the patch on 2 hours before the medicine needs to work. Remove half the liner and put the patch onto clean, dry skin on the hip area, below the waist. Peel off the rest of the liner and stick the whole patch onto the skin. Do not touch the sticky parts of the patch with the hands. Press the patch down with the palm of the hand for 30 seconds, to be sure the patch is firmly attached. It is best to alternate sides daily and to put the patch onto a different part of the skin each day. Do not use a patch more than once. After taking the patch off, fold it in half, sticky side in, and throw it away. If a young child or a pet might take it out of the trash can, flush the patch down the toilet instead of throwing it into the trash.

Some of these medicines have similar names but have different strengths or last different amounts of time (for example, Metadate ER and Metadate CD, or Ritalin LA and Ritalin SR). Be sure to check your prescription to be sure you have the correct medicine from the pharmacy.

Notes

Use this space to take notes or to write down questions you want to ask the doctor.

_____

_____

_____

_____

_____

_____

_____

_____

_____

From Dulcan MK (editor): _Helping Parents, Youth, and Teachers Understand Medications for Behavioral and Emotional Problems: A Resource Book of Medication Information Handouts,_ Third Edition. Washington, DC, American Psychiatric Publishing, 2007

Medication Information
for Youth

Methylphenidate—Methylin, Ritalin, Metadate, Concerta, Daytrana, Focalin

What the Medicine Is Called and What It Is For

The name of your medicine may be confusing. Most drugs have two names: 1) a scientific name that we call a *generic name* and 2) a trade or *brand name*. The generic name of this medicine is methylphenidate. There are a whole lot of different brand names in different forms: Ritalin, Metadate, Methylin, Concerta, Focalin, and Daytrana (a skin patch).

Although all of these medicines have methylphenidate as the active ingredient, they are made differently, so that there are many different ways to take methylphenidate. This helps the doctor to find just the right form of the medicine for each person.

Methylphenidate is called a *stimulant*. It is used to treat attention-deficit/hyperactivity disorder (ADHD or ADD), whether the person has hyperactivity (increased moving around) or not. In people who have ADHD or ADD, parts of the brain are not working as well as they should. An example is the part that controls impulsive actions ("the brakes"). Methylphenidate helps these parts of the brain work better. The medicine can help you pay attention at school and at home. It can make it easier for you to listen to and follow directions, to finish more of your schoolwork and homework with fewer mistakes, to think before you act, to sit still for longer periods, and to get into less trouble with adults or other kids.

How You Take the Medicine

Each of these medicines works for a certain length of time. Your doctor will tell you what times of the day to take the medicine. It is very important that you take it just that way. Sometimes this is at breakfast, lunch, and after school. Long-acting forms may be taken only once a day. Some kids take medicine only on school days, and others take it every day.

Do not skip doses or take extra medicine without asking an adult. If you forget a dose, ask your parent(s) what to do.

Your doctor may talk with you about times that you do not have to take your medicine, such as during school breaks, weekends, and vacations. This is different for each person, so talk to your doctor to be sure you understand this clearly.

This medicine is prescribed only for you. It should never be shared with anyone else.

Do not chew long-acting pills or capsules; you will get too much medicine all at once. If you are taking Concerta, be sure to swallow it with plenty of water.

Caffeine (coffee, tea, soft drinks) may increase the side effects of this medicine.

It is not a good idea to combine a stimulant medicine with cough or cold medicine because rapid pulse rate (heartbeat) or high blood pressure may develop. If a stuffy nose is really bad, it is better to use a nasal spray.

You do not have to tell others that you are taking this medicine, but it is not something you should feel ashamed or embarrassed about. Many young people are helped by stimulant medicines. This medicine is not habit-forming if taken as your doctor says, and you will not become "hooked" on it. It will not make you into a drug user or an addict. Myths (things that people may believe but that are not true) about these medicines usually are told by people who do not understand ADHD. You should talk to your doctor or nurse about any worries you may have.

It is important to remember that that this medicine cannot change you as a person. Successes that you have in your schoolwork or other areas are *your* achievements, not those of the medicine. The medicine cannot make you do anything; it helps you do what *you* want to do. It helps you to be yourself—only calmer, more efficient, more productive, and more successful.

How Your Doctor Will Follow Your Progress

Before giving you the medicine, your doctor or nurse will talk with you and your parent(s) and may measure your height, weight, heart rate (pulse), and blood pressure. Be sure to tell the doctor if you have had very fast or irregular heartbeat, chest pain, dizziness, fainting, shortness of breath, or severe tiredness, especially when exercising. Also tell the doctor if you have had motor or vocal tics (hard-to-control repeated movements or sounds).

Be sure to tell your doctor or nurse about any other medicines or supplements you are taking, including vitamins, herbs, or aids to weight loss or bodybuilding. Also be sure to tell the doctor or nurse if you are using alcohol or drugs. Because many medicines may affect babies, it is very important to tell the doctor if you might be pregnant or if you are at risk of becoming pregnant.

Your teachers may be asked to fill out a form about your grades and behavior in school. A psychologist may give you some tests to see how you learn best.

Most doctors have regular appointments with young people who are taking medicine. You should use these visits to share any concerns you may have about your medicine and to talk about if it has helped you. From time to time, your physician or nurse will measure your height, weight, heart rate (pulse), and blood pressure to be sure that you are in good health while you are taking the medicine. Your doctor also will ask for regular reports from your parents and maybe from your teachers (with your permission) to see how well the medicine is working.

It is hard to say how long you will need to take this medicine. It is sometimes helpful to people even when they go to college and as they become adults. Your doctor will make that decision with you as he or she watches your progress.

How the Medicine Might Affect You

In addition to the ways the medicine can help you, it may have other effects called *side effects*. Different medicines have different side effects. It is helpful to know about some of the most common side effects of your medicine so that you will understand what they are if they happen. Some people do not have any side effects. Some side effects are just uncomfortable, but others may mean a more serious problem with the medicine. Side effects are most common after starting the medicine or after a dose increase. They may go away with time, or the medicine can be adjusted or changed—ask the doctor.

You could have an allergy to any medicine, which might show up as a rash on your skin, swelling, itching, or trouble breathing. With methylphenidate, the rash happens more often under the skin patch.

Please tell your parent(s) and your doctor or nurse about any changes that you notice after taking the medicine. It is especially important to tell a responsible adult if you are feeling depressed or that you may not want to live; if you have thoughts of hurting yourself; or if you begin to feel more irritable, nervous, or restless.

You may have more trouble getting to sleep at night or suddenly have more energy when it is time to go to bed. Your doctor can help you with this problem by changing the time of day that you take your last dose of medicine.

You may not be as hungry as you used to be, and you may not want to eat at mealtimes. Try to eat a good breakfast before taking your medicine. Try to eat something at lunchtime. You also may be more hungry in the evening and want a snack after supper. Eating regularly will help prevent stomachaches and headaches, which are other side effects that some people have. If these feelings do not get better, talk to your doctor. He or she may help you work out a plan to eat many small meals during the day or change the dose of the medicine.

If you are taking Concerta, you may notice the shell of the tablet in your bowel movement. This is harmless.

You may feel slower than usual during the day, especially during the first few weeks that you are taking the medicine. This does not mean that you are sick. It is best to do the things you usually do, including sports. This medicine will not hurt your sports ability. Exercising during the day will help you sleep better at night.

If you notice repeated movements of your muscles or your body or that you are making sounds over and over again that are hard to stop ("tics"), be sure to tell your parent(s) and doctor. This effect is very uncommon and can be helped by adjusting, stopping, or changing your medicine, but your doctor should make this decision.

Tell your parent(s) and the doctor **right away** if you start seeing, hearing, or feeling unusual things or if you have very fast or irregular heartbeat, chest pain, dizziness, fainting, shortness of breath, or severe tiredness, especially when exercising.

If you feel sad or that nothing is fun for more than a few days or if you start hearing or seeing unusual things, be sure to tell your parent(s) or your doctor.

It is very important not to drink alcohol or use marijuana or street drugs. These could make your ADHD problems worse or increase the side effects of this medicine.

Notes

Use this space to take notes or to write down questions you want to ask the doctor or nurse.

_____

_____

_____

_____

_____

_____

_____

_____

_____

_____

_____

_____

_____

From Dulcan MK (editor): *Helping Parents, Youth, and Teachers Understand Medications for Behavioral and Emotional Problems: A Resource Book of Medication Information Handouts*, Third Edition. Washington, DC, American Psychiatric Publishing, 2007

Medication Information for Parents and Teachers

Mirtazapine—Remeron

General Information About Medication

Each child and adolescent is different. No one has exactly the same combination of medical and psychological problems. It is a good idea to talk with the doctor or nurse about the reasons a medicine is being used. It is very important to keep all appointments and to be in touch by telephone if you have concerns. It is important to communicate with the doctor, nurse, or therapist.

It is very important that the medicine be taken exactly as the doctor instructs. However, once in a while, everyone forgets to give a medicine on time. It is a good idea to ask the doctor or nurse what to do if this happens. Do not stop or change a medicine without asking the doctor or nurse first.

If the medicine seems to stop working, it may be because it is not being taken regularly. The youth may be "cheeking" or hiding the medicine or forgetting to take it (especially at school). The doses may be too far apart, or a different dose may be needed. Something at school, at home, or in the neighborhood may be upsetting the youth, or he or she may need special help for learning disabilities or tutoring. Please discuss your concerns with the doctor. **Do not just increase the dose.**

All medicines should be kept in a safe place, out of the reach of children, and should be supervised by an adult. If someone takes too much of a medicine, call the doctor, the poison control center, or a hospital emergency room.

Each medicine has a "generic" or chemical name. Just like laundry detergents or paper towels, some medicines are sold by more than one company under different brand names. The same medicine may be available under a generic name and several brand names. The generic medications are usually less expensive than the brand name ones. The generic medications have the same chemical formula, but they may or may not be exactly the same strength as the brand-name medications. Also, some brands of pills contain dye that can cause allergic reactions. It is a good idea to talk to the doctor and the pharmacist about whether it is important to use a specific brand of medicine.

All medicines can cause an allergic reaction. Examples are hives, itching, rashes, swelling, and trouble breathing. Even a tiny amount of a medicine can cause a reaction in patients who are allergic to that medicine. Be *sure* to talk to the doctor before restarting a medicine that has caused an allergic reaction.

Taking more than one medicine at the same time may cause more side effects or cause one of the medicines to not work as well. Always ask the doctor, nurse, or pharmacist before adding another medicine, whether prescription or over-the-counter. Be sure that each doctor knows about *all* of the medicines your child is taking. Also tell the doctor about any vitamins, herbal medicines, or supplements your child may be taking. Some of these may have side effects alone or when taken with this medication.

Everyone taking medicine should have a physical examination at least once a year.

If you suspect the youth is using drugs or alcohol, please tell the doctor right away.

443

Pregnancy requires special care in the use of medicine. Please tell the doctor immediately if you suspect the teenager is pregnant or might become pregnant.

Printed information like this applies to children and adolescents in general. If you have questions about the medicine, or if you notice changes or anything unusual, please ask the doctor or nurse. As scientific research advances, knowledge increases and advice changes. Even experts do not always agree. Many medicines have not been approved by the U.S. Food and Drug Administration (FDA) for use in children. For this reason, use of the medicine for a particular problem or age group often is not listed in the *Physicians' Desk Reference*. This does not necessarily mean that the medicine is dangerous or does not work, only that the company that makes the medicine has not received permission to advertise the medicine for use in children. Companies often do not apply for this permission because it is expensive to do the tests needed to apply for approval for use in children. Once a medication is approved by the FDA for any purpose, a doctor is allowed to prescribe it according to research and clinical experience.

Note to Teachers

It is a good idea to talk with the parent(s) about the reason(s) that a medication is being used. If the parent(s) sign consent to release information, it is often helpful to talk with the doctor. If the parent(s) give permission, the doctor may ask you to fill out rating forms about your experience with the student's behavior, feelings, academic performance, and medication side effects. This information is very useful in selecting and monitoring medication treatment. If you have observations that you think are important, do not hesitate to share these with the student's parent(s) and treating clinicians.

It is very important that the medicine be taken exactly as the doctor instructs. However, everyone forgets to give a medicine on time once in a while. It is a good idea to ask the parent(s) in advance what to do if this happens. Do not stop or change the time you are giving a medicine at school without parental permission. If a medication is to be taken with food, but lunchtime or snack time changes, be sure to notify the parent(s) so appropriate adjustments can be made.

All medicines should be kept in a secure place and should be supervised by an adult. If someone takes too much of a medicine, follow your school procedure for an urgent medical problem.

Taking medicine is a private matter and is best managed discreetly and confidentially. It is important to be sensitive to the student's feelings about taking medicine.

If you suspect that the student is using drugs or alcohol, please tell the parent(s) or a school counselor right away.

Please tell the parent(s) or school nurse if you suspect medication side effects.

Modifications of the classroom environment or assignments may be useful in addition to medication. The student may need to be evaluated for additional help or for an Individualized Education Plan for learning or behavior.

Any expression of suicidal thoughts or feelings or self-harm by a child or adolescent is a clear signal of distress and should be taken seriously. These behaviors should not be dismissed as "attention seeking."

What Is Mirtazapine (Remeron)?

Mirtazapine is called an *antidepressant*. It is sometimes called a *norepinephrine-serotonin modulator*. It comes in brand name Remeron and generic tablets. The Remeron SolTab quick-dissolving tablets can be dissolved in the mouth, for people who cannot swallow pills.

How Can This Medicine Help?

Mirtazapine has been used successfully to treat depression and anxiety (nervousness) in adults. Now it is beginning to be used to treat emotional and behavioral problems, including anxiety and depression, in children and adolescents. It may take as long as 4–8 weeks to work.

How Does This Medicine Work?

Mirtazapine works by increasing the brain chemicals *serotonin* and *norepinephrine (neurotransmitters)* to more normal activity levels in certain parts of the brain. It has a somewhat different way of working than the antidepressants called selective serotonin reuptake inhibitors (or SSRIs).

How Long Does This Medicine Last?

Mirtazapine lasts the whole day when taken only once a day.

How Will the Doctor Monitor This Medicine?

The doctor will review your child's medical history and physical examination before starting mirtazapine. The doctor may order some blood or urine tests to be sure your child does not have a hidden medical condition that would make it unsafe to use this medicine. The doctor or nurse may measure your child's height, weight, pulse, and blood pressure before starting mirtazapine. The doctor may order other tests, such as a blood cell count and levels of cholesterol and triglycerides (fats in the blood). If there is a family history of diabetes, the doctor may also want to measure sugar in the blood or urine before starting the medicine and at times afterward.

Be sure to tell the doctor if your child or anyone in the family has bipolar illness (manic-depressive illness) or has tried to kill himself or herself.

After the medicine is started, the doctor will want to have regular appointments with you and your child to see how the medicine is working, to see if a dose change is needed, to watch for side effects, to see if mirtazapine is still needed, and to see if any other treatment is needed. The doctor or nurse may check your child's height, weight, pulse, and blood pressure or order tests, such as a blood cell count and levels of cholesterol and triglycerides.

Before using medicine and at times afterward, the doctor may ask your child to fill out a rating scale about depression, to help see how your child is doing.

What Side Effects Can This Medicine Have?

Any medicine can have side effects, including an allergy to the medicine. Because each patient is different, the doctor will monitor the youth closely, especially when the medicine is started. The doctor will work with you to increase the positive effects and decrease the negative effects of the medicine. Please tell the doctor if any of the listed side effects appear or if you think that the medicine is causing any other problems. Not all of the rare or unusual side effects are listed.

445

Side effects are most common after starting the medicine or after a dose increase. Many side effects can be avoided or lessened by starting with a very low dose and increasing it slowly—ask the doctor.

Allergic Reaction

Tell the doctor in a day or two (if possible, before the next dose of medicine):

- Hives
- Itching
- Rash

    Stop the medicine and get *immediate* medical care:

- Trouble breathing or chest tightness
- Swelling of lips, tongue, or throat

Common Side Effects

Tell the doctor within a week or two:

- Daytime sleepiness—Do not allow your child to drive, ride a bicycle or motorcycle, or operate machinery if this happens. This effect may be worse at the lowest dose and get better as the dose is increased.
- Nausea
- Increased appetite and weight gain
- Dry mouth—Have your child try using sugar-free gum or candy.

Occasional Side Effects

Tell the doctor within a week or two:

- Dizziness
- Constipation—Encourage your child to drink more fluids and eat high-fiber foods; if necessary, the doctor may recommend a fiber medicine such as Benefiber or a stool softener such as Colace or mineral oil.
- Lack of energy, tiredness
- Frequent urination

Less Common, but More Serious, Side Effects

Call the doctor *immediately* or go to an emergency room:

- Confusion
- Seizure (fit, convulsion)
- Any infection, especially with sore throat and fever

Serotonin Syndrome

A very serious side effect called *serotonin syndrome* can happen when certain kinds of medicines (including trip-tans taken for migraine headaches) are taken by the same person. *Very* rarely, it can happen at high doses of just one medicine. The early signs are restlessness, confusion, shaking, skin turning red, sweating, and jerking of muscles. If your child has these symptoms, stop the medicine and go to an emergency room right away.

Some Interactions With Other Medicines or Food

Please note that the following are only the most likely interactions with food or other medicines.

Caffeine may increase side effects.

Tagamet (cimetidine) should not be used with mirtazapine, because it increases the levels of mirtazapine and may increase side effects.

Tegretol (carbamazepine) may decrease the levels of mirtazapine and make it not work as well.

It may be dangerous to take Luvox (fluvoxamine) together with mirtazapine.

It can be *very dangerous* to take mirtazapine at the same time as, or even within several weeks of, taking another type of medicine called a *monoamine oxidase inhibitor* (MAOI), such as Eldepryl (selegiline), Nardil (phenelzine), Parnate (tranylcypromine), or Marplan (isocarboxazid).

What Could Happen if This Medicine Is Stopped Suddenly?

No known serious medical withdrawal effects occur if mirtazapine is stopped suddenly, but there may be uncomfortable feelings, or the problem being treated may come back. Ask your child's doctor before stopping the medicine.

How Long Will This Medicine Be Needed?

Your child may need to keep taking the medicine for at least 6–12 months so that the emotional or behavioral problem does not come back.

What Else Should I Know About This Medicine?

In youth who have bipolar disorder (manic depression) or who are at risk for bipolar disorder, any antidepressant medicine may increase the risk of hypomania or mania (excitement, agitation, increased activity, decreased sleep).

Some people taking mirtazapine want to eat a lot more than usual and gain too much weight. It may be very important to be sure that your child has a healthy diet, without too many sweets or fast foods, and that your child has regular exercise.

Black Box Antidepressant Warning

In 2004, an advisory committee to the FDA decided that there might be an increased risk of suicidal behavior for some youth taking medicines called *antidepressants*. In the research studies that the committee reviewed, about 3%–4% of youth with depression who took an antidepressant medicine—and 1%–2% of youth with depression who took a placebo (pill without active medicine)—talked about suicidal thoughts (thinking about

447

killing themselves or wishing they were dead) or did something to harm themselves. This means that almost twice as many youth who were taking an antidepressant to treat their depression talked about suicide or had suicidal behavior compared with youth with depression who were taking inactive medicine. There were *no* completed suicides in any of these research studies, which included more than 4,000 children and adolescents. For youth being treated for anxiety, there was no difference in suicidal talking or behavior between those taking antidepressant medication and those taking placebo.

The FDA told drug companies to add a *black box warning* label to all antidepressant medicines. Because of this label, a doctor (or advanced practice nurse) prescribing one of these medicines has to warn youth and their families that there might be more suicidal thoughts and actions in youth taking these medicines.

On the other hand, in places where more youth are taking the newer antidepressant medicines, the number of adolescents who commit suicide has gotten smaller. Also, thinking about or attempting suicide is more common in surveys of teenagers in the community than it is in depressed youth treated in research studies with antidepressant medicine.

If a youth is being treated with this medicine and is doing well, then no changes are needed as a result of this warning. Increased suicidal talk or action is most likely to happen in the first few months of treatment with a medicine. If your child has recently started this medicine or is about to start, then you and your doctor (or advanced practice nurse) should watch for any changes in behavior. People who are depressed often have suicidal thoughts or actions. It is hard to know whether suicidal thoughts or actions in depressed people are caused by the depression itself or by the medicine. Also, as their depression is getting better, some people talk more about the suicidal thoughts that they had before but did not talk about. As young people get better from depression, they might be at higher risk of doing something about suicidal thoughts that they have had for some time, because they have more energy.

What Should a Parent Do?

1. Be honest with your child about possible risks and benefits of medicine.

2. Talk to your child about whether he or she is having any suicidal thoughts, and tell your child to come to you if he or she is having such thoughts.

3. You, your child, and your child's doctor or nurse should develop a safety plan. Pick adults whom your child can tell if he or she is thinking about suicide.

4. Be sure to tell your child's doctor, nurse, or therapist if you suspect that your child is using alcohol or drugs or if something has happened that might make your child feel worse, such as a family separation, breaking up with a boyfriend or girlfriend, someone close dying or attempting suicide, physical or sexual abuse, or failure in school.

5. Be sure that there are no guns in the home and that all medicines (including over-the-counter medicines like Tylenol) are closely supervised by an adult and kept in a safe place.

6. Watch for new or worse thoughts of suicide, self-harm, depression, anxiety (nerves), feeling very agitated or restless, being angry or aggressive, having more trouble sleeping, or anything else that you see for the first time, seems worse, or worries your child or you. If these appear, contact a mental health professional **right away.** Do not just stop or change the dose of the medicine on your own. If the problems are serious, and you cannot reach one of your clinicians, call a 24-hour psychiatry emergency telephone number or take your child to an emergency room.

Youth on antidepressant medicine should be watched carefully by their parent(s), clinician(s) (doctor, nurse, therapist), and other concerned adults for the first weeks of treatment. It is a good idea to have a visit or telephone call with the doctor, nurse, or therapist weekly for the first month, every 2 weeks for the second month, and after that at least once a month to check for feelings of depression or sadness, thoughts of killing or harming himself or herself, and any problems with the medication. If you have questions, be sure to ask the doctor, nurse, or therapist.

For more information, see http://www.parentsmedguide.org/ (in English and Spanish).

Notes

Use this space to take notes or to write down questions you want to ask the doctor.

_____

_____

_____

_____

_____

_____

_____

_____

_____

_____

_____

_____

_____

From Dulcan MK (editor): _Helping Parents, Youth, and Teachers Understand Medications for Behavioral and Emotional Problems: A Resource Book of Medication Information Handouts_, Third Edition. Washington, DC, American Psychiatric Publishing, 2007

Medication Information
for Youth

Mirtazapine—Remeron

What the Medicine Is Called and What It Is For

The name of your medicine may be confusing. Most drugs have two names: 1) a scientific name that we call a *generic name* and 2) a trade or *brand name*. The generic name of this medicine is mirtazapine. The brand name is Remeron.

Mirtazapine is a new kind of *antidepressant*. Mirtazapine is used to treat depression and anxiety disorders. It helps people who feel very sad or depressed, anxious (nervous), or afraid.

How You Take the Medicine

It is very important to take the medicine exactly as the doctor or nurse tells you. Do not skip doses or take extra medicine without asking an adult. If you forget a dose, ask your parent(s) what to do. It is very important that you take all the pills you are supposed to take each day. Your doctor will probably recommend that you take your medicine at the same time each day, which may be with meals or at bedtime.

It may take several weeks before you notice that the medicine is helping. Waiting for the full effect may take a month or two. You may feel discouraged and think the medicine is never going to help. You may want to give up and stop taking the medicine. Talk to your doctor and parent(s) about how you feel, but **do not stop** taking the medicine unless your doctor tells you to. It is also important not to take extra pills, hoping that you will feel better faster. Doing that could make you very sick.

Caffeine (in coffee, tea, or soft drinks) may make you feel worse.

This medicine is prescribed only for you. It should never be shared with anyone else.

You do not have to tell others that you are taking this medicine, but it is not something you should feel ashamed or embarrassed about. Many young people are helped by mirtazapine. This medicine is not habit-forming, and you cannot become "hooked" on it. You should talk to your doctor or nurse about any questions you have about the medicine. It is important to remember that the medicine *helps* you. It cannot *make* you do anything or change you as a person.

How Your Doctor Will Follow Your Progress

Before giving you the medicine, your doctor or nurse will talk with you and your parent(s) and may measure your height, weight, heart rate (pulse), and blood pressure. The doctor may order some blood or urine tests to be sure you are in good health.

Be sure to tell your doctor or nurse about any other medicines or supplements you are taking, including vitamins, herbs, or aids to weight loss or bodybuilding. Also be sure to tell the doctor or nurse if you are using alcohol or drugs. Because many medicines may affect babies, it is very important to tell the doctor if you might be pregnant or if you are at risk of becoming pregnant. Be sure to tell the doctor if you have had thoughts of hurting yourself, have tried to hurt yourself, or sometimes wish that you were not alive.

Your teachers may be asked to fill out a form about your grades and behavior in school. A psychologist may give you some tests to see how you learn best.

Before starting the medicine and afterward, the doctor may ask you to answer questions on paper about depression and anxiety.

Most doctors have regular appointments with young people who are taking medicine. You should use these visits to share any concerns you may have about your medicine and to talk about if it has helped you. From time to time, your physician or nurse may measure your height, weight, heart rate (pulse), and blood pressure to be sure that you are in good health while you are taking the medicine. Your doctor also will ask for regular reports from your parents and maybe from your teachers (with your permission) to see how well the medicine is working.

Some medicines are started at the amount you will take for as long as you are taking that medicine. Other medicines need to be increased or adjusted until your doctor decides you are taking the right amount. Starting at a low dose and increasing it slowly may lessen side effects. If the medicine helps you, your doctor will probably want you to take it for 6 months to a year if you are taking it to treat depression. If you are taking it for another problem, your doctor will decide how long you will need to take the medicine as he or she watches your progress.

It is not dangerous to stop mirtazapine suddenly, but there might be uncomfortable feelings, such as trouble sleeping, nervousness, irritability, or feeling sick. It is better to decrease it slowly. Do not stop taking a medicine unless the doctor tells you to. If you have any problems after stopping or decreasing this medicine, tell your parent(s) or doctor.

How the Medicine Might Affect You

In addition to the ways the medicine can help you, it may have other effects called *side effects*. Different medicines have different side effects. It is helpful to know about some of the most common side effects of your medicine so that you will understand what they are if they happen. Some people do not have any side effects. Some side effects are just uncomfortable, but others may mean a more serious problem with the medicine. Side effects are most common after starting the medicine or after a dose increase. They may go away with time, or the medicine can be adjusted or changed—ask the doctor.

You could have an allergy to any medicine, which might show up as a rash on your skin, swelling, itching, or trouble breathing.

Please tell your parent(s) and your doctor or nurse about any changes that you notice after taking the medicine. It is especially important to tell a responsible adult if you are feeling depressed or that you may not want to live; if you have thoughts of hurting yourself; or if you begin to feel more irritable, nervous, or restless. Also be sure to tell your parent(s) or doctor if you begin to feel "speeded up" or have trouble sleeping.

Some medicines make people feel sleepy or less coordinated. If this medicine is making you sleepy, it is very important not to drive a car or ride a bicycle or motorcycle. After starting a new medicine or increasing the dose of a medicine, please be extra careful when driving a car, riding a bike, or using machines until you can tell how the medicine affects your alertness, attention, and coordination.

One of the most common side effects of this medicine is feeling tired or sleepy during the day, even if you have had a full night's sleep. After you have been taking the medicine for a few weeks, your body will adjust, and this side effect may go away. If you have had trouble sleeping at night, the medicine can help you sleep better, especially if the doctor tells you to take a dose of medicine in the evening. Other people may feel more restless and excited. Tell your parent(s) or doctor if this is uncomfortable.

Another common side effect is dry mouth. You may be more thirsty than usual and find that you are drinking more water or other liquids. Sucking on sugar-free hard candy or cough drops usually helps. You also could try chewing sugar-free gum or sucking on ice chips. Do not chew the ice; you could hurt your teeth. Also, using lip balm will keep your lips from cracking. It is important to be especially good about brushing your teeth.

You might feel dizzy or light-headed if you stand up fast. Try standing up slowly, especially when getting out of bed in the morning.

Sometimes teenagers who take mirtazapine gain weight. The weight gain may be from increased appetite and also from ways that the medicine changes how the body processes food. It is much easier to prevent weight gain than to lose weight later. It is a good idea to eat a well-balanced diet without "junk food" and with healthy snacks like fruits and vegetables, not sweets or fried foods. It is better to drink water or skim milk, not pop, sodas, soft drinks, or sugary juices. Regular exercise is important for maintaining a healthy weight (and may also help with sleep).

Some other side effects that could happen are headache, not feeling hungry and not wanting to eat much, having an upset stomach, urinating more often, or changes in your bowel movements. You may have a change in your sexual functioning—it is OK to ask the doctor about this. This medicine may make you more likely to get sick if you get overheated, so be sure to drink plenty of liquids and rest in the shade in hot weather. Be sure to let your parent(s) and doctor know if you have a fever or a sore throat.

Please let your parent(s) and doctor know if you notice anything different or unusual about how you feel once you start taking the medicine. This includes good things, such as feeling less sad or less nervous or sleeping better at night.

Notes

Use this space to take notes or to write down questions you want to ask the doctor or nurse.

From Dulcan MK (editor): *Helping Parents, Youth, and Teachers Understand Medications for Behavioral and Emotional Problems: A Resource Book of Medication Information Handouts*, Third Edition. Washington, DC, American Psychiatric Publishing, 2007

Medication Information for Parents and Teachers

Modafinil—Provigil

General Information About Medication

Each child and adolescent is different. No one has exactly the same combination of medical and psychological problems. It is a good idea to talk with the doctor or nurse about the reasons a medicine is being used. It is very important to keep all appointments and to be in touch by telephone if you have concerns. It is important to communicate with the doctor, nurse, or therapist.

It is very important that the medicine be taken exactly as the doctor instructs. However, once in a while, everyone forgets to give a medicine on time. It is a good idea to ask the doctor or nurse what to do if this happens. Do not stop or change a medicine without asking the doctor or nurse first.

If the medicine seems to stop working, it may be because it is not being taken regularly. The youth may be "cheeking" or hiding the medicine or forgetting to take it (especially at school). The doses may be too far apart, or a different dose may be needed. Something at school, at home, or in the neighborhood may be upsetting the youth, or he or she may need special help for learning disabilities or tutoring. Please discuss your concerns with the doctor. **Do not just increase the dose.**

All medicines should be kept in a safe place, out of the reach of children, and should be supervised by an adult. If someone takes too much of a medicine, call the doctor, the poison control center, or a hospital emergency room.

Each medicine has a "generic" or chemical name. Just like laundry detergents or paper towels, some medicines are sold by more than one company under different brand names. The same medicine may be available under a generic name and several brand names. The generic medications are usually less expensive than the brand name ones. The generic medications have the same chemical formula, but they may or may not be exactly the same strength as the brand-name medications. Also, some brands of pills contain dye that can cause allergic reactions. It is a good idea to talk to the doctor and the pharmacist about whether it is important to use a specific brand of medicine.

All medicines can cause an allergic reaction. Examples are hives, itching, rashes, swelling, and trouble breathing. Even a tiny amount of a medicine can cause a reaction in patients who are allergic to that medicine. Be *sure* to talk to the doctor before restarting a medicine that has caused an allergic reaction.

Taking more than one medicine at the same time may cause more side effects or cause one of the medicines to not work as well. Always ask the doctor, nurse, or pharmacist before adding another medicine, whether prescription or over-the-counter. Be sure that each doctor knows about *all* of the medicines your child is taking. Also tell the doctor about any vitamins, herbal medicines, or supplements your child may be taking. Some of these may have side effects alone or when taken with this medication.

Everyone taking medicine should have a physical examination at least once a year.

If you suspect the youth is using drugs or alcohol, please tell the doctor right away.

Pregnancy requires special care in the use of medicine. Please tell the doctor immediately if you suspect the teenager is pregnant or might become pregnant.

Printed information like this applies to children and adolescents in general. If you have questions about the medicine, or if you notice changes or anything unusual, please ask the doctor or nurse. As scientific research advances, knowledge increases and advice changes. Even experts do not always agree. Many medicines have not been approved by the U.S. Food and Drug Administration (FDA) for use in children. For this reason, use of the medicine for a particular problem or age group often is not listed in the *Physicians' Desk Reference*. This does not necessarily mean that the medicine is dangerous or does not work, only that the company that makes the medicine has not received permission to advertise the medicine for use in children. Companies often do not apply for this permission because it is expensive to do the tests needed to apply for approval for use in children. Once a medication is approved by the FDA for any purpose, a doctor is allowed to prescribe it according to research and clinical experience.

Note to Teachers

It is a good idea to talk with the parent(s) about the reason(s) that a medication is being used. If the parent(s) sign consent to release information, it is often helpful to talk with the doctor. If the parent(s) give permission, the doctor may ask you to fill out rating forms about your experience with the student's behavior, feelings, academic performance, and medication side effects. This information is very useful in selecting and monitoring medication treatment. If you have observations that you think are important, do not hesitate to share these with the student's parent(s) and treating clinicians.

It is very important that the medicine be taken exactly as the doctor instructs. However, everyone forgets to give a medicine on time once in a while. It is a good idea to ask the parent(s) in advance what to do if this happens. Do not stop or change the time you are giving a medicine at school without parental permission. If a medication is to be taken with food, but lunchtime or snack time changes, be sure to notify the parent(s) so appropriate adjustments can be made.

All medicines should be kept in a secure place and should be supervised by an adult. If someone takes too much of a medicine, follow your school procedure for an urgent medical problem.

Taking medicine is a private matter and is best managed discreetly and confidentially. It is important to be sensitive to the student's feelings about taking medicine.

If you suspect that the student is using drugs or alcohol, please tell the parent(s) or a school counselor right away.

Please tell the parent(s) or school nurse if you suspect medication side effects.

Modifications of the classroom environment or assignments may be useful in addition to medication. The student may need to be evaluated for additional help or for an Individualized Education Plan for learning or behavior.

Any expression of suicidal thoughts or feelings or self-harm by a child or adolescent is a clear signal of distress and should be taken seriously. These behaviors should not be dismissed as "attention seeking."

What Is Modafinil (Provigil)?

Modafinil is a wake- and vigilance-promoting agent that increases alertness. It is not a stimulant medicine, and it is chemically different from methylphenidate or amphetamine. It comes in brand name Provigil tablets used for the treatment of excessive daytime sleepiness. It is sometimes used to treat attention-deficit/hyperactivity disorder (ADHD or ADD).

How Can This Medicine Help?

Modafinil is used to improve wakefulness in patients with excessive daytime sleepiness associated with narcolepsy or obstructive sleep apnea syndrome. Recently, research has shown that modafinil can improve the symptoms of ADHD, such as trouble paying attention, thinking before acting (impulsivity), and hyperactivity.

How Does This Medicine Work?

It is not known exactly how modafinil works, but it increases alertness in certain parts of the brain. It may decrease the action of some brain cells that promote sleep.

How Long Does This Medicine Last?

Modafinil is usually taken twice a day when treating excessive daytime sleepiness. The first dose is given in the morning and the second dose should be given before 2:00 P.M. because the medication stays in the body for a long time. If the medicine is given later, it can cause trouble sleeping at night. For ADHD, it can be given once a day, in the morning.

How Will the Doctor Monitor This Medicine?

The doctor will review your child's medical history and physical examination before starting modafinil. The doctor may order some blood or urine tests to be sure your child does not have a hidden medical condition. The doctor or nurse may measure your child's height, weight, pulse, and blood pressure before starting modafinil. The doctor may order a sleep study if narcolepsy or sleep apnea is suspected.

After the medicine is started, the doctor will want to have regular appointments with you and your child to see how the medicine is working, to see if a dose change is needed, to watch for side effects, to see if modafinil is still needed, and to see if any other treatment is needed. The doctor or nurse may check your child's height, weight, pulse, and blood pressure.

What Side Effects Can This Medicine Have?

Any medicine can have side effects, including an allergy to the medicine. Because each patient is different, the doctor will monitor the youth closely, especially when the medicine is started. The doctor will work with you to increase the positive effects and decrease the negative effects of the medicine. Please tell the doctor if any of the listed side effects appear or if you think that the medicine is causing any other problems. Not all of the rare or unusual side effects are listed.

Side effects are most common after starting the medicine or after a dose increase. Many side effects can be avoided or lessened by starting with a very low dose and increasing it slowly—ask the doctor.

Allergic Reaction

Tell the doctor in a day or two (if possible, before the next dose of medicine):

- Hives
- Itching
- Rash

   Stop the medicine and get *immediate* medical care:

- Trouble breathing or chest tightness
- Swelling of lips, tongue, or throat

   Overall, modafinil has few side effects. Most side effects of modafinil are not very bad, and they usually go away as soon as the medicine is stopped. Some people may have headaches, decreased appetite, nausea, diarrhea, stomachaches, nervousness (anxiety), or dizziness when taking modafinil. When modafinil is used to treat ADHD, it may cause insomnia (trouble sleeping). Studies of modafinil to treat ADHD use a higher dose than when using modafinil to treat excessive daytime sleepiness. Two youths being treated for ADHD with modafinil developed a very bad skin reaction that could be dangerous. **If your child develops a skin rash with redness or blisters, stop the medicine and call the doctor right away.**

Potentially Severe Side Effects at Very High Doses

Seek medical care *right away*:

- Excitation or agitation
- High blood pressure
- Fast heart rate (pulse), palpitations
- Anxiety or nervousness
- Irritability
- Aggression
- Confusion
- Shaking
- Increased blood clotting

Some Interactions With Other Medicines or Food

Please note that the following are only the most likely interactions with food or other medicines.

   Caution is needed if giving modafinil with medications such as carbamazepine (Tegretol) and antidepressants such as tricyclics and selective serotonin reuptake inhibitors (SSRIs). With modafinil, the levels of these medicines may decrease, and they may be less effective.

   Taking modafinil with diazepam, phenytoin, or propranolol may increase the levels of these medicines and increase the risk of side effects.

What Could Happen if This Medicine Is Stopped Suddenly?

There are no reported symptoms from stopping modafinil suddenly. The excessive daytime sleepiness or ADHD symptoms are likely to return.

How Long Will This Medicine Be Needed?

Because the problems for which modafinil is used are chronic (long lasting), the medicine is likely to be needed for years.

What Else Should I Know About This Medicine?

Modafinil is not related to drug abuse or dependency.

Notes

Use this space to take notes or to write down questions you want to ask the doctor.

_____

_____

_____

_____

_____

_____

_____

_____

_____

_____

_____

From Dulcan MK (editor): *Helping Parents, Youth, and Teachers Understand Medications for Behavioral and Emotional Problems: A Resource Book of Medication Information Handouts*, Third Edition. Washington, DC, American Psychiatric Publishing, 2007

Medication Information
for Youth

Modafinil—Provigil

What the Medicine Is Called and What It Is For

The name of your medicine may be confusing. Most drugs have two names: 1) a scientific name that we call a *generic name* and 2) a trade or *brand name*. The generic name of this medicine is modafinil. Modafinil is used to treat problems of daytime sleepiness (like narcolepsy and sleep apnea). Its brand name is Provigil.

Sometimes modafinil is used for attention-deficit/hyperactivity disorder (ADHD or ADD). It works for ADHD whether or not the person has hyperactivity (increased moving around), and it is different from the stimulant medicines (amphetamine or methylphenidate). In people who have ADHD or ADD, parts of the brain are not working as well as they should. An example is the part that controls impulsive actions ("the brakes"). Modafinil helps these parts of the brain work better. The medicine can help you pay attention at school and at home. It can make it easier for you to listen to and follow directions, to finish more of your schoolwork and homework with fewer mistakes, to think before you act, to sit still for longer periods, and to get into less trouble with adults or other kids.

How You Take the Medicine

It is very important to take the medicine exactly as the doctor or nurse tells you. Do not skip doses or take extra medicine without asking an adult. If you forget a dose, ask your parent(s) what to do.

This medicine is prescribed only for you. It should never be shared with anyone else.

You do not have to tell others that you are taking this medicine, but it is not something you should feel ashamed or embarrassed about. Many young people are helped by modafinil. This medicine is not habit-forming, and you cannot become "hooked" on it. You should talk to your doctor or nurse about any questions you have about the medicine.

It is important to remember that that this medicine cannot change you as a person. Successes that you have in your schoolwork or other areas are *your* achievements, not those of the medicine. The medicine cannot make you do anything; it helps you do what *you* want to do. It helps you to be yourself, only calmer, more efficient, more productive, and more successful.

How Your Doctor Will Follow Your Progress

Before giving you the medicine, your doctor or nurse will talk with you and your parent(s) and will measure your height, weight, heart rate (pulse), and blood pressure. There may be other tests to be sure that you are in good health.

Be sure to tell your doctor or nurse about any other medicines or supplements you are taking, including vitamins, herbs, or aids to weight loss or bodybuilding. Also be sure to tell the doctor or nurse if you are using alcohol or drugs. Because many medicines may affect babies, it is very important to tell the doctor if you might be pregnant or if you are at risk of becoming pregnant.

Your teachers may be asked to fill out a form about your grades and behavior in school. A psychologist may give you some tests to see how you learn best.

Most doctors have regular appointments with young people who are taking medicine. You should use these visits to share any concerns you may have about your medicine and to talk about if it has helped you. From time to time, your physician or nurse may measure your height, weight, heart rate (pulse), and blood pressure to be sure that you are in good health while you are taking the medicine. Your doctor also will ask for regular reports from your parents to see how well the medicine is working. With permission from you and your parent, the doctor may ask for reports from your teacher(s) to see if the medicine is helping your grades, learning, and behavior.

There is no way to know ahead of time how long you will need to take modafinil. The doctor will work together with you and your parent(s) and teachers to decide what is right for you. Sometimes the medicine is needed for a few years, but some people may need to take medicine for sleep problems or ADHD as they go to college and even as adults.

How the Medicine Might Affect You

In addition to the ways the medicine can help you, it may have other effects called *side effects*. Different medicines have different side effects. It is helpful to know about some of the most common side effects of your medicine so that you will understand what they are if they happen. Some people do not have any side effects. Some side effects are just uncomfortable, but others may mean a more serious problem with the medicine. Side effects are most common after starting the medicine or after a dose increase. They may go away with time, or the medicine can be adjusted or changed—ask the doctor.

You could have an allergy to any medicine, which might show up as a rash on your skin, swelling, itching, or trouble breathing.

Please tell your parent(s) and your doctor or nurse about any changes that you notice after taking the medicine. It is especially important to tell a responsible adult if you are feeling depressed or that you may not want to live; if you have thoughts of hurting yourself; or if you begin to feel more irritable, nervous, or restless.

When used to treat ADHD, the most common side effect of modafinil is insomnia (trouble sleeping). Tell your parent(s) and doctor if this happens—the dose of the medicine or the time that the medicine is taken can be changed to help this.

If your skin gets red or has new bumps or lots of blisters, tell your parent(s) *right away*.

Some people have stomachaches or upset stomach, headache, or feel like eating less. Usually these problems get better after your body is used to the medicine or with a lower dose. Let the doctor know if these problems do not go away.

It is very important not to drink alcohol or use marijuana or street drugs. These could make your sleep or ADHD problems worse or increase the side effects of this medicine.

Notes

Use this space to take notes or to write down questions you want to ask the doctor or nurse.

_____

_____

_____

_____

_____

_____

_____

_____

_____

_____

_____

_____

From Dulcan MK (editor): *Helping Parents, Youth, and Teachers Understand Medications for Behavioral and Emotional Problems: A Resource Book of Medication Information Handouts,* Third Edition. Washington, DC, American Psychiatric Publishing, 2007

Medication Information for Parents and Teachers

Nortriptyline—Pamelor

General Information About Medication

Each child and adolescent is different. No one has exactly the same combination of medical and psychological problems. It is a good idea to talk with the doctor or nurse about the reasons a medicine is being used. It is very important to keep all appointments and to be in touch by telephone if you have concerns. It is important to communicate with the doctor, nurse, or therapist.

It is very important that the medicine be taken exactly as the doctor instructs. However, once in a while, everyone forgets to give a medicine on time. It is a good idea to ask the doctor or nurse what to do if this happens. Do not stop or change a medicine without asking the doctor or nurse first.

If the medicine seems to stop working, it may be because it is not being taken regularly. The youth may be "cheeking" or hiding the medicine or forgetting to take it (especially at school). The doses may be too far apart, or a different dose may be needed. Something at school, at home, or in the neighborhood may be upsetting the youth, or he or she may need special help for learning disabilities or tutoring. Please discuss your concerns with the doctor. **Do not just increase the dose.**

All medicines should be kept in a safe place, out of the reach of children, and should be supervised by an adult. If someone takes too much of a medicine, call the doctor, the poison control center, or a hospital emergency room.

Each medicine has a "generic" or chemical name. Just like laundry detergents or paper towels, some medicines are sold by more than one company under different brand names. The same medicine may be available under a generic name and several brand names. The generic medications are usually less expensive than the brand name ones. The generic medications have the same chemical formula, but they may or may not be exactly the same strength as the brand-name medications. Also, some brands of pills contain dye that can cause allergic reactions. It is a good idea to talk to the doctor and the pharmacist about whether it is important to use a specific brand of medicine.

All medicines can cause an allergic reaction. Examples are hives, itching, rashes, swelling, and trouble breathing. Even a tiny amount of a medicine can cause a reaction in patients who are allergic to that medicine. Be *sure* to talk to the doctor before restarting a medicine that has caused an allergic reaction.

Taking more than one medicine at the same time may cause more side effects or cause one of the medicines to not work as well. Always ask the doctor, nurse, or pharmacist before adding another medicine, whether prescription or over-the-counter. Be sure that each doctor knows about *all* of the medicines your child is taking. Also tell the doctor about any vitamins, herbal medicines, or supplements your child may be taking. Some of these may have side effects alone or when taken with this medication.

Everyone taking medicine should have a physical examination at least once a year.

If you suspect the youth is using drugs or alcohol, please tell the doctor right away.

Pregnancy requires special care in the use of medicine. Please tell the doctor immediately if you suspect the teenager is pregnant or might become pregnant.

465

Printed information like this applies to children and adolescents in general. If you have questions about the medicine, or if you notice changes or anything unusual, please ask the doctor or nurse. As scientific research advances, knowledge increases and advice changes. Even experts do not always agree. Many medicines have not been approved by the U.S. Food and Drug Administration (FDA) for use in children. For this reason, use of the medicine for a particular problem or age group often is not listed in the *Physicians' Desk Reference*. This does not necessarily mean that the medicine is dangerous or does not work, only that the company that makes the medicine has not received permission to advertise the medicine for use in children. Companies often do not apply for this permission because it is expensive to do the tests needed to apply for approval for use in children. Once a medication is approved by the FDA for any purpose, a doctor is allowed to prescribe it according to research and clinical experience.

Note to Teachers

It is a good idea to talk with the parent(s) about the reason(s) that a medication is being used. If the parent(s) sign consent to release information, it is often helpful to talk with the doctor. If the parent(s) give permission, the doctor may ask you to fill out rating forms about your experience with the student's behavior, feelings, academic performance, and medication side effects. This information is very useful in selecting and monitoring medication treatment. If you have observations that you think are important, do not hesitate to share these with the student's parent(s) and treating clinicians.

It is very important that the medicine be taken exactly as the doctor instructs. However, everyone forgets to give a medicine on time once in a while. It is a good idea to ask the parent(s) in advance what to do if this happens. Do not stop or change the time you are giving a medicine at school without parental permission. If a medication is to be taken with food, but lunchtime or snack time changes, be sure to notify the parent(s) so appropriate adjustments can be made.

All medicines should be kept in a secure place and should be supervised by an adult. If someone takes too much of a medicine, follow your school procedure for an urgent medical problem.

Taking medicine is a private matter and is best managed discreetly and confidentially. It is important to be sensitive to the student's feelings about taking medicine.

If you suspect that the student is using drugs or alcohol, please tell the parent(s) or a school counselor right away.

Please tell the parent(s) or school nurse if you suspect medication side effects.

Modifications of the classroom environment or assignments may be useful in addition to medication. The student may need to be evaluated for additional help or for an Individualized Education Plan for learning or behavior.

Any expression of suicidal thoughts or feelings or self-harm by a child or adolescent is a clear signal of distress and should be taken seriously. These behaviors should not be dismissed as "attention seeking."

You may notice the following side effects at school:

Common Side Effects

- Dry mouth—Allow the student to chew sugar-free gum or to make extra trips to the water fountain.
- Constipation—Allow the student to drink more fluids or to use the bathroom more often.
- Daytime sleepiness—The student should not drive, ride a bicycle or motorcycle, or operate machinery.
- Dizziness (especially when standing up quickly)—This may happen in the classroom or during physical education). Suggest that the student stand up more slowly.
- Irritability

Occasional Side Effects

- Stuttering
- Increased risk of sunburn (this may be a problem if recess or physical education is outdoors in warm weather)—The student should wear sunscreen or protective clothing or stay out of the sun.

Less Common Side Effects

- Nausea—The student may need to take the medicine after a meal or snack.
- Trouble urinating—The student may need more time in the bathroom.
- Blurred vision—The student may have trouble seeing the blackboard.
- Motor tics (fast, repeated movements) or muscle twitches (jerking movements) of parts of the body
- Increased activity, rapid speech, feeling "speeded up," being very excited or irritable (cranky)
- Skin rash

Rare, but Potentially Serious, Side Effects

Call the parents(s) or follow your school's emergency procedures *immediately* **if the student experiences any of the following side effects:**

- Seizure (fit, convulsion) **(This is a medical emergency.)**
- Very fast or irregular heartbeat **(This is a medical emergency.)**
- Fainting
- Hallucinations (hearing voices or seeing things that are not there)
- Inability to urinate
- Confusion
- Severe change in behavior

What Is Nortriptyline (Pamelor)?

Nortriptyline is called a *tricyclic antidepressant.* It was first used to treat depression but is now used to treat attention-deficit/hyperactivity disorder (ADHD), school phobia, separation anxiety, panic disorder, and some sleep disorders (such as night terrors). It comes in brand name Pamelor and generic capsules and liquid.

How Can This Medicine Help?

Nortriptyline can decrease symptoms of ADHD, anxiety (nervousness), panic, and night terrors or sleepwalking. The medicine may take several weeks to work.

How Does This Medicine Work?

Tricyclic antidepressants affect *neurotransmitters*—the natural substances that are needed for certain parts of the brain to work more normally. They increase the activity of *serotonin* and *norepinephrine* to more normal levels in the parts of the brain that regulate concentration, motivation, and mood.

How Long Does This Medicine Last?

In adults and older teenagers, one dose lasts for a whole day. In younger children, several doses a day may be needed.

How Will the Doctor Monitor This Medicine?

The doctor will review your child's medical history and physical examination, paying special attention to pulse rate, blood pressure, weight, and height, before starting nortriptyline. These measurements will be taken when the dose is increased and occasionally as long as the medicine is continued. The doctor may order some blood or urine tests to be sure your child does not have a hidden medical condition that would make it unsafe to use this medicine.

Tricyclic antidepressants can slow the speed at which signals move through the heart. This effect is not dangerous if the heart is normal, which is why an ECG (electrocardiogram or heart rhythm test) is done before starting the medicine. The ECG may be repeated as the dose is increased and occasionally while the medicine is being taken. Changes in the heart from the medicine usually can be seen on the ECG before they become a problem, so your child's doctor will order an ECG every so often. To find possible hidden heart risks, it is especially important to tell the doctor if your child or anyone in the family has a history of fainting, palpitations, or irregular heartbeat or if anyone in the family died suddenly.

Be sure to tell the doctor if your child or anyone in the family has bipolar illness (manic-depressive illness) or has tried to kill himself or herself.

Because tricyclic antidepressants may increase the risk of seizures (fits, convulsions), the doctor will want to know whether your child has ever had a seizure or a head injury and if there is any family history of epilepsy. Your child's doctor may want to order an EEG (electroencephalogram or brain wave test) before starting the medicine.

Experts do not agree on whether blood tests are needed to measure the level of this medicine. Blood levels seem to be most useful when the doctor suspects that the dose of medicine is too high or too low. The most accurate level is obtained by drawing blood first thing in the morning after at least 5 days on the same dose, approximately 12 hours after the evening dose of medicine and before the morning dose.

After the medicine is started, the doctor will want to have regular appointments with you and your child to see how the medicine is working, to see if a dose change is needed, to watch for side effects, to see if nortriptyline is still needed, and to see if any other treatment is needed. The doctor or nurse may check your child's height, weight, pulse, and blood pressure or order tests, such as an ECG or blood level.

Before using medicine and at times afterward, the doctor may ask your child to fill out a rating scale about anxiety, to help see how your child is doing.

What Side Effects Can This Medicine Have?

Any medicine can have side effects, including an allergy to the medicine. Because each patient is different, the doctor will monitor the youth closely, especially when the medicine is started. The doctor will work with you to increase the positive effects and decrease the negative effects of the medicine. Please tell the doctor if any of the listed side effects appear or if you think that the medicine is causing any other problems. Not all of the rare or unusual side effects are listed.

Side effects are most common after starting the medicine or after a dose increase. Many side effects can be avoided or lessened by starting with a very low dose and increasing it slowly—ask the doctor.

Allergic Reaction

Tell the doctor in a day or two (if possible, before the next dose of medicine):

- Hives
- Itching
- Rash (may be caused by an allergy to the medicine or to a dye in the specific brand of pill)

  Stop medicine and get *immediate* medical care:

- Trouble breathing or chest tightness
- Swelling of lips, tongue, or throat

Common Side Effects

Tell the doctor within a week or two:

- Dry mouth—Have your child try using sugar-free gum or candy.
- Constipation—Encourage your child to drink more fluids and eat high-fiber foods; if necessary, the doctor may recommend a fiber medicine such as Benefiber or a stool softener such as Colace or mineral oil.
- Daytime sleepiness—Do not allow your child to drive, ride a bicycle or motorcycle, or operate machinery if this happens.
- Dizziness—This side effect is worse when the child stands up quickly, especially when getting out of bed in the morning; try having the child stand up slowly.
- Weight gain
- Loss of appetite and weight loss
- Irritability

Occasional Side Effects

Tell the doctor within a week or two:

- Nightmares
- Stuttering
- Blurred vision
- Increase in breast size, nipple discharge, or both (in girls)
- Increase in breast size (in boys)

Less Common, but More Serious, Side Effects

Call the doctor within a day or two:

- High or low blood pressure
- Nausea

- Trouble urinating
- Motor tics (fast, repeated movements) or muscle twitches (jerking movements)
- Increased activity, rapid speech, feeling "speeded up," decreased need for sleep, being very excited or irritable (cranky)

Rare, but Potentially Serious, Side Effects

Call the doctor *immediately*:

- Seizure (fit, convulsion)—**Go to an emergency room.**
- Very fast or irregular heartbeat—**Go to an emergency room.**
- Fainting
- Hallucinations (hearing voices or seeing things that are not there)
- Inability to urinate
- Confusion
- Severe change in behavior

Some Interactions With Other Medicines or Food

Please note that the following are only the most likely interactions with food or other medicines.

Check with your child's doctor before giving your child decongestants or over-the-counter cold medicine.

Taking another antidepressant or Depakote with nortriptyline may increase the level of nortriptyline and increase side effects.

Taking carbamazepine (Tegretol) with nortriptyline may decrease the positive effects of nortriptyline and increase the side effects of carbamazepine.

It can be *very dangerous* to take nortriptyline at the same time as or even within a month of taking another type of medicine called a *monoamine oxidase inhibitor* (MAOI), such as Eldepryl (selegiline), Nardil (phenelzine), Parnate (tranylcypromine), or Marplan (isocarboxazid).

Caffeine may worsen side effects on the heart or symptoms of anxiety. It is best not to drink coffee, tea, or soft drinks with caffeine while taking this medicine.

What Could Happen if This Medicine Is Stopped Suddenly?

Stopping the medicine suddenly or skipping a dose is not dangerous but can be very uncomfortable. Your child may feel like he or she has the flu—with a headache, muscle aches, stomachache, and upset stomach. Behavioral problems, sadness, nervousness, or trouble sleeping also may occur. If these feelings appear every day, the medicine may need to be given more often during each day.

How Long Will This Medicine Be Needed?

There is no way to know how long a person will need to take this medicine. Parents work together with the doctor to determine what is right for each child. The medicine may be needed for a long time. Some people may need to take the medicine even as adults.

What Else Should I Know About This Medicine?

In youth who have bipolar disorder (manic depression) or who are at risk for bipolar disorder, any antidepressant medicine may increase the risk of hypomania or mania (excitement, agitation, increased activity, decreased sleep).

An overdose by accident or on purpose with tricyclic antidepressants is *very dangerous*! You must closely supervise the medicine. You may have to lock up the medicine if your child or teenager is suicidal or if young children live in or visit your home.

Tricyclic antidepressants may cause dry mouth, which could increase the chance of tooth decay. Regular brushing of teeth and checkups with the dentist are especially important.

This medicine causes increased risk of sunburn. Be sure that your child wears sunscreen or protective clothing or stays out of the sun.

People who take tricyclic antidepressants must not drink alcohol or use tranquilizers. Severe sleepiness, loss of consciousness, or even death may result.

Black Box Antidepressant Warning

In 2004, an advisory committee to the FDA decided that there might be an increased risk of suicidal behavior for some youth taking medicines called *antidepressants*. In the research studies that the committee reviewed, about 3%–4% of youth with depression who took an antidepressant medicine—and 1%–2% of youth with depression who took a placebo (pill without active medicine)—talked about suicidal thoughts (thinking about killing themselves or wishing they were dead) or did something to harm themselves. This means that almost twice as many youth who were taking an antidepressant to treat their depression talked about suicide or had suicidal behavior compared with youth with depression who were taking inactive medicine. There were *no* completed suicides in any of these research studies, which included more than 4,000 children and adolescents. For youth being treated for anxiety, there was no difference in suicidal talking or behavior between those taking antidepressant medication and those taking placebo.

The FDA told drug companies to add a *black box warning* label to all antidepressant medicines. Because of this label, a doctor (or advanced practice nurse) prescribing one of these medicines has to warn youth and their families that there might be more suicidal thoughts and actions in youth taking these medicines.

On the other hand, in places where more youth are taking the newer antidepressant medicines, the number of adolescents who commit suicide has gotten smaller. Also, thinking about or attempting suicide is more common in surveys of teenagers in the community than it is in depressed youth treated in research studies with antidepressant medicine.

If a youth is being treated with this medicine and is doing well, then no changes are needed as a result of this warning. Increased suicidal talk or action is most likely to happen in the first few months of treatment with a medicine. If your child has recently started this medicine or is about to start, then you and your doctor (or advanced practice nurse) should watch for any changes in behavior. People who are depressed often have suicidal thoughts or actions. It is hard to know whether suicidal thoughts or actions in depressed people are caused by the depression itself or by the medicine. Also, as their depression is getting better, some people talk more about the suicidal thoughts that they had before but did not talk about. As young people get better from depression, they might be at higher risk of doing something about suicidal thoughts that they have had for some time, because they have more energy.

What Should a Parent Do?

1. Be honest with your child about possible risks and benefits of medicine.
2. Talk to your child about whether he or she is having any suicidal thoughts, and tell your child to come to you if he or she is having such thoughts.

471

3. You, your child, and your child's doctor or nurse should develop a safety plan. Pick adults whom your child can tell if he or she is thinking about suicide.

4. Be sure to tell your child's doctor, nurse, or therapist if you suspect that your child is using alcohol or drugs or if something has happened that might make your child feel worse, such as a family separation, breaking up with a boyfriend or girlfriend, someone close dying or attempting suicide, physical or sexual abuse, or failure in school.

5. Be sure that there are no guns in the home and that all medicines (including over-the-counter medicines like Tylenol) are closely supervised by an adult and kept in a safe place.

6. Watch for new or worse thoughts of suicide, self-harm, depression, anxiety (nerves), feeling very agitated or restless, being angry or aggressive, having more trouble sleeping, or anything else that you see for the first time, seems worse, or worries your child or you. If these appear, contact a mental health professional **right away.** Do not just stop or change the dose of the medicine on your own. If the problems are serious, and you cannot reach one of your clinicians, call a 24-hour psychiatry emergency telephone number or take your child to an emergency room.

Youth on antidepressant medicine should be watched carefully by their parent(s), clinician(s) (doctor, nurse, therapist), and other concerned adults for the first weeks of treatment. It is a good idea to have a visit or telephone call with the doctor, nurse, or therapist weekly for the first month, every 2 weeks for the second month, and after that at least once a month to check for feelings of depression or sadness, thoughts of killing or harming himself or herself, and any problems with the medication. If you have questions, be sure to ask the doctor, nurse, or therapist.

For more information, see http://www.parentsmedguide.org/ (in English and Spanish).

Notes

Use this space to take notes or to write down questions you want to ask the doctor.

_____

_____

_____

_____

_____

_____

_____

_____

Medication Information for Youth

Nortriptyline—Pamelor

What the Medicine Is Called and What It Is For

The name of your medicine may be confusing. Most drugs have two names: 1) a scientific name that we call a *generic name* and 2) a trade or *brand name*. The generic name of this medicine is nortriptyline. The brand name is Pamelor.

Nortriptyline is called an *antidepressant*, or *tricyclic*. Nortriptyline is used to treat depression, trouble paying attention and being too active or acting without thinking, and feeling too anxious (nervous). It can help people who have attention-deficit/hyperactivity disorder (ADHD), fear of going to school or being away from home, panic disorder, or sleep problems such as waking up at night very scared (night terrors) or sleepwalking.

How You Take the Medicine

It is very important to take the medicine exactly as the doctor or nurse tells you. Do not skip doses or take extra medicine without asking an adult. If you miss a dose, you may feel sick, as though you have the flu. It is very important that you take all the pills you are supposed to take each day. Your doctor will probably recommend that you take your medicine at the same time each day, which may be with meals or at bedtime.

It may take several weeks before you notice that the medicine is helping. Waiting for the full effect may take even longer. You may feel discouraged and think the medicine is never going to help. You may want to give up and stop taking the medicine. Talk to your doctor and parent(s) about how you feel, but **do not stop** taking the medicine unless your doctor tells you to. It is also important not to take extra pills, hoping that you will feel better faster. Doing that could make you *very* sick.

Stopping the medicine suddenly or skipping a dose can be very uncomfortable. You may feel like you have the flu—with a headache, muscle aches, stomachache, and upset stomach. If these feelings appear every day, the medicine may need to be given more often during each day.

Caffeine (in coffee, tea, or soft drinks) may make you feel worse.

Do not use any other medicines without talking to your doctor first. Do not use alcohol, marijuana, or street drugs while taking this medicine—**it can be very dangerous.** Skipping your medicine to take drugs does not work because many of the medicines stay in your body for a long time.

This medicine is prescribed only for you. It should never be shared with anyone else.

You do not have to tell others that you are taking this medicine, but it is not something you should feel ashamed or embarrassed about. Many young people are helped by nortriptyline. This medicine is not habit-forming, and you cannot become "hooked" on it. You should talk to your doctor or nurse about any questions you have about the medicine. It is important to remember that the medicine *helps* you. It cannot *make* you do anything or change you as a person.

475

How Your Doctor Will Follow Your Progress

Before giving you the medicine, your doctor or nurse will talk with you and your parent(s) and measure your height, weight, heart rate (pulse), and blood pressure. The doctor may order some blood or urine tests to be sure you are in good health. Be sure to tell the doctor if you have had very fast heartbeat, chest pain, dizziness, or fainting.

Be sure to tell your doctor or nurse about any other medicines or supplements you are taking, including vitamins, herbs, or aids to weight loss or bodybuilding. Also be sure to tell the doctor or nurse if you are using alcohol or drugs. Because many medicines may affect babies, it is very important to tell the doctor if you might be pregnant or if you are at risk of becoming pregnant. Be sure to tell the doctor if you have had thoughts of hurting yourself, have tried to hurt yourself, or sometimes wish that you were not alive.

Before starting nortriptyline, at times of increasing the dose, and every 6 months to a year after that, your doctor will ask for an ECG (electrocardiogram or heart rhythm test) to be done. This test counts your heartbeats through small wires that are taped to your chest. It takes only a few minutes.

Your teachers may be asked to fill out a form about your grades and behavior in school. A psychologist may give you some tests to see how you learn best.

Before starting the medicine and afterward, the doctor may ask you to answer questions on paper about anxiety and depression.

Most doctors have regular appointments with young people who are taking medicine. You should use these visits to share any concerns you may have about your medicine and to talk about if it has helped you. From time to time, your physician or nurse may measure your height, weight, heart rate (pulse), and blood pressure to be sure that you are in good health while you are taking the medicine. You may need to have blood tests to see if you are on the right dose of nortriptyline. Your doctor also will ask for regular reports from your parents and maybe from your teachers (with your permission) to see how well the medicine is working.

Some medicines are started at the amount you will take for as long as you are taking that medicine. Other medicines need to be increased or adjusted until your doctor decides you are taking the right amount. Starting at a low dose and increasing it slowly may lessen side effects. If the medicine helps you, your doctor will probably want you to take it for a long time, maybe even as an adult.

How the Medicine Might Affect You

In addition to the ways the medicine can help you, it may have other effects called *side effects*. Different medicines have different side effects. It is helpful to know about some of the most common side effects of your medicine so that you will understand what they are if they happen. Some people do not have any side effects. Some side effects are just uncomfortable, but others may mean a more serious problem with the medicine. Side effects are most common after starting the medicine or after a dose increase. They may go away with time, or the medicine can be adjusted or changed—ask the doctor.

You could have an allergy to any medicine, which might show up as a rash on your skin, swelling, itching, or trouble breathing.

Please tell your parent(s) and your doctor or nurse about any changes that you notice after taking the medicine. It is especially important to tell a responsible adult if you are feeling depressed or that you may not want to live; if you have thoughts of hurting yourself; or if you begin to feel more irritable, nervous, or restless. Also be sure to tell your parent(s) or doctor if you begin to feel "speeded up" or have trouble sleeping.

Some medicines make people feel sleepy or less coordinated. If this medicine is making you sleepy, it is very important not to drive a car or ride a bicycle or motorcycle. After starting a new medicine or increasing the dose of a medicine, please be extra careful when driving a car, riding a bike, or using machines until you can tell how the medicine affects your alertness, attention, and coordination.

One of the most common side effects of this medicine is feeling tired or sleepy during the day, even if you have had a full night's sleep. After you have been taking the medicine for a few weeks, your body will adjust, and this side effect may go away. If you have had trouble sleeping at night, the medicine can help you sleep better, especially if the doctor tells you to take a dose of medicine in the evening. Other people may feel more restless and excited. Tell your parent(s) or doctor if this is uncomfortable.

Another common side effect is dry mouth. You may be more thirsty than usual and find that you are drinking more water or other liquids. Sucking on sugar-free hard candy or cough drops usually helps. You also could try chewing sugar-free gum or sucking on ice chips. Do not chew the ice; you could hurt your teeth. Also, using lip balm will keep your lips from cracking. It is important to be especially good about brushing your teeth.

Sometimes people taking nortriptyline notice that their heart is beating a little faster than normal. Usually this happens within the first few weeks of taking the medicine and gets better or goes away. However, if you notice that your heart is beating very fast for more than a few minutes when you have not been exercising, if you feel light-headed or dizzy when you are sitting or standing still, or if you faint, you should let your parent(s) and doctor know right away. Some people feel dizzy or light-headed when standing up fast. If this happens, try to get up more slowly, especially first thing in the morning when getting out of bed.

Some people become constipated (have hard bowel movements) when taking this medicine. Try drinking more water and eating more fruits, vegetables, and whole grains. If that does not help, tell your parent(s) or doctor—you may need a medicine to help with this side effect.

Some other side effects that could happen are headache, blurred vision, not feeling hungry and not wanting to eat much, eating more than usual, having an upset stomach, changes in your bowel movements, or trouble passing urine. You may have a change in your sexual functioning or in your breasts—it is OK to ask the doctor about this. This medicine may make you more likely to get sick if you get overheated, so be sure to drink plenty of liquids and rest in the shade in hot weather.

Please let your parent(s) and doctor know if you notice anything different or unusual about how you feel once you start taking the medicine. This includes good things, such as feeling less sad or less nervous or sleeping better at night.

Notes

Use this space to take notes or to write down questions you want to ask the doctor or nurse.

_____

_____

_____

_____

_____

_____

_____

_____

_____

_____

_____

_____

_____

_____

From Dulcan MK (editor): _Helping Parents, Youth, and Teachers Understand Medications for Behavioral and Emotional Problems: A Resource Book of Medication Information Handouts_, Third Edition. Washington, DC, American Psychiatric Publishing, 2007

Medication Information for Parents and Teachers

Olanzapine—Zyprexa

General Information About Medication

Each child and adolescent is different. No one has exactly the same combination of medical and psychological problems. It is a good idea to talk with the doctor or nurse about the reasons a medicine is being used. It is very important to keep all appointments and to be in touch by telephone if you have concerns. It is important to communicate with the doctor, nurse, or therapist.

It is very important that the medicine be taken exactly as the doctor instructs. However, once in a while, everyone forgets to give a medicine on time. It is a good idea to ask the doctor or nurse what to do if this happens. Do not stop or change a medicine without asking the doctor or nurse first.

If the medicine seems to stop working, it may be because it is not being taken regularly. The youth may be "cheeking" or hiding the medicine or forgetting to take it (especially at school). The doses may be too far apart, or a different dose may be needed. Something at school, at home, or in the neighborhood may be upsetting the youth, or he or she may need special help for learning disabilities or tutoring. Please discuss your concerns with the doctor. **Do not just increase the dose.**

All medicines should be kept in a safe place, out of the reach of children, and should be supervised by an adult. If someone takes too much of a medicine, call the doctor, the poison control center, or a hospital emergency room.

Each medicine has a "generic" or chemical name. Just like laundry detergents or paper towels, some medicines are sold by more than one company under different brand names. The same medicine may be available under a generic name and several brand names. The generic medications are usually less expensive than the brand name ones. The generic medications have the same chemical formula, but they may or may not be exactly the same strength as the brand-name medications. Also, some brands of pills contain dye that can cause allergic reactions. It is a good idea to talk to the doctor and the pharmacist about whether it is important to use a specific brand of medicine.

All medicines can cause an allergic reaction. Examples are hives, itching, rashes, swelling, and trouble breathing. Even a tiny amount of a medicine can cause a reaction in patients who are allergic to that medicine. Be *sure* to talk to the doctor before restarting a medicine that has caused an allergic reaction.

Taking more than one medicine at the same time may cause more side effects or cause one of the medicines to not work as well. Always ask the doctor, nurse, or pharmacist before adding another medicine, whether prescription or over-the-counter. Be sure that each doctor knows about *all* of the medicines your child is taking. Also tell the doctor about any vitamins, herbal medicines, or supplements your child may be taking. Some of these may have side effects alone or when taken with this medication.

Everyone taking medicine should have a physical examination at least once a year.

If you suspect the youth is using drugs or alcohol, please tell the doctor right away.

Pregnancy requires special care in the use of medicine. Please tell the doctor immediately if you suspect the teenager is pregnant or might become pregnant.

Printed information like this applies to children and adolescents in general. If you have questions about the medicine, or if you notice changes or anything unusual, please ask the doctor or nurse. As scientific research advances, knowledge increases and advice changes. Even experts do not always agree. Many medicines have not been approved by the U.S. Food and Drug Administration (FDA) for use in children. For this reason, use of the medicine for a particular problem or age group often is not listed in the *Physicians' Desk Reference*. This does not necessarily mean that the medicine is dangerous or does not work, only that the company that makes the medicine has not received permission to advertise the medicine for use in children. Companies often do not apply for this permission because it is expensive to do the tests needed to apply for approval for use in children. Once a medication is approved by the FDA for any purpose, a doctor is allowed to prescribe it according to research and clinical experience.

Note to Teachers

It is a good idea to talk with the parent(s) about the reason(s) that a medication is being used. If the parent(s) sign consent to release information, it is often helpful to talk with the doctor. If the parent(s) give permission, the doctor may ask you to fill out rating forms about your experience with the student's behavior, feelings, academic performance, and medication side effects. This information is very useful in selecting and monitoring medication treatment. If you have observations that you think are important, do not hesitate to share these with the student's parent(s) and treating clinicians.

It is very important that the medicine be taken exactly as the doctor instructs. However, everyone forgets to give a medicine on time once in a while. It is a good idea to ask the parent(s) in advance what to do if this happens. Do not stop or change the time you are giving a medicine at school without parental permission. If a medication is to be taken with food, but lunchtime or snack time changes, be sure to notify the parent(s) so appropriate adjustments can be made.

All medicines should be kept in a secure place and should be supervised by an adult. If someone takes too much of a medicine, follow your school procedure for an urgent medical problem.

Taking medicine is a private matter and is best managed discreetly and confidentially. It is important to be sensitive to the student's feelings about taking medicine.

If you suspect that the student is using drugs or alcohol, please tell the parent(s) or a school counselor right away.

Please tell the parent(s) or school nurse if you suspect medication side effects.

Modifications of the classroom environment or assignments may be useful in addition to medication. The student may need to be evaluated for additional help or for an Individualized Education Plan for learning or behavior.

Any expression of suicidal thoughts or feelings or self-harm by a child or adolescent is a clear signal of distress and should be taken seriously. These behaviors should not be dismissed as "attention seeking."

What Is Olanzapine (Zyprexa)?

This medicine is called an *atypical* or *second-generation antipsychotic*. It is sometimes called an *atypical psychotropic agent* or simply an *atypical*. It comes in brand name Zyprexa tablets, Zyprexa Zydis rapid-dissolving tablets, and a fast-acting injection (shot). The Zydis form melts fast in the mouth.

How Can This Medicine Help?

Olanzapine is used to treat psychosis, such as in schizophrenia, mania, or very severe depression. It can reduce *positive symptoms* such as hallucinations (hearing voices or seeing things that are not there); delusions (troubling beliefs that other people do not share); agitation; and very unusual thinking, speech, and behavior. It is also used to lessen the *negative symptoms* of schizophrenia, such as lack of interest in doing things (apathy), lack of motivation, social withdrawal, and lack of energy.

Olanzapine may be used as a *mood stabilizer* in patients with bipolar disorder (manic-depressive illness) or severe mood swings. It can reduce mania and may be able to help maintain a stable mood over the long term.

Sometimes olanzapine is used to reduce severe aggression or very serious behavioral problems in young people with conduct disorder, mental retardation, autism, or pervasive developmental disorder.

Olanzapine may be used for behavior problems after a head injury.

It is also used to reduce motor and vocal tics (fast, repeated movements or sounds) and behavioral problems in people with Tourette's disorder.

This medicine is very powerful and is used to treat very serious problems or symptoms that other medicines do not help. Be patient; the positive effects of this medicine may not appear for 2–3 weeks.

How Does This Medicine Work?

Cells in the brain communicate using chemicals called *neurotransmitters*. Too much or too little of these substances in parts of the brain can cause problems. Olanzapine works by blocking the action of two of these neurotransmitters, *dopamine* and *serotonin*, in certain areas of the brain.

How Long Does This Medicine Last?

Olanzapine usually can be taken only once a day.

How Will the Doctor Monitor This Medicine?

The doctor will review your child's medical history and physical examination before starting olanzapine. The doctor may order some blood or urine tests to be sure your child does not have a hidden medical condition that would make it unsafe to use this medicine. The doctor or nurse will measure your child's height, weight, pulse, and blood pressure before starting olanzapine. The doctor may order other tests, such as baseline tests for blood sugar and cholesterol.

Be sure to tell the doctor if anyone in the family has diabetes, high blood pressure, high cholesterol, or heart disease.

Before starting olanzapine and every so often afterward, a test such as the AIMS (Abnormal Involuntary Movement Scale) may be used to check your child's tongue, legs, and arms for unusual movements that could be caused by the medicine.

After the medicine is started, the doctor will want to have regular appointments with you and your child to see how the medicine is working, to see if a dose change is needed, to watch for side effects, to see if olanzapine is still needed, and to see if any other treatment is needed. The doctor or nurse may check your child's height, weight, pulse, and blood pressure and watch for abnormal movements. Sometimes blood tests are needed to watch for diabetes or increased cholesterol.

What Side Effects Can This Medicine Have?

Any medicine can have side effects, including an allergy to the medicine. Because each patient is different, the doctor will monitor the youth closely, especially when the medicine is started. The doctor will work with you to increase the positive effects and decrease the negative effects of the medicine. Please tell the doctor if any of the listed side effects appear or if you think that the medicine is causing any other problems. Not all of the rare or unusual side effects are listed.

Side effects are most common after starting the medicine or after a dose increase. Many side effects can be avoided or lessened by starting with a very low dose and increasing it slowly—ask the doctor.

Allergic Reaction

Tell the doctor in a day or two (if possible, before the next dose of medicine):

- Hives
- Itching
- Rash

Stop the medicine and get *immediate* medical care:

- Trouble breathing or chest tightness
- Swelling of lips, tongue, or throat

Common, but Not Usually Serious, Side Effects

Discuss the following side effects with your child's doctor when convenient. Side effects often can be helped by lowering the dose of medicine, changing the times medicine is taken, or adding another medicine—ask the doctor.

- Daytime sleepiness or tiredness—Do not allow your child to drive, ride a bicycle or motorcycle, or operate machinery if this happens. This problem may be lessened by taking the medicine at bedtime.
- Dry mouth—Have your child try using sugar-free gum or candy.
- Constipation—Encourage your child to drink more fluids and eat high-fiber foods; if necessary, the doctor may recommend a fiber medicine such as Benefiber or a stool softener such as Colace or mineral oil.
- Dizziness—This side effect is worse when the child stands up quickly, especially when getting out of bed in the morning; try having the child stand up slowly.
- Increased appetite
- Weight gain—Seek nutritional counseling; provide your child with low-calorie snacks and encourage regular exercise.

Less Common, but Not Usually Serious, Side Effects

Discuss the following side effects with your child's doctor when convenient.

- Drooling
- Increased restlessness or inability to sit still
- Shaking of hands and fingers
- Decreased or slowed movement and decreased facial expressions
- Decreased sexual interest or ability
- Changes in menstrual cycle
- Increase in breast size or discharge from the breasts (in both boys and girls)—This may go away with time.

Less Common, but Potentially Serious, Side Effects

Call the doctor *immediately:*

- Stiffness of the tongue, jaw, neck, back, or legs
- Seizure (fit, convulsion)—This is more common in people with a history of seizures or head injury.
- Increased thirst, frequent urination (having to go to the bathroom often), lethargy, tiredness, dizziness, and blurred vision—These could be signs of diabetes (especially if your child is overweight or there is a family history of diabetes). **Talk to a doctor within a day.**

Very Rare, but Serious, Side Effects

- Extreme stiffness or lack of movement, very high fever, mental confusion, irregular pulse rate, or eye pain—**This is a medical emergency. Go to an emergency room right away.**
- Sudden stiffness and inability to breathe or swallow—**Go to an emergency room or call 911.** Tell the paramedics, nurses, and doctors that the patient is taking olanzapine. Other medicines can be used to treat this problem fast.

What Else Should I Know About Side Effects?

Most side effects lessen over time. If they are troublesome, talk with your child's doctor. Some side effects can be decreased by taking a smaller dose of medicine, by stopping the medicine, by changing to another medicine, or by adding another medicine.

Many people who take olanzapine gain weight. Children seem to have more problems with this than adults. The weight gain may be from increased appetite and from ways that the medicine changes how the body processes food. Olanzapine may also change the way that the body handles glucose (sugar) and cause high levels (hyperglycemia). People who take olanzapine, especially those who gain a lot of weight, are at increased risk of developing diabetes and of having increased fats (lipids—cholesterol and triglycerides) in their blood. Over time, both diabetes and increased fats in the blood may lead to heart disease, stroke, and other complications. The FDA has put warnings on all atypical agents about the increased risks of hyperglycemia, diabetes, and increased blood cholesterol and triglycerides when taking one of these medicines. It is much easier to prevent weight gain than to lose weight later. When your child first starts taking olanzapine, it is a good idea to be sure that he or she eats a well-balanced diet without "junk food" and with healthy snacks like fruits and vegetables, not sweets or fried foods. He or she should drink water or skim milk, not pop, sodas, soft drinks, or sugary juices. Regular exercise is important for maintaining a healthy weight (and may also help with sleep).

The medicine may increase the level of *prolactin*, a natural hormone made in the part of the brain called the *pituitary*. This may cause side effects such as breast tenderness or swelling or production of milk in both boys and girls. It also may interfere with sexual functioning in teenage boys and with regular menstrual cycles (periods) in teenage girls. A blood test can measure the level of prolactin. If these side effects do not go away and are troublesome, talk with your child's doctor about substituting another medicine for olanzapine.

One very rare side effect that may not go away is *tardive dyskinesia* (or TD). Patients with tardive dyskinesia have involuntary movements (movements that they cannot help making) of the body, especially the mouth and tongue. The patient may look as though he or she is making faces over and over again. Jerky movements of the arms, legs, or body may occur. There may be fine, wormlike, or sudden repeated movements of the tongue, or the person may appear to be chewing something or smacking or puckering his or her lips. The fingers may look as though they are rolling something. If you notice any unusual movements, be sure to tell the doctor. The doctor may use the AIMS test to look for these movements.

Neuroleptic malignant syndrome is a very rare side effect that can lead to death. The symptoms are severe muscle stiffness, high fever, increased heart rate and blood pressure, irregular heartbeat (pulse), and sweating. It may lead to unconsciousness. If you suspect this, **call 911 or go to an emergency room right away.**

Some Interactions With Other Medicines or Food

Please note that the following are only the most likely interactions with food or other medicines.

Olanzapine may be taken with or without food.

Fluvoxamine (Luvox), fluoxetine (Prozac), and some antibiotics such as erythromycin can increase the levels of olanzapine and increase the risk of side effects.

Carbamazepine (Tegretol) and oxcarbazepine (Trileptal) can decrease the levels of olanzapine so that it does not work as well.

Heart problems are rare with olanzapine but are more common if other medicines that affect the heart are being taken also. Be sure to tell all your child's doctors and your pharmacist about all medications your child is taking.

It is better to limit drinks with caffeine (coffee, tea, soft drinks) because caffeine works in the opposite way from this medicine, and the positive effects might be decreased.

What Could Happen if This Medicine Is Stopped Suddenly?

Involuntary movements, or *withdrawal dyskinesias*, may appear within 1–4 weeks of lowering the dose or stopping the medicine. Usually these go away, but they can last for days to months. If olanzapine is stopped suddenly, emotional disturbance (such as irritability, nervousness, moodiness, or oppositional behavior) or physical problems (such as stomachache, loss of appetite, nausea, vomiting, diarrhea, sweating, indigestion, trouble sleeping, trembling, or shaking) may appear. These problems usually last only a few days to a few weeks. If they happen, you should tell your child's doctor. The medicine dose may need to be lowered more slowly (tapered). Always check with the doctor before stopping a medicine.

How Long Will This Medicine Be Needed?

How long your child will need to take this medicine depends partly on the reason that it was prescribed. Some problems last for only a few months, whereas others last much longer. It is important to ask the doctor whether medicine is still needed, especially with medicines as powerful as this one. Every few months, you should discuss with your child's doctor the reasons for using olanzapine and whether the medicine may be stopped or the dose lowered.

What Else Should I Know About This Medicine?

There are other medicines that are used for the same kinds of problems. If your child is having bad side effects or the medicine does not seem to be working, ask the doctor if another medicine might work as well or better and have fewer side effects for your child. Each person reacts differently to medicines.

It is not a good idea to split or crush the tablets, because their coating can be very sharp when broken.

When giving Zydis, peel off the foil on both sides; do not push the tablet through the foil. The disk should be placed in the mouth right away and allowed to melt before swallowing.

Pharmacies sometimes confuse Zyprexa with Zyrtec (an antihistamine). If your child's prescription is new or the pills look different, be sure to check with the pharmacist.

Taking this medicine could make overheating or heatstroke more likely. Have your child decrease activity in hot weather, stay out of the sun, and drink water to prevent this.

Notes

Use this space to take notes or to write down questions you want to ask the doctor.

_____

_____

_____

_____

_____

_____

_____

_____

_____

_____

From Dulcan MK (editor): *Helping Parents, Youth, and Teachers Understand Medications for Behavioral and Emotional Problems: A Resource Book of Medication Information Handouts,* Third Edition. Washington, DC, American Psychiatric Publishing, 2007

Medication Information for Youth

Olanzapine—Zyprexa

What the Medicine Is Called and What It Is For

The name of your medicine may be confusing. Most drugs have two names: 1) a scientific name that we call a *generic name* and 2) a trade or *brand name*. The generic name of this medicine is olanzapine. The brand name is Zyprexa.

Olanzapine is called an *atypical* medicine. It helps people who feel very confused and have severe problems thinking clearly. It can lessen hallucinations (seeing or hearing things that are not really there) and delusions (troubling beliefs that other people do not share). The medicine also can improve *negative symptoms*, such as lack of interest in doing things, lack of motivation, loss of interest in friends, and decreased energy. It helps people who have severe depression or mood swings. This medicine also is sometimes used to help young people who have mania or severe depression or who get very angry and hit people or break things.

How You Take the Medicine

It is very important to take the medicine exactly as the doctor or nurse tells you. Do not skip doses or take extra medicine without asking an adult. If you forget a dose, ask your parent(s) what to do.

It is not a good idea to split or crush the tablets, because the coating can be very sharp when broken.

Zyprexa Zydis is a fast-dissolving tablet. Peel the foil off on both sides; do not push the tablet through the foil. Put the disk in your mouth right away and let it melt before swallowing.

Your doctor will tell you how much medicine to take and how often to take it so that it can help you the most. It is *very important* that you take all the pills you are supposed to take each day. Your doctor will probably recommend that you take your medicine at the same time each day, which may be with meals or at bedtime.

It may be several weeks or longer before you notice the full effect. You may feel discouraged and think the medicine is never going to help. You may want to give up and stop taking the medicine. Talk to your doctor and parent(s) about how you feel, but **do not stop** taking your medicine unless your doctor tells you to. It also is important not to take extra pills hoping that you will feel better faster. Doing that could make you very sick.

This medicine is prescribed only for you. It should never be shared with anyone else.

You do not have to tell others that you are taking this medicine, but it is not something you should feel ashamed or embarrassed about. Many young people are helped by olanzapine. This medicine is not habit-forming, and you cannot become "hooked" on it. You should talk to your doctor or nurse about any questions you have about the medicine. It is important to remember that the medicine *helps* you. It cannot *make* you do anything or change you as a person.

How Your Doctor Will Follow Your Progress

Before giving you the medicine, your doctor or nurse will talk with you and your parent(s) and may measure your height, weight, heart rate (pulse), and blood pressure. There may be other tests, such as blood tests for sugar and cholesterol. Before you start taking the medicine and every so often afterward, the doctor or nurse will look at your tongue, arms, and legs to check for unusual movements. This is called the AIMS (Abnormal Involuntary Movement Scale) test.

Be sure to tell your doctor or nurse about any other medicines or supplements you are taking, including vitamins, herbs, or aids to weight loss or bodybuilding. Also be sure to tell the doctor or nurse if you are using alcohol or drugs. Because many medicines may affect babies, it is very important to tell the doctor if you might be pregnant or if you are at risk of becoming pregnant.

Your teachers may be asked to fill out a form about your grades and behavior in school. A psychologist may give you some tests to see how you learn best.

Most doctors have regular appointments with young people who are taking medicine. You should use these visits to share any concerns you may have about your medicine and to talk about if it has helped you. From time to time, your physician or nurse may measure your height, weight, heart rate (pulse), and blood pressure to be sure that you are in good health while you are taking the medicine. There may be blood tests to watch for diabetes or high cholesterol. Your doctor also will ask for regular reports from your parents and maybe from your teachers (with your permission) to see how well the medicine is working.

If the medicine helps you, your doctor will probably want you to take it for several months to a year. Your doctor will decide how long you will need to take the medicine as he or she watches your progress.

How the Medicine Might Affect You

In addition to the ways the medicine can help you, it may have other effects called *side effects*. Different medicines have different side effects. It is helpful to know about some of the most common side effects of your medicine so that you will understand what they are if they happen. Some people do not have any side effects. Some side effects are just uncomfortable, but others may mean a more serious problem with the medicine. Side effects are most common after starting the medicine or after a dose increase. They may go away with time, or the medicine can be adjusted or changed—ask the doctor.

You could have an allergy to any medicine, which might show up as a rash on your skin, swelling, itching, or trouble breathing.

Please tell your parent(s) and your doctor or nurse about any changes that you notice after taking the medicine. It is especially important to tell a responsible adult if you are feeling depressed or that you may not want to live; if you have thoughts of hurting yourself; or if you begin to feel more irritable, nervous, or restless. Also be sure to tell your parent(s) or doctor if you begin to feel more "speeded up" or have more trouble sleeping.

One of the most common side effects of these medicines is feeling tired or sleepy during the day, even if you have had a full night's sleep. If this medicine is making you sleepy, it is very important not to drive a car or ride a bicycle or motorcycle. After starting the medicine or increasing the dose of medicine, please be extra careful when driving a car, riding a bike, or using machines until you can tell how the medicine affects your alertness, attention, and coordination. After you have been taking the medicine for a few weeks, your body will adjust, and this side effect will likely go away. If you had trouble sleeping at night before you began taking the medicine, it can help you sleep better, especially if the doctor tells you to take a dose of medicine in the evening.

Another common side effect is dry mouth. You may be more thirsty than usual and find that you are drinking more water or other liquids than usual. Sucking on sugar-free hard candy or cough drops usually helps.

You also could try chewing sugar-free gum or sucking on ice chips. Do not chew the ice; you could hurt your teeth. Also, using lip balm will keep your lips from cracking. It is important to be especially good about brushing your teeth.

If you get very thirsty, have to go to the bathroom a lot, feel *very* tired, or have dizziness or blurred vision, be sure to tell your parent(s) or doctor.

Taking this medicine could make you more likely to get badly sunburned or very sick in hot weather. Be sure to drink plenty of liquids and cover up or use sunscreen when you go outside in hot weather. Be careful to rest in the shade and not get overheated.

Sometimes teenagers who take olanzapine gain weight. The weight gain may be from increased appetite and also from ways that the medicine changes how the body processes food. People who take olanzapine, especially those who gain a lot of weight, might be at increased risk of developing diabetes and of having increased fats (lipids—cholesterol and triglycerides) in their blood. Over time, both diabetes and increased fats in the blood may lead to heart disease, stroke, and other complications. The U.S. Food and Drug Administration has put warnings about these problems on all medicines like olanzapine. It is much easier to prevent weight gain than to lose weight later. It is a good idea to eat a well-balanced diet without "junk food" and with healthy snacks like fruits and vegetables, not sweets or fried foods. It is better to drink water or skim milk, not pop, sodas, soft drinks, or sugary juices. Regular exercise is important for maintaining a healthy weight (and may also help with sleep).

You may notice changes in your sexual functioning or in your breasts—it is OK to ask the doctor about this.

Olanzapine is a very powerful medicine. Some side effects include feeling nervous, restless, or shaky or having stiff muscles. Talk with your doctor about these side effects. They can be helped by adding another medicine, adjusting the dose, or switching to another medicine.

Another, more serious, side effect can be longer lasting and more difficult to treat. This very rare side effect is called *tardive dyskinesia* (or TD). A person taking olanzapine may develop movements of the mouth, tongue, face, arms, legs, or body that are not being made on purpose. This side effect can go away when the medicine is stopped, but in some people it does not go away. Your doctor will explain this effect to you and your parent(s) and how he or she will watch for any signs that you are developing this problem. Be sure to ask your doctor any questions that you may have about this, but do not worry too much about it. It hardly ever happens to teenagers.

You should tell your parent(s) and doctor if you notice anything different or unusual about how you feel once you start taking the medicine. This includes good things, such as feeling less confused, feeling less sad, not hearing voices anymore, or sleeping better at night.

Notes

Use this space to take notes or to write down questions you want to ask the doctor or nurse.

_____

_____

_____

_____

_____

_____

_____

_____

_____

_____

_____

_____

_____

From Dulcan MK (editor): _Helping Parents, Youth, and Teachers Understand Medications for Behavioral and Emotional Problems: A Resource Book of Medication Information Handouts,_ Third Edition. Washington, DC, American Psychiatric Publishing, 2007

Medication Information for Parents and Teachers

Oxcarbazepine—Trileptal

General Information About Medication

Each child and adolescent is different. No one has exactly the same combination of medical and psychological problems. It is a good idea to talk with the doctor or nurse about the reasons a medicine is being used. It is very important to keep all appointments and to be in touch by telephone if you have concerns. It is important to communicate with the doctor, nurse, or therapist.

It is very important that the medicine be taken exactly as the doctor instructs. However, once in a while, everyone forgets to give a medicine on time. It is a good idea to ask the doctor or nurse what to do if this happens. Do not stop or change a medicine without asking the doctor or nurse first.

If the medicine seems to stop working, it may be because it is not being taken regularly. The youth may be "cheeking" or hiding the medicine or forgetting to take it (especially at school). The doses may be too far apart, or a different dose may be needed. Something at school, at home, or in the neighborhood may be upsetting the youth, or he or she may need special help for learning disabilities or tutoring. Please discuss your concerns with the doctor. **Do not just increase the dose.**

All medicines should be kept in a safe place, out of the reach of children, and should be supervised by an adult. If someone takes too much of a medicine, call the doctor, the poison control center, or a hospital emergency room.

Each medicine has a "generic" or chemical name. Just like laundry detergents or paper towels, some medicines are sold by more than one company under different brand names. The same medicine may be available under a generic name and several brand names. The generic medications are usually less expensive than the brand name ones. The generic medications have the same chemical formula, but they may or may not be exactly the same strength as the brand-name medications. Also, some brands of pills contain dye that can cause allergic reactions. It is a good idea to talk to the doctor and the pharmacist about whether it is important to use a specific brand of medicine.

All medicines can cause an allergic reaction. Examples are hives, itching, rashes, swelling, and trouble breathing. Even a tiny amount of a medicine can cause a reaction in patients who are allergic to that medicine. Be *sure* to talk to the doctor before restarting a medicine that has caused an allergic reaction.

Taking more than one medicine at the same time may cause more side effects or cause one of the medicines to not work as well. Always ask the doctor, nurse, or pharmacist before adding another medicine, whether prescription or over-the-counter. Be sure that each doctor knows about *all* of the medicines your child is taking. Also tell the doctor about any vitamins, herbal medicines, or supplements your child may be taking. Some of these may have side effects alone or when taken with this medication.

Everyone taking medicine should have a physical examination at least once a year.

If you suspect the youth is using drugs or alcohol, please tell the doctor right away.

Pregnancy requires special care in the use of medicine. Please tell the doctor immediately if you suspect the teenager is pregnant or might become pregnant.

491

Printed information like this applies to children and adolescents in general. If you have questions about the medicine, or if you notice changes or anything unusual, please ask the doctor or nurse. As scientific research advances, knowledge increases and advice changes. Even experts do not always agree. Many medicines have not been approved by the U.S. Food and Drug Administration (FDA) for use in children. For this reason, use of the medicine for a particular problem or age group often is not listed in the *Physicians' Desk Reference*. This does not necessarily mean that the medicine is dangerous or does not work, only that the company that makes the medicine has not received permission to advertise the medicine for use in children. Companies often do not apply for this permission because it is expensive to do the tests needed to apply for approval for use in children. Once a medication is approved by the FDA for any purpose, a doctor is allowed to prescribe it according to research and clinical experience.

Note to Teachers

It is a good idea to talk with the parent(s) about the reason(s) that a medication is being used. If the parent(s) sign consent to release information, it is often helpful to talk with the doctor. If the parent(s) give permission, the doctor may ask you to fill out rating forms about your experience with the student's behavior, feelings, academic performance, and medication side effects. This information is very useful in selecting and monitoring medication treatment. If you have observations that you think are important, do not hesitate to share these with the student's parent(s) and treating clinicians.

It is very important that the medicine be taken exactly as the doctor instructs. However, everyone forgets to give a medicine on time once in a while. It is a good idea to ask the parent(s) in advance what to do if this happens. Do not stop or change the time you are giving a medicine at school without parental permission. If a medication is to be taken with food, but lunchtime or snack time changes, be sure to notify the parent(s) so appropriate adjustments can be made.

All medicines should be kept in a secure place and should be supervised by an adult. If someone takes too much of a medicine, follow your school procedure for an urgent medical problem.

Taking medicine is a private matter and is best managed discreetly and confidentially. It is important to be sensitive to the student's feelings about taking medicine.

If you suspect that the student is using drugs or alcohol, please tell the parent(s) or a school counselor right away.

Please tell the parent(s) or school nurse if you suspect medication side effects.

Modifications of the classroom environment or assignments may be useful in addition to medication. The student may need to be evaluated for additional help or for an Individualized Education Plan for learning or behavior.

Any expression of suicidal thoughts or feelings or self-harm by a child or adolescent is a clear signal of distress and should be taken seriously. These behaviors should not be dismissed as "attention seeking."

What Is Oxcarbazepine (Trileptal)?

Oxcarbazepine was first used to treat seizures (fits, convulsions), so it is sometimes called an *anticonvulsant*. Now it is also used for behavioral problems or bipolar disorder (manic-depressive disorder) regardless of whether the patient has seizures. It also may be used when the patient has a history of severe mood changes, sometimes called *mood swings*. When used in psychiatry, this medicine is more commonly called a *mood stabilizer*.

Oxcarbazepine comes in brand name Trileptal tablets and liquid.

How Can This Medicine Help?

Oxcarbazepine can reduce aggression, anger, and severe mood swings. It also can treat mania.

How Does This Medicine Work?

Oxcarbazepine is thought to work by stabilizing a part of the brain cell (the cell membrane or envelope) and by changing the concentrations of certain *neurotransmitters* (chemicals in the brain) such as *GABA* and *glutamate*.

How Long Does This Medicine Last?

Oxcarbazepine needs to be taken twice a day.

How Will the Doctor Monitor This Medicine?

The doctor will review your child's medical history and physical examination before starting oxcarbazepine. The doctor may order some blood or urine tests to be sure your child does not have a hidden kidney condition that would make it unsafe to use this medicine. The doctor or nurse will measure your child's height, weight, pulse, and blood pressure before starting oxcarbazepine.

After the medicine is started, the doctor will want to have regular appointments with you and your child to see how the medicine is working, to see if a dose change is needed, to watch for side effects, to see if oxcarbazepine is still needed, and to see if any other treatment is needed. The doctor or nurse may check your child's height, weight, pulse, and blood pressure. The doctor will need to order blood tests every month or so to make sure that the medicine is at the right dose and to check for side effects, such as a decreased level of sodium in the blood. Blood should be drawn first thing in the morning, 10–12 hours after the evening dose and before the morning dose. Many things can change the levels of oxcarbazepine, so tests may be needed every week when the dose of this or other medicines is being changed.

What Side Effects Can This Medicine Have?

Any medicine can have side effects, including an allergy to the medicine. Because each patient is different, the doctor will monitor the youth closely, especially when the medicine is started. The doctor will work with you to increase the positive effects and decrease the negative effects of the medicine. Please tell the doctor if any of the listed side effects appear or if you think that the medicine is causing any other problems. Not all of the rare or unusual side effects are listed.

Side effects are most common after starting the medicine or after a dose increase. Many side effects can be avoided or lessened by starting with a very low dose and increasing it slowly—ask the doctor.

Allergic Reaction

Tell the doctor in a day or two (if possible, before the next dose of medicine):

- Hives
- Itching
- Rash

    Stop the medicine and get *immediate* medical care:

- Trouble breathing or chest tightness
- Swelling of lips, tongue, or throat

General Side Effects

Tell the doctor within a week or two:

    The following side effects are more common when first starting the medicine:

- Daytime sleepiness—Do not allow your child to drive, ride a bicycle or motorcycle, or operate machinery if this happens.
- Dizziness
- Nausea or upset stomach—Have your child take the medicine with food.
- Headaches

    The following side effects are more common at higher doses:

- Double or blurred vision
- Jerky, side-to-side eye movements (nystagmus)
- Clumsiness or decreased coordination

Side Effects Requiring Medical Attention

Call the doctor within a day or two:

- Problems with attention or concentration
- Anxiety or nervousness
- Moodiness
- Slowing of movements and/or speech

Very Rare, but Possibly Dangerous, Side Effects

Call the doctor *immediately*:

- Worsening or new behavioral problems
- Agitation
- Confusion
- Skin rash with fever

- Feeling sick or unusually tired
- Loss of appetite
- Persistent nausea
- Vomiting
- Yellowing of the skin or eyes
- Headaches that do not go away
- Dark urine or pale bowel movements
- Swelling of the legs or eyes
- Greatly increased thirst
- Greatly increased or decreased urination

Some Interactions With Other Medicines or Food

Please note that the following are only the most likely interactions with food or other medicines.

Caffeine may increase side effects.

Oxcarbazepine interacts with many other medicines. Taking it with another medicine may make one or both not work as well or may cause more side effects. Be sure that each doctor knows about *all* the medicines your child is taking.

Oxcarbazepine may decrease the blood levels of birth control pills (oral contraceptives) so that they do not work as well—this may lead to accidental pregnancy.

Carbamazepine (Tegretol) and divalproex (Depakote) may lower the blood levels of oxcarbazepine and make it not work as well.

What Could Happen if This Medicine Is Stopped Suddenly?

Stopping oxcarbazepine suddenly may cause uncomfortable withdrawal symptoms. If the person is taking oxcarbazepine for epilepsy (seizures), stopping the medicine suddenly could lead to an increase in very dangerous seizures (convulsions).

How Long Will This Medicine Be Needed?

The length of time a person needs to take oxcarbazepine depends on what problem is being treated. For example, someone with an impulse control disorder usually takes the medicine only until behavioral therapy begins to work. Someone with bipolar disorder may need to take the medicine for many years. Please ask the doctor about the length of treatment needed.

What Else Should I Know About This Medicine?

Oxcarbazepine increases the risk of sunburn. Be sure that your child wears sunscreen or protective clothing or stays out of the sun.

Taking oxcarbazepine with food may decrease stomach upset.

Oxcarbazepine is processed by the kidneys. Great caution should be used in patients with kidney problems.

Keep the medicine in a safe place under close supervision. An overdose can be very dangerous to small children. Keep the pill container tightly closed and in a dry place, away from bathrooms, showers, and humidifiers.

Notes

Use this space to take notes or to write down questions you want to ask the doctor.

_____

_____

_____

_____

_____

_____

_____

_____

_____

_____

_____

From Dulcan MK (editor): _Helping Parents, Youth, and Teachers Understand Medications for Behavioral and Emotional Problems: A Resource Book of Medication Information Handouts,_ Third Edition. Washington, DC, American Psychiatric Publishing, 2007

Medication Information for Youth

Oxcarbazepine—Trileptal

What the Medicine Is Called and What It Is For

The name of your medicine may be confusing. Most drugs have two names: 1) a scientific name that we call a *generic name* and 2) a trade or *brand name*. The generic name of this medicine is oxcarbazepine. The brand name is Trileptal.

Oxcarbazepine was first used to help people with epilepsy (seizures, fits, convulsions), so it is sometimes called an *anticonvulsant*. It is now also called a *mood stabilizer*, because it is used to help people who have severe mood changes, sometimes called *mood swings*, especially in children and adolescents with bipolar disorder (manic-depressive disorder), depression, or trouble controlling anger. Oxcarbazepine can reduce aggression, anger, and severe mood swings. It can treat mania or prevent relapse (mania coming back). It is thought to work by making brain cells less excitable.

How You Take the Medicine

It is very important to take the medicine exactly as the doctor or nurse tells you. Do not skip doses or take extra medicine without asking an adult. If you forget a dose, ask your parent(s) what to do.

This medicine is prescribed only for you. It should never be shared with anyone else.

You do not have to tell others that you are taking this medicine, but it is not something you should feel ashamed or embarrassed about. Many young people are helped by oxcarbazepine. This medicine is not habit-forming, and you cannot become "hooked" on it. You should talk to your doctor or nurse about any questions you have about the medicine. It is important to remember that the medicine *helps* you. It cannot *make* you do anything or change you as a person.

It is important to drink enough water so that your kidneys can process this medicine.

If your stomach is upset, taking the medicine with food may help.

Caffeine (in coffee, tea, or soft drinks) may make you feel worse.

It is very important not to stop this medicine suddenly—it could be uncomfortable or even dangerous.

How Your Doctor Will Follow Your Progress

Before starting oxcarbazepine, your doctor or nurse will talk with you and your parent(s) and may measure your height, weight, heart rate (pulse), and blood pressure. The doctor will probably order blood tests to be sure you are healthy before taking the medicine.

Be sure to tell your doctor or nurse about any other medicines or supplements you are taking, including vitamins, herbs, or aids to weight loss or bodybuilding. Also be sure to tell the doctor or nurse if you are using alcohol or drugs. Because many medicines may affect babies, it is very important to tell the doctor if you might be pregnant or if you are at risk of becoming pregnant. Oxcarbazepine may make birth control pills not work as well, so it is important to talk to the doctor if you are taking birth control pills.

Your teachers may be asked to fill out a form about your grades and behavior in school. A psychologist may give you some tests to see how you learn best.

Most doctors have regular appointments with young people who are taking medicine. You should use these visits to share any concerns you may have about your medicine and to talk about if it has helped you. From time to time, your physician or nurse may measure your height, weight, heart rate (pulse), and blood pressure to be sure that you are in good health while you are taking the medicine. There will be regular blood tests to be sure that the medicine is at the right dose and to be sure that the medicine is not causing side effects. Your doctor also will ask for regular reports from your parents and maybe from your teachers (with your permission) to see how well the medicine is working.

How the Medicine Might Affect You

In addition to the ways the medicine can help you, it may have other effects called *side effects*. Different medicines have different side effects. It is helpful to know about some of the most common side effects of your medicine so that you will understand what they are if they happen. Some people do not have any side effects. Some side effects are just uncomfortable, but others may mean a more serious problem with the medicine. Side effects are most common after starting the medicine or after a dose increase. They may go away with time, or the medicine can be adjusted or changed—ask the doctor.

You could have an allergy to any medicine, which might show up as a rash on your skin, swelling, itching, or trouble breathing.

Please tell your parent(s) and your doctor or nurse about any changes that you notice after taking the medicine. It is especially important to tell a responsible adult if you are feeling depressed or that you may not want to live; if you have thoughts of hurting yourself; or if you begin to feel more irritable, nervous, or restless. Also be sure to tell if you begin to feel more "speeded up" or have trouble sleeping.

Some medicines make people feel sleepy or less coordinated. If this medicine is making you sleepy, it is very important not to drive a car or ride a bicycle or motorcycle. After starting a new medicine or increasing the dose of a medicine, please be extra careful when driving a car, riding a bike, or using machines until you can tell how the medicine affects your alertness, attention, and coordination.

The most common side effects of oxcarbazepine are dizziness and daytime sleepiness. Other side effects that some people have are clumsiness, upset stomach, and double or blurred vision. These sometimes go away after you have been taking the medicine for a while or if the doctor lowers the dose of medicine you are taking. Your doctor will watch your blood tests closely so that the medicine can be changed if is causing problems in your body. Oxcarbazepine may make you more likely to get sunburned, so cover up or use sunscreen while outside in the sun.

Tell your parent(s) and doctor right away if you feel really sick, with a fever and a rash; if you notice any change in your urine or bowel movements; or if your skin seems to bruise easily.

Notes

Use this space to take notes or to write down questions you want to ask the doctor or nurse.

_____

_____

_____

_____

_____

_____

_____

_____

_____

_____

_____

_____

Medication Information for Parents and Teachers

Paroxetine—Paxil, Pexeva

General Information About Medication

Each child and adolescent is different. No one has exactly the same combination of medical and psychological problems. It is a good idea to talk with the doctor or nurse about the reasons a medicine is being used. It is very important to keep all appointments and to be in touch by telephone if you have concerns. It is important to communicate with the doctor, nurse, or therapist.

It is very important that the medicine be taken exactly as the doctor instructs. However, once in a while, everyone forgets to give a medicine on time. It is a good idea to ask the doctor or nurse what to do if this happens. Do not stop or change a medicine without asking the doctor or nurse first.

If the medicine seems to stop working, it may be because it is not being taken regularly. The youth may be "cheeking" or hiding the medicine or forgetting to take it (especially at school). The doses may be too far apart, or a different dose may be needed. Something at school, at home, or in the neighborhood may be upsetting the youth, or he or she may need special help for learning disabilities or tutoring. Please discuss your concerns with the doctor. **Do not just increase the dose.**

All medicines should be kept in a safe place, out of the reach of children, and should be supervised by an adult. If someone takes too much of a medicine, call the doctor, the poison control center, or a hospital emergency room.

Each medicine has a "generic" or chemical name. Just like laundry detergents or paper towels, some medicines are sold by more than one company under different brand names. The same medicine may be available under a generic name and several brand names. The generic medications are usually less expensive than the brand name ones. The generic medications have the same chemical formula, but they may or may not be exactly the same strength as the brand-name medications. Also, some brands of pills contain dye that can cause allergic reactions. It is a good idea to talk to the doctor and the pharmacist about whether it is important to use a specific brand of medicine.

All medicines can cause an allergic reaction. Examples are hives, itching, rashes, swelling, and trouble breathing. Even a tiny amount of a medicine can cause a reaction in patients who are allergic to that medicine. Be *sure* to talk to the doctor before restarting a medicine that has caused an allergic reaction.

Taking more than one medicine at the same time may cause more side effects or cause one of the medicines to not work as well. Always ask the doctor, nurse, or pharmacist before adding another medicine, whether prescription or over-the-counter. Be sure that each doctor knows about *all* of the medicines your child is taking. Also tell the doctor about any vitamins, herbal medicines, or supplements your child may be taking. Some of these may have side effects alone or when taken with this medication.

Everyone taking medicine should have a physical examination at least once a year.

If you suspect the youth is using drugs or alcohol, please tell the doctor right away.

501

Pregnancy requires special care in the use of medicine. Please tell the doctor immediately if you suspect the teenager is pregnant or might become pregnant.

Printed information like this applies to children and adolescents in general. If you have questions about the medicine, or if you notice changes or anything unusual, please ask the doctor or nurse. As scientific research advances, knowledge increases and advice changes. Even experts do not always agree. Many medicines have not been approved by the U.S. Food and Drug Administration (FDA) for use in children. For this reason, use of the medicine for a particular problem or age group often is not listed in the *Physicians' Desk Reference*. This does not necessarily mean that the medicine is dangerous or does not work, only that the company that makes the medicine has not received permission to advertise the medicine for use in children. Companies often do not apply for this permission because it is expensive to do the tests needed to apply for approval for use in children. Once a medication is approved by the FDA for any purpose, a doctor is allowed to prescribe it according to research and clinical experience.

Note to Teachers

It is a good idea to talk with the parent(s) about the reason(s) that a medication is being used. If the parent(s) sign consent to release information, it is often helpful to talk with the doctor. If the parent(s) give permission, the doctor may ask you to fill out rating forms about your experience with the student's behavior, feelings, academic performance, and medication side effects. This information is very useful in selecting and monitoring medication treatment. If you have observations that you think are important, do not hesitate to share these with the student's parent(s) and treating clinicians.

It is very important that the medicine be taken exactly as the doctor instructs. However, everyone forgets to give a medicine on time once in a while. It is a good idea to ask the parent(s) in advance what to do if this happens. Do not stop or change the time you are giving a medicine at school without parental permission. If a medication is to be taken with food, but lunchtime or snack time changes, be sure to notify the parent(s) so appropriate adjustments can be made.

All medicines should be kept in a secure place and should be supervised by an adult. If someone takes too much of a medicine, follow your school procedure for an urgent medical problem.

Taking medicine is a private matter and is best managed discreetly and confidentially. It is important to be sensitive to the student's feelings about taking medicine.

If you suspect that the student is using drugs or alcohol, please tell the parent(s) or a school counselor right away.

Please tell the parent(s) or school nurse if you suspect medication side effects.

Modifications of the classroom environment or assignments may be useful in addition to medication. The student may need to be evaluated for additional help or for an Individualized Education Plan for learning or behavior.

Any expression of suicidal thoughts or feelings or self-harm by a child or adolescent is a clear signal of distress and should be taken seriously. These behaviors should not be dismissed as "attention seeking."

What Is Paroxetine (Paxil, Pexeva)?

Paroxetine is an *antidepressant* known as a *selective serotonin reuptake inhibitor* (SSRI). It comes in brand names Paxil and Pexeva and generic tablets. Paxil also comes in controlled-release tablets (Paxil-CR) and liquid form. The controlled-release tablets do not last longer, but the medicine is released more slowly, and this may lessen side effects.

How Can This Medicine Help?

Paroxetine is used to treat depression and anxiety disorders such as obsessive-compulsive disorder (OCD), posttraumatic stress disorder (PTSD), panic disorder, and separation anxiety disorder.

How Does This Medicine Work?

People with emotional and behavioral problems, such as depression and anxiety, may have low levels of the *neurotransmitter* called *serotonin* in certain parts of the brain. SSRIs such as paroxetine help by increasing the action of brain serotonin to more normal levels.

How Long Does This Medicine Last?

Paroxetine lasts a shorter time than other antidepressants, but it can be taken only once a day.

How Will the Doctor Monitor This Medicine?

The doctor will review your child's medical history and physical examination before starting paroxetine. The doctor may order some blood or urine tests to be sure your child does not have a hidden medical condition that would make it unsafe to use this medicine. Extra care is needed when using SSRIs in youth with seizures (epilepsy), liver or kidney problems, or diabetes. The doctor or nurse will measure your child's height, weight, pulse, and blood pressure before starting the medicine.

Be sure to tell the doctor if your child or anyone in the family has bipolar illness (manic-depressive illness) or has tried to kill himself or herself.

After the medicine is started, the doctor will want to have regular appointments with you and your child to see how the medicine is working, to see if a dose change is needed, to watch for side effects, to see if paroxetine is still needed, and to see if any other treatment is needed. The doctor or nurse may check your child's height, weight, pulse, and blood pressure.

Before using medicine and at times afterward, the doctor may ask your child to fill out a rating scale about depression and anxiety, to help see how your child is doing.

What Side Effects Can This Medicine Have?

Any medicine can have side effects, including an allergy to the medicine. Because each patient is different, the doctor will monitor the youth closely, especially when the medicine is started. The doctor will work with you to increase the positive effects and decrease the negative effects of the medicine. Please tell the doctor if any of the listed side effects appear or if you think that the medicine is causing any other problems. Not all of the rare or unusual side effects are listed.

Paroxetine stays in the body for a long time, so side effects may last for days after the medicine is stopped.

Side effects are most common after starting the medicine or after a dose increase. Many side effects can be avoided or lessened by starting with a very low dose and increasing it slowly—ask the doctor. The controlled-release tablet may have fewer side effects.

Allergic Reaction

Tell the doctor in a day or two (if possible, before the next dose of medicine):

- Hives
- Itching
- Rash

  Stop the medicine and get *immediate* medical care:

- Trouble breathing or chest tightness
- Swelling of lips, tongue, or throat

Common Side Effects

Tell the doctor within a week or two:

- Nausea, upset stomach, vomiting
- Diarrhea
- Dry mouth—Have your child try using sugar-free gum or candy.
- Constipation—Encourage your child to drink more fluids and eat high-fiber foods; if necessary, the doctor may recommend a fiber medicine such as Benefiber or a stool softener such as Colace or mineral oil.
- Headache
- Anxiety or nervousness
- Insomnia (trouble sleeping)
- Restlessness, increased activity level
- Daytime sleepiness or tiredness—Do not allow your child to drive, ride a bicycle or motorcycle, or operate machinery if this side effect is present.
- Dizziness—This side effect is worse when the child stands up quickly, especially when getting out of bed in the morning; try having the child stand up slowly.
- Tremor (shakiness)
- Excessive sweating
- Apathy, lack of interest in school or friends—This may happen after a initial good response to treatment.
- Decreased sexual interest or trouble with sexual functioning
- Weight gain
- Weight loss

Less Common, but More Serious, Side Effects

Call the doctor within a day or two:

- Significant suicidal thoughts or self-injurious behavior
- Increased activity, rapid speech, feeling "speeded up," decreased need for sleep, being very excited or irritable (cranky)

Serious Side Effects

Call the doctor *immediately* or go to the nearest emergency room:

- Seizure (fit, convulsion)
- Stiffness, high fever, confusion, tremors (shaking)
- Overheating or heatstroke—Prevent by decreasing activity in hot weather, staying out of the sun, and drinking water.

Serotonin Syndrome

A very serious side effect called *serotonin syndrome* can happen when certain kinds of medicines (including some medicines for migraine headaches—triptans) are taken by the same person. *Very* rarely, it can happen at high doses of just one medicine. The early signs are restlessness, confusion, shaking, skin turning red, sweating, and jerking of muscles. If you see these symptoms, stop the medicine and send or take the youth to an emergency room right away.

Some Interactions With Other Medicines or Food

Please note that the following are only the most likely interactions with food or other medicines.

Paroxetine interacts with many other medicines, including some antibiotics and other psychiatric medicines. It is especially important to tell the doctor and pharmacist about all of the medicines your child is taking or has taken in the past few months, including over-the-counter and herbal medicines. Sometimes one medicine can increase or decrease the blood level of another medicine, so that different doses are needed. Phenytoin (Dilantin) may decrease the level of paroxetine so that it does not work as well or needs a higher dose. The herbal medicine St. John's wort also increases serotonin and can cause serious side effects if taken with paroxetine.

It can be *very dangerous* to take an SSRI at the same time as or even within a month of taking another type of medicine called a *monoamine oxidase inhibitor* (MAOI), such as Eldepryl (selegiline), Nardil (phenelzine), Parnate (tranylcypromine), or Marplan (isocarboxazid).

Paroxetine does not usually cause problems when taken with decongestant cold medicines.

Paroxetine can be taken with or without food.

Caffeine may increase side effects.

What Could Happen if This Medicine Is Stopped Suddenly?

No known serious medical effects occur if paroxetine is stopped suddenly, but there may be uncomfortable feelings, which should be avoided if possible. Your child might have trouble sleeping, nervousness, irritability, dizziness, and flu-like symptoms. Ask the doctor before stopping paroxetine or if these symptoms happen while the dose is being decreased. Because paroxetine leaves the body quickly, it may need to be tapered very slowly.

How Long Will This Medicine Be Needed?

Paroxetine may take up to 1–2 months to reach its full effect. If your child has a good response to paroxetine, it is a good idea to continue the medicine for at least 6 months.

What Else Should I Know About This Medicine?

In youth who have bipolar disorder (manic depression) or who are at risk for bipolar disorder, any antidepressant medicine may increase the risk of hypomania or mania (excitement, agitation, increased activity, decreased sleep).

In hot weather, make sure your child drinks enough water or other liquids and does not get overheated.

Sometimes, after a person has improved while taking paroxetine, he or she loses interest in school or friends or just stops trying. Please tell your child's doctor if this happens—it may be a side effect of the medication. A lower dose or a different medicine may be needed.

Store the medicine away from sunlight, heat, moisture, and humidity.

The controlled-release tablets should not be chewed, crushed, or cut but should be swallowed whole.

Black Box Antidepressant Warning

In 2004, an advisory committee to the FDA decided that there might be an increased risk of suicidal behavior for some youth taking medicines called *antidepressants*. In the research studies that the committee reviewed, about 3%–4% of youth with depression who took an antidepressant medicine—and 1%–2% of youth with depression who took a placebo (pill without active medicine)—talked about suicidal thoughts (thinking about killing themselves or wishing they were dead) or did something to harm themselves. This means that almost twice as many youth who were taking an antidepressant to treat their depression talked about suicide or had suicidal behavior compared with youth with depression who were taking inactive medicine. There were *no* completed suicides in any of these research studies, which included more than 4,000 children and adolescents. For youth being treated for anxiety, there was no difference in suicidal talking or behavior between those taking antidepressant medication and those taking placebo.

The FDA told drug companies to add a *black box warning* label to all antidepressant medicines. Because of this label, a doctor (or advanced practice nurse) prescribing one of these medicines has to warn youth and their families that there might be more suicidal thoughts and actions in youth taking these medicines.

On the other hand, in places where more youth are taking the newer antidepressant medicines, the number of adolescents who commit suicide has gotten smaller. Also, thinking about or attempting suicide is more common in surveys of teenagers in the community than it is in depressed youth treated in research studies with antidepressant medicine.

If a youth is being treated with this medicine and is doing well, then no changes are needed as a result of this warning. Increased suicidal talk or action is most likely to happen in the first few months of treatment with a medicine. If your child has recently started this medicine or is about to start, then you and your doctor (or advanced practice nurse) should watch for any changes in behavior. People who are depressed often have suicidal thoughts or actions. It is hard to know whether suicidal thoughts or actions in depressed people are caused by the depression itself or by the medicine. Also, as their depression is getting better, some people talk more about the suicidal thoughts that they had before but did not talk about. As young people get better from depression, they might be at higher risk of doing something about suicidal thoughts that they have had for some time, because they have more energy.

What Should a Parent Do?

1. Be honest with your child about possible risks and benefits of medicine.
2. Talk to your child about whether he or she is having any suicidal thoughts, and tell your child to come to you if he or she is having such thoughts.
3. You, your child, and your child's doctor or nurse should develop a safety plan. Pick adults whom your child can tell if he or she is thinking about suicide.
4. Be sure to tell your child's doctor, nurse, or therapist if you suspect that your child is using alcohol or drugs or if something has happened that might make your child feel worse, such as a family separation, breaking up with a boyfriend or girlfriend, someone close dying or attempting suicide, physical or sexual abuse, or failure in school.
5. Be sure that there are no guns in the home and that all medicines (including over-the-counter medicines like Tylenol) are closely supervised by an adult and kept in a safe place.
6. Watch for new or worse thoughts of suicide, self-harm, depression, anxiety (nerves), feeling very agitated or restless, being angry or aggressive, having more trouble sleeping, or anything else that you see for the first time, seems worse, or worries your child or you. If these appear, contact a mental health professional **right away.** Do not just stop or change the dose of the medicine on your own. If the problems are serious, and you cannot reach one of your clinicians, call a 24-hour psychiatry emergency telephone number or take your child to an emergency room.

Youth on antidepressant medicine should be watched carefully by their parent(s), clinician(s) (doctor, nurse, therapist), and other concerned adults for the first weeks of treatment. It is a good idea to have a visit or telephone call with the doctor, nurse, or therapist weekly for the first month, every 2 weeks for the second month, and after that at least once a month to check for feelings of depression or sadness, thoughts of killing or harming himself or herself, and any problems with the medication. If you have questions, be sure to ask the doctor, nurse, or therapist.

For more information, see http://www.parentsmedguide.org/ (in English and Spanish).

Notes

Use this space to take notes or to write down questions you want to ask the doctor.

_____

_____

_____

_____

_____

_____

_____

_____

_____

_____

_____

_____

_____

From Dulcan MK (editor): _Helping Parents, Youth, and Teachers Understand Medications for Behavioral and Emotional Problems: A Resource Book of Medication Information Handouts_, Third Edition. Washington, DC, American Psychiatric Publishing, 2007

Medication Information for Youth

Paroxetine—Paxil, Pexeva

What the Medicine Is Called and What It Is For

The name of your medicine may be confusing. Most drugs have two names: 1) a scientific name that we call a *generic name* and 2) a trade or *brand name.* The generic name of this medicine is paroxetine. The brand names are Paxil and Pexeva.

Paroxetine is called an *antidepressant,* or *selective serotonin reuptake inhibitor* (SSRI). Paroxetine is used to treat depression and anxiety disorders such as obsessive-compulsive disorder (OCD), posttraumatic stress disorder (PTSD), panic disorder, and separation anxiety disorder. It helps people who feel very sad or depressed, anxious (nervous), or afraid, or who have obsessions (uncomfortable thoughts that will not go away) or compulsions (habits that get in the way of daily life).

How You Take the Medicine

It is very important to take the medicine exactly as the doctor or nurse tells you. Do not skip doses or take extra medicine without asking an adult. If you forget a dose, ask your parent(s) what to do. It is very important that you take all the pills you are supposed to take each day. Your doctor will probably recommend that you take your medicine at the same time each day, which may be with meals or at bedtime.

It may take several weeks before you notice that the medicine is helping. Waiting for the full effect may take even longer. You may feel discouraged and think the medicine is never going to help. You may want to give up and stop taking the medicine. Talk to your doctor and parent(s) about how you feel, but **do not stop** taking the medicine unless your doctor tells you to. It is also important not to take extra pills, hoping that you will feel better faster. Doing that could make you very sick.

The controlled-release tablets should not be chewed, crushed, or cut. Swallow them whole.

Caffeine (in coffee, tea, or soft drinks) may make you feel worse.

This medicine is prescribed only for you. It should never be shared with anyone else.

You do not have to tell others that you are taking this medicine, but it is not something you should feel ashamed or embarrassed about. Many young people are helped by paroxetine. This medicine is not habit-forming, and you cannot become "hooked" on it. You should talk to your doctor or nurse about any questions you have about the medicine. It is important to remember that the medicine *helps* you. It cannot *make* you do anything or change you as a person.

How Your Doctor Will Follow Your Progress

Before giving you the medicine, your doctor or nurse will talk with you and your parent(s) and may measure your height, weight, heart rate (pulse), and blood pressure. The doctor may order some blood or urine tests to be sure you are in good health.

Be sure to tell your doctor or nurse about any other medicines or supplements you are taking, including vitamins, herbs, or aids to weight loss or bodybuilding. Also be sure to tell the doctor or nurse if you are using alcohol or drugs. Because many medicines may affect babies, it is very important to tell the doctor if you might be pregnant or if you are at risk of becoming pregnant. Be sure to tell the doctor if you have had thoughts of hurting yourself, have tried to hurt yourself, or sometimes wish that you were not alive.

Your teachers may be asked to fill out a form about your grades and behavior in school. A psychologist may give you some tests to see how you learn best.

Before starting the medicine and afterward, the doctor may ask you to answer questions on paper about depression and anxiety.

Most doctors have regular appointments with young people who are taking medicine. You should use these visits to share any concerns you may have about your medicine and to talk about if it has helped you. From time to time, your physician or nurse may measure your height, weight, heart rate (pulse), and blood pressure to be sure that you are in good health while you are taking the medicine. Your doctor also will ask for regular reports from your parents and maybe from your teachers (with your permission) to see how well the medicine is working.

Some medicines are started at the amount you will take for as long as you are taking that medicine. Other medicines need to be increased or adjusted until your doctor decides you are taking the right amount. Starting at a low dose and increasing it slowly may lessen side effects. If the medicine helps you, your doctor will probably want you to take it for 6 months to a year if you are taking it to treat depression. If you are taking it for another problem, your doctor will decide how long you will need to take the medicine as he or she watches your progress.

It is not dangerous to stop paroxetine suddenly, but there might be uncomfortable feelings, such as trouble sleeping, nervousness, irritability, or feeling sick. It is better to decrease it slowly. Do not stop taking a medicine unless the doctor tells you to. If you have any problems after stopping or decreasing this medicine, tell your parent(s) or doctor.

How the Medicine Might Affect You

In addition to the ways the medicine can help you, it may have other effects called *side effects*. Different medicines have different side effects. It is helpful to know about some of the most common side effects of your medicine so that you will understand what they are if they happen. Some people do not have any side effects. Some side effects are just uncomfortable, but others may mean a more serious problem with the medicine. Side effects are most common after starting the medicine or after a dose increase. They may go away with time, or the medicine can be adjusted or changed—ask the doctor.

You could have an allergy to any medicine, which might show up as a rash on your skin, swelling, itching, or trouble breathing.

Please tell your parent(s) and your doctor or nurse about any changes that you notice after taking the medicine. It is especially important to tell a responsible adult if you are feeling depressed or that you may not want to live; if you have thoughts of hurting yourself; or if you begin to feel more irritable, nervous, or restless. Also be sure to tell your parent(s) or doctor if you begin to feel "speeded up" or have trouble sleeping.

Some medicines make people feel sleepy or less coordinated. If this medicine is making you sleepy, it is very important not to drive a car or ride a bicycle or motorcycle. After starting a new medicine or increasing the dose of a medicine, please be extra careful when driving a car, riding a bike, or using machines until you can tell how the medicine affects your alertness, attention, and coordination.

One of the most common side effects of this medicine is feeling tired or sleepy during the day, even if you have had a full night's sleep. After you have been taking the medicine for a few weeks your body will adjust, and this side effect may go away. If you have had trouble sleeping at night, the medicine can help you sleep better, especially if the doctor tells you to take a dose of medicine in the evening. Other people may feel more restless and excited. Tell your parent(s) or doctor if this is uncomfortable. Sometimes after being on the medicine for a while, people do not care as much about school or friends. Changing the dose or the type of medicine can help this.

This medicine may make your mouth dry. You may be more thirsty than usual and find that you are drinking more water or other liquids. Sucking on sugar-free hard candy or cough drops usually helps. You also could try chewing sugar-free gum or sucking on ice chips. Do not chew the ice; you could hurt your teeth. Also, using lip balm will keep your lips from cracking. It is important to be especially good about brushing your teeth.

Some other side effects that could happen are headache, not feeling hungry and not wanting to eat much, eating more than usual, having an upset stomach, or changes in your bowel movements. You may have a change in your sexual functioning—it is OK to ask the doctor about this. This medicine may make you more likely to get sick if you get overheated, so be sure to drink plenty of liquids and rest in the shade in hot weather.

Please let your parent(s) and doctor know if you notice anything different or unusual about how you feel once you start taking the medicine. This includes good things, such as feeling less sad or less nervous or sleeping better at night.

Notes

Use this space to take notes or to write down questions you want to ask the doctor or nurse.

_____

_____

_____

_____

_____

_____

_____

_____

_____

_____

_____

_____

_____

From Dulcan MK (editor): _Helping Parents, Youth, and Teachers Understand Medications for Behavioral and Emotional Problems: A Resource Book of Medication Information Handouts_, Third Edition. Washington, DC, American Psychiatric Publishing, 2007

Medication Information for Parents and Teachers

Perphenazine—Trilafon

General Information About Medication

Each child and adolescent is different. No one has exactly the same combination of medical and psychological problems. It is a good idea to talk with the doctor or nurse about the reasons a medicine is being used. It is very important to keep all appointments and to be in touch by telephone if you have concerns. It is important to communicate with the doctor, nurse, or therapist.

It is very important that the medicine be taken exactly as the doctor instructs. However, once in a while, everyone forgets to give a medicine on time. It is a good idea to ask the doctor or nurse what to do if this happens. Do not stop or change a medicine without asking the doctor or nurse first.

If the medicine seems to stop working, it may be because it is not being taken regularly. The youth may be "cheeking" or hiding the medicine or forgetting to take it (especially at school). The doses may be too far apart, or a different dose may be needed. Something at school, at home, or in the neighborhood may be upsetting the youth, or he or she may need special help for learning disabilities or tutoring. Please discuss your concerns with the doctor. **Do not just increase the dose.**

All medicines should be kept in a safe place, out of the reach of children, and should be supervised by an adult. If someone takes too much of a medicine, call the doctor, the poison control center, or a hospital emergency room.

Each medicine has a "generic" or chemical name. Just like laundry detergents or paper towels, some medicines are sold by more than one company under different brand names. The same medicine may be available under a generic name and several brand names. The generic medications are usually less expensive than the brand name ones. The generic medications have the same chemical formula, but they may or may not be exactly the same strength as the brand-name medications. Also, some brands of pills contain dye that can cause allergic reactions. It is a good idea to talk to the doctor and the pharmacist about whether it is important to use a specific brand of medicine.

All medicines can cause an allergic reaction. Examples are hives, itching, rashes, swelling, and trouble breathing. Even a tiny amount of a medicine can cause a reaction in patients who are allergic to that medicine. Be *sure* to talk to the doctor before restarting a medicine that has caused an allergic reaction.

Taking more than one medicine at the same time may cause more side effects or cause one of the medicines to not work as well. Always ask the doctor, nurse, or pharmacist before adding another medicine, whether prescription or over-the-counter. Be sure that each doctor knows about *all* of the medicines your child is taking. Also tell the doctor about any vitamins, herbal medicines, or supplements your child may be taking. Some of these may have side effects alone or when taken with this medication.

Everyone taking medicine should have a physical examination at least once a year.

If you suspect the youth is using drugs or alcohol, please tell the doctor right away.

Pregnancy requires special care in the use of medicine. Please tell the doctor immediately if you suspect the teenager is pregnant or might become pregnant.

Printed information like this applies to children and adolescents in general. If you have questions about the medicine, or if you notice changes or anything unusual, please ask the doctor or nurse. As scientific research advances, knowledge increases and advice changes. Even experts do not always agree. Many medicines have not been approved by the U.S. Food and Drug Administration (FDA) for use in children. For this reason, use of the medicine for a particular problem or age group often is not listed in the *Physicians' Desk Reference*. This does not necessarily mean that the medicine is dangerous or does not work, only that the company that makes the medicine has not received permission to advertise the medicine for use in children. Companies often do not apply for this permission because it is expensive to do the tests needed to apply for approval for use in children. Once a medication is approved by the FDA for any purpose, a doctor is allowed to prescribe it according to research and clinical experience.

Note to Teachers

It is a good idea to talk with the parent(s) about the reason(s) that a medication is being used. If the parent(s) sign consent to release information, it is often helpful to talk with the doctor. If the parent(s) give permission, the doctor may ask you to fill out rating forms about your experience with the student's behavior, feelings, academic performance, and medication side effects. This information is very useful in selecting and monitoring medication treatment. If you have observations that you think are important, do not hesitate to share these with the student's parent(s) and treating clinicians.

It is very important that the medicine be taken exactly as the doctor instructs. However, everyone forgets to give a medicine on time once in a while. It is a good idea to ask the parent(s) in advance what to do if this happens. Do not stop or change the time you are giving a medicine at school without parental permission. If a medication is to be taken with food, but lunchtime or snack time changes, be sure to notify the parent(s) so appropriate adjustments can be made.

All medicines should be kept in a secure place and should be supervised by an adult. If someone takes too much of a medicine, follow your school procedure for an urgent medical problem.

Taking medicine is a private matter and is best managed discreetly and confidentially. It is important to be sensitive to the student's feelings about taking medicine.

If you suspect that the student is using drugs or alcohol, please tell the parent(s) or a school counselor right away.

Please tell the parent(s) or school nurse if you suspect medication side effects.

Modifications of the classroom environment or assignments may be useful in addition to medication. The student may need to be evaluated for additional help or for an Individualized Education Plan for learning or behavior.

Any expression of suicidal thoughts or feelings or self-harm by a child or adolescent is a clear signal of distress and should be taken seriously. These behaviors should not be dismissed as "attention seeking."

What Is Perphenazine (Trilafon)?

Perphenazine is sometimes called a *typical, conventional,* or *first-generation antipsychotic* medicine. It is also called a *neuroleptic* or *phenothiazine*. It used to be called a *major tranquilizer*. It comes in brand name Trilafon and generic tablets and liquid.

514

How Can This Medicine Help?

Perphenazine is used to treat psychosis, such as in schizophrenia, mania, or very severe depression. It can reduce hallucinations (hearing voices or seeing things that are not there) and delusions (troubling beliefs that other people do not share). Perphenazine can help the patient be less upset and agitated. It can improve the patient's ability to think clearly.

Sometimes perphenazine is used to decrease severe aggression or very serious behavioral problems in young people with conduct disorder, mental retardation, or autism.

This medicine is very powerful and should be used to treat very serious problems or symptoms that other medicines do not help. Be patient; the positive effects of this medicine may not appear for 2–3 weeks.

How Does This Medicine Work?

Cells in the brain (*neurons*) communicate using chemicals called *neurotransmitters*. Too much or too little of these substances in certain parts of the brain can cause problems. Perphenazine reduces the activity of one of these neurotransmitters, *dopamine*. Blocking the effect of dopamine in certain parts of the brain reduces what have been called *positive symptoms* of psychosis: delusions; hallucinations; disorganized and unusual thinking, speaking, and behavior; excessive activity (agitation); and lack of activity (catatonia). Blocking dopamine can also reduce tics. Reducing dopamine action in other parts of the brain may lead to the side effects of this medicine.

How Long Does This Medicine Last?

Perphenazine usually may be taken only once a day, unless divided doses are used to lessen side effects.

How Will the Doctor Monitor This Medicine?

The doctor will review your child's medical history and physical examination before starting perphenazine. The doctor may order some blood or urine tests to be sure your child does not have a hidden medical condition. The doctor or nurse may measure your child's pulse and blood pressure before starting perphenazine.

Before starting perphenazine and every so often afterward, a test such as the AIMS (Abnormal Involuntary Movement Scale) may be used to check your child's tongue, legs, and arms for unusual movements that could be caused by the medicine.

After the medicine is started, the doctor will want to have regular appointments with you and your child to see how the medicine is working, to see if a dose change is needed, to watch for side effects, to see if perphenazine is still needed, and to see if any other treatment is needed. The doctor or nurse may check your child's height, weight, pulse, and blood pressure and watch for abnormal movements.

What Side Effects Can This Medicine Have?

Any medicine can have side effects, including an allergy to the medicine. Because each patient is different, the doctor will monitor the youth closely, especially when the medicine is started. The doctor will work with you

to increase the positive effects and decrease the negative effects of the medicine. Please tell the doctor if any of the listed side effects appear or if you think that the medicine is causing any other problems. Not all of the rare or unusual side effects are listed.

Side effects are most common after starting the medicine or after a dose increase. Many side effects can be avoided or lessened by starting with a very low dose and increasing it slowly—ask the doctor.

Allergic Reaction

Tell the doctor in a day or two (if possible, before the next dose of medicine):

- Hives
- Itching
- Rash

  Stop the medicine and get *immediate* medical care:

- Trouble breathing or chest tightness
- Swelling of lips, tongue, or throat

Common, but Not Usually Serious, Side Effects

Discuss the following side effects with your child's doctor within a week or two. They often can be helped by lowering the dose of medicine, changing the times medicine is taken, or adding another medicine.

- Dry mouth—Have your child try using sugar-free gum or candy.
- Constipation—Encourage your child to drink more fluids and eat high-fiber foods; if necessary, the doctor may recommend a fiber medicine such as Benefiber or a stool softener such as Colace or mineral oil.
- Increased risk of sunburn—Have your child wear sunscreen or protective clothing or stay out of the sun.
- Mild trouble urinating
- Blurred vision
- Weight gain—Seek nutritional counseling; provide your child with low-calorie snacks and encourage regular exercise.
- Sadness, irritability, nervousness, clinginess, not wanting to go to school
- Restlessness or inability to sit still
- Shaking of hands and fingers

Less Common, but Not Usually Serious, Side Effects

Discuss the following side effects with your child's doctor within a week or two. They often can be helped by lowering the dose of medicine, changing the times medicine is taken, or adding another medicine.

- Daytime sleepiness or tiredness—Do not allow your child to drive, ride a bicycle or motorcycle, or operate machinery if this happens. This problem may be lessened by taking the medicine at bedtime.
- Dizziness—This side effect is worse when the child stands up quickly, especially when getting out of bed in the morning; try having the child stand up slowly.
- Decreased or slowed movement and decreased facial expressions
- Drooling

- Decreased sexual interest or ability
- Changes in menstrual cycle
- Increase in breast size or discharge from the breasts (in both boys and girls)—This may go away with time.

Less Common, but Potentially Serious, Side Effects

Call the doctor or go to an emergency room *right away*:

- Stiffness of the tongue, jaw, neck, back, or legs
- Overheating or heatstroke—Prevent by decreasing activity in hot weather, staying out of the sun, and drinking water.
- Seizure (fit, convulsion)—This is more likely in people with a history of seizures or head injury.
- Severe confusion

Rare, but Serious, Side Effects

- Extreme stiffness or lack of movement, very high fever, mental confusion, irregular pulse rate, or eye pain—**This is a medical emergency. Go to an emergency room right away.**
- Sudden stiffness and inability to breathe or swallow—**Go to an emergency room or call 911.** Tell the paramedics, nurses, and doctors that the patient is taking perphenazine. Other medicines can be used to treat this problem fast.
- Increased thirst, frequent urination, lethargy, tiredness, dizziness—These could be signs of diabetes (especially if your child is overweight or there is a family history of diabetes). **Talk to a doctor within a day.**

What Else Should I Know About Side Effects?

Most side effects lessen over time. If they are troublesome, talk with your child's doctor. Some side effects can be decreased by taking a smaller dose of medicine, by stopping the medicine, by changing to another medicine, or by adding another medicine (see the table).

One side effect that may not go away is *tardive dyskinesia* (or TD). Patients with tardive dyskinesia have involuntary movements of the body, especially the mouth and tongue. The patient may look as though he or she is making faces over and over again. Jerky movements of the arms, legs, or body may occur. There may be fine, wormlike, or sudden repeated movements of the tongue, or the person may appear to be chewing something or smacking or puckering his or her lips. The fingers may look as though they are rolling something. If you notice any unusual movements, be sure to tell the doctor. The doctor may use the AIMS test to look for these movements.

The medicine may increase the level of *prolactin*, a natural hormone made in the part of the brain called the *pituitary*. This may cause side effects such as breast tenderness or swelling or production of milk in both boys and girls. It also may interfere with sexual functioning in teenage boys and with regular menstrual cycles (periods) in teenage girls. A blood test can measure the level of prolactin. If these side effects do not go away and are troublesome, talk with your child's doctor about substituting another medicine for perphenazine.

Heart problems are rare with perphenazine but are more common if other medicines are being taken also. Be sure to tell all your child's doctors and your pharmacist about all medications your child is taking.

Neuroleptic malignant syndrome is a very rare side effect that can lead to death. The symptoms are severe muscle stiffness, high fever, increased heart rate and blood pressure, irregular heartbeat (pulse), and sweating. It may lead to unconsciousness. If you suspect this, **call 911 or go to an emergency room right away.**

What Medicines Are Used to Treat the Side Effects of Perphenazine?

The following medicines may be used to treat the movement side effects of perphenazine. These medicines may have their own side effects as well. Ask the doctor if you suspect a problem.

Brand name	Generic name
Akineton	Biperiden
Artane	Trihexyphenidyl
Ativan	Lorazepam*
Benadryl	Diphenhydramine*
Catapres	Clonidine*
Cogentin	Benztropine mesylate*
Inderal	Propranolol*
Klonopin	Clonazepam*
Symmetrel	Amantadine

*This medicine has its own information sheet in this book.

Some Interactions With Other Medicines or Food

Please note that the following are only the most likely interactions with food or other medicines.

Perphenazine may be taken with or without food. If the medicine causes stomach upset, taking it with food may help.

It is better to limit drinks with caffeine (coffee, tea, soft drinks) because caffeine works in the opposite way from this medicine, and the positive effects might be decreased.

What Could Happen if This Medicine Is Stopped Suddenly?

Involuntary movements, or *withdrawal dyskinesias*, may appear within 1–4 weeks of lowering the dose or stopping the medicine. Usually these go away, but they can last for days to months. If perphenazine is stopped suddenly, emotional problems such as irritability, nervousness, moodiness; behavior problems; or physical problems such as stomachache, loss of appetite, nausea, vomiting, diarrhea, sweating, indigestion, trouble sleeping, trembling, or shaking may appear. These problems usually last only a few days to a few weeks. If they happen, tell your child's doctor. The medicine dose may need to be lowered more slowly (tapered). Always check with the doctor before stopping a medicine!

How Long Will This Medicine Be Needed?

How long your child will need to be on perphenazine depends partly on the reason that it was prescribed. Some problems last for only a few months, whereas others last much longer. Sometimes perphenazine is used for only a short time until other medicines or behavioral treatments start to work. Some people need to take perphenazine for years. It is especially important with medicines as powerful as this one to ask the doctor whether it is still needed. Every few months, you should discuss with your child's doctor the reasons for using perphenazine and whether it is time for a trial of lowering the dose.

What Else Should I Know About This Medicine?

There are many older and newer medicines that are used for the same kinds of problems. If your child is having bad side effects or the medicine does not seem to be working, ask the doctor if another medicine in this group might work as well or better and have fewer side effects for your child.

Be sure to tell the doctor if there is anyone in your family who died suddenly or had a heart problem.

Notes

Use this space to take notes or to write down questions you want to ask the doctor.

_____

_____

_____

_____

_____

_____

_____

_____

_____

From Dulcan MK (editor): *Helping Parents, Youth, and Teachers Understand Medications for Behavioral and Emotional Problems: A Resource Book of Medication Information Handouts,* Third Edition. Washington, DC, American Psychiatric Publishing, 2007

Medication Information for Youth

Perphenazine—Trilafon

What the Medicine Is Called and What It Is For

The name of your medicine may be confusing. Most drugs have two names: 1) a scientific name that we call a *generic name* and 2) a trade or *brand name*. The generic name of this medicine is perphenazine. The brand name is Trilafon.

Perphenazine can help people who feel very confused and have severe problems thinking clearly. It can lessen *hallucinations* (seeing or hearing things that are not really there) and *delusions* (troubling beliefs that other people do not share). This medicine also is sometimes used to help young people who have mania or very severe depression, or who get very angry and hit people or break things.

How You Take the Medicine

It is very important to take the medicine exactly as the doctor or nurse tells you. Do not skip doses or take extra medicine without asking an adult. If you forget a dose, ask your parent(s) what to do. Your doctor will tell you how much medicine to take and how often to take it so that it can help you the most. It is *very important* that you take all the pills you are supposed to take each day. Your doctor will probably recommend that you take your medicine at the same time each day, which may be with meals or at bedtime.

It is better to limit drinks with caffeine (coffee, tea, soft drinks) because caffeine works in the opposite way from this medicine, and the positive effects might be decreased.

It may be several weeks or longer before you notice the full effect. You may feel discouraged and think the medicine is never going to help. You may want to give up and stop taking the medicine. Talk to your doctor and parent(s) about how you feel, but **do not stop** taking your medicine unless your doctor tells you to. It also is important not to take extra pills hoping that you will feel better faster. Doing that could make you very sick.

If your stomach is upset, taking the medicine with food may help.

This medicine is prescribed only for you. It should never be shared with anyone else.

You do not have to tell others that you are taking this medicine, but it is not something you should feel ashamed or embarrassed about. Many young people are helped by perphenazine. You should talk to your doctor or nurse about any questions you have about the medicine. It is important to remember that the medicine *helps* you. It cannot *make* you do anything or change you as a person.

How Your Doctor Will Follow Your Progress

Before giving you the medicine, your doctor or nurse will talk with you and your parent(s) and may measure your height, weight, heart rate (pulse), and blood pressure. There may be other tests, such as blood tests for sugar and cholesterol. Before you start taking the medicine and every so often afterward, the doctor or nurse will look at your tongue, arms, and legs to check for unusual movements. This is called the AIMS (Abnormal Involuntary Movement Scale) test.

Be sure to tell your doctor or nurse about any other medicines or supplements you are taking, including vitamins, herbs, or aids to weight loss or bodybuilding. Also be sure to tell the doctor or nurse if you are using alcohol or drugs. Because many medicines may affect babies, it is very important to tell the doctor if you might be pregnant or if you are at risk of becoming pregnant.

Your teachers may be asked to fill out a form about your grades and behavior in school. A psychologist may give you some tests to see how you learn best.

Most doctors have regular appointments with young people who are taking medicine. You should use these visits to share any concerns you may have about your medicine and to talk about if it has helped you. From time to time, your physician or nurse may measure your height, weight, heart rate (pulse), and blood pressure to be sure that you are in good health while you are taking the medicine. There may be blood tests to watch for diabetes or high cholesterol. Your doctor also will ask for regular reports from your parents and maybe from your teachers (with your permission) to see how well the medicine is working.

If the medicine helps you, your doctor will probably want you to take it for several months to a year. Your doctor will decide how long you will need to take the medicine as he or she watches your progress.

How the Medicine Might Affect You

In addition to the ways the medicine can help you, it may have other effects called *side effects*. Different medicines have different side effects. It is helpful to know about some of the most common side effects of your medicine so that you will understand what they are if they happen. Some people do not have any side effects. Some side effects are just uncomfortable, but others may mean a more serious problem with the medicine. Side effects are most common after starting the medicine or after a dose increase. They may go away with time, or the medicine can be adjusted or changed—ask the doctor.

You could have an allergy to any medicine, which might show up as a rash on your skin, swelling, itching, or trouble breathing.

Please tell your parent(s) and your doctor or nurse about any changes that you notice after taking the medicine. It is especially important to tell a responsible adult right away if you are feeling depressed or that you may not want to live; if you have thoughts of hurting yourself; or if you begin to feel more irritable, nervous, or restless.

One of the most common side effects of this medicine is feeling tired or sleepy during the day, even if you have had a full night's sleep. If this medicine is making you sleepy, it is very important not to drive a car or ride a bicycle or motorcycle. After starting the medicine or increasing the dose of medicine, please be extra careful when driving a car, riding a bike, or using machines until you can tell how the medicine affects your alertness, attention, and coordination. After you have been taking the medicine for a few weeks, your body will adjust, and this side effect will likely go away. If you had trouble sleeping at night before taking the medicine, it can help you sleep better, especially if the doctor tells you to take a dose of medicine in the evening.

You might feel dizzy or light-headed if you stand up fast. Try standing up slowly, especially when getting out of bed in the morning.

Another common side effect is dry mouth. You may be more thirsty than usual and find that you are drinking more water or other liquids than usual. Sucking on sugar-free hard candy or cough drops usually helps. You also could try chewing sugar-free gum or sucking on ice chips. Do not chew the ice; you could hurt your teeth. Also, using lip balm will keep your lips from cracking. It is important to be especially good about brushing your teeth.

Taking this medicine could make you more likely to get badly sunburned or very sick in hot weather. Be sure to drink plenty of liquids and cover up or use sunscreen when you go outside in hot weather. Be careful to rest in the shade and not get overheated.

Sometimes teenagers who take perphenazine gain weight. The weight gain may be from increased appetite and also from ways that the medicine changes how the body processes food. It is much easier to prevent weight gain than to lose weight later. It is a good idea to eat a well-balanced diet without "junk food" and with healthy snacks like fruits and vegetables, not sweets or fried foods. It is better to drink water or skim milk, not pop, sodas, soft drinks, or sugary juices. Regular exercise is important for maintaining a healthy weight (and may also help with sleep).

Some people become constipated (have hard bowel movements) when taking this medicine. Try drinking more water and eating more fruits, vegetables, and whole grains. If that does not help, tell your parent(s) or doctor—you may need a medicine to help with this side effect. Sometimes people have trouble passing urine. Tell your parent(s) or the doctor if this happens.

Perphenazine is a very powerful medicine. Some side effects include feeling nervous, restless, or shaky or having stiff muscles. Talk with your doctor about these side effects. They can be helped by adding another medicine, adjusting the dose, or switching to another medicine.

Another, more serious, side effect can be longer lasting and more difficult to treat. This very rare side effect is called *tardive dyskinesia* (or TD). A person taking perphenazine may develop movements of the mouth, tongue, face, arms, legs, or body that are not being made on purpose. This side effect can go away when the medicine is stopped, but in some people it does not go away. Your doctor will explain this effect to you and your parent(s) and how he or she will watch for any signs that you are developing this problem. Be sure to ask your doctor any questions that you may have about this, but do not worry too much about it. It hardly ever happens to teenagers.

You may notice changes in your sexual functioning or in your breasts—it is OK to ask the doctor about this.

You should tell your parent(s) and doctor if you notice anything different or unusual about how you feel once you start taking the medicine. This includes good things, such as feeling less confused, feeling less sad or angry, not hearing voices anymore, or sleeping better at night.

You cannot become addicted to this medicine, but you should not stop it suddenly. Never stop a medicine without talking to the doctor. If perphenazine is stopped or decreased suddenly you may notice more moodiness or irritability, stomachaches or upset stomach, trouble sleeping, or trembling or shaking. Let your parent(s) or doctor know if this happens—the medicine may need to be decreased more slowly.

Notes

Use this space to take notes or to write down questions you want to ask the doctor or nurse.

_____

_____

_____

_____

_____

_____

_____

_____

_____

Medication Information for Parents and Teachers

Pimozide—Orap

General Information About Medication

Each child and adolescent is different. No one has exactly the same combination of medical and psychological problems. It is a good idea to talk with the doctor or nurse about the reasons a medicine is being used. It is very important to keep all appointments and to be in touch by telephone if you have concerns. It is important to communicate with the doctor, nurse, or therapist.

It is very important that the medicine be taken exactly as the doctor instructs. However, once in a while, everyone forgets to give a medicine on time. It is a good idea to ask the doctor or nurse what to do if this happens. Do not stop or change a medicine without asking the doctor or nurse first.

If the medicine seems to stop working, it may be because it is not being taken regularly. The youth may be "cheeking" or hiding the medicine or forgetting to take it (especially at school). The doses may be too far apart, or a different dose may be needed. Something at school, at home, or in the neighborhood may be upsetting the youth, or he or she may need special help for learning disabilities or tutoring. Please discuss your concerns with the doctor. **Do not just increase the dose.**

All medicines should be kept in a safe place, out of the reach of children, and should be supervised by an adult. If someone takes too much of a medicine, call the doctor, the poison control center, or a hospital emergency room.

Each medicine has a "generic" or chemical name. Just like laundry detergents or paper towels, some medicines are sold by more than one company under different brand names. The same medicine may be available under a generic name and several brand names. The generic medications are usually less expensive than the brand name ones. The generic medications have the same chemical formula, but they may or may not be exactly the same strength as the brand-name medications. Also, some brands of pills contain dye that can cause allergic reactions. It is a good idea to talk to the doctor and the pharmacist about whether it is important to use a specific brand of medicine.

All medicines can cause an allergic reaction. Examples are hives, itching, rashes, swelling, and trouble breathing. Even a tiny amount of a medicine can cause a reaction in patients who are allergic to that medicine. Be *sure* to talk to the doctor before restarting a medicine that has caused an allergic reaction.

Taking more than one medicine at the same time may cause more side effects or cause one of the medicines to not work as well. Always ask the doctor, nurse, or pharmacist before adding another medicine, whether prescription or over-the-counter. Be sure that each doctor knows about *all* of the medicines your child is taking. Also tell the doctor about any vitamins, herbal medicines, or supplements your child may be taking. Some of these may have side effects alone or when taken with this medication.

Everyone taking medicine should have a physical examination at least once a year.

If you suspect the youth is using drugs or alcohol, please tell the doctor right away.

Pregnancy requires special care in the use of medicine. Please tell the doctor immediately if you suspect the teenager is pregnant or might become pregnant.

Printed information like this applies to children and adolescents in general. If you have questions about the medicine, or if you notice changes or anything unusual, please ask the doctor or nurse. As scientific research advances, knowledge increases and advice changes. Even experts do not always agree. Many medicines have not been approved by the U.S. Food and Drug Administration (FDA) for use in children. For this reason, use of the medicine for a particular problem or age group often is not listed in the *Physicians' Desk Reference*. This does not necessarily mean that the medicine is dangerous or does not work, only that the company that makes the medicine has not received permission to advertise the medicine for use in children. Companies often do not apply for this permission because it is expensive to do the tests needed to apply for approval for use in children. Once a medication is approved by the FDA for any purpose, a doctor is allowed to prescribe it according to research and clinical experience.

Note to Teachers

It is a good idea to talk with the parent(s) about the reason(s) that a medication is being used. If the parent(s) sign consent to release information, it is often helpful to talk with the doctor. If the parent(s) give permission, the doctor may ask you to fill out rating forms about your experience with the student's behavior, feelings, academic performance, and medication side effects. This information is very useful in selecting and monitoring medication treatment. If you have observations that you think are important, do not hesitate to share these with the student's parent(s) and treating clinicians.

It is very important that the medicine be taken exactly as the doctor instructs. However, everyone forgets to give a medicine on time once in a while. It is a good idea to ask the parent(s) in advance what to do if this happens. Do not stop or change the time you are giving a medicine at school without parental permission. If a medication is to be taken with food, but lunchtime or snack time changes, be sure to notify the parent(s) so appropriate adjustments can be made.

All medicines should be kept in a secure place and should be supervised by an adult. If someone takes too much of a medicine, follow your school procedure for an urgent medical problem.

Taking medicine is a private matter and is best managed discreetly and confidentially. It is important to be sensitive to the student's feelings about taking medicine.

If you suspect that the student is using drugs or alcohol, please tell the parent(s) or a school counselor right away.

Please tell the parent(s) or school nurse if you suspect medication side effects.

Modifications of the classroom environment or assignments may be useful in addition to medication. The student may need to be evaluated for additional help or for an Individualized Education Plan for learning or behavior.

Any expression of suicidal thoughts or feelings or self-harm by a child or adolescent is a clear signal of distress and should be taken seriously. These behaviors should not be dismissed as "attention seeking."

What Is Pimozide (Orap)?

Pimozide is sometimes called a *typical*, *conventional*, or *first-generation antipsychotic* medicine. It is also called a *neuroleptic*. It comes only in brand name Orap tablets.

How Can This Medicine Help?

Pimozide is used to decrease motor and vocal tics (fast, repeated movements or sounds) and behavioral problems in people with Tourette's disorder.

This medicine is very powerful and should be used to treat very serious problems or symptoms that other medicines do not help. Be patient; the positive effects of these medicines may not appear for 2–3 weeks.

How Does This Medicine Work?

Cells in the brain *(neurons)* communicate using chemicals called *neurotransmitters*. Too much or too little of these substances in certain parts of the brain can cause problems. Pimozide reduces the activity of one of these neurotransmitters, *dopamine*. Blocking the effect of dopamine in certain parts of the brain can also reduce tics. Reducing dopamine action in other parts of the brain may lead to the side effects of this medicine.

How Long Does This Medicine Last?

Pimozide usually is taken several times a day.

How Will the Doctor Monitor This Medicine?

The doctor will review your child's medical history and physical examination before starting pimozide. The doctor may order some blood or urine tests to be sure your child does not have a hidden medical condition. The doctor or nurse may measure your child's pulse and blood pressure before starting pimozide. An ECG (electrocardiogram or heart rhythm test) will be done before and after starting the medicine. A blood test for potassium also may be done. Be sure to tell the doctor if there is anyone in your family who died suddenly or had a heart problem.

Be sure to tell the doctor if anyone in the family is hearing impaired or has had heart problems or died suddenly.

Before your child starts taking pimozide and every so often afterward, a test such as the AIMS (Abnormal Involuntary Movement Scale) may be used to check your child's tongue, legs, and arms for unusual movements that could be caused by the medicine.

After the medicine is started, the doctor will want to have regular appointments with you and your child to see how the medicine is working, to see if a dose change is needed, to watch for side effects, to see if pimozide is still needed, and to see if any other treatment is needed. The doctor or nurse may check your child's height, weight, pulse, and blood pressure and watch for abnormal movements. Sometimes an ECG may be needed.

What Side Effects Can This Medicine Have?

Any medicine can have side effects, including an allergy to the medicine. Because each patient is different, the doctor will monitor the youth closely, especially when the medicine is started. The doctor will work with you

to increase the positive effects and decrease the negative effects of the medicine. Please tell the doctor if any of the listed side effects appear or if you think that the medicine is causing any other problems. Not all of the rare or unusual side effects are listed.

Side effects are most common after starting the medicine or after a dose increase. Many side effects can be avoided or lessened by starting with a very low dose and increasing it slowly—ask the doctor.

Allergic Reaction

Tell the doctor in a day or two (if possible, before the next dose of medicine):

- Hives
- Itching
- Rash

    Stop the medicine and get *immediate* medical care:

- Trouble breathing or chest tightness
- Swelling of lips, tongue, or throat

Common, but Not Usually Serious, Side Effects

Discuss the following side effects with your child's doctor within a week or two. They often can be helped by lowering the dose of medicine, changing the times medicine is taken, or adding another medicine.

- Dry mouth—Have your child try using sugar-free gum or candy.
- Constipation—Encourage your child to drink more fluids and eat high-fiber foods; if necessary, the doctor may recommend a fiber medicine such as Benefiber or a stool softener such as Colace or mineral oil.
- Mild trouble urinating
- Blurred vision
- Increased risk of sunburn—Have your child wear sunscreen or protective clothing or stay out of the sun.
- Weight gain—Seek nutritional counseling; provide your child with low-calorie snacks and encourage regular exercise.
- Sadness, irritability, nervousness, clinginess, not wanting to go to school
- Increased restlessness or inability to sit still
- Shaking of hands and fingers

Less Common, but Not Usually Serious, Side Effects

Discuss the following side effects with your child's doctor within a week or two. They often can be helped by lowering the dose of medicine, changing the times medicine is taken, or adding another medicine.

- Daytime sleepiness or tiredness—Do not allow your child to drive, ride a bicycle or motorcycle, or operate machinery if this happens.
- Dizziness—This side effect is worse when the child stands up quickly, especially when getting out of bed in the morning; try having the child stand up slowly.
- Drooling

- Decreased or slowed movement and decreased facial expressions
- Decreased sexual interest or ability
- Changes in menstrual cycle
- Increase in breast size or discharge from the breasts (in both boys and girls)—This may go away with time.

Less Common, but Potentially Serious, Side Effects

Call the doctor or go to an emergency room *right away:*

- Stiffness of the tongue, jaw, neck, back, or legs
- Overheating or heatstroke—Prevent by decreasing activity in hot weather, staying out of the sun, and drinking water.
- Seizure (fit, convulsion)—This is more likely in people with a history of seizures or head injury.
- Severe confusion
- Very fast or irregular heartbeat

Rare, but Serious, Side Effects

- Extreme stiffness or lack of movement, very high fever, mental confusion, irregular pulse rate, or eye pain—**This is a medical emergency. Go to an emergency room right away.**
- Sudden stiffness and inability to breathe or swallow—**Go to an emergency room or call 911.** Tell the paramedics, nurses, and doctors that the patient is taking pimozide. Other medicines can be used to treat this problem fast.
- Increased thirst, frequent urination, lethargy, tiredness, dizziness—These could be signs of diabetes (especially if your child is overweight or there is a family history of diabetes). **Talk to a doctor within a day.**

What Else Should I Know About Side Effects?

Most side effects lessen over time. If they are troublesome, talk with your child's doctor. Some side effects can be decreased by taking a smaller dose of medicine, by stopping the medicine, by changing to another medicine, or by adding another medicine.

One side effect that may not go away is *tardive dyskinesia* (or TD). Patients with tardive dyskinesia have involuntary movements of the body, especially the mouth and tongue. The patient may look as though he or she is making faces over and over again. Jerky movements of the arms, legs, or body may occur. There may be fine, wormlike, or sudden repeated movements of the tongue, or the person may appear to be chewing something or smacking or puckering his or her lips. The fingers may look as though they are rolling something. If you notice any unusual movements, be sure to tell the doctor. The doctor may use the AIMS test to look for these movements.

Heart problems are more common if other medicines are being taken also. Be sure to tell all your child's doctors and your pharmacist about all medications your child is taking.

Neuroleptic malignant syndrome is a very rare side effect that can lead to death. The symptoms are severe muscle stiffness, high fever, increased heart rate and blood pressure, irregular heartbeat (pulse), and sweating. It may lead to unconsciousness. If you suspect this, **call 911 or go to an emergency room right away.**

Some Interactions With Other Medicines or Food

Please note that the following are only the most likely interactions with food or other medicines.

Pimozide (Orap) blood levels may become dangerously high with increased side effects in the heart if the medicine is taken with grapefruit juice, fluoxetine (Prozac), paroxetine (Paxil), or some antibiotics (such as erythromycin and others) and antifungal medicines (such as ketoconazole and others).

Pimozide may be taken with or without food.

It is better to limit drinks with caffeine (coffee, tea, soft drinks) because caffeine works in the opposite way from this medicine, and the positive effects might be decreased.

What Could Happen if This Medicine Is Stopped Suddenly?

Involuntary movements, or *withdrawal dyskinesias*, may appear within 1–4 weeks of lowering the dose or stopping the medicine. Usually these go away, but they can last for days to months. If pimozide is stopped suddenly, emotional problems such as irritability, nervousness, moodiness; behavior problems; or physical problems such as stomachache, loss of appetite, nausea, vomiting, diarrhea, sweating, indigestion, trouble sleeping, trembling, or shaking may appear. These problems usually last only a few days to a few weeks. If they happen, tell your child's doctor. The medicine dose may need to be lowered more slowly (tapered). Always check with the doctor before stopping a medicine!

How Long Will This Medicine Be Needed?

How long your child will need to be on pimozide depends on how severe the tics are and whether they start to go away as your child grows up. It is especially important with medicines as powerful as this one to ask the doctor whether it is still needed. Every few months, you should discuss with your child's doctor the reasons for using pimozide and whether it is time for a trial of lowering the dose.

What Else Should I Know About This Medicine?

There are newer medicines that are used for the same kinds of problems. If your child is having bad side effects or the medicine does not seem to be working, ask the doctor if another medicine might work as well or better and have fewer side effects for your child.

Notes

Use this space to take notes or to write down questions you want to ask the doctor.

_____

_____

_____

_____

_____

_____

_____

_____

_____

_____

_____

_____

From Dulcan MK (editor): _Helping Parents, Youth, and Teachers Understand Medications for Behavioral and Emotional Problems: A Resource Book of Medication Information Handouts_, Third Edition. Washington, DC, American Psychiatric Publishing, 2007

Pimozide—Orap

What the Medicine Is Called and What It Is For

The name of your medicine may be confusing. Most drugs have two names: 1) a scientific name that we call a *generic name* and 2) a trade or *brand name*. The generic name of this medicine is pimozide. The brand name is Orap.

Pimozide is used to reduce motor and vocal tics (fast, repeated movements or sounds) in people with Tourette's disorder.

How You Take the Medicine

It is very important to take the medicine exactly as the doctor or nurse tells you. Do not skip doses or take extra medicine without asking an adult. If you forget a dose, ask your parent(s) what to do.

It is better to limit drinks with caffeine (coffee, tea, soft drinks) because caffeine works in the opposite way from this medicine, and the positive effects might be decreased.

If your stomach is upset, taking the medicine with food may help.

Do not drink grapefruit juice when taking pimozide, because grapefruit juice may increase the side effects of pimozide.

This medicine is prescribed only for you. It should never be shared with anyone else.

You do not have to tell others that you are taking this medicine, but it is not something you should feel ashamed or embarrassed about. Many young people are helped by pimozide. This medicine is not habit-forming, and you cannot become "hooked" on it. You should talk to your doctor or nurse about any questions you have about the medicine. It is important to remember that the medicine *helps* you. It cannot *make* you do anything or change you as a person.

How Your Doctor Will Follow Your Progress

Before giving you the medicine, your doctor or nurse will talk with you and your parent(s) and may measure your height, weight, heart rate (pulse), and blood pressure. There may be blood tests to be sure you are in good health. Before you start taking the medicine and every so often afterward, the doctor or nurse will look at your tongue, arms, and legs to check for unusual movements. This is called the AIMS (Abnormal Involuntary Movement Scale) test. Before starting pimozide, at times of increasing the dose, and every 6 months to a year after that, your doctor may ask for an ECG (electrocardiogram or heart rhythm test) to be done. This test counts your heartbeats through small wires that are taped to your chest. It takes only about 15 minutes.

Be sure to tell your doctor or nurse about any other medicines or supplements you are taking, including vitamins, herbs, or aids to weight loss or bodybuilding. Also be sure to tell the doctor or nurse if you are using alcohol or drugs. Because many medicines may affect babies, it is very important to tell the doctor if you might be pregnant or if you are at risk of becoming pregnant.

Your teachers may be asked to fill out a form about your grades and behavior in school. A psychologist may give you some tests to see how you learn best.

Most doctors have regular appointments with young people who are taking medicine. You should use these visits to share any concerns you may have about your medicine and to talk about if it has helped you. From time to time, your physician or nurse may measure your height, weight, heart rate (pulse), and blood pressure to be sure that you are in good health while you are taking the medicine. Your doctor also will ask for regular reports from your parent(s) and maybe from your teachers (with your permission) to see how well the medicine is working.

If the medicine helps you, your doctor will probably want you to take it for at least several months to a year. Your doctor will decide how long you will need to take the medicine as he or she watches your progress.

How the Medicine Might Affect You

In addition to the ways the medicine can help you, it may have other effects called *side effects*. Different medicines have different side effects. It is helpful to know about some of the most common side effects of your medicine so that you will understand what they are if they happen. Some people do not have any side effects. Some side effects are just uncomfortable, but others may mean a more serious problem with the medicine. Side effects are most common after starting the medicine or after a dose increase. They may go away with time, or the medicine can be adjusted or changed—ask the doctor.

You could have an allergy to any medicine, which might show up as a rash on your skin, swelling, itching, or trouble breathing.

Please tell your parent(s) and your doctor or nurse about any changes that you notice after taking the medicine. It is especially important to tell a responsible adult right away if you are feeling depressed or that you may not want to live; if you have thoughts of hurting yourself; or if you begin to feel more irritable, nervous, or restless.

One of the most common side effects of this medicine is feeling tired or sleepy during the day, even if you have had a full night's sleep. If this medicine is making you sleepy, it is very important not to drive a car or ride a bicycle or motorcycle. After starting the medicine or increasing the dose of medicine, please be extra careful when driving a car, riding a bike, or using machines until you can tell how the medicine affects your alertness, attention, and coordination. After you have been taking the medicine for a few weeks, your body will adjust, and this side effect will likely go away. If you had trouble sleeping at night before taking the medicine, it can help you sleep better, especially if the doctor tells you to take a dose of medicine in the evening.

You might feel dizzy or light-headed if you stand up fast. Try standing up slowly, especially when getting out of bed in the morning.

Another common side effect is dry mouth. You may be more thirsty than usual and find that you are drinking more water or other liquids than usual. Sucking on sugar-free hard candy or cough drops usually helps. You also could try chewing sugar-free gum or sucking on ice chips. Do not chew the ice; you could hurt your teeth. Also, using lip balm will keep your lips from cracking. It is important to be especially good about brushing your teeth.

Taking this medicine could make you more likely to get badly sunburned or very sick in hot weather. Be sure to drink plenty of liquids and cover up or use sunscreen when you go outside in hot weather. Be careful to rest in the shade and not get overheated.

Sometimes teenagers who take pimozide gain weight. The weight gain may be from increased appetite and also from ways that the medicine changes how the body processes food. It is much easier to prevent weight gain than to lose weight later. It is a good idea to eat a well-balanced diet without "junk food" and with healthy snacks like fruits and vegetables, not sweets or fried foods. It is better to drink water or skim milk, not pop, sodas, soft drinks, or sugary juices. Regular exercise is important for maintaining a healthy weight (and may also help with sleep).

Some people become constipated (have hard bowel movements) when taking this medicine. Try drinking more water and eating more fruits, vegetables, and whole grains. If that does not help, tell your parent(s) or doctor—you may need a medicine to help with this side effect. Sometimes people have trouble passing urine. Tell your parent(s) or the doctor if this happens.

This is a very powerful medicine. Some side effects include feeling nervous, restless, or shaky or having stiff muscles. Talk with your doctor about these side effects. They can be helped by adding another medicine, adjusting the dose, or switching to another medicine.

Another, more serious, side effect can be longer lasting and more difficult to treat. This very rare side effect is called *tardive dyskinesia* (or TD). A person taking pimozide may develop movements of the mouth, tongue, face, arms, legs, or body that are not being made on purpose. This side effect can go away when the medicine is stopped, but in some people it does not go away. Your doctor will explain this effect to you and your parent(s) and how he or she will watch for any signs that you are developing this problem. Be sure to ask your doctor any questions that you may have about this, but do not worry too much about it. It hardly ever happens to teenagers.

You may notice changes in your sexual functioning or in your breasts—it is OK to ask the doctor about this.

You should tell your parent(s) and doctor if you notice anything different or unusual about how you feel once you start taking the medicine. This includes good things, such as feeling less confused, feeling less sad or angry, not hearing voices anymore, or sleeping better at night.

You cannot become addicted to this medicine, but you should not stop it suddenly. Never stop a medicine without talking to the doctor. If pimozide is stopped or decreased suddenly you may notice more moodiness or irritability, stomachaches or upset stomach, trouble sleeping, or trembling or shaking. Let your parent(s) or doctor know if this happens—the medicine may need to be decreased more slowly.

Notes

Use this space to take notes or to write down questions you want to ask the doctor or nurse.

_____

_____

_____

_____

_____

_____

_____

_____

_____

_____

_____

_____

_____

Medication Information
for Parents and Teachers

Pindolol—Visken

General Information About Medication

Each child and adolescent is different. No one has exactly the same combination of medical and psychological problems. It is a good idea to talk with the doctor or nurse about the reasons a medicine is being used. It is very important to keep all appointments and to be in touch by telephone if you have concerns. It is important to communicate with the doctor, nurse, or therapist.

It is very important that the medicine be taken exactly as the doctor instructs. However, once in a while, everyone forgets to give a medicine on time. It is a good idea to ask the doctor or nurse what to do if this happens. Do not stop or change a medicine without asking the doctor or nurse first.

If the medicine seems to stop working, it may be because it is not being taken regularly. The youth may be "cheeking" or hiding the medicine or forgetting to take it (especially at school). The doses may be too far apart, or a different dose may be needed. Something at school, at home, or in the neighborhood may be upsetting the youth, or he or she may need special help for learning disabilities or tutoring. Please discuss your concerns with the doctor. **Do not just increase the dose.**

All medicines should be kept in a safe place, out of the reach of children, and should be supervised by an adult. If someone takes too much of a medicine, call the doctor, the poison control center, or a hospital emergency room.

Each medicine has a "generic" or chemical name. Just like laundry detergents or paper towels, some medicines are sold by more than one company under different brand names. The same medicine may be available under a generic name and several brand names. The generic medications are usually less expensive than the brand name ones. The generic medications have the same chemical formula, but they may or may not be exactly the same strength as the brand-name medications. Also, some brands of pills contain dye that can cause allergic reactions. It is a good idea to talk to the doctor and the pharmacist about whether it is important to use a specific brand of medicine.

All medicines can cause an allergic reaction. Examples are hives, itching, rashes, swelling, and trouble breathing. Even a tiny amount of a medicine can cause a reaction in patients who are allergic to that medicine. Be *sure* to talk to the doctor before restarting a medicine that has caused an allergic reaction.

Taking more than one medicine at the same time may cause more side effects or cause one of the medicines to not work as well. Always ask the doctor, nurse, or pharmacist before adding another medicine, whether prescription or over-the-counter. Be sure that each doctor knows about *all* of the medicines your child is taking. Also tell the doctor about any vitamins, herbal medicines, or supplements your child may be taking. Some of these may have side effects alone or when taken with this medication.

Everyone taking medicine should have a physical examination at least once a year.

If you suspect the youth is using drugs or alcohol, please tell the doctor right away.

Pregnancy requires special care in the use of medicine. Please tell the doctor immediately if you suspect the teenager is pregnant or might become pregnant.

Printed information like this applies to children and adolescents in general. If you have questions about the medicine, or if you notice changes or anything unusual, please ask the doctor or nurse. As scientific research advances, knowledge increases and advice changes. Even experts do not always agree. Many medicines have not been approved by the U.S. Food and Drug Administration (FDA) for use in children. For this reason, use of the medicine for a particular problem or age group often is not listed in the *Physicians' Desk Reference*. This does not necessarily mean that the medicine is dangerous or does not work, only that the company that makes the medicine has not received permission to advertise the medicine for use in children. Companies often do not apply for this permission because it is expensive to do the tests needed to apply for approval for use in children. Once a medication is approved by the FDA for any purpose, a doctor is allowed to prescribe it according to research and clinical experience.

Note to Teachers

It is a good idea to talk with the parent(s) about the reason(s) that a medication is being used. If the parent(s) sign consent to release information, it is often helpful to talk with the doctor. If the parent(s) give permission, the doctor may ask you to fill out rating forms about your experience with the student's behavior, feelings, academic performance, and medication side effects. This information is very useful in selecting and monitoring medication treatment. If you have observations that you think are important, do not hesitate to share these with the student's parent(s) and treating clinicians.

It is very important that the medicine be taken exactly as the doctor instructs. However, everyone forgets to give a medicine on time once in a while. It is a good idea to ask the parent(s) in advance what to do if this happens. Do not stop or change the time you are giving a medicine at school without parental permission. If a medication is to be taken with food, but lunchtime or snack time changes, be sure to notify the parent(s) so appropriate adjustments can be made.

All medicines should be kept in a secure place and should be supervised by an adult. If someone takes too much of a medicine, follow your school procedure for an urgent medical problem.

Taking medicine is a private matter and is best managed discreetly and confidentially. It is important to be sensitive to the student's feelings about taking medicine.

If you suspect that the student is using drugs or alcohol, please tell the parent(s) or a school counselor right away.

Please tell the parent(s) or school nurse if you suspect medication side effects.

Modifications of the classroom environment or assignments may be useful in addition to medication. The student may need to be evaluated for additional help or for an Individualized Education Plan for learning or behavior.

Any expression of suicidal thoughts or feelings or self-harm by a child or adolescent is a clear signal of distress and should be taken seriously. These behaviors should not be dismissed as "attention seeking."

What Is Pindolol (Visken)?

Pindolol is called a *beta-blocker*. It was first used to treat high blood pressure and irregular heartbeat. A newer use is the treatment of emotional and behavioral problems. In adults, it has been used together with an antidepressant medicine (selective serotonin reuptake inhibitors) for depression that has not gotten better with treatment or together with other medicines for bipolar disorder (manic depression) that is difficult to treat. It is also sometimes used to treat *akathisia*, which is a side effect of some antipsychotic medications. It is used for migraine headaches and a number of other medical conditions. It comes in brand name Visken and generic tablets.

How Can This Medicine Help?

Pindolol can decrease aggressive or violent behavior in children and adolescents. It may be particularly useful for patients who have developmental delays or autism. In addition, pindolol may reduce the aggression and anger that sometimes follow brain injuries. It may reduce some symptoms of anxiety (nervousness) and help children and adolescents who have experienced very frightening events and have posttraumatic stress disorder (PTSD). Pindolol may reduce the severe restlessness resulting from other medicines.

Your child may need to continue taking pindolol for at least 4 weeks before the doctor is able to decide whether the medicine is working.

How Does This Medicine Work?

When pindolol is prescribed for patients with anxiety, aggression, or other behavioral problems, these medicines stop the effect of certain chemicals on nerves in the body and possibly in the brain that are causing the symptoms. For example, pindolol can decrease the physical anxiety symptoms of shaking, sweating, and fast heartbeat. When used for treatment-resistant mood disorders, pindolol affects the functions of *serotonin*, one of the *neurotransmitters* (chemicals that the brain makes for cells to communicate).

How Will the Doctor Monitor This Medicine?

The doctor will review your child's medical history and physical examination before starting pindolol. Extreme caution is needed for children and adolescents with asthma, heart disease, diabetes, kidney disease, or thyroid disease. Please be sure to tell the doctor if your child or anyone in the family has one of these problems. The doctor may order some blood or urine tests to be sure your child does not have a hidden medical condition. The doctor or nurse will measure your child's height, weight, pulse, and blood pressure before starting pindolol. The doctor may order an ECG (electrocardiogram or heart rhythm test) before starting pindolol.

After the medicine is started, the doctor will want to have regular appointments with you and your child to see how the medicine is working, to see if a dose change is needed, to watch for side effects, to see if pindolol is still needed, and to see if any other treatment is needed. The doctor or nurse will measure pulse rate and blood pressure at each visit, particularly as the dose is increased. Sometimes these measurements are taken while the patient is both sitting or lying down and standing up. If either pulse rate or blood pressure drops too low, a pill may not be given at that time or the regular dose may be decreased.

What Side Effects Can This Medicine Have?

Any medicine can have side effects, including an allergy to the medicine. Because each patient is different, the doctor will monitor the youth closely, especially when the medicine is started. The doctor will work with you

to increase the positive effects and decrease the negative effects of the medicine. Please tell the doctor if any of the listed side effects appear or if you think that the medicine is causing any other problems. Not all of the rare or unusual side effects are listed.

Side effects are most common after starting the medicine or after a dose increase. Many side effects can be avoided or lessened by starting with a very low dose and increasing it slowly—ask the doctor.

Allergic Reaction

Tell the doctor in a day or two (if possible, before the next dose of medicine):

- Hives
- Itching
- Rash

Stop the medicine and get *immediate* medical care:

- Trouble breathing or chest tightness
- Swelling of lips, tongue, or throat

Occasional Side Effects

Tell the doctor within a week or two:

- Tingling, numbness, cold, or pain in the fingers or toes (Raynaud's phenomenon)
- Tiredness or weakness, especially with exercise
- Slow heartbeat
- Low blood pressure
- Dizziness or light-headedness—This side effect is worse when the child stands up quickly, especially when getting out of bed in the morning; try having the child stand up slowly.

Uncommon Side Effects

Call the doctor within a day or two:

- Sadness or irritability lasting more than a few days
- Nausea
- Trouble sleeping or nightmares
- Diarrhea
- Muscle cramps

Serious Side Effects

Call the doctor *immediately*:

- Wheezing
- Hallucinations (hearing voices or seeing things that are not there)

Some Interactions With Other Medicines or Food

Please note that the following are only the most likely interactions with food or other medicines.

Giving pindolol with food will decrease side effects.

Pindolol interacts with many other medicines. Be sure to tell the doctor about all medicines being taken. A doctor may use pindolol in combination with other medicines to treat a behavioral problem. Talk with your doctor and pharmacist about possible medicine interactions.

What Could Happen if This Medicine Is Stopped Suddenly?

Stopping pindolol suddenly may cause a fast or irregular heartbeat, high blood pressure, or severe emotional problems. Pindolol should be decreased slowly over at least 2 weeks under a doctor's supervision. It is especially important not to miss doses of this medicine, because withdrawal problems may occur. **Be sure not to let the prescription run out!**

How Long Will This Medicine Be Needed?

The length of time pindolol will be needed depends on how well the medicine works for your child, whether any side effects occur, and what condition is being treated. Sometimes medicine is needed for a short time to treat a particular problem. Occasionally a person may require treatment lasting for several months or may need to start the medicine again if symptoms return.

Notes

Use this space to take notes or to write down questions you want to ask the doctor.

_____

_____

_____

_____

_____

_____

_____

_____

_____

_____

_____

_____

_____

_____

Medication Information
for Youth

Pindolol—Visken

What the Medicine Is Called and What It Is For

The name of your medicine may be confusing. Most drugs have two names: 1) a scientific name that we call a *generic name* and 2) a trade or *brand name*. The generic name of this medicine is pindolol. The brand name is Visken.

Pindolol is a *beta-blocker*. These medicines work on parts of your brain and nervous system that control how your body reacts to situations in which you feel frightened, threatened, or angry. Beta-blockers were first used to treat heart and blood pressure problems. Now they are used to help young people who have too much anxiety (nervousness) or posttraumatic stress disorder (PTSD) or who fight or get angry too much. They can decrease the shaking, sweating, and fast heartbeat that come from anxiety or anger. They are also sometimes used to treat the side effects (like restlessness) of other medicines or to help other medicines work for depression or bipolar disorder (manic depression).

How You Take the Medicine

It is very important to take the medicine exactly as the doctor or nurse tells you. Do not skip doses or take extra medicine without asking an adult. If you forget a dose, ask your parent(s) what to do.

It might take as long as 4 weeks before the full effect is noticed. You may feel discouraged and think that the medicine is never going to help. You may want to give up and stop taking the medicine. Talk to your doctor and parent(s) about how you feel, but **do not stop** taking your medicine unless your doctor tells you to. It could be dangerous to stop this medicine suddenly.

This medicine is prescribed only for you. It should never be shared with anyone else.

You do not have to tell others that you are taking this medicine, but it is not something you should feel ashamed or embarrassed about. Many young people are helped by pindolol. This medicine is not habit-forming, and you cannot become "hooked" on it. You should talk to your doctor or nurse about any questions you have about the medicine. It is important to remember that the medicine *helps* you. It cannot *make* you do anything or change you as a person.

How Your Doctor Will Follow Your Progress

Before giving you the medicine, your doctor or nurse will talk with you and your parent(s) and will measure your height, weight, heart rate (pulse), and blood pressure. There may be other tests, such as blood or urine tests, or an ECG (electrocardiogram or heart rhythm test). This test counts your heartbeats through small wires that are taped to your chest. It takes only about 15 minutes.

Be sure to tell your doctor or nurse about any other medicines or supplements you are taking, including vitamins, herbs, or aids to weight loss or bodybuilding. Also be sure to tell the doctor or nurse if you are using alcohol or drugs. Because many medicines may affect babies, it is very important to tell the doctor if you might be pregnant or if you are at risk of becoming pregnant.

Your teachers may be asked to fill out a form about your grades and behavior in school. A psychologist may give you some tests to see how you learn best.

Most doctors have regular appointments with young people who are taking medicine. You should use these visits to share any concerns you may have about your medicine and to talk about if it has helped you. At the appointments, your doctor or nurse will measure your pulse rate (heartbeat) and blood pressure, particularly as the dose of medication is increased. Sometimes these measurements are taken while you are sitting or lying down and then standing up. There may be other tests, such as repeating the ECG. Your doctor also will ask for regular reports from your parents and maybe from your teachers (with your permission) to see how well the medicine is working.

How long you will need to take this medicine depends on how well it works for you, whether there are any side effects, and what problems are being treated. Sometimes medicine is needed for only a short time to treat a particular problem. Some people need it for months or years or may need to start the medicine again if symptoms return.

How the Medicine Might Affect You

In addition to the ways the medicine can help you, it may have other effects called *side effects*. Different medicines have different side effects. It is helpful to know about some of the most common side effects of your medicine so that you will understand what they are if they happen. Some people do not have any side effects. Some side effects are just uncomfortable, but others may mean a more serious problem with the medicine. Side effects are most common after starting the medicine or after a dose increase. They may go away with time, or the medicine can be adjusted or changed—ask the doctor.

You could have an allergy to any medicine, which might show up as a rash on your skin, swelling, itching, or trouble breathing.

Please tell your parent(s) and your doctor or nurse about any changes that you notice after taking the medicine. It is especially important to tell a responsible adult if you are feeling depressed or that you may not want to live; if you have thoughts of hurting yourself; or if you begin to feel more irritable, nervous, or restless.

Some medicines make people feel sleepy or less coordinated. If this medicine is making you sleepy, it is very important not to drive a car or ride a bicycle or motorcycle. After starting a new medicine or increasing the dose of a medicine, please be extra careful when driving a car, riding a bike, or using machines until you can tell how the medicine affects your alertness, attention, and coordination.

You might feel dizzy, tired, or even faint when you stand up fast. Try standing up slowly, especially first thing in the morning when getting out of bed.

You might notice that your fingers or toes feel very cold or tingly, that they look pale, or that they hurt. These are signs of *Raynaud's phenomenon*, which happens when the blood vessels to your fingers or toes tighten. Tell the doctor if you have these symptoms, and the dose of medicine can be adjusted or a different medicine can be used so that the problem will go away.

Other side effects (that hardly ever happen) are hallucinations (hearing voices or seeing things that are not there), upset stomach, nausea, trouble sleeping, nightmares, and sadness or irritability. You should talk to your parent(s) or doctor if you think you may be having any of these side effects.

If you are having trouble breathing, tell your parent(s) or doctor **right away.**

It is *very* important not to miss a dose or to stop this medicine suddenly—it could make you very sick.

Notes

Use this space to take notes or to write down questions you want to ask the doctor or nurse.

_____

_____

_____

_____

_____

_____

_____

_____

_____

_____

_____

_____

From Dulcan MK (editor): *Helping Parents, Youth, and Teachers Understand Medications for Behavioral and Emotional Problems: A Resource Book of Medication Information Handouts,* Third Edition. Washington, DC, American Psychiatric Publishing, 2007

Medication Information for Parents and Teachers

Propranolol—Inderal

General Information About Medication

Each child and adolescent is different. No one has exactly the same combination of medical and psychological problems. It is a good idea to talk with the doctor or nurse about the reasons a medicine is being used. It is very important to keep all appointments and to be in touch by telephone if you have concerns. It is important to communicate with the doctor, nurse, or therapist.

It is very important that the medicine be taken exactly as the doctor instructs. However, once in a while, everyone forgets to give a medicine on time. It is a good idea to ask the doctor or nurse what to do if this happens. Do not stop or change a medicine without asking the doctor or nurse first.

If the medicine seems to stop working, it may be because it is not being taken regularly. The youth may be "cheeking" or hiding the medicine or forgetting to take it (especially at school). The doses may be too far apart, or a different dose may be needed. Something at school, at home, or in the neighborhood may be upsetting the youth, or he or she may need special help for learning disabilities or tutoring. Please discuss your concerns with the doctor. **Do not just increase the dose.**

All medicines should be kept in a safe place, out of the reach of children, and should be supervised by an adult. If someone takes too much of a medicine, call the doctor, the poison control center, or a hospital emergency room.

Each medicine has a "generic" or chemical name. Just like laundry detergents or paper towels, some medicines are sold by more than one company under different brand names. The same medicine may be available under a generic name and several brand names. The generic medications are usually less expensive than the brand name ones. The generic medications have the same chemical formula, but they may or may not be exactly the same strength as the brand-name medications Also, some brands of pills contain dye that can cause allergic reactions. It is a good idea to talk to the doctor and the pharmacist about whether it is important to use a specific brand of medicine.

All medicines can cause an allergic reaction. Examples are hives, itching, rashes, swelling, and trouble breathing. Even a tiny amount of a medicine can cause a reaction in patients who are allergic to that medicine. Be *sure* to talk to the doctor before restarting a medicine that has caused an allergic reaction.

Taking more than one medicine at the same time may cause more side effects or cause one of the medicines to not work as well. Always ask the doctor, nurse, or pharmacist before adding another medicine, whether prescription or over-the-counter. Be sure that each doctor knows about *all* of the medicines your child is taking. Also tell the doctor about any vitamins, herbal medicines, or supplements your child may be taking. Some of these may have side effects alone or when taken with this medication.

Everyone taking medicine should have a physical examination at least once a year.

If you suspect the youth is using drugs or alcohol, please tell the doctor right away.

Pregnancy requires special care in the use of medicine. Please tell the doctor immediately if you suspect the teenager is pregnant or might become pregnant.

Printed information like this applies to children and adolescents in general. If you have questions about the medicine, or if you notice changes or anything unusual, please ask the doctor or nurse. As scientific research advances, knowledge increases and advice changes. Even experts do not always agree. Many medicines have not been approved by the U.S. Food and Drug Administration (FDA) for use in children. For this reason, use of the medicine for a particular problem or age group often is not listed in the *Physicians' Desk Reference*. This does not necessarily mean that the medicine is dangerous or does not work, only that the company that makes the medicine has not received permission to advertise the medicine for use in children. Companies often do not apply for this permission because it is expensive to do the tests needed to apply for approval for use in children. Once a medication is approved by the FDA for any purpose, a doctor is allowed to prescribe it according to research and clinical experience.

Note to Teachers

It is a good idea to talk with the parent(s) about the reason(s) that a medication is being used. If the parent(s) sign consent to release information, it is often helpful to talk with the doctor. If the parent(s) give permission, the doctor may ask you to fill out rating forms about your experience with the student's behavior, feelings, academic performance, and medication side effects. This information is very useful in selecting and monitoring medication treatment. If you have observations that you think are important, do not hesitate to share these with the student's parent(s) and treating clinicians.

It is very important that the medicine be taken exactly as the doctor instructs. However, everyone forgets to give a medicine on time once in a while. It is a good idea to ask the parent(s) in advance what to do if this happens. Do not stop or change the time you are giving a medicine at school without parental permission. If a medication is to be taken with food, but lunchtime or snack time changes, be sure to notify the parent(s) so appropriate adjustments can be made.

All medicines should be kept in a secure place and should be supervised by an adult. If someone takes too much of a medicine, follow your school procedure for an urgent medical problem.

Taking medicine is a private matter and is best managed discreetly and confidentially. It is important to be sensitive to the student's feelings about taking medicine.

If you suspect that the student is using drugs or alcohol, please tell the parent(s) or a school counselor right away.

Please tell the parent(s) or school nurse if you suspect medication side effects.

Modifications of the classroom environment or assignments may be useful in addition to medication. The student may need to be evaluated for additional help or for an Individualized Education Plan for learning or behavior.

Any expression of suicidal thoughts or feelings or self-harm by a child or adolescent is a clear signal of distress and should be taken seriously. These behaviors should not be dismissed as "attention seeking."

What Is Propranolol (Inderal)?

Propranolol is called a *beta-blocker*. It was first used to treat high blood pressure and irregular heartbeat. A newer use is the treatment of emotional and behavioral problems. It is also sometimes used to treat *akathisia*, which is a side effect of some antipsychotic medications, or to reduce tremor (shaking) in people taking lithium. It is used for migraine headaches and a number of other medical conditions.

Propranolol comes in generic propranolol and brand name Inderal tablets and liquid, Inderal LA sustained-release capsules, and InnoPranXL extended-release capsules.

How Can This Medicine Help?

Propranolol can decrease aggressive or violent behavior in children and adolescents. It may be particularly useful for patients who have developmental delays or autism. In addition, propranolol may reduce the aggression and anger that sometimes follow brain injuries. It may reduce some symptoms of anxiety (nervousness) and help children and adolescents who have experienced very frightening events and have posttraumatic stress disorder (PTSD). Propranolol may reduce the severe restlessness or shaking resulting from other medicines.

Your child may need to continue taking propranolol for at least 4 weeks before the doctor is able to decide whether the medicine is working.

How Does This Medicine Work?

When propranolol is prescribed for patients with anxiety, aggression, or other behavioral problems, it stops the effects of certain chemicals on nerves in the body and possibly in the brain that are causing the symptoms. For example, propranolol can decrease the physical anxiety symptoms of shaking, sweating, and fast heartbeat.

How Long Does This Medicine Last?

Propranolol is usually taken three times a day.

How Will the Doctor Monitor This Medicine?

The doctor will review your child's medical history and physical examination before starting propranolol. Extreme caution is needed for children and adolescents with asthma, heart disease, diabetes, kidney disease, or thyroid disease. Please be sure to tell the doctor if your child or anyone in the family has one of these problems. The doctor may order some blood or urine tests to be sure your child does not have a hidden medical condition that would make it unsafe to use this medicine. The doctor or nurse will measure your child's height, weight, pulse, and blood pressure before starting propranolol. The doctor may order an ECG (electrocardiogram or heart rhythm test) before starting propranolol.

After the medicine is started, the doctor will want to have regular appointments with you and your child to see how the medicine is working, to see if a dose change is needed, to watch for side effects, to see if propranolol is still needed, and to see if any other treatment is needed. The doctor or nurse will measure pulse rate and blood pressure at each visit, particularly as the dose is increased. Sometimes these measurements are taken while the patient is both sitting or lying down and standing up. If either pulse rate or blood pressure drops too low, a pill may not be given at that time or the regular dose may be decreased.

549

What Side Effects Can This Medicine Have?

Any medicine can have side effects, including an allergy to the medicine. Because each patient is different, the doctor will monitor the youth closely, especially when the medicine is started. The doctor will work with you to increase the positive effects and decrease the negative effects of the medicine. Please tell the doctor if any of the listed side effects appear or if you think that the medicine is causing any other problems. Not all of the rare or unusual side effects are listed.

Side effects are most common after starting the medicine or after a dose increase. Many side effects can be avoided or lessened by starting with a very low dose and increasing it slowly—ask the doctor.

Allergic Reaction

Tell the doctor in a day or two (if possible, before the next dose of medicine):

- Hives
- Itching
- Rash

  Stop the medicine and get *immediate* medical care:

- Trouble breathing or chest tightness
- Swelling of lips, tongue, or throat

Occasional Side Effects

Tell the doctor within a week or two:

- Tingling, numbness, cold, or pain in the fingers or toes (Raynaud's phenomenon)
- Tiredness or weakness, especially with exercise
- Slow heartbeat
- Low blood pressure
- Dizziness—This side effect is worse when the child stands up quickly, especially when getting out of bed in the morning; try having the child stand up slowly.

Uncommon Side Effects

Call the doctor within a day or two:

- Sadness or irritability lasting more than a few days
- Nausea
- Trouble sleeping or nightmares
- Diarrhea
- Muscle cramps

Serious Side Effects

Call the doctor *immediately*:

- Wheezing
- Hallucinations (hearing voices or seeing things that are not there)

Some Interactions With Other Medicines or Food

Please note that the following are only the most likely interactions with food or other medicines.

Giving propranolol with food will decrease side effects. The extended-release capsule should be taken the same way each time, either always with food or always without food.

Propranolol interacts with many other medicines. Be sure to tell the doctor about all medicines being taken. A doctor may use propranolol in combination with other medicines to treat a behavioral problem. The blood level of certain drugs (such as chlorpromazine [Thorazine]) increases when taken with beta-blockers. Talk with your doctor and pharmacist about possible medicine interactions.

What Could Happen if This Medicine Is Stopped Suddenly?

Stopping propranolol suddenly may cause a fast or irregular heartbeat, high blood pressure, or severe emotional problems. Propranolol should be decreased slowly over at least 2 weeks under a doctor's supervision. It is especially important not to miss doses of this medicine, because withdrawal problems may occur. **Be sure not to let the prescription run out!**

How Long Will This Medicine Be Needed?

The length of time propranolol will be needed depends on how well the medicine works for your child, whether any side effects occur, and what condition is being treated. Sometimes medicine is needed for a short time to treat a particular problem. Occasionally a person may require treatment lasting for several months or may need to start the medicine again if symptoms return.

What Else Should I Know About This Medicine?

The extended-release capsule should not be chewed or crushed; it should always be swallowed whole.

The oral solution should be mixed with water, fruit juice, or food such as applesauce before giving.

Inderal may be confused with Adderall. Be sure to check the prescription when you get it from the pharmacy.

Notes

Use this space to take notes or to write down questions you want to ask the doctor.

_____

_____

_____

_____

_____

_____

_____

_____

_____

_____

_____

_____

From Dulcan MK (editor): _Helping Parents, Youth, and Teachers Understand Medications for Behavioral and Emotional Problems: A Resource Book of Medication Information Handouts_, Third Edition. Washington, DC, American Psychiatric Publishing, 2007

Propranolol—Inderal

What the Medicine Is Called and What It Is For

The name of your medicine may be confusing. Most drugs have two names: 1) a scientific name that we call a *generic name* and 2) a trade or *brand name*. The generic name of this medicine is propranolol. The brand name is Inderal.

Propranolol is called a *beta-blocker*. These medicines work on parts of your brain and nervous system that control how your body reacts to situations in which you feel frightened, threatened, or angry. Beta-blockers were first used to treat heart and blood pressure problems. Now they are used to help young people who have too much anxiety (nervousness) or posttraumatic stress disorder (PTSD) or who fight or get angry too much. They can decrease shaking, sweating, and fast heartbeat that come from anxiety or anger. Propranolol is also sometimes used to treat restlessness caused by other medicines or to help stop shaking caused by lithium.

How You Take the Medicine

It is very important to take the medicine exactly as the doctor or nurse tells you. Do not skip doses or take extra medicine without asking an adult. If you forget a dose, ask your parent(s) what to do.

It might take as long as 4 weeks before the full effect is noticed. You may feel discouraged and think that the medicine is never going to help. You may want to give up and stop taking the medicine. Talk to your doctor and parent(s) about how you feel, but **do not stop** taking your medicine unless your doctor tells you to. It could be dangerous to stop this medicine suddenly.

Taking the medicine with food will help make side effects less. The extended-release capsule should be swallowed whole, not crushed or chewed, and always taken the same way—with or without food.

This medicine is prescribed only for you. It should never be shared with anyone else.

You do not have to tell others that you are taking this medicine, but it is not something you should feel ashamed or embarrassed about. Many young people are helped by propranolol. This medicine is not habit-forming, and you cannot become "hooked" on it. You should talk to your doctor or nurse about any questions you have about the medicine. It is important to remember that the medicine *helps* you. It cannot *make* you do anything or change you as a person.

How Your Doctor Will Follow Your Progress

Before giving you the medicine, your doctor or nurse will talk with you and your parent(s) and will measure your height, weight, heart rate (pulse), and blood pressure. Be sure to tell the doctor if you have had chest pain, very fast heartbeat, dizziness, or fainting. There may be other tests, such as blood or urine tests, or an ECG (electrocardiogram or heart rhythm test). This test counts your heartbeats through small wires that are taped to your chest. It takes only about 15 minutes.

Be sure to tell your doctor or nurse about any other medicines or supplements you are taking, including vitamins, herbs, or aids to weight loss or bodybuilding. Also be sure to tell the doctor or nurse if you are using alcohol or drugs. Because many medicines may affect babies, it is very important to tell the doctor if you might be pregnant or if you are at risk of becoming pregnant.

Your teachers may be asked to fill out a form about your grades and behavior in school. A psychologist may give you some tests to see how you learn best.

Most doctors have regular appointments with young people who are taking medicine. You should use these visits to share any concerns you may have about your medicine and to talk about if it has helped you. At the appointments, your doctor or nurse will measure your pulse rate (heartbeat) and blood pressure, particularly as the dose is increased. Sometimes these measurements are taken while you are sitting or lying down and then standing up. There may be other tests, such as repeating the ECG. Your doctor also will ask for regular reports from your parents and maybe from your teachers (with your permission) to see how well the medicine is working.

How long you will need to take this medicine depends on how well it works for you, whether there are any side effects, and what problems are being treated. Sometimes medicine is needed for only a short time to treat a particular problem. Some people need it for months or years or may need to start the medicine again if symptoms come back.

How the Medicine Might Affect You

In addition to the ways the medicine can help you, it may have other effects called *side effects*. Different medicines have different side effects. It is helpful to know about some of the most common side effects of your medicine so that you will understand what they are if they happen. Some people do not have any side effects. Some side effects are just uncomfortable, but others may mean a more serious problem with the medicine. Side effects are most common after starting the medicine or after a dose increase. They may go away with time, or the medicine can be adjusted or changed—ask the doctor.

You could have an allergy to any medicine, which might show up as a rash on your skin, swelling, itching, or trouble breathing.

Please tell your parent(s) and your doctor or nurse about any changes that you notice after taking the medicine. It is especially important to tell a responsible adult if you are feeling depressed or that you may not want to live; if you have thoughts of hurting yourself; or if you begin to feel more irritable, nervous, or restless.

Some medicines make people feel sleepy or less coordinated. If this medicine is making you sleepy, it is very important not to drive a car or ride a bicycle or motorcycle. After starting a new medicine or increasing the dose of a medicine, please be extra careful when driving a car, riding a bike, or using machines until you can tell how the medicine affects your alertness, attention, and coordination.

You might feel dizzy, tired, or even faint when you stand up fast. Try standing up slowly, especially first thing in the morning when getting out of bed.

You might notice that your fingers or toes feel very cold or tingly, that they look pale, or that they hurt. These are signs of *Raynaud's phenomenon*, which happens when the blood vessels to your fingers or toes tighten. Tell the doctor if you have these symptoms, and the dose of medicine can be adjusted or a different medicine can be used so that the problem will go away.

Other side effects (that hardly ever happen) are hallucinations (hearing voices or seeing things that are not there), upset stomach, nausea, trouble sleeping, nightmares, and sadness or irritability. You should talk to your parent(s) or doctor if you think you may be having any of these side effects.

If you are having trouble breathing, tell your parent(s) or doctor **right away.**

It is *very* important not to miss a dose or to stop this medicine suddenly—it could make you very sick.

Notes

Use this space to take notes or to write down questions you want to ask the doctor or nurse.

_____

_____

_____

_____

_____

_____

_____

_____

_____

_____

_____

_____

_____

Medication Information for Parents and Teachers

Quetiapine—Seroquel

General Information About Medication

Each child and adolescent is different. No one has exactly the same combination of medical and psychological problems. It is a good idea to talk with the doctor or nurse about the reasons a medicine is being used. It is very important to keep all appointments and to be in touch by telephone if you have concerns. It is important to communicate with the doctor, nurse, or therapist.

It is very important that the medicine be taken exactly as the doctor instructs. However, once in a while, everyone forgets to give a medicine on time. It is a good idea to ask the doctor or nurse what to do if this happens. Do not stop or change a medicine without asking the doctor or nurse first.

If the medicine seems to stop working, it may be because it is not being taken regularly. The youth may be "cheeking" or hiding the medicine or forgetting to take it (especially at school). The doses may be too far apart, or a different dose may be needed. Something at school, at home, or in the neighborhood may be upsetting the youth, or he or she may need special help for learning disabilities or tutoring. Please discuss your concerns with the doctor. **Do not just increase the dose.**

All medicines should be kept in a safe place, out of the reach of children, and should be supervised by an adult. If someone takes too much of a medicine, call the doctor, the poison control center, or a hospital emergency room.

Each medicine has a "generic" or chemical name. Just like laundry detergents or paper towels, some medicines are sold by more than one company under different brand names. The same medicine may be available under a generic name and several brand names. The generic medications are usually less expensive than the brand name ones. The generic medications have the same chemical formula, but they may or may not be exactly the same strength as the brand-name medications. Also, some brands of pills contain dye that can cause allergic reactions. It is a good idea to talk to the doctor and the pharmacist about whether it is important to use a specific brand of medicine.

All medicines can cause an allergic reaction. Examples are hives, itching, rashes, swelling, and trouble breathing. Even a tiny amount of a medicine can cause a reaction in patients who are allergic to that medicine. Be *sure* to talk to the doctor before restarting a medicine that has caused an allergic reaction.

Taking more than one medicine at the same time may cause more side effects or cause one of the medicines to not work as well. Always ask the doctor, nurse, or pharmacist before adding another medicine, whether prescription or over-the-counter. Be sure that each doctor knows about *all* of the medicines your child is taking. Also tell the doctor about any vitamins, herbal medicines, or supplements your child may be taking. Some of these may have side effects alone or when taken with this medication.

Everyone taking medicine should have a physical examination at least once a year.

If you suspect the youth is using drugs or alcohol, please tell the doctor right away.

557

Pregnancy requires special care in the use of medicine. Please tell the doctor immediately if you suspect the teenager is pregnant or might become pregnant.

Printed information like this applies to children and adolescents in general. If you have questions about the medicine, or if you notice changes or anything unusual, please ask the doctor or nurse. As scientific research advances, knowledge increases and advice changes. Even experts do not always agree. Many medicines have not been approved by the U.S. Food and Drug Administration (FDA) for use in children. For this reason, use of the medicine for a particular problem or age group often is not listed in the *Physicians' Desk Reference*. This does not necessarily mean that the medicine is dangerous or does not work, only that the company that makes the medicine has not received permission to advertise the medicine for use in children. Companies often do not apply for this permission because it is expensive to do the tests needed to apply for approval for use in children. Once a medication is approved by the FDA for any purpose, a doctor is allowed to prescribe it according to research and clinical experience.

Note to Teachers

It is a good idea to talk with the parent(s) about the reason(s) that a medication is being used. If the parent(s) sign consent to release information, it is often helpful to talk with the doctor. If the parent(s) give permission, the doctor may ask you to fill out rating forms about your experience with the student's behavior, feelings, academic performance, and medication side effects. This information is very useful in selecting and monitoring medication treatment. If you have observations that you think are important, do not hesitate to share these with the student's parent(s) and treating clinicians.

It is very important that the medicine be taken exactly as the doctor instructs. However, everyone forgets to give a medicine on time once in a while. It is a good idea to ask the parent(s) in advance what to do if this happens. Do not stop or change the time you are giving a medicine at school without parental permission. If a medication is to be taken with food, but lunchtime or snack time changes, be sure to notify the parent(s) so appropriate adjustments can be made.

All medicines should be kept in a secure place and should be supervised by an adult. If someone takes too much of a medicine, follow your school procedure for an urgent medical problem.

Taking medicine is a private matter and is best managed discreetly and confidentially. It is important to be sensitive to the student's feelings about taking medicine.

If you suspect that the student is using drugs or alcohol, please tell the parent(s) or a school counselor right away.

Please tell the parent(s) or school nurse if you suspect medication side effects.

Modifications of the classroom environment or assignments may be useful in addition to medication. The student may need to be evaluated for additional help or for an Individualized Education Plan for learning or behavior.

Any expression of suicidal thoughts or feelings or self-harm by a child or adolescent is a clear signal of distress and should be taken seriously. These behaviors should not be dismissed as "attention seeking."

What Is Quetiapine (Seroquel)?

This medicine is called an *atypical* or *second-generation antipsychotic*. It is sometimes called an *atypical psychotropic agent* or simply an *atypical*. It comes in brand name Seroquel tablets.

How Can This Medicine Help?

Quetiapine is used to treat psychosis, such as in schizophrenia, mania, or very severe depression. It can reduce *positive symptoms* such as hallucinations (hearing voices or seeing things that are not there); delusions (troubling beliefs that other people do not share); agitation; and very unusual thinking, speech, and behavior. It is also used to lessen the *negative symptoms* of schizophrenia, such as lack of interest in doing things (apathy), lack of motivation, social withdrawal, and lack of energy.

Quetiapine may be used as a *mood stabilizer* in patients with bipolar disorder (manic-depressive illness) or severe mood swings. It can reduce mania and may be able to help maintain a stable mood over the long term.

Sometimes quetiapine is used to reduce severe aggression or very serious behavioral problems in young people with conduct disorder, mental retardation, autism, or pervasive developmental disorder.

Quetiapine may be used for behavior problems that arise after a head injury.

It is also used to reduce motor and vocal tics (fast, repeated movements or sounds) and behavioral problems in people with Tourette's disorder.

This medicine is very powerful and is used to treat very serious problems or symptoms that other medicines do not help. Be patient; the positive effects of this medicine may not appear for 2–3 weeks.

How Does This Medicine Work?

Cells in the brain communicate using chemicals called *neurotransmitters*. Too much or too little of these substances in parts of the brain can cause problems. Quetiapine works by blocking the action of two of these neurotransmitters, *dopamine* and *serotonin*, in certain areas of the brain.

How Long Does This Medicine Last?

Quetiapine is usually taken two or three times a day.

How Will the Doctor Monitor This Medicine?

The doctor will review your child's medical history and physical examination before starting quetiapine. The doctor may order some blood or urine tests to be sure your child does not have a hidden medical condition that would make it unsafe to use this medicine. The doctor or nurse may measure your child's pulse and blood pressure before starting quetiapine. The doctor may order other tests, such as baseline tests for blood sugar and cholesterol.

Be sure to tell the doctor if anyone in the family has diabetes, high blood pressure, high cholesterol, heart disease, or thyroid problems.

Before starting quetiapine and every so often afterward, a test such as the AIMS (Abnormal Involuntary Movement Scale) may be used to check your child's tongue, legs, and arms for unusual movements that could be caused by the medicine.

After the medicine is started, the doctor will want to have regular appointments with you and your child to see how the medicine is working, to see if a dose change is needed, to watch for side effects, to see if quetiapine is still needed, and to see if any other treatment is needed. The doctor or nurse may check your child's height, weight, pulse, and blood pressure and watch for abnormal movements. Sometimes blood tests are needed to watch for diabetes or increased cholesterol.

What Side Effects Can This Medicine Have?

Any medicine can have side effects, including an allergy to the medicine. Because each patient is different, the doctor will monitor the youth closely, especially when the medicine is started. The doctor will work with you to increase the positive effects and decrease the negative effects of the medicine. Please tell the doctor if any of the listed side effects appear or if you think that the medicine is causing any other problems. Not all of the rare or unusual side effects are listed.

Side effects are most common after starting the medicine or after a dose increase. Many side effects can be avoided or lessened by starting with a very low dose and increasing it slowly—ask the doctor.

Allergic Reaction

Tell the doctor in a day or two (if possible, before the next dose of medicine):

- Hives
- Itching
- Rash

    Stop the medicine and get *immediate* medical care:

- Trouble breathing or chest tightness
- Swelling of lips, tongue, or throat

Common, but Not Usually Serious, Side Effects

Discuss the following side effects with your child's doctor when convenient. These side effects often can be helped by lowering the dose of medicine, changing the times medicine is taken, or adding another medicine.

- Daytime sleepiness or tiredness—Do not allow your child to drive, ride a bicycle or motorcycle, or operate machinery if this happens. This problem may be lessened by taking the medicine at bedtime.
- Dry mouth—Have your child try using sugar-free gum or candy.
- Constipation—Encourage your child to drink more fluids and eat high-fiber foods; if necessary, the doctor may recommend a fiber medicine such as Benefiber or a stool softener such as Colace or mineral oil.
- Dizziness—This side effect is worse when the child stands up quickly, especially when getting out of bed in the morning; try having the child stand up slowly.
- Increased appetite
- Weight gain—Seek nutritional counseling; provide your child with low-calorie snacks and encourage regular exercise.

Less Common, but Not Usually Serious, Side Effects

Discuss the following side effects with your child's doctor when convenient. These side effects often can be helped by lowering the dose of medicine, changing the times medicine is taken, or adding another medicine.

- Increased restlessness or inability to sit still
- Shaking of hands and fingers
- Decreased or slowed movement and decreased facial expressions

Less Common, but Potentially Serious, Side Effects

Call the doctor *immediately*:

- Stiffness of the tongue, jaw, neck, back, or legs
- Seizure (fit, convulsion)—This is more common in people with a history of seizures or head injury.
- Increased thirst, frequent urination (having to go to the bathroom often), lethargy, tiredness, dizziness, and blurred vision—These could be signs of diabetes (especially if your child is overweight or there is a family history of diabetes). **Talk to a doctor within a day.**

Very Rare, but Serious, Side Effects

- Extreme stiffness or lack of movement, very high fever, mental confusion, irregular pulse rate, or eye pain—**This is a medical emergency. Go to an emergency room right away.**
- Sudden stiffness and inability to breathe or swallow—**Go to an emergency room or call 911.** Tell the paramedics, nurses, and doctors that the patient is taking quetiapine. Other medicines can be used to treat this problem fast.
- Illness, yellowing of eyes or skin, stomach pain—This may mean damage to the liver. **Call the doctor within a day or two.**

What Else Should I Know About Side Effects?

Most side effects lessen over time. If they are troublesome, talk with your child's doctor. Some side effects can be decreased by taking a smaller dose of medicine, by stopping the medicine, by changing to another medicine, or by adding another medicine.

Many people who take quetiapine gain weight. Children seem to have more problems with this than adults. The weight gain may be from increased appetite and from ways that the medicine changes how the body processes food. Quetiapine may also change the way that the body handles glucose (sugar) and cause high levels (hyperglycemia). People who take quetiapine, especially those who gain a lot of weight, are at increased risk of developing diabetes and of having increased fats (lipids—cholesterol and triglycerides) in their blood. Over time, both diabetes and increased fats in the blood may lead to heart disease, stroke, and other complications. The FDA has put warnings on all atypical agents about the increased risks of hyperglycemia, diabetes, and increased blood cholesterol and triglycerides when taking one of these medicines. It is much easier to prevent weight gain than to lose weight later. When your child first starts taking quetiapine, it is a good idea to be sure that he or she eats a well-balanced diet without "junk food" and with healthy snacks like fruits and vegetables, not sweets or fried foods. He or she should drink water or skim milk, not pop, sodas, soft drinks, or sugary juices. Regular exercise is important for maintaining a healthy weight (and may also help with sleep).

One very rare side effect that may not go away is *tardive dyskinesia* (or TD). Patients with tardive dyskinesia have involuntary movements (movements that they cannot help making) of the body, especially the mouth and tongue. The patient may look as though he or she is making faces over and over again. Jerky movements of the arms, legs, or body may occur. There may be fine, wormlike, or sudden repeated movements of the tongue, or the person may appear to be chewing something or smacking or puckering his or her lips. The fingers may look as though they are rolling something. If you notice any unusual movements, be sure to tell the doctor. The doctor may use the AIMS test to look for these movements.

Neuroleptic malignant syndrome is a very rare side effect that can lead to death. The symptoms are severe muscle stiffness, high fever, increased heart rate and blood pressure, irregular heartbeat (pulse), and sweating. It may lead to unconsciousness. If you suspect this, **call 911 or go to an emergency room right away.**

Some Interactions With Other Medicines or Food

Please note that the following are only the most likely interactions with food or other medicines.

Quetiapine may be taken with or without food.

Carbamazepine (Tegretol) and phenytoin (Dilantin) may decrease levels of quetiapine, making it not work as well.

It is better to limit drinks with caffeine (coffee, tea, soft drinks) because caffeine works in the opposite way from this medicine, and the positive effects might be decreased.

What Could Happen if This Medicine Is Stopped Suddenly?

Involuntary movements, or *withdrawal dyskinesias*, may appear within 1–4 weeks of lowering the dose or stopping the medicine. Usually these go away, but they can last for days to months. If quetiapine is stopped suddenly, emotional disturbance (such as irritability, nervousness, moodiness, or oppositional behavior) or physical problems (such as stomachache, loss of appetite, nausea, vomiting, diarrhea, sweating, indigestion, trouble sleeping, trembling, or shaking) may appear. These problems usually last only a few days to a few weeks. If they happen, you should tell your child's doctor. The medicine dose may need to be lowered more slowly (tapered). Always check with the doctor before stopping a medicine.

How Long Will This Medicine Be Needed?

How long your child will need to take this medicine depends partly on the reason that it was prescribed. Some problems last for only a few months, whereas others last much longer. It is important to ask the doctor whether medicine is still needed, especially with medicines as powerful as this one. Every few months, you should discuss with your child's doctor the reasons for using quetiapine and whether it may be stopped or the dose lowered.

What Else Should I Know About This Medicine?

There are other medicines that are used for the same kinds of problems. If your child is having bad side effects or the medicine does not seem to be working, ask the doctor if another medicine might work as well or better and have fewer side effects for your child. Each person reacts differently to medicines.

Taking this medicine could make overheating or heatstroke more likely. Have your child decrease activity in hot weather, stay out of the sun, and drink water to prevent this.

Notes

Use this space to take notes or to write down questions you want to ask the doctor.

_____

_____

_____

_____

_____

_____

_____

_____

_____

_____

_____

From Dulcan MK (editor): _Helping Parents, Youth, and Teachers Understand Medications for Behavioral and Emotional Problems: A Resource Book of Medication Information Handouts_, Third Edition. Washington, DC, American Psychiatric Publishing, 2007

Medication Information
for Youth

Quetiapine—Seroquel

What the Medicine Is Called and What It Is For

The name of your medicine may be confusing. Most drugs have two names: 1) a scientific name that we call a *generic name* and 2) a trade or *brand name*. The generic name of this medicine is quetiapine. The brand name is Seroquel.

Quetiapine is called an *atypical* medicine. It helps people who feel very confused and have severe problems thinking clearly. It can lessen hallucinations (seeing or hearing things that are not really there) and delusions (troubling beliefs that other people do not share). The medicine also can improve *negative symptoms*, such as lack of interest in doing things, lack of motivation, loss of interest in friends, and decreased energy. It helps people who have severe depression or mood swings. This medicine also is sometimes used to help young people who have mania or severe depression or who get very angry and hit people or break things. Quetiapine can reduce motor and vocal tics (fast, repeated movements or sounds) in people with Tourette's disorder.

How You Take the Medicine

It is very important to take the medicine exactly as the doctor or nurse tells you. Do not skip doses or take extra medicine without asking an adult. If you forget a dose, ask your parent(s) what to do.

It is better to limit drinks with caffeine (coffee, tea, soft drinks) because caffeine works in the opposite way from this medicine, and the positive effects might be decreased.

Your doctor will tell you how much medicine to take and how often to take it so that it can help you the most. It is *very important* that you take all the pills you are supposed to take each day. Your doctor will probably recommend that you take your medicine at the same time each day, which may be with meals or at bedtime.

It may be several weeks or longer before you notice the full effect. You may feel discouraged and think the medicine is never going to help. You may want to give up and stop taking the medicine. Talk to your doctor and parent(s) about how you feel, but **do not stop** taking your medicine unless your doctor tells you to. It also is important not to take extra pills hoping that you will feel better faster. Doing that could make you very sick.

This medicine is prescribed only for you. It should never be shared with anyone else.

You do not have to tell others that you are taking this medicine, but it is not something you should feel ashamed or embarrassed about. Many young people are helped by quetiapine. This medicine is not habit-forming, and you cannot become "hooked" on it. You should talk to your doctor or nurse about any questions you have about the medicine. It is important to remember that the medicine *helps* you. It cannot *make* you do anything or change you as a person.

565

How Your Doctor Will Follow Your Progress

Before giving you the medicine, your doctor or nurse will talk with you and your parent(s) and may measure your height, weight, heart rate (pulse), and blood pressure. There may be other tests, such as blood tests for sugar and cholesterol. Before you start taking the medicine and every so often afterward, the doctor or nurse will look at your tongue, arms, and legs to check for unusual movements. This is called the AIMS (Abnormal Involuntary Movement Scale) test.

Be sure to tell your doctor or nurse about any other medicines or supplements you are taking, including vitamins, herbs, or aids to weight loss or bodybuilding. Also be sure to tell the doctor or nurse if you are using alcohol or drugs. Because many medicines may affect babies, it is very important to tell the doctor if you might be pregnant or if you are at risk of becoming pregnant.

Your teachers may be asked to fill out a form about your grades and behavior in school. A psychologist may give you some tests to see how you learn best.

Most doctors have regular appointments with young people who are taking medicine. You should use these visits to share any concerns you may have about your medicine and to talk about if it has helped you. From time to time, your physician or nurse may measure your height, weight, heart rate (pulse), and blood pressure to be sure that you are in good health while you are taking the medicine. There may be blood tests to watch for diabetes or high cholesterol. Your doctor also will ask for regular reports from your parents and maybe from your teachers (with your permission) to see how well the medicine is working.

If the medicine helps you, your doctor will probably want you to take it for several months to a year. Your doctor will decide how long you will need to take the medicine as he or she watches your progress.

How the Medicine Might Affect You

In addition to the ways the medicine can help you, it may have other effects called *side effects*. Different medicines have different side effects. It is helpful to know about some of the most common side effects of your medicine so that you will understand what they are if they happen. Some people do not have any side effects. Some side effects are just uncomfortable, but others may mean a more serious problem with the medicine. Side effects are most common after starting the medicine or after a dose increase. They may go away with time, or the medicine can be adjusted or changed—ask the doctor.

You could have an allergy to any medicine, which might show up as a rash on your skin, swelling, itching, or trouble breathing.

Please tell your parent(s) and your doctor or nurse about any changes that you notice after taking the medicine. It is especially important to tell a responsible adult if you are feeling depressed or that you may not want to live; if you have thoughts of hurting yourself; or if you begin to feel more irritable, nervous, or restless. Also be sure to tell your parent(s) or doctor if you begin to feel "speeded up" or have trouble sleeping.

One of the most common side effects of this medicine is feeling tired or sleepy during the day, even if you have had a full night's sleep. If this medicine is making you sleepy, it is very important not to drive a car or ride a bicycle or motorcycle. After starting the medicine or increasing the dose of medicine, please be extra careful when driving a car, riding a bike, or using machines until you can tell how the medicine affects your alertness, attention, and coordination. After you have been taking the medicine for a few weeks, your body will adjust, and this side effect will likely go away. If you had trouble sleeping at night before taking the medicine, it can help you sleep better, especially if the doctor tells you to take a dose of medicine in the evening.

Another common side effect is dry mouth. You may be more thirsty than usual and find that you are drinking more water or other liquids than usual. Sucking on sugar-free hard candy or cough drops usually helps. You also could try chewing sugar-free gum or sucking on ice chips. Do not chew the ice; you could hurt your teeth. Also, using lip balm will keep your lips from cracking. It is important to be especially good about brushing your teeth.

If you get very thirsty, have to go to the bathroom a lot, feel *very* tired, or have dizziness or blurred vision, be sure to tell your parent(s) or doctor.

Taking this medicine could make you more likely to get badly sunburned or very sick in hot weather. Be sure to drink plenty of liquids and cover up or use sunscreen when you go outside in hot weather. Be careful to rest in the shade and not get overheated.

Sometimes teenagers who take quetiapine gain weight. The weight gain may be from increased appetite and also from ways that the medicine changes how the body processes food. People who take quetiapine, especially those who gain a lot of weight, might be at increased risk of developing diabetes and of having increased fats (lipids—cholesterol and triglycerides) in their blood. Over time, both diabetes and increased fats in the blood may lead to heart disease, stroke, and other complications. U.S. Food and Drug Administration has put warnings about these problems on all medicines like quetiapine. It is much easier to prevent weight gain than to lose weight later. It is a good idea to eat a well-balanced diet without "junk food" and with healthy snacks like fruits and vegetables, not sweets or fried foods. It is better to drink water or skim milk, not pop, sodas, soft drinks, or sugary juices. Regular exercise is important for maintaining a healthy weight (and may also help with sleep).

You may notice changes in your sexual functioning—it is OK to ask the doctor about this.

Quetiapine is a very powerful medicine. Some side effects include feeling nervous, restless, or shaky or having stiff muscles. Talk with your doctor about these side effects. They can be helped by adding another medicine, adjusting the dose, or switching to another medicine.

Another, more serious, side effect can be longer lasting and more difficult to treat. This very rare side effect is called *tardive dyskinesia* (or TD). A person taking quetiapine may develop movements of the mouth, tongue, face, arms, legs, or body that are not being made on purpose. This side effect can go away when the medicine is stopped, but in some people it does not go away. Your doctor will explain this effect to you and your parent(s) and how he or she will watch for any signs that you are developing this problem. Be sure to ask your doctor any questions that you may have about this, but do not worry too much about it. It hardly ever happens to teenagers.

You should tell your parent(s) and doctor if you notice anything different or unusual about how you feel once you start taking the medicine. This includes good things, such as feeling less confused, feeling less sad, not hearing voices anymore, or sleeping better at night.

Notes

Use this space to take notes or to write down questions you want to ask the doctor or nurse.

_____

_____

_____

_____

_____

_____

_____

_____

_____

_____

_____

_____

_____

From Dulcan MK (editor): *Helping Parents, Youth, and Teachers Understand Medications for Behavioral and Emotional Problems: A Resource Book of Medication Information Handouts*, Third Edition. Washington, DC, American Psychiatric Publishing, 2007

Medication Information for Parents and Teachers

Ramelteon—Rozerem

General Information About Medication

Each child and adolescent is different. No one has exactly the same combination of medical and psychological problems. It is a good idea to talk with the doctor or nurse about the reasons a medicine is being used. It is very important to keep all appointments and to be in touch by telephone if you have concerns. It is important to communicate with the doctor, nurse, or therapist.

It is very important that the medicine be taken exactly as the doctor instructs. However, once in a while, everyone forgets to give a medicine on time. It is a good idea to ask the doctor or nurse what to do if this happens. Do not stop or change a medicine without asking the doctor or nurse first.

If the medicine seems to stop working, it may be because it is not being taken regularly. The youth may be "cheeking" or hiding the medicine or forgetting to take it. A different dose may be needed. Something at school, at home, or in the neighborhood may be upsetting the youth, or he or she may need special help for learning disabilities or tutoring. Please discuss your concerns with the doctor. **Do not just increase the dose.**

All medicines should be kept in a safe place, out of the reach of children, and should be supervised by an adult. If someone takes too much of a medicine, call the doctor, the poison control center, or a hospital emergency room.

Each medicine has a "generic" or chemical name. Just like laundry detergents or paper towels, some medicines are sold by more than one company under different brand names. The same medicine may be available under a generic name and several brand names. The generic medications are usually less expensive than the brand name ones. The generic medications have the same chemical formula, but they may or may not be exactly the same strength as the brand-name medications. Also, some brands of pills contain dye that can cause allergic reactions. It is a good idea to talk to the doctor and the pharmacist about whether it is important to use a specific brand of medicine.

All medicines can cause an allergic reaction. Examples are hives, itching, rashes, swelling, and trouble breathing. Even a tiny amount of a medicine can cause a reaction in patients who are allergic to that medicine. Be *sure* to talk to the doctor before restarting a medicine that has caused an allergic reaction.

Taking more than one medicine at the same time may cause more side effects or cause one of the medicines to not work as well. Always ask the doctor, nurse, or pharmacist before adding another medicine, whether prescription or over-the-counter. Be sure that each doctor knows about *all* of the medicines your child is taking. Also tell the doctor about any vitamins, herbal medicines, or supplements your child may be taking. Some of these may have side effects alone or when taken with this medication.

Everyone taking medicine should have a physical examination at least once a year.

If you suspect the youth is using drugs or alcohol, please tell the doctor right away.

Pregnancy requires special care in the use of medicine. Please tell the doctor immediately if you suspect the teenager is pregnant or might become pregnant.

Printed information like this applies to children and adolescents in general. If you have questions about the medicine, or if you notice changes or anything unusual, please ask the doctor or nurse. As scientific research advances, knowledge increases and advice changes. Even experts do not always agree. Many medicines have not been approved by the U.S. Food and Drug Administration (FDA) for use in children. For this reason, use of the medicine for a particular problem or age group often is not listed in the *Physicians' Desk Reference*. This does not necessarily mean that the medicine is dangerous or does not work, only that the company that makes the medicine has not received permission to advertise the medicine for use in children. Companies often do not apply for this permission because it is expensive to do the tests needed to apply for approval for use in children. Once a medication is approved by the FDA for any purpose, a doctor is allowed to prescribe it according to research and clinical experience.

Note to Teachers

It is a good idea to talk with the parent(s) about the reason(s) that a medication is being used. If the parent(s) sign consent to release information, it is often helpful to talk with the doctor. If the parent(s) give permission, the doctor may ask you to fill out rating forms about your experience with the student's behavior, feelings, academic performance, and medication side effects. This information is very useful in selecting and monitoring medication treatment. If you have observations that you think are important, do not hesitate to share these with the student's parent(s) and treating clinicians.

All medicines should be kept in a secure place and should be supervised by an adult. If someone takes too much of a medicine, follow your school procedure for an urgent medical problem.

Taking medicine is a private matter and is best managed discreetly and confidentially. It is important to be sensitive to the student's feelings about taking medicine.

If you suspect that the student is using drugs or alcohol, please tell the parent(s) or a school counselor right away.

Please tell the parent(s) or school nurse if you suspect medication side effects.

Any expression of suicidal thoughts or feelings or self-harm by a child or adolescent is a clear signal of distress and should be taken seriously. These behaviors should not be dismissed as "attention seeking."

What Is Ramelteon (Rozerem)?

Ramelteon is a *hypnotic* or *sedative-hypnotic* medicine. It is *not* a *benzodiazepine*. It comes in Rozerem brand name tablets.

How Can This Medicine Help?

Ramelteon is used to treat insomnia (problems falling asleep or staying asleep).

How Does This Medicine Work?

Ramelteon works in the same way as a natural substance called *melatonin* that is produced by the body. It helps regulate the sleep-wake cycle (circadian rhythm).

How Long Does This Medicine Last?

Ramelteon is taken before bedtime and starts working within an hour.

How Will the Doctor Monitor This Medicine?

The doctor will review your child's medical history and physical examination before starting ramelteon. Be sure to tell the doctor if your child has liver disease.

After the medicine is started, the doctor will want to have regular appointments with you and your child to see how the medicine is working, to see if a dose change is needed, to watch for side effects, to see if ramelteon is still needed, and to see if any other treatment is needed.

What Side Effects Can This Medicine Have?

Any medicine can have side effects, including an allergy to the medicine. Because each patient is different, the doctor will monitor the youth closely, especially when the medicine is started. The doctor will work with you to increase the positive effects and decrease the negative effects of the medicine. Please tell the doctor if any of the listed side effects appear or if you think that the medicine is causing any other problems. Not all of the rare or unusual side effects are listed.

Side effects are most common after starting the medicine or after a dose increase. Many side effects can be avoided or lessened by starting with a very low dose and increasing it slowly—ask the doctor.

Allergic Reaction

Tell the doctor in a day or two (if possible, before the next dose of medicine):

- Hives
- Itching
- Rash

    Stop the medicine and get *immediate* medical care:

- Trouble breathing or chest tightness
- Swelling of lips, tongue, or throat

Common Side Effects

Tell the doctor within a week or two:

- Daytime sleepiness—Do not allow your child to drive a car, ride a bicycle or motorcycle, or operate machinery if this happens.
- Dizziness, feeling "spacey," or decreased coordination
- Low energy or tiredness
- Headache

Less Common Side Effects

Tell the doctor within a week or two:

- More trouble sleeping
- Nausea
- Diarrhea

Rare, but Potentially Serious, Side Effects

Tell the doctor within a week or two:

- Missed menstrual periods
- Fluid discharge from the breasts

Rare, but Serious, Side Effects

Stop the medicine and call the doctor right away:

- Depression
- Thoughts of harming oneself

Some Interactions With Other Medicines or Food

Please note that the following are only the most likely interactions with food or other medicines.

Caffeine may cause trouble sleeping and make ramelteon less effective. If caffeine is eliminated, less ramelteon may be needed, or ramelteon may not be needed at all.

Do not take ramelteon with or immediately after a high-fat meal because fat can affect how well this drug works.

Do not take ramelteon with fluvoxamine (Luvox).

It is important not to use other sedatives, tranquilizers, or sleeping pills or antihistamines (such as Benadryl) when taking ramelteon because of increased side effects.

What Could Happen if This Medicine Is Stopped Suddenly?

There are no known medical withdrawal effects, but the sleep problem may come back.

How Long Will This Medicine Be Needed?

Ramelteon is usually prescribed for a short time, but some people may need to take it for longer. A behavioral program, such as regular soothing routines at bedtime and increased exercise in the daytime, should be used along with the medicine to improve sleep. Finding developmentally appropriate bed- and wake-times and sticking to them is very important. These strategies should be continued after the medicine is stopped or when the medicine is used only occasionally.

What Else Should I Know About This Medicine?

People who take ramelteon must not drink alcohol. Severe sleepiness or even loss of consciousness may result.

People with sleep apnea (breathing stops while they are asleep) should not take ramelteon. Tell the doctor if your child snores very loudly.

Notes

Use this space to take notes or to write down questions you want to ask the doctor.

_____

_____

_____

_____

_____

_____

_____

_____

_____

_____

From Dulcan MK (editor): _Helping Parents, Youth, and Teachers Understand Medications for Behavioral and Emotional Problems: A Resource Book of Medication Information Handouts_, Third Edition. Washington, DC, American Psychiatric Publishing, 2007

Medication Information for Youth

Ramelteon—Rozerem

What the Medicine Is Called and What It Is For

The name of your medicine may be confusing. Most drugs have two names: 1) a scientific name that we call a *generic name* and 2) a trade or *brand name*. The generic name of this medicine is ramelteon. The brand name is Rozerem.

Ramelteon works like *melatonin*, which is a natural hormone made by a gland in the brain. Ramelteon is not a sedative or a tranquilizer. It is not like other sleeping pills, but it can improve sleep by helping a person have a more natural sleep cycle. It can help with falling asleep and staying asleep long enough to feel rested. Some teenagers do not get sleepy until later and later at night and have more and more trouble getting up in the morning for school. Ramelteon can help shift sleep to a more regular schedule.

How You Take the Medicine

It is very important to take the medicine exactly as the doctor or nurse tells you. Do not skip doses or take extra medicine without asking an adult. If you forget a dose, ask your parent(s) what to do.

Ramelteon works best if combined with a regular bedtime, calming routines before bedtime, and physical exercise during the day. Getting up on time is also important in keeping a regular sleep schedule.

Caffeine (in coffee, tea, or soft drinks) may make it harder to fall asleep and make the ramelteon not work as well.

This medicine does not work as well when taken after a high-fat meal. Take it several hours after eating.

This medicine is prescribed only for you. It should never be shared with anyone else.

You do not have to tell others that you are taking this medicine, but it is not something you should feel ashamed or embarrassed about. Many young people are helped by ramelteon. This medicine is not habit-forming, and you cannot become "hooked" on it. You should talk to your doctor or nurse about any questions you have about the medicine. It is important to remember that the medicine *helps* you. It cannot *make* you do anything or change you as a person.

How Your Doctor Will Follow Your Progress

Before giving you the medicine, your doctor or nurse will talk with you and your parent(s) and may measure your height, weight, heart rate (pulse), and blood pressure.

Be sure to tell your doctor or nurse about any other medicines or supplements you are taking, including vitamins, herbs, or aids to weight loss or bodybuilding. Also be sure to tell the doctor or nurse if you are using alcohol or drugs. Because many medicines may affect babies, it is very important to tell the doctor if you might be pregnant or if you are at risk of becoming pregnant.

Most doctors have regular appointments with young people who are taking medicine. You should use these visits to share any concerns you may have about your medicine and to talk about if it has helped you. From time to time, your physician or nurse may measure your height, weight, heart rate (pulse), and blood pressure to be sure that you are in good health while you are taking the medicine. Your doctor also will ask for regular reports from your parents to see how well the medicine is working.

How the Medicine Might Affect You

In addition to the ways the medicine can help you, it may have other effects called *side effects*. Different medicines have different side effects. It is helpful to know about some of the most common side effects of your medicine so that you will understand what they are if they happen. Some people do not have any side effects. Some side effects are just uncomfortable, but others may mean a more serious problem with the medicine. Side effects are most common after starting the medicine or after a dose increase. They may go away with time, or the medicine can be adjusted or changed—ask the doctor.

You could have an allergy to any medicine, which might show up as a rash on your skin, swelling, itching, or trouble breathing.

Please tell your parent(s) and doctor or nurse about any changes that you notice after taking the medicine. It is especially important to tell a responsible adult right away if you are feeling depressed or that you may not want to live; if you have thoughts of hurting yourself; or if you begin to feel more irritable, nervous, or restless.

Some medicines make people feel sleepy or less coordinated. If this medicine is making you sleepy, it is very important not to drive a car or ride a bicycle or motorcycle. After starting a new medicine or increasing the dose of a medicine, please be extra careful when driving a car, riding a bike, or using machines until you can tell how the medicine affects your alertness, attention, and coordination.

The most common side effects of ramelteon are daytime sleepiness, tiredness, low energy, dizziness, feeling "spacey," headache, or clumsiness. Some people have nausea or diarrhea. In girls, ramelteon may change the timing of menstrual periods and in both boys and girls there may be changes in the breasts—it is OK to ask the doctor about this.

Notes

Use this space to take notes or to write down questions you want to ask the doctor or nurse.

_____

_____

_____

_____

_____

_____

_____

_____

_____

_____

_____

_____

_____

Medication Information for Parents and Teachers

Risperidone—Risperdal

General Information About Medication

Each child and adolescent is different. No one has exactly the same combination of medical and psychological problems. It is a good idea to talk with the doctor or nurse about the reasons a medicine is being used. It is very important to keep all appointments and to be in touch by telephone if you have concerns. It is important to communicate with the doctor, nurse, or therapist.

It is very important that the medicine be taken exactly as the doctor instructs. However, once in a while, everyone forgets to give a medicine on time. It is a good idea to ask the doctor or nurse what to do if this happens. Do not stop or change a medicine without asking the doctor or nurse first.

If the medicine seems to stop working, it may be because it is not being taken regularly. The youth may be "cheeking" or hiding the medicine or forgetting to take it (especially at school). The doses may be too far apart, or a different dose may be needed. Something at school, at home, or in the neighborhood may be upsetting the youth, or he or she may need special help for learning disabilities or tutoring. Please discuss your concerns with the doctor. **Do not just increase the dose.**

All medicines should be kept in a safe place, out of the reach of children, and should be supervised by an adult. If someone takes too much of a medicine, call the doctor, the poison control center, or a hospital emergency room.

Each medicine has a "generic" or chemical name. Just like laundry detergents or paper towels, some medicines are sold by more than one company under different brand names. The same medicine may be available under a generic name and several brand names. The generic medications are usually less expensive than the brand name ones. The generic medications have the same chemical formula, but they may or may not be exactly the same strength as the brand-name medications. Also, some brands of pills contain dye that can cause allergic reactions. It is a good idea to talk to the doctor and the pharmacist about whether it is important to use a specific brand of medicine.

All medicines can cause an allergic reaction. Examples are hives, itching, rashes, swelling, and trouble breathing. Even a tiny amount of a medicine can cause a reaction in patients who are allergic to that medicine. Be *sure* to talk to the doctor before restarting a medicine that has caused an allergic reaction.

Taking more than one medicine at the same time may cause more side effects or cause one of the medicines to not work as well. Always ask the doctor, nurse, or pharmacist before adding another medicine, whether prescription or over-the-counter. Be sure that each doctor knows about *all* of the medicines your child is taking. Also tell the doctor about any vitamins, herbal medicines, or supplements your child may be taking. Some of these may have side effects alone or when taken with this medication.

Everyone taking medicine should have a physical examination at least once a year.

If you suspect the youth is using drugs or alcohol, please tell the doctor right away.

Pregnancy requires special care in the use of medicine. Please tell the doctor immediately if you suspect the teenager is pregnant or might become pregnant.

Printed information like this applies to children and adolescents in general. If you have questions about the medicine, or if you notice changes or anything unusual, please ask the doctor or nurse. As scientific research advances, knowledge increases and advice changes. Even experts do not always agree. Many medicines have not been approved by the U.S. Food and Drug Administration (FDA) for use in children. For this reason, use of the medicine for a particular problem or age group often is not listed in the *Physicians' Desk Reference*. This does not necessarily mean that the medicine is dangerous or does not work, only that the company that makes the medicine has not received permission to advertise the medicine for use in children. Companies often do not apply for this permission because it is expensive to do the tests needed to apply for approval for use in children. Once a medication is approved by the FDA for any purpose, a doctor is allowed to prescribe it according to research and clinical experience.

Note to Teachers

It is a good idea to talk with the parent(s) about the reason(s) that a medication is being used. If the parent(s) sign consent to release information, it is often helpful to talk with the doctor. If the parent(s) give permission, the doctor may ask you to fill out rating forms about your experience with the student's behavior, feelings, academic performance, and medication side effects. This information is very useful in selecting and monitoring medication treatment. If you have observations that you think are important, do not hesitate to share these with the student's parent(s) and treating clinicians.

It is very important that the medicine be taken exactly as the doctor instructs. However, everyone forgets to give a medicine on time once in a while. It is a good idea to ask the parent(s) in advance what to do if this happens. Do not stop or change the time you are giving a medicine at school without parental permission. If a medication is to be taken with food, but lunchtime or snack time changes, be sure to notify the parent(s) so appropriate adjustments can be made.

All medicines should be kept in a secure place and should be supervised by an adult. If someone takes too much of a medicine, follow your school procedure for an urgent medical problem.

Taking medicine is a private matter and is best managed discreetly and confidentially. It is important to be sensitive to the student's feelings about taking medicine.

If you suspect that the student is using drugs or alcohol, please tell the parent(s) or a school counselor right away.

Please tell the parent(s) or school nurse if you suspect medication side effects.

Modifications of the classroom environment or assignments may be useful in addition to medication. The student may need to be evaluated for additional help or for an Individualized Education Plan for learning or behavior.

Any expression of suicidal thoughts or feelings or self-harm by a child or adolescent is a clear signal of distress and should be taken seriously. These behaviors should not be dismissed as "attention seeking."

What Is Risperidone (Risperdal)?

This medicine is called an *atypical* or *second-generation antipsychotic*. It is sometimes called an *atypical psychotropic agent* or simply an *atypical*. It comes in brand name Risperdal tablets, Risperdal M-Tab rapid-disintegrating tablets, liquid, and Risperdal Consta long-acting injection (shot). The peppermint-flavored M-Tab melts fast in the mouth.

How Can This Medicine Help?

Risperidone is used to treat psychosis, such as in schizophrenia, mania, or very severe depression. It can reduce *positive symptoms* such as hallucinations (hearing voices or seeing things that are not there); delusions (troubling beliefs that other people do not share); agitation; and very unusual thinking, speech, and behavior. It is also used to lessen the *negative symptoms* of schizophrenia, such as lack of interest in doing things (apathy), lack of motivation, social withdrawal, and lack of energy.

Risperidone may be used as a *mood stabilizer* in patients with bipolar disorder (manic-depressive illness) or severe mood swings. It can reduce mania and may be able to help maintain a stable mood over the long term.

Sometimes risperidone is used to reduce severe aggression or very serious behavioral problems in young people with conduct disorder, mental retardation, autism, or pervasive developmental disorder.

Risperidone may be used for behavior problems after a head injury.

It is also used to reduce motor and vocal tics (fast, repeated movements or sounds) and behavioral problems in people with Tourette's disorder.

This medicine is very powerful and is used to treat very serious problems or symptoms that other medicines do not help. Be patient; the positive effects of this medicine may not appear for 2–3 weeks.

How Does This Medicine Work?

Cells in the brain communicate using chemicals called *neurotransmitters*. Too much or too little of these substances in parts of the brain can cause problems. Risperidone works by blocking the action of two of these neurotransmitters, *dopamine* and *serotonin*, in certain areas of the brain.

How Long Does This Medicine Last?

Risperidone is usually taken once or twice a day. Risperdal Consta lasts for 2 weeks, but when it is first started, an oral antipsychotic medicine must be taken as well for about 3 weeks, until enough Consta builds up in the blood to work.

How Will the Doctor Monitor This Medicine?

The doctor will review your child's medical history and physical examination before starting risperidone. The doctor may order some blood or urine tests to be sure your child does not have a hidden medical condition that would make it unsafe to use this medicine. The doctor or nurse will measure your child's height, weight, pulse, and blood pressure before starting risperidone. The doctor may order other tests, such as baseline tests for blood sugar and cholesterol or an ECG (electrocardiogram or heart rhythm test).

Be sure to tell the doctor if anyone in the family has diabetes, high blood pressure, high cholesterol, or heart disease.

Before your child starts taking risperidone and every so often afterward, a test such as the AIMS (Abnormal Involuntary Movement Scale) may be used to check your child's tongue, legs, and arms for unusual movements that could be caused by the medicine.

After the medicine is started, the doctor will want to have regular appointments with you and your child to see how the medicine is working, to see if a dose change is needed, to watch for side effects, to see if risperidone is still needed, and to see if any other treatment is needed. The doctor or nurse will check your child's height, weight, pulse, and blood pressure, and watch for abnormal movements. Sometimes blood tests are needed to watch for diabetes or increased cholesterol.

What Side Effects Can This Medicine Have?

Any medicine can have side effects, including an allergy to the medicine. Because each patient is different, the doctor will monitor the youth closely, especially when the medicine is started. The doctor will work with you to increase the positive effects and decrease the negative effects of the medicine. Please tell the doctor if any of the listed side effects appear or if you think that the medicine is causing any other problems. Not all of the rare or unusual side effects are listed.

Side effects are most common after starting the medicine or after a dose increase. Many side effects can be avoided or lessened by starting with a very low dose and increasing it slowly—ask the doctor.

Allergic Reaction

Tell the doctor in a day or two (if possible, before the next dose of medicine):

- Hives
- Itching
- Rash

Stop the medicine and get *immediate* medical care:

- Trouble breathing or chest tightness
- Swelling of lips, tongue, or throat

Common, but Not Usually Serious, Side Effects

Discuss the following side effects with your child's doctor when convenient. These side effects often can be helped by lowering the dose of medicine, changing the times medicine is taken, or adding another medicine.

- Daytime sleepiness or tiredness—Do not allow your child to drive, ride a bicycle or motorcycle, or operate machinery if this happens. This problem may be lessened by taking the medicine at bedtime.
- Dry mouth—Have your child try using sugar-free gum or candy.
- Constipation—Encourage your child to drink more fluids and eat high-fiber foods; if necessary, the doctor may recommend a fiber medicine such as Benefiber or a stool softener such as Colace or mineral oil.
- Dizziness—This side effect is worse when the child stands up quickly, especially when getting out of bed in the morning; try having the child stand up slowly.
- Increased appetite
- Weight gain—Seek nutritional counseling; provide your child with low-calorie snacks and encourage regular exercise.
- Increased risk of sunburn—Have your child wear sunscreen or protective clothing or stay out of the sun.
- Nausea
- Vomiting
- Insomnia (trouble sleeping)

Less Common, but Not Usually Serious, Side Effects

Discuss the following side effects with your child's doctor when convenient. These side effects often can be helped by lowering the dose of medicine, changing the times medicine is taken, or adding another medicine.

- Drooling
- Increased restlessness or inability to sit still
- Shaking of hands and fingers
- Decreased or slowed movement and decreased facial expressions
- Decreased sexual interest or ability
- Changes in menstrual cycle
- Increase in breast size or discharge from the breasts (in both boys and girls)—This may go away with time.

Less Common, but Potentially Serious, Side Effects

Call the doctor *immediately*:

- Stiffness of the tongue, jaw, neck, back, or legs
- Seizure (fit, convulsion)—This is more common in people with a history of seizures or head injury.
- Increased thirst, frequent urination (having to go to the bathroom often), lethargy, tiredness, dizziness, and blurred vision—These could be signs of diabetes, especially if your child is overweight or there is a family history of diabetes. **Talk to a doctor within a day.**

Very Rare, but Serious, Side Effects

- Extreme stiffness or lack of movement, very high fever, mental confusion, irregular pulse rate, or eye pain—**This is a medical emergency. Go to an emergency room right away.**
- Sudden stiffness and inability to breathe or swallow—**Go to an emergency room or call 911.** Tell the paramedics, nurses, and doctors that the patient is taking risperidone. Other medicines can be used to treat this problem fast.

What Else Should I Know About Side Effects?

Most side effects lessen over time. If they are troublesome, talk with your child's doctor. Some side effects can be decreased by taking a smaller dose of medicine, by stopping the medicine, by changing to another medicine, or by adding another medicine.

Many young people who take risperidone gain weight. The weight gain may be from increased appetite and from ways that the medicine changes how the body processes food. Risperidone may also change the way that the body handles glucose (sugar) and cause high levels (hyperglycemia). People who take risperidone, especially those who gain a lot of weight, are at increased risk of developing diabetes and of having increased fats (lipids—cholesterol and triglycerides) in their blood. Over time, both diabetes and increased fats in the blood may lead to heart disease, stroke, and other complications. The FDA has put warnings on all atypical agents about the increased risks of hyperglycemia, diabetes, and increased blood cholesterol and triglycerides when taking one of these medicines. It is much easier to prevent weight gain than to lose weight later. When your child first starts taking risperidone, it is a good idea to be sure that he or she eats a well-balanced diet without "junk food" and with healthy snacks like fruits and vegetables, not sweets or fried foods. He or she should drink water or skim milk, not pop, sodas, soft drinks, or sugary juices. Regular exercise is important for maintaining a healthy weight (and may also help with sleep).

The medicine may increase the level of *prolactin*, a natural hormone made in the part of the brain called the *pituitary*. This may cause side effects such as breast tenderness or swelling or production of milk in both boys and girls. It also may interfere with sexual functioning in teenage boys and with regular menstrual cycles (periods) in teenage girls. A blood test can measure the level of prolactin. If these side effects do not go away and are troublesome, talk with your child's doctor about substituting another medicine for risperidone.

One very rare side effect that may not go away is *tardive dyskinesia* (or TD). Patients with tardive dyskinesia have involuntary movements (movements that they cannot help making) of the body, especially the mouth and tongue. The patient may look as though he or she is making faces over and over again. Jerky movements of the arms, legs, or body may occur. There may be fine, wormlike, or sudden repeated movements of the tongue, or the person may appear to be chewing something or smacking or puckering his or her lips. The fingers may look as though they are rolling something. If you notice any unusual movements, be sure to tell the doctor. The doctor may use the AIMS test to look for these movements.

Neuroleptic malignant syndrome is a very rare side effect that can lead to death. The symptoms are severe muscle stiffness, high fever, increased heart rate and blood pressure, irregular heartbeat (pulse), and sweating. It may lead to unconsciousness. If you suspect this, **call 911 or go to an emergency room right away.**

Some Interactions With Other Medicines or Food

Please note that the following are only the most likely interactions with food or other medicines.

Risperidone may be taken with or without food.

Risperidone liquid should *not* be taken with tea or cola. It may be taken with water, orange juice, coffee, or low-fat milk.

Paroxetine (Paxil), fluoxetine (Prozac), and other selective serotonin reuptake inhibitor (SSRI) antidepressants can increase the levels of risperidone and increase the risk of side effects.

Carbamazepine (Tegretol) can decrease the levels of risperidone so that it does not work as well.

Heart problems are more common if other medicines that affect the heart are being taken as well. Be sure to tell all your child's doctors and your pharmacist about all medications your child is taking.

It is better to limit drinks with caffeine (coffee, tea, soft drinks) because caffeine works in the opposite way from this medicine, and the positive effects might be decreased.

What Could Happen if This Medicine Is Stopped Suddenly?

Involuntary movements, or *withdrawal dyskinesias*, may appear within 1–4 weeks of lowering the dose or stopping the medicine. Usually these go away, but they can last for days to months. If this medicine is stopped suddenly, emotional disturbance (such as irritability, nervousness, moodiness, or oppositional behavior) or physical problems (such as stomachache, loss of appetite, nausea, vomiting, diarrhea, sweating, indigestion, trouble sleeping, trembling, or shaking) may appear. These problems usually last only a few days to a few weeks. If they happen, you should tell your child's doctor. The medicine dose may need to be lowered more slowly (tapered). Always check with the doctor before stopping a medicine.

How Long Will This Medicine Be Needed?

How long your child will need to take this medicine depends partly on the reason that it was prescribed. Some problems last for only a few months, whereas others last much longer. It is important to ask the doctor whether medicine is still needed, especially with medicines as powerful as this one. Every few months, you should discuss with your child's doctor the reasons for using the medicine and whether the medicine may be stopped or the dose lowered.

What Else Should I Know About This Medicine?

There are other medicines that are used for the same kinds of problems. If your child is having bad side effects or the medicine does not seem to be working, ask the doctor if another medicine might work as well or better and have fewer side effects for your child. Each person reacts differently to medicines.

Taking this medicine could make overheating or heatstroke more likely. Have your child decrease activity in hot weather, stay out of the sun, and drink water to prevent this.

Notes

Use this space to take notes or to write down questions you want to ask the doctor.

_____

_____

_____

_____

_____

_____

_____

_____

_____

_____

_____

_____

_____

Medication Information
for Youth

Risperidone—Risperdal

What the Medicine Is Called and What It Is For

The name of your medicine may be confusing. Most drugs have two names: 1) a scientific name that we call a *generic name* and 2) a trade or *brand name*. The generic name of this medicine is risperidone. The brand name is Risperdal.

Risperidone is called an *atypical* medicine. This medicine helps people who feel very confused and have severe problems thinking clearly. It can lessen hallucinations (seeing or hearing things that are not really there) and delusions (troubling beliefs that other people do not share). The medicine also can improve *negative symptoms*, such as lack of interest in doing things, lack of motivation, loss of interest in friends, and decreased energy. It helps people who have severe depression or mood swings. This medicine also is sometimes used to help young people who have mania or severe depression or who get very angry and hit people or break things. It can help with motor and vocal tics (fast, repeated movements or sounds) in people with Tourette's disorder.

How You Take the Medicine

It is very important to take the medicine exactly as the doctor or nurse tells you. Do not skip doses or take extra medicine without asking an adult. If you forget a dose, ask your parent(s) what to do.

The Risperdal M-Tab is a fast-dissolving, peppermint-flavored tablet. Put it in your mouth and let it melt before swallowing.

If you are taking the liquid form of the medicine, it may be taken with water, orange juice, or low-fat milk. Do not take it with tea or cola.

It is better to limit drinks with caffeine (coffee, tea, soft drinks) because caffeine works in the opposite way from this medicine, and the positive effects might be decreased.

Your doctor will tell you how much medicine to take and how often to take it so that it can help you the most. It is *very important* that you take all the pills you are supposed to take each day. Your doctor will probably recommend that you take your medicine at the same time each day, which may be with meals or at bedtime.

It may be several weeks or longer before you notice the full effect. You may feel discouraged and think the medicine is never going to help. You may want to give up and stop taking the medicine. Talk to your doctor and parent(s) about how you feel, but **do not stop** taking your medicine unless your doctor tells you to. Stopping suddenly could cause uncomfortable feelings. It also is important not to take extra pills hoping that you will feel better faster. Doing that could make you very sick.

This medicine is prescribed only for you. It should never be shared with anyone else.

You do not have to tell others that you are taking this medicine, but it is not something you should feel ashamed or embarrassed about. Many young people are helped by risperidone. This medicine is not habit-forming, and you cannot become "hooked" on it. You should talk to your doctor or nurse about any questions you have about the medicine. It is important to remember that the medicine *helps* you. It cannot *make* you do anything or change you as a person.

How Your Doctor Will Follow Your Progress

Before giving you the medicine, your doctor or nurse will talk with you and your parent(s) and will measure your height, weight, heart rate (pulse), and blood pressure. There may be other tests, such as blood tests for sugar and cholesterol. Before you start taking the medicine and every so often afterward, the doctor or nurse will look at your tongue, arms, and legs to check for unusual movements. This is called the AIMS (Abnormal Involuntary Movement Scale) test.

Be sure to tell your doctor or nurse about any other medicines or supplements you are taking, including vitamins, herbs, or aids to weight loss or bodybuilding. Also be sure to tell the doctor or nurse if you are using alcohol or drugs. Because many medicines may affect babies, it is very important to tell the doctor if you might be pregnant or if you are at risk of becoming pregnant.

Your teachers may be asked to fill out a form about your grades and behavior in school. A psychologist may give you some tests to see how you learn best.

Most doctors have regular appointments with young people who are taking medicine. You should use these visits to share any concerns you may have about your medicine and to talk about if it has helped you. From time to time, your physician or nurse may measure your height, weight, heart rate (pulse), and blood pressure to be sure that you are in good health while you are taking the medicine. There may be blood tests to watch for diabetes or high cholesterol. Your doctor also will ask for regular reports from your parents and maybe from your teachers (with your permission) to see how well the medicine is working.

If the medicine helps you, your doctor will probably want you to take it for several months to a year. Your doctor will decide how long you will need to take the medicine as he or she watches your progress.

How the Medicine Might Affect You

In addition to the ways the medicine can help you, it may have other effects called *side effects*. Different medicines have different side effects. It is helpful to know about some of the most common side effects of your medicine so that you will understand what they are if they happen. Some people do not have any side effects. Some side effects are just uncomfortable, but others may mean a more serious problem with the medicine. Side effects are most common after starting the medicine or after a dose increase. They may go away with time, or the medicine can be adjusted or changed—ask the doctor.

You could have an allergy to any medicine, which might show up as a rash on your skin, swelling, itching, or trouble breathing.

Please tell your parent(s) and doctor or nurse about any changes that you notice after taking the medicine. It is especially important to tell a responsible adult right away if you are feeling depressed or that you may not want to live; if you have thoughts of hurting yourself; or if you begin to feel more irritable, nervous, or restless. Also be sure to tell your parent(s) or doctor if you begin to feel more "speeded up" or have more trouble sleeping.

One of the most common side effects of this medicine is feeling tired or sleepy during the day, even if you have had a full night's sleep. If this medicine is making you sleepy, it is very important not to drive a car or ride a bicycle or motorcycle. After starting the medicine or increasing the dose of medicine, please be extra careful when driving a car, riding a bike, or using machines until you can tell how the medicine affects your alertness, attention, and coordination. After you have been taking the medicine for a few weeks, your body will adjust, and this side effect will likely go away. If you had trouble sleeping at night before taking the medicine, it can help you sleep better, especially if the doctor tells you to take a dose of medicine in the evening.

Another common side effect is dry mouth. You may be more thirsty than usual and find that you are drinking more water or other liquids than usual. Sucking on sugar-free hard candy or cough drops usually helps. You also could try chewing sugar-free gum or sucking on ice chips. Do not chew the ice; you could hurt your teeth. Also, using lip balm will keep your lips from cracking. It is important to be especially good about brushing your teeth.

If you get very thirsty, have to go to the bathroom a lot, feel *very* tired, or have dizziness or blurred vision, be sure to tell your parent(s) or doctor.

Taking this medicine could make you more likely to get badly sunburned or very sick in hot weather. Be sure to drink plenty of liquids and cover up or use sunscreen when you go outside in hot weather. Be careful to rest in the shade and not get overheated.

Sometimes teenagers who take risperidone gain weight. The weight gain may be from increased appetite and also from ways that the medicine changes how the body processes food. People who take risperidone, especially those who gain a lot of weight, might be at increased risk of developing diabetes and of having increased fats (lipids—cholesterol and triglycerides) in their blood. Over time, both diabetes and increased fats in the blood may lead to heart disease, stroke, and other complications. The U.S. Food and Drug Administration has put warnings about these problems on all medicines like risperidone. It is much easier to prevent weight gain than to lose weight later. It is a good idea to eat a well-balanced diet without "junk food" and with healthy snacks like fruits and vegetables, not sweets or fried foods. It is better to drink water or skim milk, not pop, sodas, soft drinks, or sugary juices. Regular exercise is important for maintaining a healthy weight (and may also help with sleep).

You may notice changes in your sexual functioning or in your breasts—it is OK to ask the doctor about this.

This is a very powerful medicine. Some side effects include feeling nervous, restless, or shaky or having stiff muscles. Talk with your doctor about these side effects. They can be helped by adding another medicine, adjusting the dose, or switching to another medicine.

Another, more serious, side effect can be longer lasting and more difficult to treat. This very rare side effect is called *tardive dyskinesia* (or TD). A person taking risperidone may develop movements of the mouth, tongue, face, arms, legs, or body that are not being made on purpose. This side effect can go away when the medicine is stopped, but in some people it does not go away. Your doctor will explain this effect to you and your parent(s) and how he or she will watch for any signs that you are developing this problem. Be sure to ask your doctor any questions that you may have about this, but do not worry too much about it. It hardly ever happens to teenagers.

You should tell your parent(s) and doctor if you notice anything different or unusual about how you feel once you start taking the medicine. This includes good things, such as feeling less confused, feeling less sad, not hearing voices anymore, or sleeping better at night.

Notes

Use this space to take notes or to write down questions you want to ask the doctor or nurse.

_____

_____

_____

_____

_____

_____

_____

_____

_____

_____

_____

_____

_____

From Dulcan MK (editor): _Helping Parents, Youth, and Teachers Understand Medications for Behavioral and Emotional Problems: A Resource Book of Medication Information Handouts_, Third Edition. Washington, DC, American Psychiatric Publishing, 2007

Medication Information for Parents and Teachers

Sertraline—Zoloft

General Information About Medication

Each child and adolescent is different. No one has exactly the same combination of medical and psychological problems. It is a good idea to talk with the doctor or nurse about the reasons a medicine is being used. It is very important to keep all appointments and to be in touch by telephone if you have concerns. It is important to communicate with the doctor, nurse, or therapist.

It is very important that the medicine be taken exactly as the doctor instructs. However, once in a while, everyone forgets to give a medicine on time. It is a good idea to ask the doctor or nurse what to do if this happens. Do not stop or change a medicine without asking the doctor or nurse first.

If the medicine seems to stop working, it may be because it is not being taken regularly. The youth may be "cheeking" or hiding the medicine or forgetting to take it (especially at school). The doses may be too far apart, or a different dose may be needed. Something at school, at home, or in the neighborhood may be upsetting the youth, or he or she may need special help for learning disabilities or tutoring. Please discuss your concerns with the doctor. **Do not just increase the dose.**

All medicines should be kept in a safe place, out of the reach of children, and should be supervised by an adult. If someone takes too much of a medicine, call the doctor, the poison control center, or a hospital emergency room.

Each medicine has a "generic" or chemical name. Just like laundry detergents or paper towels, some medicines are sold by more than one company under different brand names. The same medicine may be available under a generic name and several brand names. The generic medications are usually less expensive than the brand name ones. The generic medications have the same chemical formula, but they may or may not be exactly the same strength as the brand-name medications. Also, some brands of pills contain dye that can cause allergic reactions. It is a good idea to talk to the doctor and the pharmacist about whether it is important to use a specific brand of medicine.

All medicines can cause an allergic reaction. Examples are hives, itching, rashes, swelling, and trouble breathing. Even a tiny amount of a medicine can cause a reaction in patients who are allergic to that medicine. Be *sure* to talk to the doctor before restarting a medicine that has caused an allergic reaction.

Taking more than one medicine at the same time may cause more side effects or cause one of the medicines to not work as well. Always ask the doctor, nurse, or pharmacist before adding another medicine, whether prescription or over-the-counter. Be sure that each doctor knows about *all* of the medicines your child is taking. Also tell the doctor about any vitamins, herbal medicines, or supplements your child may be taking. Some of these may have side effects alone or when taken with this medication.

Everyone taking medicine should have a physical examination at least once a year.

If you suspect the youth is using drugs or alcohol, please tell the doctor right away.

Pregnancy requires special care in the use of medicine. Please tell the doctor immediately if you suspect the teenager is pregnant or might become pregnant.

Printed information like this applies to children and adolescents in general. If you have questions about the medicine, or if you notice changes or anything unusual, please ask the doctor or nurse. As scientific research advances, knowledge increases and advice changes. Even experts do not always agree. Many medicines have not been approved by the U.S. Food and Drug Administration (FDA) for use in children. For this reason, use of the medicine for a particular problem or age group often is not listed in the *Physicians' Desk Reference*. This does not necessarily mean that the medicine is dangerous or does not work, only that the company that makes the medicine has not received permission to advertise the medicine for use in children. Companies often do not apply for this permission because it is expensive to do the tests needed to apply for approval for use in children. Once a medication is approved by the FDA for any purpose, a doctor is allowed to prescribe it according to research and clinical experience.

Note to Teachers

It is a good idea to talk with the parent(s) about the reason(s) that a medication is being used. If the parent(s) sign consent to release information, it is often helpful to talk with the doctor. If the parent(s) give permission, the doctor may ask you to fill out rating forms about your experience with the student's behavior, feelings, academic performance, and medication side effects. This information is very useful in selecting and monitoring medication treatment. If you have observations that you think are important, do not hesitate to share these with the student's parent(s) and treating clinicians.

It is very important that the medicine be taken exactly as the doctor instructs. However, everyone forgets to give a medicine on time once in a while. It is a good idea to ask the parent(s) in advance what to do if this happens. Do not stop or change the time you are giving a medicine at school without parental permission. If a medication is to be taken with food, but lunchtime or snack time changes, be sure to notify the parent(s) so appropriate adjustments can be made.

All medicines should be kept in a secure place and should be supervised by an adult. If someone takes too much of a medicine, follow your school procedure for an urgent medical problem.

Taking medicine is a private matter and is best managed discreetly and confidentially. It is important to be sensitive to the student's feelings about taking medicine.

If you suspect that the student is using drugs or alcohol, please tell the parent(s) or a school counselor right away.

Please tell the parent(s) or school nurse if you suspect medication side effects.

Modifications of the classroom environment or assignments may be useful in addition to medication. The student may need to be evaluated for additional help or for an Individualized Education Plan for learning or behavior.

Any expression of suicidal thoughts or feelings or self-harm by a child or adolescent is a clear signal of distress and should be taken seriously. These behaviors should not be dismissed as "attention seeking."

What Is Sertraline (Zoloft)?

Sertraline is an *antidepressant* known as a *selective serotonin reuptake inhibitor* (SSRI). It comes in brand name Zoloft and generic tablets and liquid.

How Can This Medicine Help?

Sertraline is used to treat depression and anxiety disorders such as obsessive-compulsive disorder (OCD), posttraumatic stress disorder (PTSD), panic disorder, and separation anxiety disorder.

How Does This Medicine Work?

Sertraline increases the amount of a *neurotransmitter* called *serotonin* in certain parts of the brain. People with emotional and behavioral problems, such as depression and anxiety, may have low levels of serotonin in certain parts of the brain. SSRIs such as sertraline help by increasing the action of brain serotonin to more normal levels.

How Long Does This Medicine Last?

Sertraline can be taken only once a day.

How Will the Doctor Monitor This Medicine?

The doctor will review your child's medical history and physical examination before starting sertraline. The doctor may order some blood or urine tests to be sure your child does not have a hidden medical condition that would make it unsafe to use this medicine. Extra care is needed when using SSRIs in youth with seizures (epilepsy), liver or kidney problems, or diabetes. The doctor or nurse will measure your child's height, weight, pulse, and blood pressure before starting the medicine.

Be sure to tell the doctor if your child or anyone in the family has bipolar illness (manic-depressive illness) or has tried to kill himself or herself.

After the medicine is started, the doctor will want to have regular appointments with you and your child to see how the medicine is working, to see if a dose change is needed, to watch for side effects, to see if sertraline is still needed, and to see if any another treatment is needed. The doctor or nurse will check your child's height, weight, pulse, and blood pressure.

Before using medicine and at times afterward, the doctor may ask your child to fill out a rating scale about depression and anxiety, to help see how your child is doing.

What Side Effects Can This Medicine Have?

Any medicine can have side effects, including an allergy to the medicine. Because each patient is different, the doctor will monitor the youth closely, especially when the medicine is started. The doctor will work with you to increase the positive effects and decrease the negative effects of the medicine. Please tell the doctor if any of the listed side effects appear or if you think that the medicine is causing any other problems. Not all of the rare or unusual side effects are listed.

Side effects are most common after starting the medicine or after a dose increase. Many side effects can be avoided or lessened by starting with a very low dose and increasing it slowly—ask the doctor.

Allergic Reaction

Tell the doctor in a day or two (if possible, before the next dose of medicine):

- Hives
- Itching
- Rash

  Stop the medicine and get *immediate* medical care:

- Trouble breathing or chest tightness
- Swelling of lips, tongue, or throat

Common Side Effects

Tell the doctor within a week or two:

- Nausea, upset stomach, vomiting
- Diarrhea
- Constipation—Encourage your child to drink more fluids and eat high-fiber foods; if necessary, the doctor may recommend a fiber medicine such as Benefiber or a stool softener such as Colace or mineral oil.
- Headache
- Anxiety or nervousness
- Insomnia (trouble sleeping)
- Restlessness, increased activity level
- Daytime sleepiness or tiredness—Do not allow your child to drive, ride a bicycle or motorcycle, or operate machinery if this side effect is present.
- Dizziness—This side effect is worse when the child stands up quickly, especially when getting out of bed in the morning; try having the child stand up slowly.
- Tremor (shakiness)
- Excessive sweating
- Apathy, lack of interest in school or friends—This may happen after a initial good response to treatment.
- Decreased sexual interest, trouble with sexual functioning
- Weight gain
- Weight loss

Less Common, but More Serious, Side Effects

Call the doctor within a day:

- Significant suicidal thoughts or self-injurious behavior
- Increased activity, rapid speech, feeling "speeded up," decreased need for sleep, being very excited or irritable (cranky)

Serious Side Effects

Call the doctor *immediately* or go to the nearest emergency room:

- Seizure (fit, convulsion)
- Stiffness, high fever, confusion, tremors (shaking)
- Overheating or heatstroke—Prevent by decreasing activity in hot weather, staying out of the sun, and drinking water.

Serotonin Syndrome

A very serious side effect called *serotonin syndrome* can happen when certain kinds of medicines (including some medicines for migraine headaches—triptans) are taken by the same person. *Very* rarely, it can happen at high doses of just one medicine. The early signs are restlessness, confusion, shaking, skin turning red, sweating, and jerking of muscles. If you see these symptoms, stop the medicine and send or take the youth to an emergency room right away.

Some Interactions With Other Medicines or Food

Please note that the following are only the most likely interactions with food or other medicines.

Sertraline interacts with many other medicines, including some antibiotics and other psychiatric medicines. It is especially important to tell the doctor and pharmacist about all of the medicines your child is taking or has taken in the past few months, including over-the-counter and herbal medicines. Sometimes one medicine can increase or decrease the blood level of another medicine so that different doses are needed. The herbal medicine St. John's wort also increases serotonin and can cause serious side effects if taken with sertraline.

It can be very dangerous to take an SSRI at the same time as or even within a month of taking another type of medicine called a *monoamine oxidase inhibitor* (MAOI), such as Eldepryl (selegiline), Nardil (phenelzine), Parnate (tranylcypromine), or Marplan (isocarboxazid).

Sertraline should not be taken with pimozide.

Sertraline does not usually cause problems when taken with decongestant cold medicines.

Sertraline can be taken with or without food.

Caffeine may increase side effects.

What Could Happen if This Medicine Is Stopped Suddenly?

No known serious medical effects occur if sertraline is stopped suddenly, but there may be uncomfortable feelings, which should be avoided if possible. Your child might have trouble sleeping, nervousness, irritability, dizziness, and flu-like symptoms. Ask the doctor before stopping sertraline or if these symptoms happen while the dose is being decreased.

How Long Will This Medicine Be Needed?

Sertraline may take up to 1–2 months to reach its full effect. If your child has a good response to sertraline, it is a good idea to continue the medicine for at least 6 months.

What Else Should I Know About This Medicine?

In youth who have bipolar disorder (manic depression) or who are at risk for bipolar disorder, any antidepressant medicine may increase the risk of hypomania or mania (excitement, agitation, increased activity, decreased sleep).

In hot weather, make sure your child drinks enough water or other liquids and does not get overheated.

Sometimes, after a person has improved while taking sertraline, he or she loses interest in school or friends or just stops trying. Please tell your child's doctor if this happens—it may be a side effect of the medication. A lower dose or a different medicine may be needed.

This medicine may cause the child to have a dry mouth. Have the child try using sugar-free gum or candy.

Store the medicine away from sunlight, heat, moisture, and humidity.

Black Box Antidepressant Warning

In 2004, an advisory committee to the FDA decided that there might be an increased risk of suicidal behavior for some youth taking medicines called *antidepressants*. In the research studies that the committee reviewed, about 3%–4% of youth with depression who took an antidepressant medicine—and 1%–2% of youth with depression who took a placebo (pill without active medicine)—talked about suicidal thoughts (thinking about killing themselves or wishing they were dead) or did something to harm themselves. This means that almost twice as many youth who were taking an antidepressant to treat their depression talked about suicide or had suicidal behavior compared with youth with depression who were taking inactive medicine. There were *no* completed suicides in any of these research studies, which included more than 4,000 children and adolescents. For youth being treated for anxiety, there was no difference in suicidal talking or behavior between those taking antidepressant medication and those taking placebo.

The FDA told drug companies to add a *black box warning* label to all antidepressant medicines. Because of this label, a doctor (or advanced practice nurse) prescribing one of these medicines has to warn youth and their families that there might be more suicidal thoughts and actions in youth taking these medicines.

On the other hand, in places where more youth are taking the newer antidepressant medicines, the number of adolescents who commit suicide has gotten smaller. Also, thinking about or attempting suicide is more common in surveys of teenagers in the community than it is in depressed youth treated in research studies with antidepressant medicine.

If a youth is being treated with this medicine and is doing well, then no changes are needed as a result of this warning. Increased suicidal talk or action is most likely to happen in the first few months of treatment with a medicine. If your child has recently started this medicine or is about to start, then you and your doctor (or advanced practice nurse) should watch for any changes in behavior. People who are depressed often have suicidal thoughts or actions. It is hard to know whether suicidal thoughts or actions in depressed people are caused by the depression itself or by the medicine. Also, as their depression is getting better, some people talk more about the suicidal thoughts that they had before but did not talk about. As young people get better from depression, they might be at higher risk of doing something about suicidal thoughts that they have had for some time, because they have more energy.

What Should a Parent Do?

1. Be honest with your child about possible risks and benefits of medicine.
2. Talk to your child about whether he or she is having any suicidal thoughts, and tell your child to come to you if he or she is having such thoughts.
3. You, your child, and your child's doctor or nurse should develop a safety plan. Pick adults whom your child can tell if he or she is thinking about suicide.

4. Be sure to tell your child's doctor, nurse, or therapist if you suspect that your child is using alcohol or drugs or if something has happened that might make your child feel worse, such as a family separation, breaking up with a boyfriend or girlfriend, someone close dying or attempting suicide, physical or sexual abuse, or failure in school.

5. Be sure that there are no guns in the home and that all medicines (including over-the-counter medicines like Tylenol) are closely supervised by an adult and kept in a safe place.

6. Watch for new or worse thoughts of suicide, self-harm, depression, anxiety (nerves), feeling very agitated or restless, being angry or aggressive, having more trouble sleeping, or anything else that you see for the first time, seems worse, or worries your child or you. If these appear, contact a mental health professional **right away.** Do not just stop or change the dose of the medicine on your own. If the problems are serious, and you cannot reach one of your clinicians, call a 24-hour psychiatry emergency telephone number or take your child to an emergency room.

Youth on antidepressant medicine should be watched carefully by their parent(s), clinician(s) (doctor, nurse, therapist), and other concerned adults for the first weeks of treatment. It is a good idea to have a visit or telephone call with the doctor, nurse, or therapist weekly for the first month, every 2 weeks for the second month, and after that at least once a month to check for feelings of depression or sadness, thoughts of killing or harming himself or herself, and any problems with the medication. If you have questions, be sure to ask the doctor, nurse, or therapist.

For more information, see http://www.parentsmedguide.org/ (in English and Spanish).

Notes

Use this space to take notes or to write down questions you want to ask the doctor.

_____

_____

_____

_____

_____

_____

_____

_____

_____

_____

_____

_____

From Dulcan MK (editor): *Helping Parents, Youth, and Teachers Understand Medications for Behavioral and Emotional Problems: A Resource Book of Medication Information Handouts*, Third Edition. Washington, DC, American Psychiatric Publishing, 2007

Medication Information for Youth

Sertraline—Zoloft

What the Medicine Is Called and What It Is For

The name of your medicine may be confusing. Most drugs have two names: 1) a scientific name that we call a *generic name* and 2) a trade or *brand name*. The generic name of this medicine is sertraline. The brand name is Zoloft.

Sertraline is called an *antidepressant* or *selective serotonin reuptake inhibitor* (SSRI). Sertraline is used to treat depression and anxiety disorders such as obsessive-compulsive disorder (OCD), posttraumatic stress disorder (PTSD), panic disorder, and separation anxiety disorder. It helps people who feel very sad or depressed, anxious (nervous), or afraid, or who have obsessions (uncomfortable thoughts that won't go away) or compulsions (habits that get in the way of daily life).

How You Take the Medicine

It is very important to take the medicine exactly as the doctor or nurse tells you. Do not skip doses or take extra medicine without asking an adult. If you forget a dose, ask your parent(s) what to do. It is very important that you take all the pills you are supposed to take each day. Your doctor will probably recommend that you take your medicine at the same time each day, which may be with meals or at bedtime.

It may take several weeks before you notice that the medicine is helping. Waiting for the full effect may take even longer. You may feel discouraged and think the medicine is never going to help. You may want to give up and stop taking the medicine. Talk to your doctor and parent(s) about how you feel, but **do not stop** taking the medicine unless your doctor tells you to. It is also important not to take extra pills, hoping that you will feel better faster. Doing that could make you very sick.

Caffeine (in coffee, tea, or soft drinks) may make you feel worse.

This medicine is prescribed only for you. It should never be shared with anyone else.

You do not have to tell others that you are taking this medicine, but it is not something you should feel ashamed or embarrassed about. Many young people are helped by sertraline. This medicine is not habit-forming, and you cannot become "hooked" on it. You should talk to your doctor or nurse about any questions you have about the medicine. It is important to remember that the medicine *helps* you. It cannot *make* you do anything or change you as a person.

How Your Doctor Will Follow Your Progress

Before giving you the medicine, your doctor or nurse will talk with you and your parent(s) and may measure your height, weight, heart rate (pulse), and blood pressure. The doctor may order some blood or urine tests to be sure you are in good health.

Be sure to tell your doctor or nurse about any other medicines or supplements you are taking, including vitamins, herbs, or aids to weight loss or bodybuilding. Also be sure to tell the doctor or nurse if you are using alcohol or drugs. Because many medicines may affect babies, it is very important to tell the doctor if you might be pregnant or if you are at risk of becoming pregnant. Be sure to tell the doctor if you have had thoughts of hurting yourself, have tried to hurt yourself, or sometimes wish that you were not alive.

Your teachers may be asked to fill out a form about your grades and behavior in school. A psychologist may give you some tests to see how you learn best.

Before starting the medicine and afterward, the doctor may ask you to answer questions on paper about depression and anxiety.

Most doctors have regular appointments with young people who are taking medicine. You should use these visits to share any concerns you may have about your medicine and to talk about if it has helped you. From time to time, your physician or nurse may measure your height, weight, heart rate (pulse), and blood pressure to be sure that you are in good health while you are taking the medicine. Your doctor also will ask for regular reports from your parents and maybe from your teachers (with your permission) to see how well the medicine is working.

Some medicines are started at the amount you will take for as long as you are taking that medicine. Other medicines need to be increased or adjusted until your doctor decides you are taking the right amount. Starting at a low dose and increasing it slowly may lessen side effects. If the medicine helps you, your doctor will probably want you to take it for 6 months to a year if you are taking it to treat depression. If you are taking it for another problem, your doctor will decide how long you will need to take the medicine as he or she watches your progress.

It is not dangerous to stop sertraline suddenly, but there might be uncomfortable feelings, such as trouble sleeping, nervousness, irritability, or feeling sick. It is better to decrease it slowly. Do not stop taking a medicine unless the doctor tells you to. If you have any problems after stopping or decreasing this medicine, tell your parent(s) or doctor.

How the Medicine Might Affect You

In addition to the ways the medicine can help you, it may have other effects called *side effects*. Different medicines have different side effects. It is helpful to know about some of the most common side effects of your medicine so that you will understand what they are if they happen. Some people do not have any side effects. Some side effects are just uncomfortable, but others may mean a more serious problem with the medicine. Side effects are most common after starting the medicine or after a dose increase. They may go away with time, or the medicine can be adjusted or changed—ask the doctor.

You could have an allergy to any medicine, which might show up as a rash on your skin, swelling, itching, or trouble breathing.

Please tell your parent(s) and your doctor or nurse about any changes that you notice after taking the medicine. It is especially important to tell a responsible adult if you are feeling depressed or that you may not want to live; if you have thoughts of hurting yourself; or if you begin to feel more irritable, nervous, or restless. Also be sure to tell your parent(s) or doctor if you begin to feel "speeded up" or have trouble sleeping.

Some medicines make people feel sleepy or less coordinated. If this medicine is making you sleepy, it is very important not to drive a car or ride a bicycle or motorcycle. After starting a new medicine or increasing the dose of a medicine, please be extra careful when driving a car, riding a bike, or using machines until you can tell how the medicine affects your alertness, attention, and coordination.

One of the most common side effects of this medicine is feeling tired or sleepy during the day, even if you have had a full night's sleep. After you have been taking the medicine for a few weeks, your body will adjust, and this side effect may go away. If you have had trouble sleeping at night, the medicine can help you sleep better, especially if the doctor tells you to take a dose of medicine in the evening. Other people may feel more restless and excited. Tell your parent(s) or doctor if this is uncomfortable. Sometimes after being on the medicine for a while, people do not care as much about school or friends. Changing the dose or the type of medicine can help this.

This medicine may make your mouth dry. You may be more thirsty than usual and find that you are drinking more water or other liquids. Sucking on sugar-free hard candy or cough drops usually helps. You also could try chewing sugar-free gum or sucking on ice chips. Do not chew the ice; you could hurt your teeth. Also, using lip balm will keep your lips from cracking. It is important to be especially good about brushing your teeth.

Some other side effects that could happen are headache, not feeling hungry and not wanting to eat much, eating more than usual, having an upset stomach, or changes in your bowel movements. You may have a change in your sexual functioning—it is OK to ask the doctor about this. This medicine may make you more likely to get sick if you get overheated, so be sure to drink plenty of liquids and rest in the shade in hot weather.

Please let your parent(s) and doctor know if you notice anything different or unusual about how you feel once you start taking the medicine. This includes good things, such as feeling less sad or less nervous or sleeping better at night.

Notes

Use this space to take notes or to write down questions you want to ask the doctor or nurse.

_____

_____

_____

_____

_____

_____

_____

_____

_____

_____

_____

_____

_____

Medication Information for Parents and Teachers

Temazepam—Restoril

General Information About Medication

Each child and adolescent is different. No one has exactly the same combination of medical and psychological problems. It is a good idea to talk with the doctor or nurse about the reasons a medicine is being used. It is very important to keep all appointments and to be in touch by telephone if you have concerns. It is important to communicate with the doctor, nurse, or therapist.

It is very important that the medicine be taken exactly as the doctor instructs. However, once in a while, everyone forgets to give a medicine on time. It is a good idea to ask the doctor or nurse what to do if this happens. Do not stop or change a medicine without asking the doctor or nurse first.

If the medicine seems to stop working, it may be because it is not being taken regularly. The youth may be "cheeking" or hiding the medicine or forgetting to take it (especially at school). The doses may be too far apart, or a different dose may be needed. Something at school, at home, or in the neighborhood may be upsetting the youth, or he or she may need special help for learning disabilities or tutoring. Please discuss your concerns with the doctor. **Do not just increase the dose.**

All medicines should be kept in a safe place, out of the reach of children, and should be supervised by an adult. If someone takes too much of a medicine, call the doctor, the poison control center, or a hospital emergency room.

Each medicine has a "generic" or chemical name. Just like laundry detergents or paper towels, some medicines are sold by more than one company under different brand names. The same medicine may be available under a generic name and several brand names. The generic medications are usually less expensive than the brand name ones. The generic medications have the same chemical formula, but they may or may not be exactly the same strength as the brand-name medications. Also, some brands of pills contain dye that can cause allergic reactions. It is a good idea to talk to the doctor and the pharmacist about whether it is important to use a specific brand of medicine.

All medicines can cause an allergic reaction. Examples are hives, itching, rashes, swelling, and trouble breathing. Even a tiny amount of a medicine can cause a reaction in patients who are allergic to that medicine. Be *sure* to talk to the doctor before restarting a medicine that has caused an allergic reaction.

Taking more than one medicine at the same time may cause more side effects or cause one of the medicines to not work as well. Always ask the doctor, nurse, or pharmacist before adding another medicine, whether prescription or over-the-counter. Be sure that each doctor knows about *all* of the medicines your child is taking. Also tell the doctor about any vitamins, herbal medicines, or supplements your child may be taking. Some of these may have side effects alone or when taken with this medication.

Everyone taking medicine should have a physical examination at least once a year.

If you suspect the youth is using drugs or alcohol, please tell the doctor right away.

Pregnancy requires special care in the use of medicine. Please tell the doctor immediately if you suspect the teenager is pregnant or might become pregnant.

Printed information like this applies to children and adolescents in general. If you have questions about the medicine, or if you notice changes or anything unusual, please ask the doctor or nurse. As scientific research advances, knowledge increases and advice changes. Even experts do not always agree. Many medicines have not been approved by the U.S. Food and Drug Administration (FDA) for use in children. For this reason, use of the medicine for a particular problem or age group often is not listed in the *Physicians' Desk Reference*. This does not necessarily mean that the medicine is dangerous or does not work, only that the company that makes the medicine has not received permission to advertise the medicine for use in children. Companies often do not apply for this permission because it is expensive to do the tests needed to apply for approval for use in children. Once a medication is approved by the FDA for any purpose, a doctor is allowed to prescribe it according to research and clinical experience.

Note to Teachers

It is a good idea to talk with the parent(s) about the reason(s) that a medication is being used. If the parent(s) sign consent to release information, it is often helpful to talk with the doctor. If the parent(s) give permission, the doctor may ask you to fill out rating forms about your experience with the student's behavior, feelings, academic performance, and medication side effects. This information is very useful in selecting and monitoring medication treatment. If you have observations that you think are important, do not hesitate to share these with the student's parent(s) and treating clinicians.

It is very important that the medicine be taken exactly as the doctor instructs. However, everyone forgets to give a medicine on time once in a while. It is a good idea to ask the parent(s) in advance what to do if this happens. Do not stop or change the time you are giving a medicine at school without parental permission. If a medication is to be taken with food, but lunchtime or snack time changes, be sure to notify the parent(s) so appropriate adjustments can be made.

All medicines should be kept in a secure place and should be supervised by an adult. If someone takes too much of a medicine, follow your school procedure for an urgent medical problem.

Taking medicine is a private matter and is best managed discreetly and confidentially. It is important to be sensitive to the student's feelings about taking medicine.

If you suspect that the student is using drugs or alcohol, please tell the parent(s) or a school counselor right away.

Please tell the parent(s) or school nurse if you suspect medication side effects.

Modifications of the classroom environment or assignments may be useful in addition to medication. The student may need to be evaluated for additional help or for an Individualized Education Plan for learning or behavior.

Any expression of suicidal thoughts or feelings or self-harm by a child or adolescent is a clear signal of distress and should be taken seriously. These behaviors should not be dismissed as "attention seeking."

What Is Temazepam (Restoril)?

Temazepam is a *benzodiazepine* medicine. It is called a *hypnotic* or *sedative-hypnotic*. It comes in brand name Restoril and generic capsules.

How Can This Medicine Help?

Temazepam is used to treat insomnia—problems falling asleep or staying asleep—when used for a short time along with a behavioral program. It can also be used for problem sleep behaviors, called *parasomnias*, such as night terrors (sudden waking up from sleep with great fear), sleepwalking, or sleeptalking, when these put the youth at risk of an accident or make it impossible for other family members to get enough sleep.

How Does This Medicine Work?

Temazepam works on *receptors* (special places on brain cells) in certain parts of the brain to change the action of *GABA*, a *neurotransmitter*—a chemical that the brain makes for brain cells to communicate with each other.

How Long Does This Medicine Last?

Temazepam is taken an hour before bedtime and starts working within an hour. There may still be some effects in the morning.

How Will the Doctor Monitor This Medicine?

The doctor will review your child's medical history and physical examination before starting temazepam.

After the medicine is started, the doctor will want to have regular appointments with you and your child to see how the medicine is working, to see if a dose change is needed, to watch for side effects, to see if temazepam is still needed, and to see if any other treatment is needed.

What Side Effects Can This Medicine Have?

Any medicine can have side effects, including an allergy to the medicine. Because each patient is different, the doctor will monitor the youth closely, especially when the medicine is started. The doctor will work with you to increase the positive effects and decrease the negative effects of the medicine. Please tell the doctor if any of the listed side effects appear or if you think that the medicine is causing any other problems. Not all of the rare or unusual side effects are listed.

Side effects are most common after starting the medicine or after a dose increase. Many side effects can be avoided or lessened by starting with a very low dose and increasing it slowly—ask the doctor.

Allergic Reaction

Tell the doctor in a day or two (if possible, before the next dose of medicine):

- Hives
- Itching
- Rash

Stop the medicine and get *immediate* medical care:

- Trouble breathing or chest tightness
- Swelling of lips, tongue, or throat

Temazepam is usually very safe when used for short periods as the doctor prescribes.

The most common side effect is daytime sleepiness. Temazepam can also cause dizziness, feeling "spacey," or decreased coordination. If the medicine is causing any of these problems it is very important not to drive a car, ride a bicycle or motorcycle, or operate machinery.

Temazepam can cause decreased concentration and memory. These problems, along with daytime sleepiness, may decrease learning and performance in school.

People who take temazepam must not drink alcohol. Severe sleepiness or even loss of consciousness may result.

It is possible to become psychologically and physically dependent on temazepam, but that is not a common problem for patients who see their doctors regularly. Because some people abuse benzodiazepines, it is illegal to give or sell these medicines to someone other than the patient for whom they were prescribed.

Very rarely, temazepam causes excitement, irritability, anger, aggression, agitation, trouble sleeping, nightmares, uncontrollable behavior, or memory loss. This is called *disinhibition* or a *paradoxical effect*. This may be more common in younger children. Stop the medicine and call the doctor if this happens.

Some Interactions With Other Medicines or Food

Please note that the following are only the most likely interactions with food or other medicines.

Caffeine may cause trouble sleeping and make temazepam less effective. If caffeine is eliminated, less temazepam may be needed, or temazepam may not be needed at all.

Oral contraceptives (birth control pills) may increase the levels of temazepam and increase side effects.

It is important not to use other sedatives, tranquilizers, or sleeping pills or antihistamines (such as Benadryl) when taking temazepam because of greatly increased side effects.

What Could Happen if This Medicine Is Stopped Suddenly?

Many medicines cause problems if stopped suddenly. Temazepam must be decreased slowly (tapered) rather than stopped suddenly. When temazepam is stopped suddenly, there are withdrawal symptoms that are uncomfortable and may even be dangerous. Problems are more likely in patients taking high doses of temazepam for 2 months or longer, but even after taking temazepam for just a few weeks, it is important to stop it slowly. Withdrawal symptoms may include anxiety, irritability, shaking, sweating, aches and pains, muscle cramps, vomiting, confusion, and trouble sleeping. If large doses taken for a long time are stopped suddenly, seizures (fits, convulsions), hallucinations (hearing voices or seeing things that are not there), or out-of-control behavior may result.

How Long Will This Medicine Be Needed?

The length of time depends on why temazepam is being used. When used for sleep, it is usually prescribed for only a week or so. A behavioral program, such as regular soothing routines at bedtime and increased exercise in the daytime, should be used along with the medicine to improve sleep. This program can be continued after the medicine is tapered (stopped slowly) or when the medicine is used only occasionally.

When used for night terrors or other parasomnias, the medicine may be needed for months or years.

What Else Should I Know About This Medicine?

Because benzodiazepines can be abused (especially by people who abuse alcohol or drugs) and can cause psychological dependence or physical dependence (addiction), they are regulated by special state and federal laws as *controlled substances*. These laws place limitations on telephone prescriptions and refills, and prescriptions expire if they are not filled promptly.

People with sleep apnea (breathing stops while they are asleep) should not take temazepam. Tell the doctor if your child snores very loudly.

Temazepam should be avoided during pregnancy, especially in the first 3 months, because it may cause birth defects in the baby. If taken regularly at the end of pregnancy, temazepam may cause withdrawal symptoms in the baby.

Notes

Use this space to take notes or to write down questions you want to ask the doctor.

_____

_____

_____

_____

_____

_____

_____

_____

_____

_____

_____

From Dulcan MK (editor): *Helping Parents, Youth, and Teachers Understand Medications for Behavioral and Emotional Problems: A Resource Book of Medication Information Handouts,* Third Edition. Washington, DC, American Psychiatric Publishing, 2007

Medication Information for Youth

Temazepam—Restoril

What the Medicine Is Called and What It Is For

The name of your medicine may be confusing. Most drugs have two names: 1) a scientific name that we call a *generic name* and 2) a trade or *brand name*. The generic name of this medicine is temazepam. The brand name is Restoril.

Temazepam is a *benzodiazepine* medicine. It works by calming the parts of the brain that are too excitable. Temazepam can help with insomnia (difficulty falling asleep or staying asleep) when used for a short time along with routines that help you to relax and fall asleep. Temazepam also can be used for sleep problems such as night terrors (sudden waking up from sleep very scared) or sleepwalking.

How You Take the Medicine

It is very important to take the medicine exactly as the doctor or nurse tells you. Do not skip doses or take extra medicine without asking an adult. If you forget a dose, ask your parent(s) what to do.

It is better to limit drinks with caffeine (coffee, tea, soft drinks) because caffeine works in the opposite way from this medicine, and the positive effects might be decreased.

This medicine is prescribed only for you. It should never be shared with anyone else.

You do not have to tell others that you are taking this medicine, but it is not something you should feel ashamed or embarrassed about. Many young people are helped by temazepam. You should talk to your doctor or nurse about any questions you have about the medicine. It is important to remember that the medicine *helps* you. It cannot *make* you do anything or change you as a person.

Many medicines cause problems if stopped suddenly. Always ask your doctor before stopping a medicine. Problems are more likely to happen in patients taking high doses of temazepam for 2 months or longer, but it is important to decrease the medicine slowly (taper) even after a few weeks. If you notice anxiety, irritability, shaking, sweating, aches and pains, muscle cramps, vomiting, or trouble sleeping, you may need to decrease the medicine more slowly. If large doses are stopped suddenly, seizures (fits, convulsions), hallucinations (hearing voices or seeing things that are not there), or out-of-control behavior may result.

How Your Doctor Will Follow Your Progress

Before giving you the medicine, your doctor or nurse will talk with you and your parent(s) and may measure your height, weight, heart rate (pulse), and blood pressure.

Be sure to tell your doctor or nurse about any other medicines or supplements you are taking, including vitamins, herbs, or aids to weight loss or bodybuilding. Also be sure to tell the doctor or nurse if you are using alcohol or drugs. Because many medicines may affect babies, it is very important to tell the doctor if you might be pregnant or if you are at risk of becoming pregnant.

Most doctors have regular appointments with young people who are taking medicine. You should use these visits to share any concerns you may have about your medicine and to talk about if it has helped you. From time to time, your physician or nurse may measure your height, weight, heart rate (pulse), and blood pressure to be sure that you are in good health while you are taking the medicine. Your doctor also will ask for regular reports from your parents to see how well the medicine is working.

Temazepam is usually prescribed for only a week or so to allow you to develop better sleep habits. Regular exercise in the daytime usually helps with sleep at night.

Each person is unique, and some people may need this medicine for months or years.

How the Medicine Might Affect You

In addition to the ways the medicine can help you, it may have other effects called *side effects*. Different medicines have different side effects. It is helpful to know about some of the most common side effects of your medicine so that you will understand what they are if they happen. Some people do not have any side effects. Some side effects are just uncomfortable, but others may mean a more serious problem with the medicine. Side effects are most common after starting the medicine or after a dose increase. They may go away with time, or the medicine can be adjusted or changed—ask the doctor.

You could have an allergy to any medicine, which might show up as a rash on your skin, swelling, itching, or trouble breathing.

Please tell your parent(s) and doctor or nurse about any changes that you notice after taking the medicine. It is especially important to tell a responsible adult right away if you are feeling depressed or that you may not want to live; if you have thoughts of hurting yourself; or if you begin to feel more irritable, nervous, or restless.

The most common side effect of temazepam is daytime sleepiness. If this medicine is making you sleepy, it is very important not to drive a car or ride a bicycle or motorcycle. After starting temazepam or increasing the dose, please be extra careful when driving a car, riding a bike, or using machines until you can tell how the medicine affects your alertness, attention, and coordination.

Sometimes sleep medicines seem to work in the opposite way, causing excitement, irritability, anger, aggression, and other problems. If this happens, tell your parent(s) or your doctor.

Drinking alcohol while taking this medicine can cause severe drowsiness or even passing out. **Don't do it!** Do not use marijuana or street drugs while taking this medicine. They can cause serious side effects. Skipping your medicine to take drugs does not work because many medicines stay in your body for a long time.

Temazepam can be habit-forming, but that is not a common problem for people who take their medicine as the doctor says.

Notes

Use this space to take notes or to write down questions you want to ask the doctor or nurse.

_____

_____

_____

_____

_____

_____

_____

_____

_____

_____

_____

_____

_____

From Dulcan MK (editor): *Helping Parents, Youth, and Teachers Understand Medications for Behavioral and Emotional Problems: A Resource Book of Medication Information Handouts,* Third Edition. Washington, DC, American Psychiatric Publishing, 2007

Medication Information
for Parents and Teachers

Thiothixene—Navane

General Information About Medication

Each child and adolescent is different. No one has exactly the same combination of medical and psychological problems. It is a good idea to talk with the doctor or nurse about the reasons a medicine is being used. It is very important to keep all appointments and to be in touch by telephone if you have concerns. It is important to communicate with the doctor, nurse, or therapist.

It is very important that the medicine be taken exactly as the doctor instructs. However, once in a while, everyone forgets to give a medicine on time. It is a good idea to ask the doctor or nurse what to do if this happens. Do not stop or change a medicine without asking the doctor or nurse first.

If the medicine seems to stop working, it may be because it is not being taken regularly. The youth may be "cheeking" or hiding the medicine or forgetting to take it (especially at school). The doses may be too far apart, or a different dose may be needed. Something at school, at home, or in the neighborhood may be upsetting the youth, or he or she may need special help for learning disabilities or tutoring. Please discuss your concerns with the doctor. **Do not just increase the dose.**

All medicines should be kept in a safe place, out of the reach of children, and should be supervised by an adult. If someone takes too much of a medicine, call the doctor, the poison control center, or a hospital emergency room.

Each medicine has a "generic" or chemical name. Just like laundry detergents or paper towels, some medicines are sold by more than one company under different brand names. The same medicine may be available under a generic name and several brand names. The generic medications are usually less expensive than the brand name ones. The generic medications have the same chemical formula, but they may or may not be exactly the same strength as the brand-name medications. Also, some brands of pills contain dye that can cause allergic reactions. It is a good idea to talk to the doctor and the pharmacist about whether it is important to use a specific brand of medicine.

All medicines can cause an allergic reaction. Examples are hives, itching, rashes, swelling, and trouble breathing. Even a tiny amount of a medicine can cause a reaction in patients who are allergic to that medicine. Be *sure* to talk to the doctor before restarting a medicine that has caused an allergic reaction.

Taking more than one medicine at the same time may cause more side effects or cause one of the medicines to not work as well. Always ask the doctor, nurse, or pharmacist before adding another medicine, whether prescription or over-the-counter. Be sure that each doctor knows about *all* of the medicines your child is taking. Also tell the doctor about any vitamins, herbal medicines, or supplements your child may be taking. Some of these may have side effects alone or when taken with this medication.

Everyone taking medicine should have a physical examination at least once a year.

If you suspect the youth is using drugs or alcohol, please tell the doctor right away.

Pregnancy requires special care in the use of medicine. Please tell the doctor immediately if you suspect the teenager is pregnant or might become pregnant.

Printed information like this applies to children and adolescents in general. If you have questions about the medicine, or if you notice changes or anything unusual, please ask the doctor or nurse. As scientific research advances, knowledge increases and advice changes. Even experts do not always agree. Many medicines have not been approved by the U.S. Food and Drug Administration (FDA) for use in children. For this reason, use of the medicine for a particular problem or age group often is not listed in the *Physicians' Desk Reference*. This does not necessarily mean that the medicine is dangerous or does not work, only that the company that makes the medicine has not received permission to advertise the medicine for use in children. Companies often do not apply for this permission because it is expensive to do the tests needed to apply for approval for use in children. Once a medication is approved by the FDA for any purpose, a doctor is allowed to prescribe it according to research and clinical experience.

Note to Teachers

It is a good idea to talk with the parent(s) about the reason(s) that a medication is being used. If the parent(s) sign consent to release information, it is often helpful to talk with the doctor. If the parent(s) give permission, the doctor may ask you to fill out rating forms about your experience with the student's behavior, feelings, academic performance, and medication side effects. This information is very useful in selecting and monitoring medication treatment. If you have observations that you think are important, do not hesitate to share these with the student's parent(s) and treating clinicians.

It is very important that the medicine be taken exactly as the doctor instructs. However, everyone forgets to give a medicine on time once in a while. It is a good idea to ask the parent(s) in advance what to do if this happens. Do not stop or change the time you are giving a medicine at school without parental permission. If a medication is to be taken with food, but lunchtime or snack time changes, be sure to notify the parent(s) so appropriate adjustments can be made.

All medicines should be kept in a secure place and should be supervised by an adult. If someone takes too much of a medicine, follow your school procedure for an urgent medical problem.

Taking medicine is a private matter and is best managed discreetly and confidentially. It is important to be sensitive to the student's feelings about taking medicine.

If you suspect that the student is using drugs or alcohol, please tell the parent(s) or a school counselor right away.

Please tell the parent(s) or school nurse if you suspect medication side effects.

Modifications of the classroom environment or assignments may be useful in addition to medication. The student may need to be evaluated for additional help or for an Individualized Education Plan for learning or behavior.

Any expression of suicidal thoughts or feelings or self-harm by a child or adolescent is a clear signal of distress and should be taken seriously. These behaviors should not be dismissed as "attention seeking."

What Is Thiothixene (Navane)?

Thiothixene is sometimes called a *typical*, *conventional*, or *first-generation antipsychotic* medicine. It is also called a *neuroleptic*. It used to be called a *major tranquilizer*. It comes in brand name Navane and generic capsules and liquid.

How Can This Medicine Help?

Thiothixene is used to treat psychosis, such as in schizophrenia, mania, or very severe depression. It can reduce hallucinations (hearing voices or seeing things that are not there) and delusions (troubling beliefs that other people do not share). It can help the patient be less upset and agitated. It can improve the patient's ability to think clearly.

Sometimes thiothixene is used to decrease severe aggression or very serious behavioral problems in young people with conduct disorder, mental retardation, or autism.

This medicine is very powerful and should be used to treat very serious problems or symptoms that other medicines do not help. Be patient; the positive effects of this medicine may not appear for 2–3 weeks.

How Does This Medicine Work?

Cells in the brain (neurons) communicate using chemicals called *neurotransmitters*. Too much or too little of these substances in certain parts of the brain can cause problems. Thiothixene reduces the activity of one of these neurotransmitters, *dopamine*. Blocking the effect of dopamine in certain parts of the brain reduces what have been called *positive symptoms* of psychosis: delusions; hallucinations; disorganized and unusual thinking, speaking, and behavior; excessive activity (agitation); and lack of activity (catatonia). Blocking dopamine can also reduce tics. Reducing dopamine action in other parts of the brain may lead to the side effects of this medicine.

How Long Does This Medicine Last?

Thiothixene is usually taken twice a day.

How Will the Doctor Monitor This Medicine?

The doctor will review your child's medical history and physical examination before starting thiothixene. The doctor may order some blood or urine tests to be sure your child does not have a hidden medical condition. The doctor or nurse may measure your child's pulse and blood pressure before starting thiothixene.

Before starting thiothixene and every so often afterward, a test such as the AIMS (Abnormal Involuntary Movement Scale) may be used to check your child's tongue, legs, and arms for unusual movements that could be caused by the medicine.

After the medicine is started, the doctor will want to have regular appointments with you and your child to see how the medicine is working, to see if a dose change is needed, to watch for side effects, to see if thiothixene is still needed, and to see if any other treatment is needed. The doctor or nurse may check your child's height, weight, pulse, and blood pressure and watch for abnormal movements.

What Side Effects Can This Medicine Have?

Any medicine can have side effects, including an allergy to the medicine. Because each patient is different, the doctor will monitor the youth closely, especially when the medicine is started. The doctor will work with you

to increase the positive effects and decrease the negative effects of the medicine. Please tell the doctor if any of the listed side effects appear or if you think that the medicine is causing any other problems. Not all of the rare or unusual side effects are listed.

Side effects are most common after starting the medicine or after a dose increase. Many side effects can be avoided or lessened by starting with a very low dose and increasing it slowly—ask the doctor.

Allergic Reaction

Tell the doctor in a day or two (if possible, before the next dose of medicine):

- Hives
- Itching
- Rash

Stop the medicine and get *immediate* medical care:

- Trouble breathing or chest tightness
- Swelling of lips, tongue, or throat

Common, but Not Usually Serious, Side Effects

Discuss the following side effects with your child's doctor within a week or two. They often can be helped by lowering the dose of medicine, changing the times medicine is taken, or adding another medicine.

- Dry mouth—Have your child try using sugar-free gum or candy.
- Constipation—Encourage your child to drink more fluids and eat high-fiber foods; if necessary, the doctor may recommend a fiber medicine such as Benefiber or a stool softener such as Colace or mineral oil.
- Increased risk of sunburn—Have your child wear sunscreen or protective clothing or stay out of the sun.
- Mild trouble urinating
- Blurred vision
- Weight gain—Seek nutritional counseling; provide your child with low-calorie snacks and encourage regular exercise.
- Sadness, irritability, nervousness, clinginess, not wanting to go to school
- Restlessness or inability to sit still
- Shaking of hands and fingers

Less Common, but Not Usually Serious, Side Effects

Discuss the following side effects with your child's doctor within a week or two. They often can be helped by lowering the dose of medicine, changing the times medicine is taken, or adding another medicine.

- Daytime sleepiness or tiredness—Do not allow your child to drive, ride a bicycle or motorcycle, or operate machinery if this happens. This problem may be lessened by taking the medicine at bedtime.
- Dizziness—This side effect is worse when the child stands up quickly, especially when getting out of bed in the morning; try having the child stand up slowly.
- Decreased or slowed movement and decreased facial expressions
- Drooling

- Decreased sexual interest or ability
- Changes in menstrual cycle
- Increase in breast size or discharge from the breasts (in both boys and girls)—This may go away with time.

Less Common, but Potentially Serious, Side Effects

Call the doctor or go to an emergency room *right away:*

- Stiffness of the tongue, jaw, neck, back, or legs
- Overheating or heatstroke—Prevent by decreasing activity in hot weather, staying out of the sun, and drinking water.
- Seizure (fit, convulsion)—This is more likely in people with a history of seizures or head injury.
- Severe confusion

Rare, but Serious, Side Effects

- Extreme stiffness or lack of movement, very high fever, mental confusion, irregular pulse rate, or eye pain—**This is a medical emergency. Go to an emergency room right away.**
- Sudden stiffness and inability to breathe or swallow—**Go to an emergency room or call 911.** Tell the paramedics, nurses, and doctors that the patient is taking thiothixene. Other medicines can be used to treat this problem fast.
- Increased thirst, frequent urination, lethargy, tiredness, dizziness—These could be signs of diabetes, especially if your child is overweight or there is a family history of diabetes. **Talk to a doctor within a day.**

What Else Should I Know About Side Effects?

Most side effects lessen over time. If they are troublesome, talk with your child's doctor. Some side effects can be decreased by taking a smaller dose of medicine, by stopping the medicine, by changing to another medicine, or by adding another medicine (see the table).

One side effect that may not go away is *tardive dyskinesia* (or TD). Patients with tardive dyskinesia have involuntary movements of the body, especially the mouth and tongue. The patient may look as though he or she is making faces over and over again. Jerky movements of the arms, legs, or body may occur. There may be fine, wormlike, or sudden repeated movements of the tongue, or the person may appear to be chewing something or smacking or puckering his or her lips. The fingers may look as though they are rolling something. If you notice any unusual movements, be sure to tell the doctor. The doctor may use the AIMS test to look for these movements.

The medicine may increase the level of *prolactin*, a natural hormone made in the part of the brain called the *pituitary*. This may cause side effects such as breast tenderness or swelling or production of milk, in both boys and girls. It also may interfere with sexual functioning in teenage boys and with regular menstrual cycles (periods) in teenage girls. A blood test can measure the level of prolactin. If these side effects do not go away and are troublesome, talk with your child's doctor about substituting another medicine for thiothixene.

Heart problems are more common if other medicines are being taken also. Be sure to tell all your child's doctors and your pharmacist about all medications your child is taking.

Neuroleptic malignant syndrome is a very rare side effect that can lead to death. The symptoms are severe muscle stiffness, high fever, increased heart rate and blood pressure, irregular heartbeat (pulse), and sweating. It may lead to unconsciousness. If you suspect this, **call 911 or go to an emergency room right away.**

What Medicines Are Used to Treat Side Effects of Thiothixene?

The following medicines may be used to treat the movement side effects of thiothixene. These medicines may have their own side effects as well. Ask the doctor if you suspect a problem.

Brand name	Generic name
Akineton	Biperiden
Artane	Trihexyphenidyl
Ativan	Lorazepam*
Benadryl	Diphenhydramine*
Catapres	Clonidine*
Cogentin	Benztropine mesylate*
Inderal	Propranolol*
Klonopin	Clonazepam*
Symmetrel	Amantadine

*This medicine has its own information sheet in this book.

Some Interactions With Other Medicines or Food

Please note that the following are only the most likely interactions with food or other medicines.

Thiothixene may be taken with or without food. If the medicine causes stomach upset, taking it with food may help.

It is better to limit drinks with caffeine (coffee, tea, soft drinks) because caffeine works in the opposite way from this medicine, and the positive effects might be decreased.

What Could Happen if This Medicine Is Stopped Suddenly?

Involuntary movements, or *withdrawal dyskinesias*, may appear within 1–4 weeks of lowering the dose or stopping the medicine. Usually these go away, but they can last for days to months. If thiothixene is stopped suddenly, emotional problems such as irritability, nervousness, moodiness; behavior problems; or physical problems such as stomachache, loss of appetite, nausea, vomiting, diarrhea, sweating, indigestion, trouble sleeping, trembling, or shaking may appear. These problems usually last only a few days to a few weeks. If they happen, tell your child's doctor. The medicine dose may need to be lowered more slowly (tapered). Always check with the doctor before stopping a medicine!

How Long Will This Medicine Be Needed?

How long your child will need to be on thiothixene depends partly on the reason that it was prescribed. Some problems last for only a few months, whereas others last much longer. Sometimes thiothixene is used for only a short time until other medicines or behavioral treatments start to work. Some people need to take thiothixene for years. It is especially important with medicines as powerful as this one to ask the doctor whether it is still needed. Every few months, you should discuss with your child's doctor the reasons for using thiothixene and whether it is time for a trial of lowering the dose.

What Else Should I Know About This Medicine?

There are many older and newer medicines that are used for the same kinds of problems. If your child is having bad side effects or the medicine does not seem to be working, ask the doctor if another medicine in this group might work as well or better and have fewer side effects for your child.

Be sure to tell the doctor if there is anyone in your family who died suddenly or had a heart problem.

Notes

Use this space to take notes or to write down questions you want to ask the doctor.

_____

_____

_____

_____

_____

_____

_____

_____

_____

From Dulcan MK (editor): *Helping Parents, Youth, and Teachers Understand Medications for Behavioral and Emotional Problems: A Resource Book of Medication Information Handouts,* Third Edition. Washington, DC, American Psychiatric Publishing, 2007

Medication Information for Youth

Thiothixene—Navane

What the Medicine Is Called and What It Is For

The name of your medicine may be confusing. Most drugs have two names: 1) a scientific name that we call a *generic name* and 2) a trade or *brand name*. The generic name of this medicine is thiothixene. The brand name is Navane.

Thiothixene can help people who feel very confused and have severe problems thinking clearly. It can lessen *hallucinations* (seeing or hearing things that are not really there) and *delusions* (troubling beliefs that other people do not share). This medicine also is sometimes used to help young people who have mania or very severe depression or who get very angry and hit people or break things.

How You Take the Medicine

It is very important to take the medicine exactly as the doctor or nurse tells you. Do not skip doses or take extra medicine without asking an adult. If you forget a dose, ask your parent(s) what to do. Your doctor will tell you how much medicine to take and how often to take it so that it can help you the most. It is *very important* that you take all the pills you are supposed to take each day. Your doctor will probably recommend that you take your medicine at the same time each day, which may be with meals or at bedtime.

It is better to limit drinks with caffeine (coffee, tea, soft drinks) because caffeine works in the opposite way from this medicine, and the positive effects might be decreased.

It may be several weeks or longer before you notice the full effect. You may feel discouraged and think the medicine is never going to help. You may want to give up and stop taking the medicine. Talk to your doctor and parent(s) about how you feel, but **do not stop** taking your medicine unless your doctor tells you to. It also is important not to take extra pills hoping that you will feel better faster. Doing that could make you very sick.

If your stomach is upset, taking the medicine with food may help.

This medicine is prescribed only for you. It should never be shared with anyone else.

You do not have to tell others that you are taking this medicine, but it is not something you should feel ashamed or embarrassed about. Many young people are helped by thiothixene. You should talk to your doctor or nurse about any questions you have about the medicine. It is important to remember that the medicine *helps* you. It cannot *make* you do anything or change you as a person.

How Your Doctor Will Follow Your Progress

Before giving you the medicine, your doctor or nurse will talk with you and your parent(s) and may measure your height, weight, heart rate (pulse), and blood pressure. There may be other tests, such as blood tests for sugar and cholesterol. Before you start taking the medicine and every so often afterward, the doctor or nurse will look at your tongue, arms, and legs to check for unusual movements. This is called the AIMS (Abnormal Involuntary Movement Scale) test.

Be sure to tell your doctor or nurse about any other medicines or supplements you are taking, including vitamins, herbs, or aids to weight loss or bodybuilding. Also be sure to tell the doctor or nurse if you are using alcohol or drugs. Because many medicines may affect babies, it is very important to tell the doctor if you might be pregnant or if you are at risk of becoming pregnant.

Your teachers may be asked to fill out a form about your grades and behavior in school. A psychologist may give you some tests to see how you learn best.

Most doctors have regular appointments with young people who are taking medicine. You should use these visits to share any concerns you may have about your medicine and to talk about if it has helped you. From time to time, your physician or nurse may measure your height, weight, heart rate (pulse), and blood pressure to be sure that you are in good health while you are taking the medicine. There may be blood tests to watch for diabetes or high cholesterol. Your doctor also will ask for regular reports from your parents and maybe from your teachers (with your permission) to see how well the medicine is working.

If the medicine helps you, your doctor will probably want you to take it for several months to a year. Your doctor will decide how long you will need to take the medicine as he or she watches your progress.

How the Medicine Might Affect You

In addition to the ways the medicine can help you, it may have other effects called *side effects*. Different medicines have different side effects. It is helpful to know about some of the most common side effects of your medicine so that you will understand what they are if they happen. Some people do not have any side effects. Some side effects are just uncomfortable, but others may mean a more serious problem with the medicine. Side effects are most common after starting the medicine or after a dose increase. They may go away with time, or the medicine can be adjusted or changed—ask the doctor.

You could have an allergy to any medicine, which might show up as a rash on your skin, swelling, itching, or trouble breathing.

Please tell your parent(s) and your doctor or nurse about any changes that you notice after taking the medicine. It is especially important to tell a responsible adult right away if you are feeling depressed or that you may not want to live; if you have thoughts of hurting yourself; or if you begin to feel more irritable, nervous, or restless.

One of the most common side effects of this medicine is feeling tired or sleepy during the day, even if you have had a full night's sleep. If this medicine is making you sleepy, it is very important not to drive a car or ride a bicycle or motorcycle. After starting the medicine or increasing the dose of medicine, please be extra careful when driving a car, riding a bike, or using machines until you can tell how the medicine affects your alertness, attention, and coordination. After you have been taking the medicine for a few weeks, your body will adjust, and this side effect will likely go away. If you had trouble sleeping at night before taking the medicine, it can help you sleep better, especially if the doctor tells you to take a dose of medicine in the evening.

You might feel dizzy or light-headed if you stand up fast. Try standing up slowly, especially when getting out of bed in the morning.

Another common side effect is dry mouth. You may be more thirsty than usual and find that you are drinking more water or other liquids than usual. Sucking on sugar-free hard candy or cough drops usually helps. You also could try chewing sugar-free gum or sucking on ice chips. Do not chew the ice; you could hurt your teeth. Also, using lip balm will keep your lips from cracking. It is important to be especially good about brushing your teeth.

Taking this medicine could make you more likely to get badly sunburned or very sick in hot weather. Be sure to drink plenty of liquids and cover up or use sunscreen when you go outside in hot weather. Be careful to rest in the shade and not get overheated.

Sometimes teenagers who take thiothixene gain weight. The weight gain may be from increased appetite and also from ways that the medicine changes how the body processes food. It is much easier to prevent weight gain than to lose weight later. It is a good idea to eat a well-balanced diet without "junk food" and with healthy snacks like fruits and vegetables, not sweets or fried foods. It is better to drink water or skim milk, not pop, sodas, soft drinks, or sugary juices. Regular exercise is important for maintaining a healthy weight (and may also help with sleep).

Some people become constipated (have hard bowel movements) when taking this medicine. Try drinking more water and eating more fruits, vegetables, and whole grains. If that does not help, tell your parent(s) or doctor—you may need a medicine to help with this side effect. Sometimes people have trouble passing urine. Tell your parent(s) or the doctor if this happens.

Thiothixene is a very powerful medicine. Some side effects include feeling nervous, restless, or shaky or having stiff muscles. Talk with your doctor about these side effects. They can be helped by adding another medicine, adjusting the dose, or switching to another medicine.

Another, more serious, side effect can be longer lasting and more difficult to treat. This very rare side effect is called *tardive dyskinesia* (or TD). A person taking thiothixene may develop movements of the mouth, tongue, face, arms, legs, or body that are not being made on purpose. This side effect can go away when the medicine is stopped, but in some people it does not go away. Your doctor will explain this effect to you and your parent(s) and how he or she will watch for any signs that you are developing this problem. Be sure to ask your doctor any questions that you may have about this, but do not worry too much about it. It hardly ever happens to teenagers.

You may notice changes in your sexual functioning or in your breasts—it is OK to ask the doctor about this.

You should tell your parent(s) and doctor if you notice anything different or unusual about how you feel once you start taking the medicine. This includes good things, such as feeling less confused, feeling less sad or angry, not hearing voices anymore, or sleeping better at night.

You cannot become addicted to this medicine, but you should not stop it suddenly. Never stop a medicine without talking to the doctor. If thiothixene is stopped or decreased suddenly you may notice more moodiness or irritability, stomachaches or upset stomach, trouble sleeping, or trembling or shaking. Let your parent(s) or doctor know if this happens—the medicine may need to be decreased more slowly.

Notes

Use this space to take notes or to write down questions you want to ask the doctor or nurse.

_____

_____

_____

_____

_____

_____

_____

_____

_____

_____

Medication Information for Parents and Teachers

Topiramate—Topamax

General Information About Medication

Each child and adolescent is different. No one has exactly the same combination of medical and psychological problems. It is a good idea to talk with the doctor or nurse about the reasons a medicine is being used. It is very important to keep all appointments and to be in touch by telephone if you have concerns. It is important to communicate with the doctor, nurse, or therapist.

It is very important that the medicine be taken exactly as the doctor instructs. However, once in a while, everyone forgets to give a medicine on time. It is a good idea to ask the doctor or nurse what to do if this happens. Do not stop or change a medicine without asking the doctor or nurse first.

If the medicine seems to stop working, it may be because it is not being taken regularly. The youth may be "cheeking" or hiding the medicine or forgetting to take it (especially at school). The doses may be too far apart, or a different dose may be needed. Something at school, at home, or in the neighborhood may be upsetting the youth, or he or she may need special help for learning disabilities or tutoring. Please discuss your concerns with the doctor. **Do not just increase the dose.**

All medicines should be kept in a safe place, out of the reach of children, and should be supervised by an adult. If someone takes too much of a medicine, call the doctor, the poison control center, or a hospital emergency room.

Each medicine has a "generic" or chemical name. Just like laundry detergents or paper towels, some medicines are sold by more than one company under different brand names. The same medicine may be available under a generic name and several brand names. The generic medications are usually less expensive than the brand name ones. The generic medications have the same chemical formula, but they may or may not be exactly the same strength as the brand-name medications. Also, some brands of pills contain dye that can cause allergic reactions. It is a good idea to talk to the doctor and the pharmacist about whether it is important to use a specific brand of medicine.

All medicines can cause an allergic reaction. Examples are hives, itching, rashes, swelling, and trouble breathing. Even a tiny amount of a medicine can cause a reaction in patients who are allergic to that medicine. Be *sure* to talk to the doctor before restarting a medicine that has caused an allergic reaction.

Taking more than one medicine at the same time may cause more side effects or cause one of the medicines to not work as well. Always ask the doctor, nurse, or pharmacist before adding another medicine, whether prescription or over-the-counter. Be sure that each doctor knows about *all* of the medicines your child is taking. Also tell the doctor about any vitamins, herbal medicines, or supplements your child may be taking. Some of these may have side effects alone or when taken with this medication.

Everyone taking medicine should have a physical examination at least once a year.

If you suspect the youth is using drugs or alcohol, please tell the doctor right away.

Pregnancy requires special care in the use of medicine. Please tell the doctor immediately if you suspect the teenager is pregnant or might become pregnant.

Printed information like this applies to children and adolescents in general. If you have questions about the medicine, or if you notice changes or anything unusual, please ask the doctor or nurse. As scientific research advances, knowledge increases and advice changes. Even experts do not always agree. Many medicines have not been approved by the U.S. Food and Drug Administration (FDA) for use in children. For this reason, use of the medicine for a particular problem or age group often is not listed in the *Physicians' Desk Reference*. This does not necessarily mean that the medicine is dangerous or does not work, only that the company that makes the medicine has not received permission to advertise the medicine for use in children. Companies often do not apply for this permission because it is expensive to do the tests needed to apply for approval for use in children. Once a medication is approved by the FDA for any purpose, a doctor is allowed to prescribe it according to research and clinical experience.

Note to Teachers

It is a good idea to talk with the parent(s) about the reason(s) that a medication is being used. If the parent(s) sign consent to release information, it is often helpful to talk with the doctor. If the parent(s) give permission, the doctor may ask you to fill out rating forms about your experience with the student's behavior, feelings, academic performance, and medication side effects. This information is very useful in selecting and monitoring medication treatment. If you have observations that you think are important, do not hesitate to share these with the student's parent(s) and treating clinicians.

It is very important that the medicine be taken exactly as the doctor instructs. However, everyone forgets to give a medicine on time once in a while. It is a good idea to ask the parent(s) in advance what to do if this happens. Do not stop or change the time you are giving a medicine at school without parental permission. If a medication is to be taken with food, but lunchtime or snack time changes, be sure to notify the parent(s) so appropriate adjustments can be made.

All medicines should be kept in a secure place and should be supervised by an adult. If someone takes too much of a medicine, follow your school procedure for an urgent medical problem.

Taking medicine is a private matter and is best managed discreetly and confidentially. It is important to be sensitive to the student's feelings about taking medicine.

If you suspect that the student is using drugs or alcohol, please tell the parent(s) or a school counselor right away.

Please tell the parent(s) or school nurse if you suspect medication side effects.

Modifications of the classroom environment or assignments may be useful in addition to medication. The student may need to be evaluated for additional help or for an Individualized Education Plan for learning or behavior.

Any expression of suicidal thoughts or feelings or self-harm by a child or adolescent is a clear signal of distress and should be taken seriously. These behaviors should not be dismissed as "attention seeking."

What Is Topiramate (Topamax)?

Topiramate was first used to treat seizures (fits, convulsions), so it is sometimes called an *anticonvulsant*. Now it is also used for behavioral problems or bipolar disorder (manic-depressive disorder) regardless of whether the patient has seizures. It also may be used when the patient has a history of severe mood changes, sometimes called *mood swings*. When used in psychiatry, this medicine is more commonly called a *mood stabilizer*.

Topiramate comes in brand name Topamax tablets and sprinkle capsules.

How Can This Medicine Help?

Topiramate can reduce aggression, anger, and severe mood swings. It can treat mania or prevent relapse (mania coming back).

How Does This Medicine Work?

Topiramate is thought to work by stabilizing a part of the brain cell (the cell membrane or envelope) and by changing the concentrations of certain *neurotransmitters* (chemicals in the brain) such as *GABA* and *glutamate*.

How Long Does This Medicine Last?

Topiramate needs to be taken twice a day.

How Will the Doctor Monitor This Medicine?

The doctor will review your child's medical history and physical examination before starting topiramate. The doctor or nurse may measure your child's pulse and blood pressure before starting topiramate. The doctor may order a baseline blood test of liver and kidney functions.

After the medicine is started, the doctor will want to have regular appointments with you and your child to see how the medicine is working, to see if a dose change is needed, to watch for side effects, to see if topiramate is still needed, and to see if any other treatment is needed. The doctor or nurse may check your child's height, weight, pulse, and blood pressure.

What Side Effects Can This Medicine Have?

Any medicine can have side effects, including an allergy to the medicine. Because each patient is different, the doctor will monitor the youth closely, especially when the medicine is started. The doctor will work with you to increase the positive effects and decrease the negative effects of the medicine. Please tell the doctor if any of the listed side effects appear or if you think that the medicine is causing any other problems. Not all of the rare or unusual side effects are listed.

Side effects are most common after starting the medicine or after a dose increase. Many side effects can be avoided or lessened by starting with a very low dose and increasing it slowly—ask the doctor.

Allergic Reaction

Tell the doctor in a day or two (if possible, before the next dose of medicine):

- Hives
- Itching
- Rash

Stop the medicine and get *immediate* medical care:

- Trouble breathing or chest tightness
- Swelling of lips, tongue, or throat

Allergic reaction to topiramate may be more common in people who are allergic to sulfa drugs.

General Side Effects

These side effects are more common when first starting the medicine. Tell the doctor within a week or two:

- Daytime sleepiness—Do not allow your child to drive, ride a bicycle or motorcycle, or operate machinery if this happens.
- Dizziness
- Vision problems
- Unsteadiness when walking
- Speech problems
- Slowed movements
- Skin feeling like "pins and needles"
- Decreased sweating
- Decreased appetite, weight loss
- Nausea, vomiting
- Stomach cramps
- Tremor (shakiness)
- Decreased concentration or attention

Thinking and Emotional Side Effects

Call the doctor within a day or two:

- Nervousness, anxiety
- Irritability
- Memory problems
- Confusion

Possibly Dangerous Side Effects

Call the doctor *immediately*:

- Clumsiness or poor coordination
- Bloody or cloudy urine (could be from a kidney stone)
- Unexplained fever or chills
- Sharp back pain (could be a kidney stone)
- Blurred vision or eye pain

Some Interactions With Other Medicines or Food

Please note that the following are only the most likely interactions with food or other medicines.

Caffeine may increase side effects.

Topiramate interacts with many other medicines. Taking it with another medicine may make one or both not work as well or may cause more side effects. Be sure that each doctor knows about *all* of the medicines being taken.

Topiramate may decrease the blood levels of birth control pills (oral contraceptives) so that they do not work as well—this may lead to accidental pregnancy.

What Could Happen if This Medicine Is Stopped Suddenly?

Stopping topiramate suddenly could cause an increase in very dangerous seizures (convulsions) if your child is being treated for epilepsy (seizures).

How Long Will This Medicine Be Needed?

The length of time a person needs to take topiramate depends on what problem is being treated. For example, someone with an impulse control disorder usually takes the medicine only until behavioral therapy begins to work. Someone with bipolar disorder may need to take the medicine for many years. Please ask the doctor about the length of treatment needed.

What Else Should I Know About This Medicine?

Taking topiramate with food may decrease stomach upset.

While taking topiramate, diets low in carbohydrates (such as Atkins, South Beach, or ketogenic diet [used to treat severe epilepsy]) should be avoided to prevent kidney stones. It is also important to drink plenty of liquids to decrease the risk of kidney stones.

Keep the medicine in a safe place under close supervision. Keep the pill container tightly closed and in a dry place, away from bathrooms, showers, and humidifiers.

Notes

Use this space to take notes or to write down questions you want to ask the doctor.

_____

_____

_____

_____

_____

_____

_____

_____

_____

_____

_____

_____

_____

Medication Information for Youth

Topiramate—Topamax

What the Medicine Is Called and What It Is For

The name of your medicine may be confusing. Most drugs have two names: 1) a scientific name that we call a *generic name* and 2) a trade or *brand name*. The generic name of this medicine is topiramate. The brand name is Topamax.

Topiramate was first used to help people with epilepsy (seizures, fits, convulsions), so it is sometimes called an *anticonvulsant*. It is now also called a *mood stabilizer*, because it is used to help people who have severe mood changes, sometimes called *mood swings*, especially in children and adolescents with bipolar disorder (manic-depressive disorder), depression, or trouble controlling anger. Topiramate can reduce aggression, anger, and severe mood swings. It can treat mania or prevent relapse (mania coming back). It is thought to work by making brain cells less excitable.

How You Take the Medicine

It is very important to take the medicine exactly as the doctor or nurse tells you. Do not skip doses or take extra medicine without asking an adult. If you forget a dose, ask your parent(s) what to do.

This medicine is prescribed only for you. It should never be shared with anyone else.

You do not have to tell others that you are taking this medicine, but it is not something you should feel ashamed or embarrassed about. Many young people are helped by topiramate. This medicine is not habit-forming, and you cannot become "hooked" on it. You should talk to your doctor or nurse about any questions you have about the medicine. It is important to remember that the medicine *helps* you. It cannot *make* you do anything or change you as a person.

If your stomach is upset, taking the medicine with food may help.

Caffeine (in coffee, tea, or soft drinks) may make you feel worse.

To be sure that your kidneys keep working well, drink plenty of water and do not go on any low carbohydrate diets (such as Atkins or South Beach).

Topiramate may make birth control pills not work as well, increasing the risk of pregnancy. Be sure to talk with the doctor if you are on birth control pills.

It is very important not to stop this medicine suddenly—it could be uncomfortable or even dangerous.

How Your Doctor Will Follow Your Progress

Before giving you the medicine, your doctor or nurse will talk with you and your parent(s) and may measure your height, weight, heart rate (pulse), and blood pressure. The doctor may order blood tests to be sure you are healthy before taking the medicine.

Be sure to tell your doctor or nurse about any other medicines or supplements you are taking, including vitamins, herbs, or aids to weight loss or bodybuilding. Also be sure to tell the doctor or nurse if you are using alcohol or drugs. Because many medicines may affect babies, it is very important to tell the doctor if you might be pregnant or if you are at risk of becoming pregnant.

Your teachers may be asked to fill out a form about your grades and behavior in school. A psychologist may give you some tests to see how you learn best.

Most doctors have regular appointments with young people who are taking medicine. You should use these visits to share any concerns you may have about your medicine and to talk about if it has helped you. From time to time, your physician or nurse may measure your height, weight, heart rate (pulse), and blood pressure to be sure that you are in good health while you are taking the medicine and that your kidneys are working well. Your doctor also will ask for regular reports from your parents and maybe from your teachers (with your permission) to see how well the medicine is working.

How the Medicine Might Affect You

In addition to the ways the medicine can help you, it may have other effects called *side effects*. Different medicines have different side effects. It is helpful to know about some of the most common side effects of your medicine so that you will understand what they are if they happen. Some people do not have any side effects. Some side effects are just uncomfortable, but others may mean a more serious problem with the medicine. Side effects are most common after starting the medicine or after a dose increase. They may go away with time, or the medicine can be adjusted or changed—ask the doctor.

You could have an allergy to any medicine, which might show up as a rash on your skin, swelling, itching, or trouble breathing.

Please tell your parent(s) and doctor or nurse about any changes that you notice after taking the medicine. It is especially important to tell a responsible adult right away if you are feeling depressed or that you may not want to live; if you have thoughts of hurting yourself; or if you begin to feel more irritable, nervous, or restless. Also be sure to tell your parent(s) or doctor if you begin to feel more "speeded up" or have trouble sleeping.

Some medicines make people feel sleepy or less coordinated. If this medicine is making you sleepy, it is very important not to drive a car or ride a bicycle or motorcycle. After starting a new medicine or increasing the dose of a medicine, please be extra careful when driving a car, riding a bike, or using machines until you can tell how the medicine affects your alertness, attention, and coordination.

The most common side effects of topiramate are dizziness, daytime sleepiness, feeling tired, and slowing of movements or speech. Less common side effects are decreased appetite; problems with paying attention; confusion or trouble with memory; feeling anxious (nervous), irritable, or angry; clumsiness; muscle pain; shaking; and double or blurred vision. These sometimes go away after you have been taking the medicine for a while or if the doctor lowers the dose of medicine you are taking. Tell your parent(s) or the doctor if you are having trouble with any of these side effects.

Tell your parent(s) or doctor right away if there are any changes in your urine or if you have fever or chills, back pain, or pain in your eye.

Notes

Use this space to take notes or to write down questions you want to ask the doctor or nurse.

_____

_____

_____

_____

_____

_____

_____

_____

_____

_____

_____

_____

Medication Information for Parents and Teachers

Trazodone—Desyrel

General Information About Medication

Each child and adolescent is different. No one has exactly the same combination of medical and psychological problems. It is a good idea to talk with the doctor or nurse about the reasons a medicine is being used. It is very important to keep all appointments and to be in touch by telephone if you have concerns. It is important to communicate with the doctor, nurse, or therapist.

It is very important that the medicine be taken exactly as the doctor instructs. However, once in a while, everyone forgets to give a medicine on time. It is a good idea to ask the doctor or nurse what to do if this happens. Do not stop or change a medicine without asking the doctor or nurse first.

If the medicine seems to stop working, it may be because it is not being taken regularly. The youth may be "cheeking" or hiding the medicine or forgetting to take it. A different dose may be needed. Something at school, at home, or in the neighborhood may be upsetting the youth, or he or she may need special help for learning disabilities or tutoring. Please discuss your concerns with the doctor. **Do not just increase the dose.**

All medicines should be kept in a safe place, out of the reach of children, and should be supervised by an adult. If someone takes too much of a medicine, call the doctor, the poison control center, or a hospital emergency room.

Each medicine has a "generic" or chemical name. Just like laundry detergents or paper towels, some medicines are sold by more than one company under different brand names. The same medicine may be available under a generic name and several brand names. The generic medications are usually less expensive than the brand name ones. The generic medications have the same chemical formula, but they may or may not be exactly the same strength as the brand-name medications. Also, some brands of pills contain dye that can cause allergic reactions. It is a good idea to talk to the doctor and the pharmacist about whether it is important to use a specific brand of medicine.

All medicines can cause an allergic reaction. Examples are hives, itching, rashes, swelling, and trouble breathing. Even a tiny amount of a medicine can cause a reaction in patients who are allergic to that medicine. Be *sure* to talk to the doctor before restarting a medicine that has caused an allergic reaction.

Taking more than one medicine at the same time may cause more side effects or cause one of the medicines to not work as well. Always ask the doctor, nurse, or pharmacist before adding another medicine, whether prescription or over-the-counter. Be sure that each doctor knows about *all* of the medicines your child is taking. Also tell the doctor about any vitamins, herbal medicines, or supplements your child may be taking. Some of these may have side effects alone or when taken with this medication.

Everyone taking medicine should have a physical examination at least once a year.

If you suspect the youth is using drugs or alcohol, please tell the doctor right away.

Pregnancy requires special care in the use of medicine. Please tell the doctor immediately if you suspect the teenager is pregnant or might become pregnant.

Printed information like this applies to children and adolescents in general. If you have questions about the medicine, or if you notice changes or anything unusual, please ask the doctor or nurse. As scientific research advances, knowledge increases and advice changes. Even experts do not always agree. Many medicines have not been approved by the U.S. Food and Drug Administration (FDA) for use in children. For this reason, use of the medicine for a particular problem or age group often is not listed in the *Physicians' Desk Reference*. This does not necessarily mean that the medicine is dangerous or does not work, only that the company that makes the medicine has not received permission to advertise the medicine for use in children. Companies often do not apply for this permission because it is expensive to do the tests needed to apply for approval for use in children. Once a medication is approved by the FDA for any purpose, a doctor is allowed to prescribe it according to research and clinical experience.

Note to Teachers

It is a good idea to talk with the parent(s) about the reason(s) that a medication is being used. If the parent(s) sign consent to release information, it is often helpful to talk with the doctor. If the parent(s) give permission, the doctor may ask you to fill out rating forms about your experience with the student's behavior, feelings, academic performance, and medication side effects. This information is very useful in selecting and monitoring medication treatment. If you have observations that you think are important, do not hesitate to share these with the student's parent(s) and treating clinicians.

All medicines should be kept in a secure place and should be supervised by an adult. If someone takes too much of a medicine, follow your school procedure for an urgent medical problem.

Taking medicine is a private matter and is best managed discreetly and confidentially. It is important to be sensitive to the student's feelings about taking medicine.

If you suspect that the student is using drugs or alcohol, please tell the parent(s) or a school counselor right away.

Please tell the parent(s) or school nurse if you suspect medication side effects.

Any expression of suicidal thoughts or feelings or self-harm by a child or adolescent is a clear signal of distress and should be taken seriously. These behaviors should not be dismissed as "attention seeking."

What Is Trazodone (Desyrel)?

Trazodone is called an *antidepressant*. It is most often used for insomnia (trouble falling asleep) in people who are on other medicines for emotional or behavioral problems. It comes in brand name Desyrel and generic tablets.

How Can This Medicine Help?

Trazodone can help people fall asleep at night. It may also decrease depression, anxiety (nervousness), irritability (crankiness), and aggression.

How Does This Medicine Work?

People with emotional and behavior problems may have low levels of a brain chemical *(neurotransmitter)* called *serotonin*. Trazodone is believed to help by increasing brain serotonin to more normal activity.

How Long Does This Medicine Last?

The medicine lasts about a day, but the sleepiness effect should be gone by morning if the medicine is taken at bedtime. If your child is still sleepy in the morning, talk with the doctor.

How Will the Doctor Monitor This Medicine?

The doctor will review your child's medical history and physical examination before starting trazodone. The doctor or nurse may measure your child's pulse and blood pressure.

Be sure to tell the doctor if your child or anyone in the family has bipolar illness (manic-depressive illness) or has tried to kill himself or herself.

After the medicine is started, the doctor will want to have regular appointments with you and your child to see how the medicine is working, to see if a dose change is needed, to watch for side effects, to see if trazodone is still needed, and to see if any other treatment is needed. The doctor or nurse may check your child's height, weight, pulse, and blood pressure.

Before using medicine and at times afterward, the doctor may ask your child to fill out a rating scale about depression, to help see how your child is doing. The doctor may ask you and your child to keep a log of sleep and awake times.

What Side Effects Can This Medicine Have?

Any medicine can have side effects, including an allergy to the medicine. Because each patient is different, the doctor will monitor the youth closely, especially when the medicine is started. The doctor will work with you to increase the positive effects and decrease the negative effects of the medicine. Please tell the doctor if any of the listed side effects appear or if you think that the medicine is causing any other problems. Not all of the rare or unusual side effects are listed.

Side effects are most common after starting the medicine or after a dose increase. Many side effects can be avoided or lessened by starting with a very low dose and increasing it slowly—ask the doctor.

Allergic Reaction

Tell the doctor in a day or two (if possible, before the next dose of medicine):

- Hives
- Itching
- Rash

Stop the medicine and get *immediate* medical care:

- Trouble breathing or chest tightness
- Swelling of lips, tongue, or throat

Common Side Effects

Tell the doctor within a week or two:

- Daytime drowsiness or sleepiness—Do not allow your child to drive, ride a bicycle or motorcycle, or operate machinery if this happens.
- Dry mouth—Have your child try using sugar-free gum or candy.
- Dizziness or light-headedness, especially when standing or sitting up fast
- Headache
- Blurred vision
- Nausea
- Decreased appetite
- Seeing trails or shadows that are not there
- Tremors (shaking)
- More frequent erections (in boys)

Rare, but Serious, Side Effect (boys only)

Go to an emergency room *right away:*

- Erection of the penis lasting more than 1 hour—This may be painful and could cause permanent damage.

Serotonin Syndrome

A very serious side effect called *serotonin syndrome* can happen when certain kinds of medicines are taken by the same person. *Very* rarely, it can happen at high doses of just one medicine. The early signs are restlessness, confusion, shaking, skin turning red, sweating, and jerking of muscles. If your child has these symptoms, stop the medicine and go to an emergency room right away.

Some Interactions With Other Medicines or Food

Please note that the following are only the most likely interactions with food or other medicines.

It is better to limit drinks with caffeine (coffee, tea, soft drinks) because caffeine works in the opposite way from trazodone, may increase the side effects of the medicine, and might decrease the positive effects.

Other antidepressant medicines may increase the levels of trazodone, increasing side effects.

When carbamazepine (Tegretol) is combined with trazodone, Tegretol levels and side effects may increase, and trazodone levels may decrease, causing it to not work as well.

It can be *very dangerous* to take trazodone at the same time as, or even within several weeks of, taking another type of medicine called a *monoamine oxidase inhibitor* (MAOI), such as Eldepryl (selegiline), Nardil (phenelzine), Parnate (tranylcypromine), or Marplan (isocarboxazid).

What Could Happen if This Medicine Is Stopped Suddenly?

There are no known medical problems from stopping this medicine, although there may be uncomfortable feelings, or the original problems may come back. Always talk to the doctor before stopping a medication.

How Long Will This Medicine Be Needed?

Trazodone may not reach its full effect for several weeks. Your child may need to keep taking the medicine for at least several months.

When trazodone is used to improve sleep, a behavioral program, such as regular soothing routines at bedtime and increased exercise in the daytime, should be used in combination with the medicine. Finding developmentally appropriate bed- and wake-times and sticking to them is very important. These strategies should be continued after the medicine is stopped or when the medicine is used only occasionally.

What Else Should I Know About This Medicine?

In youth who have bipolar disorder (manic depression) or are at risk for bipolar disorder, any antidepressant medicine may increase the risk of hypomania or mania (excitement agitation, increased activity, decreased sleep).

Priapism, or erection of the penis lasting for a very long time, is a very rare but serious side effect that may require surgery. If there is any sign of this, **the boy should go to an emergency room right away.**

Black Box Antidepressant Warning

In 2004, an advisory committee to the FDA decided that there might be an increased risk of suicidal behavior for some youth taking medicines called *antidepressants*. In the research studies that the committee reviewed, about 3%–4% of youth with depression who took an antidepressant medicine—and 1%–2% of youth with depression who took a placebo (pill without active medicine)—talked about suicidal thoughts (thinking about killing themselves or wishing they were dead) or did something to harm themselves. This means that almost twice as many youth who were taking an antidepressant to treat their depression talked about suicide or had suicidal behavior compared with youth with depression who were taking inactive medicine. There were *no* completed suicides in any of these research studies, which included more than 4,000 children and adolescents. For youth being treated for anxiety, there was no difference in suicidal talking or behavior between those taking antidepressant medication and those taking placebo.

The FDA told drug companies to add a *black box warning* label to all antidepressant medicines. Because of this label, a doctor (or advanced practice nurse) prescribing one of these medicines has to warn youth and their families that there might be more suicidal thoughts and actions in youth taking these medicines.

On the other hand, in places where more youth are taking the newer antidepressant medicines, the number of adolescents who commit suicide has gotten smaller. Also, thinking about or attempting suicide is more common in surveys of teenagers in the community than it is in depressed youth treated in research studies with antidepressant medicine.

If a youth is being treated with this medicine and is doing well, then no changes are needed as a result of this warning. Increased suicidal talk or action is most likely to happen in the first few months of treatment with a medicine. If your child has recently started this medicine or is about to start, then you and your doctor (or advanced practice nurse) should watch for any changes in behavior. People who are depressed often have suicidal thoughts or actions. It is hard to know whether suicidal thoughts or actions in depressed people are caused by the depression itself or by the medicine. Also, as their depression is getting better, some people talk more about the suicidal thoughts that they had before but did not talk about. As young people get better from depression, they might be at higher risk of doing something about suicidal thoughts that they have had for some time, because they have more energy.

What Should a Parent Do?

1. Be honest with your child about possible risks and benefits of medicine.
2. Talk to your child about whether he or she is having any suicidal thoughts, and tell your child to come to you if he or she is having such thoughts.
3. You, your child, and your child's doctor or nurse should develop a safety plan. Pick adults whom your child can tell if he or she is thinking about suicide.
4. Be sure to tell your child's doctor, nurse, or therapist if you suspect that your child is using alcohol or drugs or if something has happened that might make your child feel worse, such as a family separation, breaking up with a boyfriend or girlfriend, someone close dying or attempting suicide, physical or sexual abuse, or failure in school.
5. Be sure that there are no guns in the home and that all medicines (including over-the-counter medicines like Tylenol) are closely supervised by an adult and kept in a safe place.
6. Watch for new or worse thoughts of suicide, self-harm, depression, anxiety (nerves), feeling very agitated or restless, being angry or aggressive, having more trouble sleeping, or anything else that you see for the first time, seems worse, or worries your child or you. If these appear, contact a mental health professional **right away.** Do not just stop or change the dose of the medicine on your own. If the problems are serious, and you cannot reach one of your clinicians, call a 24-hour psychiatry emergency telephone number or take your child to an emergency room.

Youth on antidepressant medicine should be watched carefully by their parent(s), clinician(s) (doctor, nurse, therapist), and other concerned adults for the first weeks of treatment. It is a good idea to have a visit or telephone call with the doctor, nurse, or therapist weekly for the first month, every 2 weeks for the second month, and after that at least once a month to check for feelings of depression or sadness, thoughts of killing or harming himself or herself, and any problems with the medication. If you have questions, be sure to ask the doctor, nurse, or therapist.

For more information, see http://www.parentsmedguide.org/ (in English and Spanish).

Notes

Use this space to take notes or to write down questions you want to ask the doctor.

_____

_____

_____

_____

_____

_____

_____

_____

_____

_____

_____

_____

_____

From Dulcan MK (editor): _Helping Parents, Youth, and Teachers Understand Medications for Behavioral and Emotional Problems: A Resource Book of Medication Information Handouts,_ Third Edition. Washington, DC, American Psychiatric Publishing, 2007

Medication Information
for Youth

Trazodone—Desyrel

What the Medicine Is Called and What It Is For

The name of your medicine may be confusing. Most drugs have two names: 1) a scientific name that we call a *generic name* and 2) a trade or *brand name*. The generic name of this medicine is trazodone. The brand name is Desyrel.

Trazodone is an *antidepressant*. Trazodone is used to treat depression and anxiety disorders. It helps people who feel very sad or depressed, anxious (nervous), or afraid. It is also used to help people who are on other medicines sleep better at night.

How You Take the Medicine

It is very important to take the medicine exactly as the doctor or nurse tells you. Do not skip doses or take extra medicine without asking an adult. If you forget a dose, ask your parent(s) what to do. It is *very important* that you take all the pills you are supposed to take each day. Your doctor will probably recommend that you take your medicine at bedtime.

You may feel discouraged and think the medicine is not going to help. You may want to give up and stop taking the medicine. Talk to your doctor and parent(s) about how you feel, but **do not stop** taking the medicine unless your doctor tells you to. It is also important *not* to take extra pills, hoping that you will feel better faster. Doing that could make you very sick.

Trazodone works best if combined with a regular bedtime, calming routines before bedtime, and physical exercise during the day. Getting up on time is also important in keeping a regular sleep schedule.

Caffeine (in coffee, tea, or soft drinks) may make it harder to fall asleep and make the trazodone not work as well.

This medicine is prescribed only for you. It should never be shared with anyone else.

You do not have to tell others that you are taking this medicine, but it is not something you should feel ashamed or embarrassed about. Many young people are helped by trazodone. This medicine is not habit-forming, and you cannot become "hooked" on it. You should talk to your doctor or nurse about any questions you have about the medicine. It is important to remember that the medicine *helps* you. It cannot *make* you do anything or change you as a person.

How Your Doctor Will Follow Your Progress

Before giving you the medicine, your doctor or nurse will talk with you and your parent(s) and may measure your height, weight, heart rate (pulse), and blood pressure.

Be sure to tell your doctor or nurse about any other medicines or supplements you are taking, including vitamins, herbs, or aids to weight loss or bodybuilding. Also be sure to tell the doctor or nurse if you are using alcohol or drugs. Because many medicines may affect babies, it is very important to tell the doctor if you might be pregnant or if you are at risk of becoming pregnant. Be sure to tell the doctor if you have had thoughts of hurting yourself, have tried to hurt yourself, or sometimes wish that you were not alive.

Your teachers may be asked to fill out a form about your grades and behavior in school. A psychologist may give you some tests to see how you learn best.

Before starting the medicine and afterward, the doctor may ask you to answer questions on paper about depression and anxiety. The doctor may ask you to keep a diary about your sleep.

Most doctors have regular appointments with young people who are taking medicine. You should use these visits to share any concerns you may have about your medicine and to talk about if it has helped you. From time to time, your physician or nurse may measure your height, weight, heart rate (pulse), and blood pressure to be sure that you are in good health while you are taking the medicine. Your doctor also will ask for regular reports from your parents to see how well the medicine is working.

Some medicines are started at the amount you will take for as long as you are taking that medicine. Other medicines need to be increased or adjusted until your doctor decides you are taking the right amount. Starting at a low dose and increasing it slowly may lessen side effects. Your doctor will decide how long you will need to take the medicine as he or she watches your progress.

It is not dangerous to stop trazodone suddenly, but there might be uncomfortable feelings, such as trouble sleeping, nervousness, irritability, or feeling sick. It is better to decrease trazodone slowly. Do not stop taking a medicine unless the doctor tells you to. If you have any problems after stopping or decreasing this medicine, tell your parent(s) or doctor.

How the Medicine Might Affect You

In addition to the ways the medicine can help you, it may have other effects called *side effects*. Different medicines have different side effects. It is helpful to know about some of the most common side effects of your medicine so that you will understand what they are if they happen. Some people do not have any side effects. Some side effects are just uncomfortable, but others may mean a more serious problem with the medicine. Side effects are most common after starting the medicine or after a dose increase. They may go away with time, or the medicine can be adjusted or changed—ask the doctor.

You could have an allergy to any medicine, which might show up as a rash on your skin, swelling, itching, or trouble breathing.

Please tell your parent(s) and doctor or nurse about any changes that you notice after taking the medicine. It is especially important to tell a responsible adult right away if you are feeling depressed or that you may not want to live; if you have thoughts of hurting yourself; or if you begin to feel more irritable, nervous, or restless. Also be sure to tell your parent(s) or doctor if you begin to feel "speeded up" or have trouble sleeping.

Some medicines make people feel sleepy or less coordinated. If this medicine is making you sleepy, it is very important not to drive a car or ride a bicycle or motorcycle. After starting a new medicine or increasing the dose of a medicine, please be extra careful when driving a car, riding a bike, or using machines until you can tell how the medicine affects your alertness, attention, and coordination.

One of the most common side effects of this medicine is feeling tired or sleepy during the day, even if you have had a full night's sleep. After you have been taking the medicine for a few weeks, your body will adjust, and this side effect may go away. If you have had trouble sleeping at night, the medicine can help you sleep better. Other people may feel more restless and excited. Tell your parent(s) or doctor if this is uncomfortable.

Another common side effect is dry mouth. You may be more thirsty than usual and find that you are drinking more water or other liquids. Sucking on sugar-free hard candy or cough drops usually helps. You also could try chewing sugar-free gum or sucking on ice chips. Do not chew the ice; you could hurt your teeth. Also, using lip balm will keep your lips from cracking. It is important to be especially good about brushing your teeth.

You might feel dizzy or light-headed if you stand up fast. Try standing up slowly, especially when getting out of bed in the morning.

Some people become constipated (have hard bowel movements). Try drinking more water and eating more fruits, vegetables, and whole grains. If that does not help, tell your parent(s) or doctor—you may need a medicine to help with this side effect.

Some other side effects that could happen are headache, blurry vision, not feeling hungry and not wanting to eat much, or having an upset stomach.

Very rarely, boys who are taking trazodone may have an erection of the penis that does not go away. It is OK to ask the doctor questions about this. If you get an erection that lasts longer than usual or hurts, **tell a responsible adult right away.** You need to go to an emergency room if this happens.

Please let your parent(s) and doctor know if you notice anything different or unusual about how you feel once you start taking the medicine. This includes good things, such as feeling less sad or less nervous or sleeping better at night.

Notes

Use this space to take notes or to write down questions you want to ask the doctor or nurse.

_____

_____

_____

_____

_____

_____

_____

_____

_____

_____

_____

_____

_____

From Dulcan MK (editor): *Helping Parents, Youth, and Teachers Understand Medications for Behavioral and Emotional Problems: A Resource Book of Medication Information Handouts*, Third Edition. Washington, DC, American Psychiatric Publishing, 2007

Triazolam—Halcion

General Information About Medication

Each child and adolescent is different. No one has exactly the same combination of medical and psychological problems. It is a good idea to talk with the doctor or nurse about the reasons a medicine is being used. It is very important to keep all appointments and to be in touch by telephone if you have concerns. It is important to communicate with the doctor, nurse, or therapist.

It is very important that the medicine be taken exactly as the doctor instructs. However, once in a while, everyone forgets to give a medicine on time. It is a good idea to ask the doctor or nurse what to do if this happens. Do not stop or change a medicine without asking the doctor or nurse first.

If the medicine seems to stop working, it may be because it is not being taken regularly. The youth may be "cheeking" or hiding the medicine or forgetting to take it (especially at school). The doses may be too far apart, or a different dose may be needed. Something at school, at home, or in the neighborhood may be upsetting the youth, or he or she may need special help for learning disabilities or tutoring. Please discuss your concerns with the doctor. **Do not just increase the dose.**

All medicines should be kept in a safe place, out of the reach of children, and should be supervised by an adult. If someone takes too much of a medicine, call the doctor, the poison control center, or a hospital emergency room.

Each medicine has a "generic" or chemical name. Just like laundry detergents or paper towels, some medicines are sold by more than one company under different brand names. The same medicine may be available under a generic name and several brand names. The generic medications are usually less expensive than the brand name ones. The generic medications have the same chemical formula, but they may or may not be exactly the same strength as the brand-name medications. Also, some brands of pills contain dye that can cause allergic reactions. It is a good idea to talk to the doctor and the pharmacist about whether it is important to use a specific brand of medicine.

All medicines can cause an allergic reaction. Examples are hives, itching, rashes, swelling, and trouble breathing. Even a tiny amount of a medicine can cause a reaction in patients who are allergic to that medicine. Be *sure* to talk to the doctor before restarting a medicine that has caused an allergic reaction.

Taking more than one medicine at the same time may cause more side effects or cause one of the medicines to not work as well. Always ask the doctor, nurse, or pharmacist before adding another medicine, whether prescription or over-the-counter. Be sure that each doctor knows about *all* of the medicines your child is taking. Also tell the doctor about any vitamins, herbal medicines, or supplements your child may be taking. Some of these may have side effects alone or when taken with this medication.

Everyone taking medicine should have a physical examination at least once a year.

If you suspect the youth is using drugs or alcohol, please tell the doctor right away.

Pregnancy requires special care in the use of medicine. Please tell the doctor immediately if you suspect the teenager is pregnant or might become pregnant.

Printed information like this applies to children and adolescents in general. If you have questions about the medicine, or if you notice changes or anything unusual, please ask the doctor or nurse. As scientific research advances, knowledge increases and advice changes. Even experts do not always agree. Many medicines have not been approved by the U.S. Food and Drug Administration (FDA) for use in children. For this reason, use of the medicine for a particular problem or age group often is not listed in the *Physicians' Desk Reference*. This does not necessarily mean that the medicine is dangerous or does not work, only that the company that makes the medicine has not received permission to advertise the medicine for use in children. Companies often do not apply for this permission because it is expensive to do the tests needed to apply for approval for use in children. Once a medication is approved by the FDA for any purpose, a doctor is allowed to prescribe it according to research and clinical experience.

Note to Teachers

It is a good idea to talk with the parent(s) about the reason(s) that a medication is being used. If the parent(s) sign consent to release information, it is often helpful to talk with the doctor. If the parent(s) give permission, the doctor may ask you to fill out rating forms about your experience with the student's behavior, feelings, academic performance, and medication side effects. This information is very useful in selecting and monitoring medication treatment. If you have observations that you think are important, do not hesitate to share these with the student's parent(s) and treating clinicians.

It is very important that the medicine be taken exactly as the doctor instructs. However, everyone forgets to give a medicine on time once in a while. It is a good idea to ask the parent(s) in advance what to do if this happens. Do not stop or change the time you are giving a medicine at school without parental permission. If a medication is to be taken with food, but lunchtime or snack time changes, be sure to notify the parent(s) so appropriate adjustments can be made.

All medicines should be kept in a secure place and should be supervised by an adult. If someone takes too much of a medicine, follow your school procedure for an urgent medical problem.

Taking medicine is a private matter and is best managed discreetly and confidentially. It is important to be sensitive to the student's feelings about taking medicine.

If you suspect that the student is using drugs or alcohol, please tell the parent(s) or a school counselor right away.

Please tell the parent(s) or school nurse if you suspect medication side effects.

Modifications of the classroom environment or assignments may be useful in addition to medication. The student may need to be evaluated for additional help or for an Individualized Education Plan for learning or behavior.

Any expression of suicidal thoughts or feelings or self-harm by a child or adolescent is a clear signal of distress and should be taken seriously. These behaviors should not be dismissed as "attention seeking."

What Is Triazolam (Halcion)?

Triazolam is a *benzodiazepine* medicine. It is called a *hypnotic* or *sedative-hypnotic*. It comes in Halcion brand name and generic tablets.

How Can This Medicine Help?

Triazolam is used to treat insomnia—problems falling asleep—when used for a short time along with a behavioral program.

How Does This Medicine Work?

Triazolam works on *receptors* (special places on brain cells) in certain parts of the brain to change the action of *GABA*, a *neurotransmitter*—a chemical that the brain makes for brain cells to communicate with each other.

How Long Does This Medicine Last?

Triazolam is taken before bedtime and starts working within 15–30 minutes. There may still be some effects in the morning. Benzodiazepine sleeping pills differ in how long they last. Triazolam is a short-acting benzodiazepine (4–6 hours), so it is less likely to cause sleepiness and memory problems the next day or to build up in the body if taken every day.

How Will the Doctor Monitor This Medicine?

The doctor will review your child's medical history and physical examination before starting triazolam.

After the medicine is started, the doctor will want to have regular appointments with you and your child to see how the medicine is working, to see if a dose change is needed, to watch for side effects, to see if triazolam is still needed, and to see if any other treatment is needed.

What Side Effects Can This Medicine Have?

Any medicine can have side effects, including an allergy to the medicine. Because each patient is different, the doctor will monitor the youth closely, especially when the medicine is started. The doctor will work with you to increase the positive effects and decrease the negative effects of the medicine. Please tell the doctor if any of the listed side effects appear or if you think that the medicine is causing any other problems. Not all of the rare or unusual side effects are listed.

Side effects are most common after starting the medicine or after a dose increase. Many side effects can be avoided or lessened by starting with a very low dose and increasing it slowly—ask the doctor.

Allergic Reaction

Tell the doctor in a day or two (if possible, before the next dose of medicine):

- Hives
- Itching
- Rash

Stop the medicine and get *immediate* medical care:

- Trouble breathing or chest tightness
- Swelling of lips, tongue, or throat

Triazolam is usually safe when used for short periods as the doctor prescribes.

The most common side effect is daytime sleepiness. Triazolam can also cause dizziness, feeling "spacey," or decreased coordination. If the medicine is causing any of these problems it is very important not to drive a car, ride a bicycle or motorcycle, or operate machinery.

Triazolam can cause decreased concentration and memory. These problems, along with daytime sleepiness, may decrease learning and performance in school.

People who take triazolam must not drink alcohol. Severe sleepiness or even loss of consciousness may result.

It is possible to become psychologically and physically dependent on triazolam, but that is not a common problem for patients who see their doctors regularly. Because some people abuse benzodiazepines, it is illegal to give or sell these medicines to someone other than the patient for whom they were prescribed.

At higher doses, triazolam may be associated with dangerous and unusual behaviors and loss of memory for the period of time after taking the pill.

Very rarely, even low doses of triazolam cause excitement, irritability, anger, aggression, agitation, trouble sleeping, nightmares, uncontrollable behavior, or memory loss. This is called *disinhibition* or a *paradoxical effect*. This may be more common in younger children. Stop the medicine and call the doctor if this happens.

Some Interactions With Other Medicines or Food

Please note that the following are only the most likely interactions with food or other medicines.

Caffeine may cause trouble sleeping and make triazolam less effective. If caffeine is eliminated, less triazolam may be needed, or triazolam may not be needed at all.

Grapefruit juice can increase levels of triazolam and increase side effects.

Oral contraceptives (birth control pills), fluoxetine (Prozac), fluvoxamine (Luvox), and other medicines may increase the levels of triazolam and increase side effects.

It is important not to use other sedatives, tranquilizers, or sleeping pills or antihistamines (such as Benadryl) when taking triazolam because of greatly increased side effects.

What Could Happen if This Medicine Is Stopped Suddenly?

Many medicines cause problems if stopped suddenly. Triazolam must be decreased slowly (tapered) rather than stopped suddenly. When triazolam is stopped suddenly, there are withdrawal symptoms that are uncomfortable and may even be dangerous. Problems are more likely in patients taking high doses of triazolam for 2 months or longer, but even after taking triazolam for just a few weeks, it is important to stop it slowly. Withdrawal symptoms may include anxiety, irritability, shaking, sweating, aches and pains, muscle cramps, vomiting, confusion, and trouble sleeping. If large doses taken for a long time are stopped suddenly, seizures (fits, convulsions), hallucinations (hearing voices or seeing things that are not there), or out-of-control behavior may result.

How Long Will This Medicine Be Needed?

Triazolam is usually prescribed for only a week or so or for occasional use. A behavioral program, such as regular soothing routines at bedtime and increased exercise in the daytime, should be used along with the medicine to improve sleep. This program can be continued after the medicine is tapered (stopped slowly) or when the medicine is used only occasionally.

What Else Should I Know About This Medicine?

Because benzodiazepines can be abused (especially by people who abuse alcohol or drugs) and can cause psychological dependence or physical dependence (addiction), they are regulated by special state and federal laws as *controlled substances*. These laws place limitations on telephone prescriptions and refills, and prescriptions expire if they are not filled promptly.

People with sleep apnea (breathing stops while they are asleep) should not take triazolam. Tell the doctor if your child snores very loudly.

Triazolam should be avoided during pregnancy, especially in the first 3 months, because it may cause birth defects in the baby. If taken regularly at the end of pregnancy, triazolam may cause withdrawal symptoms in the baby.

Notes

Use this space to take notes or to write down questions you want to ask the doctor.

_____

_____

_____

_____

_____

_____

_____

_____

_____

_____

_____

_____

_____

Medication Information for Youth

Triazolam—Halcion

What the Medicine Is Called and What It Is For

The name of your medicine may be confusing. Most drugs have two names: 1) a scientific name that we call a *generic name* and 2) a trade or *brand name*. The generic name of this medicine is triazolam. The brand name is Halcion.

Triazolam is a *benzodiazepine* medicine. It works by calming the parts of the brain that are too excitable. Triazolam can help with insomnia (difficulty falling asleep or staying asleep) when used for a short time along with routines that help you to relax and fall asleep.

How You Take the Medicine

It is very important to take the medicine exactly as the doctor or nurse tells you. Do not skip doses or take extra medicine without asking an adult. If you forget a dose, ask your parent(s) what to do.

It is better to limit drinks with caffeine (coffee, tea, soft drinks) because caffeine works in the opposite way from this medicine, and the positive effects might be decreased.

Drinking a lot of grapefruit juice can increase the side effects of triazolam.

This medicine is prescribed only for you. It should never be shared with anyone else.

You do not have to tell others that you are taking this medicine, but it is not something you should feel ashamed or embarrassed about. Many young people are helped by triazolam. You should talk to your doctor or nurse about any questions you have about the medicine. It is important to remember that the medicine *helps* you. It cannot *make* you do anything or change you as a person.

Many medicines cause problems if stopped suddenly. Always ask your doctor before stopping a medicine. Problems are more likely to happen in patients taking high doses of triazolam for 2 months or longer, but it is important to decrease the medicine slowly (taper) even after a few weeks. If you notice anxiety, irritability, shaking, sweating, aches and pains, muscle cramps, vomiting, or trouble sleeping, you may need to decrease the medicine more slowly. If large doses are stopped suddenly, seizures (fits, convulsions), hallucinations (hearing voices or seeing things that are not there), or out-of-control behavior may result.

How Your Doctor Will Follow Your Progress

Before giving you the medicine, your doctor or nurse will talk with you and your parent(s). Be sure to tell your doctor or nurse about any other medicines or supplements you are taking, including vitamins, herbs, or aids

653

to weight loss or bodybuilding. Also be sure to tell the doctor or nurse if you are using alcohol or drugs. Because triazolam may affect babies, it is very important to tell the doctor if you might be pregnant or if you are at risk of becoming pregnant.

Most doctors have regular appointments with young people who are taking medicine. You should use these visits to share any concerns you may have about your medicine and to talk about if it has helped you. From time to time, your physician or nurse may measure your height, weight, heart rate (pulse), and blood pressure to be sure that you are in good health while you are taking the medicine. Your doctor also will ask for regular reports from your parents to see how well the medicine is working.

Triazolam is usually prescribed for only a week or so to allow you to develop better sleep habits. A regular bedtime, a relaxing routine before bedtime, and physical exercise in the daytime usually help with sleep at night.

Each person is unique, and some people may need this medicine for months or years.

How the Medicine Might Affect You

In addition to the ways the medicine can help you, it may have other effects called *side effects*. Different medicines have different side effects. It is helpful to know about some of the most common side effects of your medicine so that you will understand what they are if they happen. Some people do not have any side effects. Some side effects are just uncomfortable, but others may mean a more serious problem with the medicine. Side effects are most common after starting the medicine or after a dose increase. They may go away with time, or the medicine can be adjusted or changed—ask the doctor.

You could have an allergy to any medicine, which might show up as a rash on your skin, swelling, itching, or trouble breathing.

Please tell your parent(s) and doctor or nurse about any changes that you notice after taking the medicine. It is especially important to tell a responsible adult if you are feeling depressed or that you may not want to live; if you have thoughts of hurting yourself; or if you begin to feel more irritable, nervous, or restless.

The most common side effect of triazolam is daytime sleepiness. If this medicine is making you sleepy, it is very important not to drive a car or ride a bicycle or motorcycle. After starting triazolam or increasing the dose, please be extra careful when driving a car, riding a bike, or using machines until you can tell how the medicine affects your alertness, attention, and coordination.

Sometimes sleep medicines seem to work in the opposite way, causing excitement, irritability, anger, aggression, and other problems. If this happens, tell your parent(s) or your doctor.

Drinking alcohol while taking this medicine can cause severe drowsiness or even passing out. **Don't do it!** Do not use marijuana or street drugs while taking this medicine. They can cause serious side effects. Skipping your medicine to take drugs does not work because many medicines stay in your body for a long time.

Triazolam can be habit-forming, but that is not a common problem for people who take their medicine as the doctor says.

Notes

Use this space to take notes or to write down questions you want to ask the doctor or nurse.

_____

_____

_____

_____

_____

_____

_____

_____

_____

_____

_____

_____

_____

From Dulcan MK (editor): _Helping Parents, Youth, and Teachers Understand Medications for Behavioral and Emotional Problems: A Resource Book of Medication Information Handouts,_ Third Edition. Washington, DC, American Psychiatric Publishing, 2007

Medication Information for Parents and Teachers

Trifluoperazine—Stelazine

General Information About Medication

Each child and adolescent is different. No one has exactly the same combination of medical and psychological problems. It is a good idea to talk with the doctor or nurse about the reasons a medicine is being used. It is very important to keep all appointments and to be in touch by telephone if you have concerns. It is important to communicate with the doctor, nurse, or therapist.

It is very important that the medicine be taken exactly as the doctor instructs. However, once in a while, everyone forgets to give a medicine on time. It is a good idea to ask the doctor or nurse what to do if this happens. Do not stop or change a medicine without asking the doctor or nurse first.

If the medicine seems to stop working, it may be because it is not being taken regularly. The youth may be "cheeking" or hiding the medicine or forgetting to take it (especially at school). The doses may be too far apart, or a different dose may be needed. Something at school, at home, or in the neighborhood may be upsetting the youth, or he or she may need special help for learning disabilities or tutoring. Please discuss your concerns with the doctor. **Do not just increase the dose.**

All medicines should be kept in a safe place, out of the reach of children, and should be supervised by an adult. If someone takes too much of a medicine, call the doctor, the poison control center, or a hospital emergency room.

Each medicine has a "generic" or chemical name. Just like laundry detergents or paper towels, some medicines are sold by more than one company under different brand names. The same medicine may be available under a generic name and several brand names. The generic medications are usually less expensive than the brand name ones. The generic medications have the same chemical formula, but they may or may not be exactly the same strength as the brand-name medications. Also, some brands of pills contain dye that can cause allergic reactions. It is a good idea to talk to the doctor and the pharmacist about whether it is important to use a specific brand of medicine.

All medicines can cause an allergic reaction. Examples are hives, itching, rashes, swelling, and trouble breathing. Even a tiny amount of a medicine can cause a reaction in patients who are allergic to that medicine. Be *sure* to talk to the doctor before restarting a medicine that has caused an allergic reaction.

Taking more than one medicine at the same time may cause more side effects or cause one of the medicines to not work as well. Always ask the doctor, nurse, or pharmacist before adding another medicine, whether prescription or over-the-counter. Be sure that each doctor knows about *all* of the medicines your child is taking. Also tell the doctor about any vitamins, herbal medicines, or supplements your child may be taking. Some of these may have side effects alone or when taken with this medication.

Everyone taking medicine should have a physical examination at least once a year.

If you suspect the youth is using drugs or alcohol, please tell the doctor right away.

Pregnancy requires special care in the use of medicine. Please tell the doctor immediately if you suspect the teenager is pregnant or might become pregnant.

Printed information like this applies to children and adolescents in general. If you have questions about the medicine, or if you notice changes or anything unusual, please ask the doctor or nurse. As scientific research advances, knowledge increases and advice changes. Even experts do not always agree. Many medicines have not been approved by the U.S. Food and Drug Administration (FDA) for use in children. For this reason, use of the medicine for a particular problem or age group often is not listed in the *Physicians' Desk Reference*. This does not necessarily mean that the medicine is dangerous or does not work, only that the company that makes the medicine has not received permission to advertise the medicine for use in children. Companies often do not apply for this permission because it is expensive to do the tests needed to apply for approval for use in children. Once a medication is approved by the FDA for any purpose, a doctor is allowed to prescribe it according to research and clinical experience.

Note to Teachers

It is a good idea to talk with the parent(s) about the reason(s) that a medication is being used. If the parent(s) sign consent to release information, it is often helpful to talk with the doctor. If the parent(s) give permission, the doctor may ask you to fill out rating forms about your experience with the student's behavior, feelings, academic performance, and medication side effects. This information is very useful in selecting and monitoring medication treatment. If you have observations that you think are important, do not hesitate to share these with the student's parent(s) and treating clinicians.

It is very important that the medicine be taken exactly as the doctor instructs. However, everyone forgets to give a medicine on time once in a while. It is a good idea to ask the parent(s) in advance what to do if this happens. Do not stop or change the time you are giving a medicine at school without parental permission. If a medication is to be taken with food, but lunchtime or snack time changes, be sure to notify the parent(s) so appropriate adjustments can be made.

All medicines should be kept in a secure place and should be supervised by an adult. If someone takes too much of a medicine, follow your school procedure for an urgent medical problem.

Taking medicine is a private matter and is best managed discreetly and confidentially. It is important to be sensitive to the student's feelings about taking medicine.

If you suspect that the student is using drugs or alcohol, please tell the parent(s) or a school counselor right away.

Please tell the parent(s) or school nurse if you suspect medication side effects.

Modifications of the classroom environment or assignments may be useful in addition to medication. The student may need to be evaluated for additional help or for an Individualized Education Plan for learning or behavior.

Any expression of suicidal thoughts or feelings or self-harm by a child or adolescent is a clear signal of distress and should be taken seriously. These behaviors should not be dismissed as "attention seeking."

What Is Trifluoperazine (Stelazine)?

Trifluoperazine is sometimes called a *typical*, *conventional*, or *first-generation antipsychotic* medicine. It is also called a *neuroleptic* or *phenothiazine*. It used to be called a *major tranquilizer*. It comes in brand name Stelazine and generic tablets and liquid.

How Can This Medicine Help?

Trifluoperazine is used to treat psychosis, such as in schizophrenia, mania, or very severe depression. It can reduce hallucinations (hearing voices or seeing things that are not there) and delusions (troubling beliefs that other people do not share). It can help the patient be less upset and agitated. It can improve the patient's ability to think clearly.

Sometimes trifluoperazine is used to decrease severe aggression or very serious behavioral problems in young people with conduct disorder, mental retardation, or autism.

This medicine is very powerful and should be used to treat very serious problems or symptoms that other medicines do not help. Be patient; the positive effects of this medicine may not appear for 2–3 weeks.

How Does This Medicine Work?

Cells in the brain (neurons) communicate using chemicals called *neurotransmitters*. Too much or too little of these substances in certain parts of the brain can cause problems. Trifluoperazine reduces the activity of one of these neurotransmitters, *dopamine*. Blocking the effect of dopamine in certain parts of the brain reduces what have been called *positive symptoms* of psychosis: delusions; hallucinations; disorganized and unusual thinking, speaking, and behavior; excessive activity (agitation); and lack of activity (catatonia). Blocking dopamine can also reduce tics. Reducing dopamine action in other parts of the brain may lead to the side effects of this medicine.

How Long Does This Medicine Last?

Trifluoperazine usually may be taken only once a day, unless divided doses are used to lessen side effects.

How Will the Doctor Monitor This Medicine?

The doctor will review your child's medical history and physical examination before starting trifluoperazine. The doctor may order some blood or urine tests to be sure your child does not have a hidden medical condition. The doctor or nurse may measure your child's pulse and blood pressure before starting trifluoperazine.

Before starting trifluoperazine and every so often afterward, a test such as the AIMS (Abnormal Involuntary Movement Scale) may be used to check your child's tongue, legs, and arms for unusual movements that could be caused by the medicine.

After the medicine is started, the doctor will want to have regular appointments with you and your child to see how the medicine is working, to see if a dose change is needed, to watch for side effects, to see if trifluoperazine is still needed, and to see if any other treatment is needed. The doctor or nurse may check your child's height, weight, pulse, and blood pressure and watch for abnormal movements.

What Side Effects Can This Medicine Have?

Any medicine can have side effects, including an allergy to the medicine. Because each patient is different, the doctor will monitor the youth closely, especially when the medicine is started. The doctor will work with you

to increase the positive effects and decrease the negative effects of the medicine. Please tell the doctor if any of the listed side effects appear or if you think that the medicine is causing any other problems. Not all of the rare or unusual side effects are listed.

Side effects are most common after starting the medicine or after a dose increase. Many side effects can be avoided or lessened by starting with a very low dose and increasing it slowly—ask the doctor.

Allergic Reaction

Tell the doctor in a day or two (if possible, before the next dose of medicine):

- Hives
- Itching
- Rash

Stop the medicine and get *immediate* medical care:

- Trouble breathing or chest tightness
- Swelling of lips, tongue, or throat

Common, but Not Usually Serious, Side Effects

Discuss the following side effects with your child's doctor within a week or two. They often can be helped by lowering the dose of medicine, changing the times medicine is taken, or adding another medicine.

- Dry mouth—Have your child try using sugar-free gum or candy.
- Constipation—Encourage your child to drink more fluids and eat high-fiber foods; if necessary, the doctor may recommend a fiber medicine such as Benefiber or a stool softener such as Colace or mineral oil.
- Increased risk of sunburn—Have your child wear sunscreen or protective clothing or stay out of the sun.
- Mild trouble urinating
- Blurred vision
- Weight gain—Seek nutritional counseling; provide your child with low-calorie snacks and encourage regular exercise.
- Sadness, irritability, nervousness, clinginess, not wanting to go to school
- Restlessness or inability to sit still
- Shaking of hands and fingers

Less Common, but Not Usually Serious, Side Effects

Discuss the following side effects with your child's doctor within a week or two. They often can be helped by lowering the dose of medicine, changing the times medicine is taken, or adding another medicine.

- Daytime sleepiness or tiredness—Do not allow your child to drive, ride a bicycle or motorcycle, or operate machinery if this happens. This problem may be lessened by taking the medicine at bedtime.
- Dizziness—This side effect is worse when the child stands up quickly, especially when getting out of bed in the morning; try having the child stand up slowly.
- Decreased or slowed movement and decreased facial expressions
- Drooling

- Decreased sexual interest or ability
- Changes in menstrual cycle
- Increase in breast size or discharge from the breasts (in both boys and girls)—This may go away with time.

Less Common, but Potentially Serious, Side Effects

Call the doctor or go to an emergency room *right away:*

- Stiffness of the tongue, jaw, neck, back, or legs
- Overheating or heatstroke—Prevent by decreasing activity in hot weather, staying out of the sun, and drinking water.
- Seizure (fit, convulsion)—This is more likely in people with a history of seizures or head injury.
- Severe confusion

Rare, but Serious, Side Effects

- Extreme stiffness or lack of movement, very high fever, mental confusion, irregular pulse rate, or eye pain—**This is a medical emergency. Go to an emergency room right away.**
- Sudden stiffness and inability to breathe or swallow—**Go to an emergency room or call 911.** Tell the paramedics, nurses, and doctors that the patient is taking trifluoperazine. Other medicines can be used to treat this problem fast.
- Increased thirst, frequent urination, lethargy, tiredness, dizziness—These could be signs of diabetes, especially if your child is overweight or there is a family history of diabetes. **Talk to a doctor within a day.**

What Else Should I Know About Side Effects?

Most side effects lessen over time. If they are troublesome, talk with your child's doctor. Some side effects can be decreased by taking a smaller dose of medicine, by stopping the medicine, by changing to another medicine, or by adding another medicine (see the table).

One side effect that may not go away is *tardive dyskinesia* (or TD). Patients with tardive dyskinesia have involuntary movements of the body, especially the mouth and tongue. The patient may look as though he or she is making faces over and over again. Jerky movements of the arms, legs, or body may occur. There may be fine, wormlike, or sudden repeated movements of the tongue, or the person may appear to be chewing something or smacking or puckering his or her lips. The fingers may look as though they are rolling something. If you notice any unusual movements, be sure to tell the doctor. The doctor may use the AIMS test to look for these movements.

The medicine may increase the level of *prolactin*, a natural hormone made in the part of the brain called the *pituitary*. This may cause side effects such as breast tenderness or swelling or production of milk, in both boys and girls. It also may interfere with sexual functioning in teenage boys and with regular menstrual cycles (periods) in teenage girls. A blood test can measure the level of prolactin. If these side effects do not go away and are troublesome, talk with your child's doctor about substituting another medicine for trifluoperazine.

Heart problems are more common if other medicines are being taken as well. Be sure to tell all your child's doctors and your pharmacist about all medications your child is taking.

Neuroleptic malignant syndrome is a very rare side effect that can lead to death. The symptoms are severe muscle stiffness, high fever, increased heart rate and blood pressure, irregular heartbeat (pulse), and sweating. It may lead to unconsciousness. If you suspect this, **call 911 or go to an emergency room right away.**

What Medicines Are Used to Treat the Side Effects of Trifluoperazine?

The following medicines may be used to treat the movement side effects of trifluoperazine. These medicines may have their own side effects as well. Ask the doctor if you suspect a problem.

Brand name	Generic name
Akineton	Biperiden
Artane	Trihexyphenidyl
Ativan	Lorazepam*
Benadryl	Diphenhydramine*
Catapres	Clonidine*
Cogentin	Benztropine mesylate*
Inderal	Propranolol*
Klonopin	Clonazepam*
Symmetrel	Amantadine

*This medicine has its own information sheet in this book.

Some Interactions With Other Medicines or Food

Please note that the following are only the most likely interactions with food or other medicines.

Trifluoperazine may be taken with or without food. If the medicine causes stomach upset, taking it with food may help.

It is better to limit drinks with caffeine (coffee, tea, soft drinks) because caffeine works in the opposite way from this medicine, and the positive effects might be decreased.

What Could Happen if This Medicine Is Stopped Suddenly?

Involuntary movements, or *withdrawal dyskinesias*, may appear within 1–4 weeks of lowering the dose or stopping the medicine. Usually these go away, but they can last for days to months. If trifluoperazine is stopped suddenly, emotional problems such as irritability, nervousness, moodiness; behavior problems; or physical problems such as stomachache, loss of appetite, nausea, vomiting, diarrhea, sweating, indigestion, trouble sleeping, trembling, or shaking may appear. These problems usually last only a few days to a few weeks. If they happen, tell your child's doctor. The medicine dose may need to be lowered more slowly (tapered). Always check with the doctor before stopping a medicine!

How Long Will This Medicine Be Needed?

How long your child will need to be on trifluoperazine depends partly on the reason that it was prescribed. Some problems last for only a few months, whereas others last much longer. Sometimes trifluoperazine is used for only a short time until other medicines or behavioral treatments start to work. Some people need to take trifluoperazine for years. It is especially important with medicines as powerful as this one to ask the doctor whether it is still needed. Every few months, you should discuss with your child's doctor the reasons for using trifluoperazine and whether it is time for a trial of lowering the dose.

What Else Should I Know About This Medicine?

There are many older and newer medicines that are used for the same kinds of problems. If your child is having bad side effects or the medicine does not seem to be working, ask the doctor if another medicine in this group might work as well or better and have fewer side effects for your child.

Be sure to tell the doctor if there is anyone in your family who died suddenly or had a heart problem.

Notes

Use this space to take notes or to write down questions you want to ask the doctor.

_____

_____

_____

_____

_____

_____

_____

_____

_____

_____

_____

_____

_____

_____

_____

From Dulcan MK (editor): *Helping Parents, Youth, and Teachers Understand Medications for Behavioral and Emotional Problems: A Resource Book of Medication Information Handouts*, Third Edition. Washington, DC, American Psychiatric Publishing, 2007

Medication Information for Youth

Trifluoperazine—Stelazine

What the Medicine Is Called and What It Is For

The name of your medicine may be confusing. Most drugs have two names: 1) a scientific name that we call a *generic name* and 2) a trade or *brand name*. The generic name of this medicine is trifluoperazine. The brand name is Stelazine.

Trifluoperazine can help people who feel very confused and have severe problems thinking clearly. It can lessen *hallucinations* (seeing or hearing things that are not really there) and *delusions* (troubling beliefs that other people do not share). This medicine also is sometimes used to help young people who have mania or very severe depression or who get very angry and hit people or break things.

How You Take the Medicine

It is very important to take the medicine exactly as the doctor or nurse tells you. Do not skip doses or take extra medicine without asking an adult. If you forget a dose, ask your parent(s) what to do. Your doctor will tell you how much medicine to take and how often to take it so that it can help you the most. It is *very important* that you take all the pills you are supposed to take each day. Your doctor will probably recommend that you take your medicine at the same time each day, which may be with meals or at bedtime.

It is better to limit drinks with caffeine (coffee, tea, soft drinks) because caffeine works in the opposite way from this medicine, and the positive effects might be decreased.

It may be several weeks or longer before you notice the full effect. You may feel discouraged and think the medicine is never going to help. You may want to give up and stop taking the medicine. Talk to your doctor and parent(s) about how you feel, but **do not stop** taking your medicine unless your doctor tells you to. It also is important not to take extra pills hoping that you will feel better faster. Doing that could make you very sick.

If your stomach is upset, taking the medicine with food may help.

This medicine is prescribed only for you. It should never be shared with anyone else.

You do not have to tell others that you are taking this medicine, but it is not something you should feel ashamed or embarrassed about. Many young people are helped by trifluoperazine. You should talk to your doctor or nurse about any questions you have about the medicine. It is important to remember that the medicine *helps* you. It cannot *make* you do anything or change you as a person.

How Your Doctor Will Follow Your Progress

Before giving you the medicine, your doctor or nurse will talk with you and your parent(s) and may measure your height, weight, heart rate (pulse), and blood pressure. There may be other tests, such as blood tests for sugar and cholesterol. Before you start taking the medicine and every so often afterward, the doctor or nurse will look at your tongue, arms, and legs to check for unusual movements. This is called the AIMS (Abnormal Involuntary Movement Scale) test.

Be sure to tell your doctor or nurse about any other medicines or supplements you are taking, including vitamins, herbs, or aids to weight loss or bodybuilding. Also be sure to tell the doctor or nurse if you are using alcohol or drugs. Because many medicines may affect babies, it is very important to tell the doctor if you might be pregnant or if you are at risk of becoming pregnant.

Your teachers may be asked to fill out a form about your grades and behavior in school. A psychologist may give you some tests to see how you learn best.

Most doctors have regular appointments with young people who are taking medicine. You should use these visits to share any concerns you may have about your medicine and to talk about if it has helped you. From time to time, your physician or nurse may measure your height, weight, heart rate (pulse), and blood pressure to be sure that you are in good health while you are taking the medicine. There may be blood tests to watch for diabetes or high cholesterol. Your doctor also will ask for regular reports from your parents and maybe from your teachers (with your permission) to see how well the medicine is working.

If the medicine helps you, your doctor will probably want you to take it for several months to a year. Your doctor will decide how long you will need to take the medicine as he or she watches your progress.

How the Medicine Might Affect You

In addition to the ways the medicine can help you, it may have other effects called *side effects*. Different medicines have different side effects. It is helpful to know about some of the most common side effects of your medicine so that you will understand what they are if they happen. Some people do not have any side effects. Some side effects are just uncomfortable, but others may mean a more serious problem with the medicine. Side effects are most common after starting the medicine or after a dose increase. They may go away with time, or the medicine can be adjusted or changed—ask the doctor.

You could have an allergy to any medicine, which might show up as a rash on your skin, swelling, itching, or trouble breathing.

Please tell your parent(s) and your doctor or nurse about any changes that you notice after taking the medicine. It is especially important to tell a responsible adult right away if you are feeling depressed or that you may not want to live; if you have thoughts of hurting yourself; or if you begin to feel more irritable, nervous, or restless.

One of the most common side effects of this medicine is feeling tired or sleepy during the day, even if you have had a full night's sleep. If this medicine is making you sleepy, it is very important not to drive a car or ride a bicycle or motorcycle. After starting the medicine or increasing the dose of medicine, please be extra careful when driving a car, riding a bike, or using machines until you can tell how the medicine affects your alertness, attention, and coordination. After you have been taking the medicine for a few weeks, your body will adjust, and this side effect will likely go away. If you had trouble sleeping at night before taking the medicine, it can help you sleep better, especially if the doctor tells you to take a dose of medicine in the evening.

You might feel dizzy or light-headed if you stand up fast. Try standing up slowly, especially when getting out of bed in the morning.

Another common side effect is dry mouth. You may be more thirsty than usual and find that you are drinking more water or other liquids than usual. Sucking on sugar-free hard candy or cough drops usually helps. You also could try chewing sugar-free gum or sucking on ice chips. Do not chew the ice; you could hurt your teeth. Also, using lip balm will keep your lips from cracking. It is important to be especially good about brushing your teeth.

Taking this medicine could make you more likely to get badly sunburned or very sick in hot weather. Be sure to drink plenty of liquids and cover up or use sunscreen when you go outside in hot weather. Be careful to rest in the shade and not get overheated.

Sometimes teenagers who take trifluoperazine gain weight. The weight gain may be from increased appetite and also from ways that the medicine changes how the body processes food. It is much easier to prevent weight gain than to lose weight later. It is a good idea to eat a well-balanced diet without "junk food" and with healthy snacks like fruits and vegetables, not sweets or fried foods. It is better to drink water or skim milk, not pop, sodas, soft drinks, or sugary juices. Regular exercise is important for maintaining a healthy weight (and may also help with sleep).

Some people become constipated (have hard bowel movements) when taking this medicine. Try drinking more water and eating more fruits, vegetables, and whole grains. If that does not help, tell your parent(s) or doctor—you may need a medicine to help with this side effect. Sometimes people have trouble passing urine. Tell your parent(s) or the doctor if this happens.

This is a very powerful medicine. Some side effects include feeling nervous, restless, or shaky or having stiff muscles. Talk with your doctor about these side effects. They can be helped by adding another medicine, adjusting the dose, or switching to another medicine.

Another, more serious, side effect can be longer lasting and more difficult to treat. This very rare side effect is called *tardive dyskinesia* (or TD). A person taking trifluoperazine may develop movements of the mouth, tongue, face, arms, legs, or body that are not being made on purpose. This side effect can go away when the medicine is stopped, but in some people it does not go away. Your doctor will explain this effect to you and your parent(s) and how he or she will watch for any signs that you are developing this problem. Be sure to ask your doctor any questions that you may have about this, but do not worry too much about it. It hardly ever happens to teenagers.

You may notice changes in your sexual functioning or in your breasts—it is OK to ask the doctor about this.

You should tell your parent(s) and doctor if you notice anything different or unusual about how you feel once you start taking the medicine. This includes good things, such as feeling less confused, feeling less sad or angry, not hearing voices anymore, or sleeping better at night.

You cannot become addicted to this medicine, but you should not stop it suddenly. Never stop a medicine without talking to the doctor. If trifluoperazine is stopped or decreased suddenly you may notice more moodiness or irritability, stomachaches or upset stomach, trouble sleeping, or trembling or shaking. Let your parent(s) or doctor know if this happens—the medicine may need to be decreased more slowly.

Notes

Use this space to take notes or to write down questions you want to ask the doctor or nurse.

_____

_____

_____

_____

_____

_____

_____

_____

_____

_____

_____

_____

Medication Information for Parents and Teachers

Valproic Acid—Depakene
Divalproex Sodium—Depakote

General Information About Medication

Each child and adolescent is different. No one has exactly the same combination of medical and psychological problems. It is a good idea to talk with the doctor or nurse about the reasons a medicine is being used. It is very important to keep all appointments and to be in touch by telephone if you have concerns. It is important to communicate with the doctor, nurse, or therapist.

It is very important that the medicine be taken exactly as the doctor instructs. However, once in a while, everyone forgets to give a medicine on time. It is a good idea to ask the doctor or nurse what to do if this happens. Do not stop or change a medicine without asking the doctor or nurse first.

If the medicine seems to stop working, it may be because it is not being taken regularly. The youth may be "cheeking" or hiding the medicine or forgetting to take it (especially at school). The doses may be too far apart, or a different dose may be needed. Something at school, at home, or in the neighborhood may be upsetting the youth, or he or she may need special help for learning disabilities or tutoring. Please discuss your concerns with the doctor. **Do not just increase the dose.**

All medicines should be kept in a safe place, out of the reach of children, and should be supervised by an adult. If someone takes too much of a medicine, call the doctor, the poison control center, or a hospital emergency room.

Each medicine has a "generic" or chemical name. Just like laundry detergents or paper towels, some medicines are sold by more than one company under different brand names. The same medicine may be available under a generic name and several brand names. The generic medications are usually less expensive than the brand name ones. The generic medications have the same chemical formula, but they may or may not be exactly the same strength as the brand-name medications. Also, some brands of pills contain dye that can cause allergic reactions. It is a good idea to talk to the doctor and the pharmacist about whether it is important to use a specific brand of medicine.

All medicines can cause an allergic reaction. Examples are hives, itching, rashes, swelling, and trouble breathing. Even a tiny amount of a medicine can cause a reaction in patients who are allergic to that medicine. Be *sure* to talk to the doctor before restarting a medicine that has caused an allergic reaction.

Taking more than one medicine at the same time may cause more side effects or cause one of the medicines to not work as well. Always ask the doctor, nurse, or pharmacist before adding another medicine, whether prescription or over-the-counter. Be sure that each doctor knows about *all* of the medicines your child is taking. Also tell the doctor about any vitamins, herbal medicines, or supplements your child may be taking. Some of these may have side effects alone or when taken with this medication.

669

Everyone taking medicine should have a physical examination at least once a year.

If you suspect the youth is using drugs or alcohol, please tell the doctor right away.

Pregnancy requires special care in the use of medicine. Please tell the doctor immediately if you suspect the teenager is pregnant or might become pregnant.

Printed information like this applies to children and adolescents in general. If you have questions about the medicine, or if you notice changes or anything unusual, please ask the doctor or nurse. As scientific research advances, knowledge increases and advice changes. Even experts do not always agree. Many medicines have not been approved by the U.S. Food and Drug Administration (FDA) for use in children. For this reason, use of the medicine for a particular problem or age group often is not listed in the *Physicians' Desk Reference*. This does not necessarily mean that the medicine is dangerous or does not work, only that the company that makes the medicine has not received permission to advertise the medicine for use in children. Companies often do not apply for this permission because it is expensive to do the tests needed to apply for approval for use in children. Once a medication is approved by the FDA for any purpose, a doctor is allowed to prescribe it according to research and clinical experience.

Note to Teachers

It is a good idea to talk with the parent(s) about the reason(s) that a medication is being used. If the parent(s) sign consent to release information, it is often helpful to talk with the doctor. If the parent(s) give permission, the doctor may ask you to fill out rating forms about your experience with the student's behavior, feelings, academic performance, and medication side effects. This information is very useful in selecting and monitoring medication treatment. If you have observations that you think are important, do not hesitate to share these with the student's parent(s) and treating clinicians.

It is very important that the medicine be taken exactly as the doctor instructs. However, everyone forgets to give a medicine on time once in a while. It is a good idea to ask the parent(s) in advance what to do if this happens. Do not stop or change the time you are giving a medicine at school without parental permission. If a medication is to be taken with food, but lunchtime or snack time changes, be sure to notify the parent(s) so appropriate adjustments can be made.

All medicines should be kept in a secure place and should be supervised by an adult. If someone takes too much of a medicine, follow your school procedure for an urgent medical problem.

Taking medicine is a private matter and is best managed discreetly and confidentially. It is important to be sensitive to the student's feelings about taking medicine.

If you suspect that the student is using drugs or alcohol, please tell the parent(s) or a school counselor right away.

Please tell the parent(s) or school nurse if you suspect medication side effects.

Modifications of the classroom environment or assignments may be useful in addition to medication. The student may need to be evaluated for additional help or for an Individualized Education Plan for learning or behavior.

Any expression of suicidal thoughts or feelings or self-harm by a child or adolescent is a clear signal of distress and should be taken seriously. These behaviors should not be dismissed as "attention seeking."

What Are Valproic Acid (Depakene) and Divalproex Sodium (Depakote)?

Valproic acid and divalproex sodium come in many forms, but the active ingredient in all of them is valproic acid. All of the forms can be referred to as *valproate*. It was first used to treat seizures (fits, convulsions), so it is sometimes called an *anticonvulsant*. Now it is also used for behavioral problems or bipolar disorder (manic-depressive disorder), whether or not the patient has seizures. It also may be used when the patient has a history of severe mood changes, sometimes called *mood swings*. When used in psychiatry, this medicine is more commonly called a *mood stabilizer*.

Valproate comes in tablets (Depakote), gel capsules, liquid syrup, sprinkle capsules, and extended-release tablets (Depakote-ER). Depakote and Depakote-ER tablets have a coating that decreases stomach irritation. A generic valproate capsule (not sprinkle) and liquid are also available. Valproic acid comes in Depakene capsules.

How Can This Medicine Help?

Valproate can reduce aggression, anger, and severe mood swings. It can treat mania or prevent relapse (mania coming back).

How Does This Medicine Work?

Valproate is thought to work by stabilizing a part of the brain cell (the cell membrane or envelope) and by changing the concentrations of certain *neurotransmitters* (chemicals in the brain) such as *GABA* and *glutamate*.

How Long Does This Medicine Last?

Most forms of valproate are taken two to four times a day. Depakote may be taken twice a day. Depakote-ER can be taken only once a day.

How Will the Doctor Monitor This Medicine?

The doctor will review your child's medical history and physical examination before starting valproate. The doctor may order some blood tests to be sure your child does not have a hidden medical condition that would make it unsafe to use this medicine. The doctor or nurse will measure your child's height, weight, pulse, and blood pressure before starting valproate. The doctor may order a baseline blood test of liver functions.

After the medicine is started, the doctor will want to have regular appointments with you and your child to see how the medicine is working, to see if a dose change is needed, to watch for side effects, to see if valproate is still needed, and to see if any other treatment is needed. The doctor or nurse will check your child's height, weight, pulse, and blood pressure. The doctor will need to order blood tests every month or so to make sure that the medicine is at the right dose as well as to look for any side effects in the liver. To see if the medicine is at the right dose, blood should be drawn first thing in the morning, 10–12 hours after the last dose and before the morning dose.

What Side Effects Can This Medicine Have?

Any medicine can have side effects, including an allergy to the medicine. Because each patient is different, the doctor will monitor the youth closely, especially when the medicine is started. The doctor will work with you to increase the positive effects and decrease the negative effects of the medicine. Please tell the doctor if any of the listed side effects appear or if you think that the medicine is causing any other problems. Not all of the rare or unusual side effects are listed.

Side effects are most common after starting the medicine or after a dose increase. Many side effects can be avoided or lessened by starting with a very low dose and increasing it slowly—ask the doctor.

Allergic Reaction

Tell the doctor in a day or two (if possible, before the next dose of medicine):

- Hives
- Itching
- Rash

Stop the medicine and get *immediate* medical care:

- Trouble breathing or chest tightness
- Swelling of lips, tongue, or throat

General Side Effects

Tell the doctor within a week or two:

- Upset stomach—This can be helped by taking medicine with food, or ask the doctor about a different form of the medicine.
- Stomach cramps
- Increased appetite
- Weight gain
- Hand tremor (shakiness)
- Clumsiness and difficulty walking
- Daytime drowsiness, sleepiness, or tiredness—Do not allow your child to drive, ride a bicycle or motor-cycle, or operate machinery if this happens.
- Increased facial or body hair
- Irregular menstrual periods
- Severe acne

Behavioral and Emotional Side Effects

Call the doctor within a day or two:

- Increased aggression
- Increased irritability

Possibly Dangerous Side Effects

Call the doctor *immediately:*

- Weakness or feels sick or is unusually tired for no reason
- Loss of appetite (for more than a few hours)
- Yellowing of skin or eyes
- Dark urine or pale bowel movements
- Swelling of the legs, feet, or face
- Greatly increased or decreased urination
- Unusual bruising or bleeding
- Sore throat or fever
- Mouth ulcers
- Vomiting (for more than a few hours)
- Persistent stomachache (more than 20 minutes)
- Skin rash
- Seizure (fit, convulsion)
- Severe behavioral problems
- Mental confusion

Some Interactions With Other Medicines or Food

Please note that the following are only the most likely interactions with food or other medicines.

Caffeine may increase side effects.

Valproate interacts with many other medicines. Taking it with another medicine may make one or both not work as well or may cause more side effects. Be sure that each doctor knows about *all* of the medicines being taken.

These medicines (and many others) increase the levels of valproate and increase the risk of serious side effects:

- Tagamet (cimetidine)
- Prozac (fluoxetine)
- Luvox (fluvoxamine)
- Motrin (ibuprofen) or aspirin
- Erythromycin and similar antibiotics
- Ketoconazole and similar antifungal agents

Taking valproate with Lamictal (lamotrigine) increases the risk of dangerous skin rash.

What Could Happen if This Medicine Is Stopped Suddenly?

Stopping valproate suddenly causes uncomfortable withdrawal symptoms. If the person is taking valproate for epilepsy (seizures), stopping the medicine suddenly could lead to an increase in very dangerous seizures (convulsions).

How Long Will This Medicine Be Needed?

The length of time a person needs to take valproate depends on what problem is being treated. For example, someone with an impulse control disorder usually takes the medicine only until behavioral therapy begins to work. Someone with bipolar disorder may need to take the medicine for many years. Please ask the doctor about the length of treatment needed.

What Else Should I Know About This Medicine?

Taking valproate with food may decrease stomach upset. The liquid may be mixed with another liquid or with food.

Your child should not chew the Depakene capsules or the Depakote tablets; chewing these medicines will irritate the mouth, throat, and stomach. Do not crush or chew Depakote-ER tablets; doing so will destroy the protective coating of the tablet.

Some people taking valproate want to eat a lot more than usual and gain too much weight. It may be very important to be sure that your child has a healthy diet without too many sweets or fast food and that your child has regular exercise.

Valproate may cause hair loss. Taking a daily multivitamin with minerals may stop this. The hair usually grows back when the valproate is stopped.

When taken during pregnancy, valproate may cause birth defects in the baby, so it is important to avoid pregnancy when taking this medicine.

Young women taking valproate may develop polycystic ovary syndrome. This very rare condition shows itself as a combination of obesity, acne, excess body hair, and infertility.

People with certain genetic metabolic diseases should not take Depakene or Depakote. Please ask your doctor about this if your child has a genetic disorder.

Liver failure and inflammation of the pancreas may occur with valproate, but this almost never happens except in children younger than 6 years old who are taking more than one medicine.

Keep the medicine in a safe place, under close supervision. **Valproate is very dangerous in overdose.** Keep the pill container tightly closed and in a dry place, away from bathrooms, showers, and humidifiers.

The names of the different forms can be confusing. When you get the medicine from the pharmacy, check to be sure you got the right medicine.

Notes

Use this space to take notes or to write down questions you want to ask the doctor.

_____

_____

_____

_____

_____

_____

_____

_____

_____

_____

_____

_____

From Dulcan MK (editor): _Helping Parents, Youth, and Teachers Understand Medications for Behavioral and Emotional Problems: A Resource Book of Medication Information Handouts_, Third Edition. Washington, DC, American Psychiatric Publishing, 2007

Medication Information
for Youth

Valproic Acid—Depakene
Divalproex Sodium—Depakote

What the Medicine Is Called and What It Is For

The name of your medicine may be confusing. Most drugs have two names: 1) a scientific name that we call a *generic name* and 2) a trade or *brand name*. This medicine comes in two chemical forms—the generic names are valproic acid and divalproex sodium. The active ingredient in the body for all the forms of this medicine is valproic acid. The brand names are Depakene and Depakote. In this information sheet, the name *valproate* will be used.

Valproate was first used to help people with epilepsy (seizures, fits, convulsions), so it is sometimes called an *anticonvulsant*. It is now also called a *mood stabilizer*, because it is used to help people who have severe mood changes, sometimes called *mood swings*, especially in children and adolescents with bipolar disorder (manic-depressive disorder), depression, or trouble controlling anger. Valproate can reduce aggression, anger, and severe mood swings. It can treat mania or prevent relapse (mania coming back). It is thought to work by making brain cells less excitable.

How You Take the Medicine

It is very important to take the medicine exactly as the doctor or nurse tells you. Do not skip doses or take extra medicine without asking an adult. If you forget a dose, ask your parent(s) what to do.

This medicine is prescribed only for you. It should never be shared with anyone else.

You do not have to tell others that you are taking this medicine, but it is not something you should feel ashamed or embarrassed about. Many young people are helped by valproate. This medicine is not habit-forming, and you cannot become "hooked" on it. You should talk to your doctor or nurse about any questions you have about the medicine. It is important to remember that the medicine *helps* you. It cannot *make* you do anything or change you as a person.

Do not chew or crush this medicine—swallow it whole. If you cannot swallow pills, ask about the sprinkles or liquid forms.

If your stomach is upset, taking the medicine with food may help.

Caffeine (in coffee, tea, or soft drinks) may make you feel worse.

It is very important not to stop this medicine suddenly—it could be uncomfortable or even dangerous.

677

How Your Doctor Will Follow Your Progress

Before giving you the medicine, your doctor or nurse will talk with you and your parent(s) and may measure your height, weight, heart rate (pulse), and blood pressure. The doctor will probably order blood tests to be sure you are healthy before taking the medicine.

Be sure to tell your doctor or nurse about any other medicines or supplements you are taking, including vitamins, herbs, or aids to weight loss or bodybuilding. Also be sure to tell the doctor or nurse if you are using alcohol or drugs. Because this medicine can cause birth defects, it is very important to tell the doctor if you might be pregnant or if you are at risk of becoming pregnant.

Your teachers may be asked to fill out a form about your grades and behavior in school. A psychologist may give you some tests to see how you learn best.

Most doctors have regular appointments with young people who are taking medicine. You should use these visits to share any concerns you may have about your medicine and to talk about if it has helped you. From time to time, your physician or nurse may measure your height, weight, heart rate (pulse), and blood pressure to be sure that you are in good health while you are taking the medicine. There will be regular blood tests to be sure that the medicine is at the right dose and to be sure that the medicine is not affecting your liver. Your doctor also will ask for regular reports from your parents and maybe from your teachers (with your permission) to see how well the medicine is working.

How the Medicine Might Affect You

In addition to the ways the medicine can help you, it may have other effects called *side effects*. Different medicines have different side effects. It is helpful to know about some of the most common side effects of your medicine so that you will understand what they are if they happen. Some people do not have any side effects. Some side effects are just uncomfortable, but others may mean a more serious problem with the medicine. Side effects are most common after starting the medicine or after a dose increase. They may go away with time, or the medicine can be adjusted or changed—ask the doctor.

You could have an allergy to any medicine, which might show up as a rash on your skin, swelling, itching, or trouble breathing.

Please tell your parent(s) and doctor or nurse about any changes that you notice after taking the medicine. It is especially important to tell a responsible adult if you are feeling depressed or that you may not want to live; if you have thoughts of hurting yourself; or if you begin to feel more irritable, nervous, or restless. Also be sure to tell your parent(s) or doctor if you begin to feel more "speeded up" or have trouble sleeping.

Some medicines make people feel sleepy or less coordinated. If this medicine is making you sleepy, it is very important not to drive a car or ride a bicycle or motorcycle. After starting a new medicine or increasing the dose of a medicine, please be extra careful when driving a car, riding a bike, or using machines until you can tell how the medicine affects your alertness, attention, and coordination.

The most common side effects of valproate are dizziness, daytime sleepiness, clumsiness, shakiness, and upset stomach. These sometimes go away after you have been taking the medicine for a while or if the doctor lowers the dose of medicine you are taking. Other side effects are increased facial or body hair, acne, and (in girls) irregular periods. Your doctor will watch your blood tests closely so that the medicine can be changed if the level is too high or too low or if you have problems with your liver.

Many teenagers who take valproate gain too much weight. It is much easier to prevent weight gain than to lose weight later. It is a good idea to eat a well-balanced diet without "junk food" and with healthy snacks like fruits and vegetables, not sweets or fried foods. It is better to drink water or skim milk, not pop, sodas, soft drinks, or sugary juices. Regular exercise is important for maintaining a healthy weight (and may also help with sleep).

Tell the doctor right away if you notice any change in your skin, urine, or bowel movements; if your skin seems to bruise easily; if you have a sore throat, mouth sores, or a fever; or if you have nausea, vomiting, and stomach pain.

Notes

Use this space to take notes or to write down questions you want to ask the doctor or nurse.

_____

_____

_____

_____

_____

_____

_____

_____

_____

_____

_____

_____

From Dulcan MK (editor): _Helping Parents, Youth, and Teachers Understand Medications for Behavioral and Emotional Problems: A Resource Book of Medication Information Handouts_, Third Edition. Washington, DC, American Psychiatric Publishing, 2007

Venlafaxine—Effexor

General Information About Medication

Each child and adolescent is different. No one has exactly the same combination of medical and psychological problems. It is a good idea to talk with the doctor or nurse about the reasons a medicine is being used. It is very important to keep all appointments and to be in touch by telephone if you have concerns. It is important to communicate with the doctor, nurse, or therapist.

It is very important that the medicine be taken exactly as the doctor instructs. However, once in a while, everyone forgets to give a medicine on time. It is a good idea to ask the doctor or nurse what to do if this happens. Do not stop or change a medicine without asking the doctor or nurse first.

If the medicine seems to stop working, it may be because it is not being taken regularly. The youth may be "cheeking" or hiding the medicine or forgetting to take it (especially at school). The doses may be too far apart, or a different dose may be needed. Something at school, at home, or in the neighborhood may be upsetting the youth, or he or she may need special help for learning disabilities or tutoring. Please discuss your concerns with the doctor. **Do not just increase the dose.**

All medicines should be kept in a safe place, out of the reach of children, and should be supervised by an adult. If someone takes too much of a medicine, call the doctor, the poison control center, or a hospital emergency room.

Each medicine has a "generic" or chemical name. Just like laundry detergents or paper towels, some medicines are sold by more than one company under different brand names. The same medicine may be available under a generic name and several brand names. The generic medications are usually less expensive than the brand name ones. The generic medications have the same chemical formula, but they may or may not be exactly the same strength as the brand-name medications. Also, some brands of pills contain dye that can cause allergic reactions. It is a good idea to talk to the doctor and the pharmacist about whether it is important to use a specific brand of medicine.

All medicines can cause an allergic reaction. Examples are hives, itching, rashes, swelling, and trouble breathing. Even a tiny amount of a medicine can cause a reaction in patients who are allergic to that medicine. Be *sure* to talk to the doctor before restarting a medicine that has caused an allergic reaction.

Taking more than one medicine at the same time may cause more side effects or cause one of the medicines to not work as well. Always ask the doctor, nurse, or pharmacist before adding another medicine, whether prescription or over-the-counter. Be sure that each doctor knows about *all* of the medicines your child is taking. Also tell the doctor about any vitamins, herbal medicines, or supplements your child may be taking. Some of these may have side effects alone or when taken with this medication.

Everyone taking medicine should have a physical examination at least once a year.

If you suspect the youth is using drugs or alcohol, please tell the doctor right away.

Pregnancy requires special care in the use of medicine. Please tell the doctor immediately if you suspect the teenager is pregnant or might become pregnant.

Printed information like this applies to children and adolescents in general. If you have questions about the medicine, or if you notice changes or anything unusual, please ask the doctor or nurse. As scientific research advances, knowledge increases and advice changes. Even experts do not always agree. Many medicines have not been approved by the U.S. Food and Drug Administration (FDA) for use in children. For this reason, use of the medicine for a particular problem or age group often is not listed in the *Physicians' Desk Reference*. This does not necessarily mean that the medicine is dangerous or does not work, only that the company that makes the medicine has not received permission to advertise the medicine for use in children. Companies often do not apply for this permission because it is expensive to do the tests needed to apply for approval for use in children. Once a medication is approved by the FDA for any purpose, a doctor is allowed to prescribe it according to research and clinical experience.

Note to Teachers

It is a good idea to talk with the parent(s) about the reason(s) that a medication is being used. If the parent(s) sign consent to release information, it is often helpful to talk with the doctor. If the parent(s) give permission, the doctor may ask you to fill out rating forms about your experience with the student's behavior, feelings, academic performance, and medication side effects. This information is very useful in selecting and monitoring medication treatment. If you have observations that you think are important, do not hesitate to share these with the student's parent(s) and treating clinicians.

It is very important that the medicine be taken exactly as the doctor instructs. However, everyone forgets to give a medicine on time once in a while. It is a good idea to ask the parent(s) in advance what to do if this happens. Do not stop or change the time you are giving a medicine at school without parental permission. If a medication is to be taken with food, but lunchtime or snack time changes, be sure to notify the parent(s) so appropriate adjustments can be made.

All medicines should be kept in a secure place and should be supervised by an adult. If someone takes too much of a medicine, follow your school procedure for an urgent medical problem.

Taking medicine is a private matter and is best managed discreetly and confidentially. It is important to be sensitive to the student's feelings about taking medicine.

If you suspect that the student is using drugs or alcohol, please tell the parent(s) or a school counselor right away.

Please tell the parent(s) or school nurse if you suspect medication side effects.

Modifications of the classroom environment or assignments may be useful in addition to medication. The student may need to be evaluated for additional help or for an Individualized Education Plan for learning or behavior.

Any expression of suicidal thoughts or feelings or self-harm by a child or adolescent is a clear signal of distress and should be taken seriously. These behaviors should not be dismissed as "attention seeking."

What Is Venlafaxine (Effexor)?

Venlafaxine is called an *antidepressant*. It is sometimes called a *serotonin-norepinephrine reuptake inhibitor* (SNRI). It comes in brand name Effexor-IR tablets and Effexor-XR controlled-release capsules.

How Can This Medicine Help?

Venlafaxine has been used successfully to treat depression and anxiety (nervousness) in adults. Now it is beginning to be used to treat emotional and behavioral problems, including anxiety and depression, in children and adolescents. Venlafaxine may take as long as 4–8 weeks to reach its full effect.

How Does This Medicine Work?

Venlafaxine works by increasing the brain chemicals *serotonin* and *norepinephrine (neurotransmitters)* to more normal activity levels in certain parts of the brain. It has a somewhat different way of working than the antidepressants that are called selective serotonin reuptake inhibitors (or SSRIs).

How Long Does This Medicine Last?

The immediate-release Effexor IR tablets must be taken two or three times a day. The controlled-release Effexor-XR lasts the whole day when taken only once a day.

How Will the Doctor Monitor This Medicine?

The doctor will review your child's medical history and physical examination before starting venlafaxine. The doctor may order some blood or urine tests to be sure your child does not have a hidden medical condition that would make it unsafe to use this medicine. The doctor or nurse may measure your child's height, weight, pulse, and blood pressure before starting venlafaxine.

Be sure to tell the doctor if your child or anyone in the family has bipolar illness (manic-depressive illness) or has tried to kill himself or herself.

After the medicine is started, the doctor will want to have regular appointments with you and your child to see how the medicine is working, to see if a dose change is needed, to watch for side effects, to see if venlafaxine is still needed, and to see if any other treatment is needed. The doctor or nurse may check your child's height, weight, pulse, and blood pressure.

Before using medicine and at times afterward, the doctor may ask your child to fill out a rating scale about depression and anxiety, to help see how your child is doing.

What Side Effects Can This Medicine Have?

Any medicine can have side effects, including an allergy to the medicine. Because each patient is different, the doctor will monitor the youth closely, especially when the medicine is started. The doctor will work with you to increase the positive effects and decrease the negative effects of the medicine. Please tell the doctor if any of the listed side effects appear or if you think that the medicine is causing any other problems. Not all of the rare or unusual side effects are listed.

Side effects are most common after starting the medicine or after a dose increase. Many side effects can be avoided or lessened by starting with a very low dose and increasing it slowly—ask the doctor.

Allergic Reaction

Tell the doctor in a day or two (if possible, before the next dose of medicine):

- Hives
- Itching
- Rash

Stop the medicine and get *immediate* medical care:

- Trouble breathing or chest tightness
- Swelling of lips, tongue, or throat

Common Side Effects

Tell the doctor within a week or two:

- Anxiety and nervousness
- Nausea
- Daytime sleepiness—Do not allow your child to drive, ride a bicycle or motorcycle, or operate machinery if this happens.
- Insomnia (trouble sleeping)
- Decreased appetite
- Weight loss
- Dry mouth—Have your child try using sugar-free gum or candy.

Occasional Side Effects

Tell the doctor within a week or two:

- Yawning
- Blurred vision
- Dizziness
- Constipation—Encourage your child to drink more fluids and eat high-fiber foods; if necessary, the doctor may recommend a fiber medicine such as Benefiber or a stool softener such as Colace or mineral oil.
- Lack of energy, tiredness
- Excessive sweating
- Trouble with sexual functioning

Less Common, but More Serious, Side Effects

Call the doctor *immediately*:

- Increased blood pressure
- Seizure (fit, convulsion)

Serotonin Syndrome

A very serious side effect called *serotonin syndrome* can happen when certain kinds of medicines (including some medicines for migraine headaches—triptans) are taken by the same person. *Very* rarely, it can happen at high doses of just one medicine. The early signs are restlessness, confusion, shaking, skin turning red, sweating, and jerking of muscles. If you see these symptoms, stop the medicine and send or take the youth to an emergency room right away.

Some Interactions With Other Medicines or Food

Please note that the following are only the most likely interactions with food or other medicines.

Caffeine may increase side effects.

Tagamet (cimetidine) should not be used with venlafaxine, because it increases the levels of venlafaxine and may increase side effects.

If venlafaxine is taken with haloperidol (Haldol), the levels of haloperidol and its side effects may increase.

It can be *very dangerous* to take venlafaxine at the same time as, or even within several weeks of, taking another type of medicine called a *monoamine oxidase inhibitor* (MAOI), such as Eldepryl (selegiline), Nardil (phenelzine), Parnate (tranylcypromine), or Marplan (isocarboxazid).

What Could Happen if This Medicine Is Stopped Suddenly?

No known serious medical withdrawal effects occur if venlafaxine is stopped suddenly, but there may be uncomfortable feelings such as dizziness, insomnia, nausea, or nervousness, or the problem being treated may come back. Ask the doctor before stopping the medicine.

How Long Will This Medicine Be Needed?

Your child may need to keep taking the medicine for at least 6–12 months so that the emotional or behavioral problem does not come back.

What Else Should I Know About This Medicine?

In youth who have bipolar disorder (manic depression) or who are at risk for bipolar disorder, any antidepressant medicine may increase the risk of hypomania or mania (excitement, agitation, increased activity, decreased sleep).

Black Box Antidepressant Warning

In 2004, an advisory committee to the FDA decided that there might be an increased risk of suicidal behavior for some youth taking medicines called *antidepressants*. In the research studies that the committee reviewed, about 3%–4% of youth with depression who took an antidepressant medicine—and 1%–2% of youth with depression who took a placebo (pill without active medicine)—talked about suicidal thoughts (thinking about killing themselves or wishing they were dead) or did something to harm themselves. This means that almost twice as many youth who were taking an antidepressant to treat their depression talked about suicide or had suicidal behavior compared with youth with depression who were taking inactive medicine. There were *no* completed suicides in any of these research studies, which included more than 4,000 children and adolescents. For youth being treated for anxiety, there was no difference in suicidal talking or behavior between those taking antidepressant medication and those taking placebo.

The FDA told drug companies to add a *black box warning* label to all antidepressant medicines. Because of this label, a doctor (or advanced practice nurse) prescribing one of these medicines has to warn youth and their families that there might be more suicidal thoughts and actions in youth taking these medicines.

On the other hand, in places where more youth are taking the newer antidepressant medicines, the number of adolescents who commit suicide has gotten smaller. Also, thinking about or attempting suicide is more common in surveys of teenagers in the community than it is in depressed youth treated in research studies with antidepressant medicine.

If a youth is being treated with this medicine and is doing well, then no changes are needed as a result of this warning. Increased suicidal talk or action is most likely to happen in the first few months of treatment with a medicine. If your child has recently started this medicine or is about to start, then you and your doctor (or advanced practice nurse) should watch for any changes in behavior. People who are depressed often have suicidal thoughts or actions. It is hard to know whether suicidal thoughts or actions in depressed people are caused by the depression itself or by the medicine. Also, as their depression is getting better, some people talk more about the suicidal thoughts that they had before but did not talk about. As young people get better from depression, they might be at higher risk of doing something about suicidal thoughts that they have had for some time, because they have more energy.

What Should a Parent Do?

1. Be honest with your child about possible risks and benefits of medicine.

2. Talk to your child about whether he or she is having any suicidal thoughts, and tell your child to come to you if he or she is having such thoughts.

3. You, your child, and your child's doctor or nurse should develop a safety plan. Pick adults whom your child can tell if he or she is thinking about suicide.

4. Be sure to tell your child's doctor, nurse, or therapist if you suspect that your child is using alcohol or drugs or if something has happened that might make your child feel worse, such as a family separation, breaking up with a boyfriend or girlfriend, someone close dying or attempting suicide, physical or sexual abuse, or failure in school.

5. Be sure that there are no guns in the home and that all medicines (including over-the-counter medicines like Tylenol) are closely supervised by an adult and kept in a safe place.

6. Watch for new or worse thoughts of suicide, self-harm, depression, anxiety (nerves), feeling very agitated or restless, being angry or aggressive, having more trouble sleeping, or anything else that you see for the first time, seems worse, or worries your child or you. If these appear, contact a mental health professional **right away.** Do not just stop or change the dose of the medicine on your own. If the problems are serious, and you cannot reach one of your clinicians, call a 24-hour psychiatry emergency telephone number or take your child to an emergency room.

Youth on antidepressant medicine should be watched carefully by their parent(s), clinician(s) (doctor, nurse, therapist), and other concerned adults for the first weeks of treatment. It is a good idea to have a visit or telephone call with the doctor, nurse, or therapist weekly for the first month, every 2 weeks for the second month, and after that at least once a month to check for feelings of depression or sadness, thoughts of killing or harming himself or herself, and any problems with the medication. If you have questions, be sure to ask the doctor, nurse, or therapist.

For more information, see http://www.parentsmedguide.org/ (in English and Spanish).

Notes

Use this space to take notes or to write down questions you want to ask the doctor.

_____

_____

_____

_____

_____

_____

_____

_____

_____

_____

_____

_____

_____

From Dulcan MK (editor): *Helping Parents, Youth, and Teachers Understand Medications for Behavioral and Emotional Problems: A Resource Book of Medication Information Handouts*, Third Edition. Washington, DC, American Psychiatric Publishing, 2007

Medication Information for Youth

Venlafaxine—Effexor

What the Medicine Is Called and What It Is For

The name of your medicine may be confusing. Most drugs have two names: 1) a scientific name that we call a *generic name* and 2) a trade or *brand name*. The generic name of this medicine is venlafaxine. The brand name is Effexor.

Venlafaxine is called an *antidepressant*. It is used to treat depression and anxiety disorders. It helps people who feel very sad or depressed, anxious (nervous), or afraid.

How You Take the Medicine

It is very important to take the medicine exactly as the doctor or nurse tells you. Do not skip doses or take extra medicine without asking an adult. If you forget a dose, ask your parent(s) what to do. It is very important that you take all the pills you are supposed to take each day. Your doctor will probably recommend that you take your medicine at the same time each day, which may be with meals or at bedtime.

It may take a month before you notice that the medicine is helping. Waiting for the full effect may take another month. You may feel discouraged and think the medicine is never going to help. You may want to give up and stop taking the medicine. Talk to your doctor and parent(s) about how you feel, but **do not stop** taking the medicine unless your doctor tells you to. It is also important not to take extra pills, hoping that you will feel better faster. Doing that could make you very sick.

Caffeine (in coffee, tea, or soft drinks) may make you feel worse.

This medicine is prescribed only for you. It should never be shared with anyone else.

You do not have to tell others that you are taking this medicine, but it is not something you should feel ashamed or embarrassed about. Many young people are helped by venlafaxine. This medicine is not habit-forming, and you cannot become "hooked" on it. You should talk to your doctor or nurse about any questions you have about the medicine. It is important to remember that the medicine *helps* you. It cannot *make* you do anything or change you as a person.

How Your Doctor Will Follow Your Progress

Before giving you the medicine, your doctor or nurse will talk with you and your parent(s) and may measure your height, weight, heart rate (pulse), and blood pressure. The doctor may order some blood or urine tests to be sure you are in good health.

Be sure to tell your doctor or nurse about any other medicines or supplements you are taking, including vitamins, herbs, or aids to weight loss or bodybuilding. Also be sure to tell the doctor or nurse if you are using alcohol or drugs. Because many medicines may affect babies, it is very important to tell the doctor if you might be pregnant or if you are at risk of becoming pregnant. Be sure to tell the doctor if you have had thoughts of hurting yourself, have tried to hurt yourself, or sometimes wish that you were not alive.

Your teachers may be asked to fill out a form about your grades and behavior in school. A psychologist may give you some tests to see how you learn best.

Before starting the medicine and afterward, the doctor may ask you to answer questions on paper about depression and anxiety.

Most doctors have regular appointments with young people who are taking medicine. You should use these visits to share any concerns you may have about your medicine and to talk about if it has helped you. From time to time, your physician or nurse may measure your height, weight, heart rate (pulse), and blood pressure to be sure that you are in good health while you are taking the medicine. Your doctor also will ask for regular reports from your parents and maybe from your teachers (with your permission) to see how well the medicine is working.

Some medicines are started at the amount you will take for as long as you are taking that medicine. Other medicines need to be increased or adjusted until your doctor decides you are taking the right amount. Starting at a low dose and increasing it slowly may lessen side effects. If the medicine helps you, your doctor will probably want you to take it for 6 months to a year if you are taking it to treat depression. If you are taking it for another problem, your doctor will decide how long you will need to take the medicine as he or she watches your progress.

It is not dangerous to stop venlafaxine suddenly, but there might be uncomfortable feelings, such as trouble sleeping, nervousness, irritability, or feeling sick. It is better to decrease it slowly. Do not stop taking a medicine unless the doctor tells you to. If you have any problems after stopping or decreasing this medicine, tell your parent(s) or doctor.

How the Medicine Might Affect You

In addition to the ways the medicine can help you, it may have other effects called *side effects*. Different medicines have different side effects. It is helpful to know about some of the most common side effects of your medicine so that you will understand what they are if they happen. Some people do not have any side effects. Some side effects are just uncomfortable, but others may mean a more serious problem with the medicine. Side effects are most common after starting the medicine or after a dose increase. They may go away with time, or the medicine can be adjusted or changed—ask the doctor.

You could have an allergy to any medicine, which might show up as a rash on your skin, swelling, itching, or trouble breathing.

Please tell your parent(s) and doctor or nurse about any changes that you notice after taking the medicine. It is especially important to tell a responsible adult right away if you are feeling depressed or that you may not want to live; if you have thoughts of hurting yourself; or if you begin to feel more irritable, nervous, or restless. Also be sure to tell your parent(s) or doctor if you begin to feel "speeded up" or have trouble sleeping.

Some medicines make people feel sleepy or less coordinated. If this medicine is making you sleepy, it is very important not to drive a car or ride a bicycle or motorcycle. After starting a new medicine or increasing the dose of a medicine, please be extra careful when driving a car, riding a bike, or using machines until you can tell how the medicine affects your alertness, attention, and coordination.

One of the most common side effects of this medicine is feeling tired or sleepy during the day, even if you have had a full night's sleep. After you have been taking the medicine for a few weeks, your body will adjust, and this side effect may go away. If you have had trouble sleeping at night, the medicine can help you sleep better, especially if the doctor tells you to take a dose of medicine in the evening. Other people may feel more restless and excited. Tell your parent(s) or doctor if this is uncomfortable.

Another common side effect is dry mouth. You may be more thirsty than usual and find that you are drinking more water or other liquids. Sucking on sugar-free hard candy or cough drops usually helps. You also could try chewing sugar-free gum or sucking on ice chips. Do not chew the ice; you could hurt your teeth. Also, using lip balm will keep your lips from cracking. It is important to be especially good about brushing your teeth.

Some people become constipated (have hard bowel movements) when taking this medicine. Try drinking more water and eating more fruits, vegetables, and whole grains. If that does not help, tell your parent(s) or doctor—you may need a medicine to help with this side effect.

Some other side effects that could happen are trouble sleeping, headache, not feeling hungry and not wanting to eat much, having an upset stomach, or blurred vision. You may have a change in your sexual functioning—it is OK to ask the doctor about this.

Please let your parent(s) and doctor know if you notice anything different or unusual about how you feel once you start taking the medicine.

Notes

Use this space to take notes or to write down questions you want to ask the doctor or nurse.

_____

_____

_____

_____

_____

_____

_____

_____

_____

_____

_____

_____

_____

Medication Information
for Parents and Teachers

Zaleplon—Sonata

General Information About Medication

Each child and adolescent is different. No one has exactly the same combination of medical and psychological problems. It is a good idea to talk with the doctor or nurse about the reasons a medicine is being used. It is very important to keep all appointments and to be in touch by telephone if you have concerns. It is important to communicate with the doctor, nurse, or therapist.

It is very important that the medicine be taken exactly as the doctor instructs. However, once in a while, everyone forgets to give a medicine on time. It is a good idea to ask the doctor or nurse what to do if this happens. Do not stop or change a medicine without asking the doctor or nurse first.

If the medicine seems to stop working, it may be because it is not being taken regularly. The youth may be "cheeking" or hiding the medicine or forgetting to take it. A different dose may be needed. Something at school, at home, or in the neighborhood may be upsetting the youth, or he or she may need special help for learning disabilities or tutoring. Please discuss your concerns with the doctor. **Do not just increase the dose.**

All medicines should be kept in a safe place, out of the reach of children, and should be supervised by an adult. If someone takes too much of a medicine, call the doctor, the poison control center, or a hospital emergency room.

Each medicine has a "generic" or chemical name. Just like laundry detergents or paper towels, some medicines are sold by more than one company under different brand names. The same medicine may be available under a generic name and several brand names. The generic medications are usually less expensive than the brand name ones. The generic medications have the same chemical formula, but they may or may not be exactly the same strength as the brand-name medications. Also, some brands of pills contain dye that can cause allergic reactions. It is a good idea to talk to the doctor and the pharmacist about whether it is important to use a specific brand of medicine.

All medicines can cause an allergic reaction. Examples are hives, itching, rashes, swelling, and trouble breathing. Even a tiny amount of a medicine can cause a reaction in patients who are allergic to that medicine. Be *sure* to talk to the doctor before restarting a medicine that has caused an allergic reaction.

Taking more than one medicine at the same time may cause more side effects or cause one of the medicines to not work as well. Always ask the doctor, nurse, or pharmacist before adding another medicine, whether prescription or over-the-counter. Be sure that each doctor knows about *all* of the medicines your child is taking. Also tell the doctor about any vitamins, herbal medicines, or supplements your child may be taking. Some of these may have side effects alone or when taken with this medication.

Everyone taking medicine should have a physical examination at least once a year.

If you suspect the youth is using drugs or alcohol, please tell the doctor right away.

Pregnancy requires special care in the use of medicine. Please tell the doctor immediately if you suspect the teenager is pregnant or might become pregnant.

693

Printed information like this applies to children and adolescents in general. If you have questions about the medicine, or if you notice changes or anything unusual, please ask the doctor or nurse. As scientific research advances, knowledge increases and advice changes. Even experts do not always agree. Many medicines have not been approved by the U.S. Food and Drug Administration (FDA) for use in children. For this reason, use of the medicine for a particular problem or age group often is not listed in the *Physicians' Desk Reference*. This does not necessarily mean that the medicine is dangerous or does not work, only that the company that makes the medicine has not received permission to advertise the medicine for use in children. Companies often do not apply for this permission because it is expensive to do the tests needed to apply for approval for use in children. Once a medication is approved by the FDA for any purpose, a doctor is allowed to prescribe it according to research and clinical experience.

Note to Teachers

It is a good idea to talk with the parent(s) about the reason(s) that a medication is being used. If the parent(s) sign consent to release information, it is often helpful to talk with the doctor. If the parent(s) give permission, the doctor may ask you to fill out rating forms about your experience with the student's behavior, feelings, academic performance, and medication side effects. This information is very useful in selecting and monitoring medication treatment. If you have observations that you think are important, do not hesitate to share these with the student's parent(s) and treating clinicians.

All medicines should be kept in a secure place and should be supervised by an adult. If someone takes too much of a medicine, follow your school procedure for an urgent medical problem.

Taking medicine is a private matter and is best managed discreetly and confidentially. It is important to be sensitive to the student's feelings about taking medicine.

If you suspect that the student is using drugs or alcohol, please tell the parent(s) or a school counselor right away.

Please tell the parent(s) or school nurse if you suspect medication side effects.

Any expression of suicidal thoughts or feelings or self-harm by a child or adolescent is a clear signal of distress and should be taken seriously. These behaviors should not be dismissed as "attention seeking."

What Is Zaleplon (Sonata)?

Zaleplon is a *hypnotic* or *sedative-hypnotic* medicine. It is *not* a *benzodiazepine*. It comes in brand name Sonata tablets.

How Can This Medicine Help?

Zaleplon is used to treat insomnia—problems falling asleep or staying asleep—when used for a short time along with a behavioral program.

How Does This Medicine Work?

Zaleplon works in certain parts of the brain to help people fall asleep. It works in a different way than other sleep medicines.

How Long Does This Medicine Last?

Zaleplon is taken within 30 minutes before bedtime and starts working in 30–60 minutes. It leaves the body very quickly, so it is less likely to cause daytime sleepiness or memory problems than other kinds of sleep medicines. It is very short acting, so it can be given in the middle of the night if the youth wakes up and cannot fall back to sleep.

How Will the Doctor Monitor This Medicine?

The doctor will review your child's medical history and physical examination before starting zaleplon.

After the medicine is started, the doctor will want to have regular appointments with you and your child to see how the medicine is working, to see if a dose change is needed, to watch for side effects, to see if zaleplon is still needed, and to see if any other treatment is needed.

What Side Effects Can This Medicine Have?

Any medicine can have side effects, including an allergy to the medicine. Because each patient is different, the doctor will monitor the youth closely, especially when the medicine is started. The doctor will work with you to increase the positive effects and decrease the negative effects of the medicine. Please tell the doctor if any of the listed side effects appear or if you think that the medicine is causing any other problems. Not all of the rare or unusual side effects are listed.

Side effects are most common after starting the medicine or after a dose increase. Many side effects can be avoided or lessened by starting with a very low dose and increasing it slowly—ask the doctor.

Allergic Reaction

Tell the doctor in a day or two (if possible, before the next dose of medicine):

- Hives
- Itching
- Rash

Stop the medicine and get *immediate* medical care:

- Trouble breathing or chest tightness
- Swelling of lips, tongue, or throat

Zaleplon is usually very safe when used for short periods as the doctor prescribes.

The most common side effect is daytime sleepiness. Zaleplon can also cause dizziness, feeling "spacey," or decreased coordination. If the medicine is causing any of these problems it is very important not to drive a car, ride a bicycle or motorcycle, or operate machinery.

Zaleplon can cause decreased concentration and memory. These problems, along with daytime sleepiness, may decrease learning and performance in school.

People who take zaleplon must not drink alcohol. Severe sleepiness or even loss of consciousness may result.

It is possible to become psychologically and physically dependent on zaleplon, but that is not a common problem for patients who see their doctors regularly. It is less common for zaleplon than for other types of sleep medicines.

Some Interactions With Other Medicines or Food

Please note that the following are only the most likely interactions with food or other medicines.

Caffeine may cause trouble sleeping and make zaleplon less effective. If caffeine is eliminated, less zaleplon may be needed, or zaleplon may not be needed at all.

It is important not to use other sedatives, tranquilizers, or sleeping pills or antihistamines (such as Benadryl) when taking zaleplon because of greatly increased side effects.

What Could Happen if This Medicine Is Stopped Suddenly?

Many medicines cause problems if stopped suddenly. Zaleplon must be decreased slowly (tapered) rather than stopped suddenly. When zaleplon is stopped suddenly, there are withdrawal symptoms that are uncomfortable. Problems are more likely in patients taking high doses of zaleplon for 2 months or longer, but even after taking zaleplon for just a few weeks, it is important to stop it slowly. Withdrawal symptoms may include anxiety, irritability, shaking, sweating, aches and pains, muscle cramps, vomiting, confusion, and trouble sleeping.

How Long Will This Medicine Be Needed?

Zaleplon is usually prescribed for only a week or so or for occasional use. A behavioral program, such as regular soothing routines at bedtime and increased exercise in the daytime, should be used along with the medicine to improve sleep. Finding developmentally appropriate bed- and wake-times and sticking to them is very important. These strategies should be continued after the medicine is tapered (stopped slowly) or when the medicine is used only occasionally.

What Else Should I Know About This Medicine?

Because zaleplon can be abused (especially by people who abuse alcohol or drugs) and can cause psychological dependence or physical dependence (addiction), it is regulated by special state and federal laws as a *controlled substance*. These laws place limitations on telephone prescriptions and refills, and prescriptions expire if they are not filled promptly.

People with sleep apnea (breathing stops while they are asleep) should not take zaleplon. Tell the doctor if your child snores very loudly.

Notes

Use this space to take notes or to write down questions you want to ask the doctor.

_____

_____

_____

_____

_____

_____

_____

_____

_____

_____

_____

_____

From Dulcan MK (editor): _Helping Parents, Youth, and Teachers Understand Medications for Behavioral and Emotional Problems: A Resource Book of Medication Information Handouts_, Third Edition. Washington, DC, American Psychiatric Publishing, 2007

Zaleplon—Sonata

What the Medicine Is Called and What It Is For

The name of your medicine may be confusing. Most drugs have two names: 1) a scientific name that we call a *generic name* and 2) a trade or *brand name*. The generic name of this medicine is zaleplon. The brand name is Sonata.

Zaleplon works by calming the parts of the brain that are too excitable. Zaleplon can help with insomnia (difficulty falling asleep or staying asleep) when used for a short time along with routines that help you to relax and fall asleep.

How You Take the Medicine

It is very important to take the medicine exactly as the doctor or nurse tells you. Do not skip doses or take extra medicine without asking an adult. If you forget a dose, ask your parent(s) what to do.

Zaleplon works best if combined with a regular bedtime, calming routines before bedtime, and physical exercise during the day. Getting up on time is also important in keeping a regular sleep schedule.

It is better to limit drinks with caffeine (coffee, tea, soft drinks) because caffeine works in the opposite way from zaleplon, and the positive effects might be decreased.

This medicine is prescribed only for you. It should never be shared with anyone else.

You do not have to tell others that you are taking this medicine, but it is not something you should feel ashamed or embarrassed about. Many young people are helped by zaleplon. You should talk to your doctor or nurse about any questions you have about the medicine. It is important to remember that the medicine *helps* you. It cannot *make* you do anything or change you as a person.

Many medicines cause problems if stopped suddenly. Always ask your doctor before stopping a medicine. Problems are more likely to happen in patients taking high doses of zaleplon for 2 months or longer, but it is important to decrease the medicine slowly (taper) even after a few weeks. If you notice anxiety, irritability, shaking, sweating, aches and pains, muscle cramps, vomiting, or trouble sleeping, you may need to decrease the medicine more slowly.

How Your Doctor Will Follow Your Progress

Before giving you the medicine, your doctor or nurse will talk with you and your parent(s) and may measure your height, weight, heart rate (pulse), and blood pressure.

Be sure to tell your doctor or nurse about any other medicines or supplements you are taking, including vitamins, herbs, or aids to weight loss or bodybuilding. Also be sure to tell the doctor or nurse if you are using alcohol or drugs. Because many medicines may affect babies, it is very important to tell the doctor if you might be pregnant or if you are at risk of becoming pregnant.

Most doctors have regular appointments with young people who are taking medicine. You should use these visits to share any concerns you may have about your medicine and to talk about if it has helped you. From time to time, your physician or nurse may measure your height, weight, heart rate (pulse), and blood pressure to be sure that you are in good health while you are taking the medicine. Your doctor also will ask for regular reports from your parents to see how well the medicine is working.

Zaleplon is usually prescribed for only a week or so to allow you to develop better sleep habits. A regular bedtime, a relaxing routine before bedtime, and physical exercise in the daytime usually help with sleep at night.

Each person is unique, and some people may need this medicine for months or years.

How the Medicine Might Affect You

In addition to the ways the medicine can help you, it may have other effects called *side effects*. Different medicines have different side effects. It is helpful to know about some of the most common side effects of your medicine so that you will understand what they are if they happen. Some people do not have any side effects. Some side effects are just uncomfortable, but others may mean a more serious problem with the medicine. Side effects are most common after starting the medicine or after a dose increase. They may go away with time, or the medicine can be adjusted or changed—ask the doctor.

You could have an allergy to any medicine, which might show up as a rash on your skin, swelling, itching, or trouble breathing.

Please tell your parent(s) and doctor or nurse about any changes that you notice after taking the medicine. It is especially important to tell a responsible adult if you are feeling depressed or that you may not want to live; if you have thoughts of hurting yourself; or if you begin to feel more irritable, nervous, or restless.

The most common side effect of zaleplon is daytime sleepiness. If this medicine is making you sleepy, it is very important not to drive a car or ride a bicycle or motorcycle. After starting zaleplon or increasing the dose, please be extra careful when driving a car, riding a bike, or using machines until you can tell how the medicine affects your alertness, attention, and coordination.

Sometimes sleep medicines seem to work in the opposite way, causing more trouble sleeping, nightmares, excitement, irritability, anger, aggression, or other problems. If this happens, tell your parent(s) or your doctor.

Some people feel dizzy, clumsy, or "spacey" or have more trouble remembering things when taking this medicine. Be sure to tell your parent(s) or doctor if any of these happen.

Drinking alcohol while taking this medicine can cause severe drowsiness or even passing out. **Don't do it!** Do not use marijuana or street drugs while taking this medicine. They can cause serious side effects. Skipping your medicine to take drugs does not work because many medicines stay in your body for a long time.

Zaleplon can be habit-forming, but that is not a common problem for people who take their medicine as the doctor says.

Notes

Use this space to take notes or to write down questions you want to ask the doctor or nurse.

_____

_____

_____

_____

_____

_____

_____

_____

_____

_____

_____

_____

_____

From Dulcan MK (editor): _Helping Parents, Youth, and Teachers Understand Medications for Behavioral and Emotional Problems: A Resource Book of Medication Information Handouts,_ Third Edition. Washington, DC, American Psychiatric Publishing, 2007

Medication Information for Parents and Teachers

Ziprasidone—Geodon

General Information About Medication

Each child and adolescent is different. No one has exactly the same combination of medical and psychological problems. It is a good idea to talk with the doctor or nurse about the reasons a medicine is being used. It is very important to keep all appointments and to be in touch by telephone if you have concerns. It is important to communicate with the doctor, nurse, or therapist.

It is very important that the medicine be taken exactly as the doctor instructs. However, once in a while, everyone forgets to give a medicine on time. It is a good idea to ask the doctor or nurse what to do if this happens. Do not stop or change a medicine without asking the doctor or nurse first.

If the medicine seems to stop working, it may be because it is not being taken regularly. The youth may be "cheeking" or hiding the medicine or forgetting to take it (especially at school). The doses may be too far apart, or a different dose may be needed. Something at school, at home, or in the neighborhood may be upsetting the youth, or he or she may need special help for learning disabilities or tutoring. Please discuss your concerns with the doctor. **Do not just increase the dose.**

All medicines should be kept in a safe place, out of the reach of children, and should be supervised by an adult. If someone takes too much of a medicine, call the doctor, the poison control center, or a hospital emergency room.

Each medicine has a "generic" or chemical name. Just like laundry detergents or paper towels, some medicines are sold by more than one company under different brand names. The same medicine may be available under a generic name and several brand names. The generic medications are usually less expensive than the brand name ones. The generic medications have the same chemical formula, but they may or may not be exactly the same strength as the brand-name medications. Also, some brands of pills contain dye that can cause allergic reactions. It is a good idea to talk to the doctor and the pharmacist about whether it is important to use a specific brand of medicine.

All medicines can cause an allergic reaction. Examples are hives, itching, rashes, swelling, and trouble breathing. Even a tiny amount of a medicine can cause a reaction in patients who are allergic to that medicine. Be *sure* to talk to the doctor before restarting a medicine that has caused an allergic reaction.

Taking more than one medicine at the same time may cause more side effects or cause one of the medicines to not work as well. Always ask the doctor, nurse, or pharmacist before adding another medicine, whether prescription or over-the-counter. Be sure that each doctor knows about *all* of the medicines your child is taking. Also tell the doctor about any vitamins, herbal medicines, or supplements your child may be taking. Some of these may have side effects alone or when taken with this medication.

Everyone taking medicine should have a physical examination at least once a year.

If you suspect the youth is using drugs or alcohol, please tell the doctor right away.

Pregnancy requires special care in the use of medicine. Please tell the doctor immediately if you suspect the teenager is pregnant or might become pregnant.

Printed information like this applies to children and adolescents in general. If you have questions about the medicine, or if you notice changes or anything unusual, please ask the doctor or nurse. As scientific research advances, knowledge increases and advice changes. Even experts do not always agree. Many medicines have not been approved by the U.S. Food and Drug Administration (FDA) for use in children. For this reason, use of the medicine for a particular problem or age group often is not listed in the *Physicians' Desk Reference*. This does not necessarily mean that the medicine is dangerous or does not work, only that the company that makes the medicine has not received permission to advertise the medicine for use in children. Companies often do not apply for this permission because it is expensive to do the tests needed to apply for approval for use in children. Once a medication is approved by the FDA for any purpose, a doctor is allowed to prescribe it according to research and clinical experience.

Note to Teachers

It is a good idea to talk with the parent(s) about the reason(s) that a medication is being used. If the parent(s) sign consent to release information, it is often helpful to talk with the doctor. If the parent(s) give permission, the doctor may ask you to fill out rating forms about your experience with the student's behavior, feelings, academic performance, and medication side effects. This information is very useful in selecting and monitoring medication treatment. If you have observations that you think are important, do not hesitate to share these with the student's parent(s) and treating clinicians.

It is very important that the medicine be taken exactly as the doctor instructs. However, everyone forgets to give a medicine on time once in a while. It is a good idea to ask the parent(s) in advance what to do if this happens. Do not stop or change the time you are giving a medicine at school without parental permission. If a medication is to be taken with food, but lunchtime or snack time changes, be sure to notify the parent(s) so appropriate adjustments can be made.

All medicines should be kept in a secure place and should be supervised by an adult. If someone takes too much of a medicine, follow your school procedure for an urgent medical problem.

Taking medicine is a private matter and is best managed discreetly and confidentially. It is important to be sensitive to the student's feelings about taking medicine.

If you suspect that the student is using drugs or alcohol, please tell the parent(s) or a school counselor right away.

Please tell the parent(s) or school nurse if you suspect medication side effects.

Modifications of the classroom environment or assignments may be useful in addition to medication. The student may need to be evaluated for additional help or for an Individualized Education Plan for learning or behavior.

Any expression of suicidal thoughts or feelings or self-harm by a child or adolescent is a clear signal of distress and should be taken seriously. These behaviors should not be dismissed as "attention seeking."

What Is Ziprasidone (Geodon)?

This medicine is called an *atypical* or *second-generation antipsychotic*. It is sometimes called an *atypical psychotropic agent* or simply an *atypical*. It comes in brand name Geodon capsules and a fast-acting injection (shot).

How Can This Medicine Help?

Ziprasidone is used to treat psychosis, such as in schizophrenia, mania, or very severe depression. It can reduce *positive symptoms* such as hallucinations (hearing voices or seeing things that are not there); delusions (troubling beliefs that other people do not share); agitation; and very unusual thinking, speech, and behavior. It is also used to lessen the *negative symptoms* of schizophrenia, such as lack of interest in doing things (apathy), lack of motivation, social withdrawal, and lack of energy.

Ziprasidone may be used as a *mood stabilizer* in patients with bipolar disorder (manic-depressive illness) or severe mood swings. It can reduce mania and may be able to help maintain a stable mood over the long term.

Sometimes ziprasidone is used to reduce severe aggression or very serious behavioral problems in young people with conduct disorder, mental retardation, autism, or pervasive developmental disorder.

Ziprasidone may be used for behavior problems after a head injury.

It may be used for severe obsessive-compulsive disorder (OCD).

This medicine is very powerful and is used to treat very serious problems or symptoms that other medicines do not help. Be patient; the positive effects of this medicine may not appear for 2–3 weeks.

How Does This Medicine Work?

Cells in the brain communicate using chemicals called *neurotransmitters*. Too much or too little of these substances in parts of the brain can cause problems. Ziprasidone works by blocking the action of two of these neurotransmitters, *dopamine* and *serotonin*, in certain areas of the brain.

How Long Does This Medicine Last?

Ziprasidone is usually taken twice a day.

How Will the Doctor Monitor This Medicine?

The doctor will review your child's medical history and physical examination before starting ziprasidone. The doctor may order some blood or urine tests to be sure your child does not have a hidden medical condition that would make it unsafe to use this medicine. The doctor or nurse may measure your child's height, weight, pulse, and blood pressure before starting ziprasidone. The doctor may order other tests, such as baseline tests for blood sugar and cholesterol. An ECG (electrocardiogram or heart rhythm test) may be done before and after starting the medicine. A blood test for potassium also may be done.

Be sure to tell the doctor if anyone in the family has diabetes, high blood pressure, high cholesterol, or heart disease or if a family member died suddenly.

Before starting ziprasidone and every so often afterward, a test such as the AIMS (Abnormal Involuntary Movement Scale) may be used to check your child's tongue, legs, and arms for unusual movements that could be caused by the medicine.

After the medicine is started, the doctor will want to have regular appointments with you and your child to see how the medicine is working, to see if a dose change is needed, to watch for side effects, to see if ziprasidone is still needed, and to see if any other treatment is needed. The doctor or nurse may check your child's height, weight, pulse, and blood pressure, and watch for abnormal movements. Sometimes blood tests are needed to watch for diabetes or increased cholesterol.

What Side Effects Can This Medicine Have?

Any medicine can have side effects, including an allergy to the medicine. Because each patient is different, the doctor will monitor the youth closely, especially when the medicine is started. The doctor will work with you to increase the positive effects and decrease the negative effects of the medicine. Please tell the doctor if any of the listed side effects appear or if you think that the medicine is causing any other problems. Not all of the rare or unusual side effects are listed.

Side effects are most common after starting the medicine or after a dose increase. Many side effects can be avoided or lessened by starting with a very low dose and increasing it slowly—ask the doctor.

Allergic Reaction

Tell the doctor in a day or two (if possible, before the next dose of medicine):

- Hives
- Itching
- Rash

  Stop the medicine and get *immediate* medical care:

- Trouble breathing or chest tightness
- Swelling of lips, tongue, or throat

Common, but Not Usually Serious, Side Effects

Discuss the following side effects with your child's doctor when convenient. These side effects often can be helped by lowering the dose of medicine, changing the times medicine is taken, or adding another medicine.

- Daytime sleepiness or tiredness—Do not allow your child to drive, ride a bicycle or motorcycle, or operate machinery if this happens. This problem may be lessened by taking the medicine at bedtime.
- Dry mouth—Have your child try using sugar-free gum or candy.
- Constipation—Encourage your child to drink more fluids and eat high-fiber foods; if necessary, the doctor may recommend a fiber medicine such as Benefiber or a stool softener such as Colace or mineral oil.
- Upset stomach
- Increased appetite
- Weight gain—Seek nutritional counseling; provide your child with low-calorie snacks and encourage regular exercise.

Rare, but Not Usually Serious, Side Effects

Discuss the following side effects with your child's doctor when convenient. These side effects often can be helped by lowering the dose of medicine, changing the times medicine is taken, or adding another medicine.

- Dizziness—This side effect is worse when the child stands up quickly, especially when getting out of bed in the morning; try having the child stand up slowly.
- Increased restlessness or inability to sit still
- Shaking of hands and fingers
- Decreased or slowed movement and decreased facial expressions

Less Common, but Potentially Serious, Side Effects

Call the doctor *immediately:*

- Stiffness of the tongue, jaw, neck, back, or legs
- Seizure (fit, convulsion)—This is more common in people with a history of seizures or head injury.
- Irregular heartbeat (pulse), palpitations, or fainting
- Increased thirst, frequent urination (having to go to the bathroom often), lethargy, tiredness, dizziness, and blurred vision—These could be signs of diabetes, especially if your child is overweight or there is a family history of diabetes. **Talk to a doctor within a day.**

Very Rare, but Serious, Side Effects

- Extreme stiffness or lack of movement, very high fever, mental confusion, irregular pulse rate, or eye pain—**This is a medical emergency. Go to an emergency room right away.**
- Sudden stiffness and inability to breathe or swallow—**Go to an emergency room or call 911.** Tell the paramedics, nurses, and doctors that the patient is taking ziprasidone. Other medicines can be used to treat this problem fast.

What Else Should I Know About Side Effects?

Most side effects lessen over time. If they are troublesome, talk with your child's doctor. Some side effects can be decreased by taking a smaller dose of medicine, by stopping the medicine, by changing to another medicine, or by adding another medicine.

Sometimes people who take ziprasidone gain weight. Children seem to have more problems with this than adults. This is less a problem with ziprasidone than with other atypical antipsychotics. The weight gain may be from increased appetite and from ways that the medicine changes how the body processes food. Ziprasidone may also change the way that the body handles glucose (sugar) and cause high levels (hyperglycemia). People who take ziprasidone, especially those who gain a lot of weight, are at increased risk of developing diabetes and of having increased fats (lipids—cholesterol and triglycerides) in their blood. Over time, both diabetes and increased fats in the blood may lead to heart disease, stroke, and other complications. The FDA has put warnings on all atypical agents about the increased risks of hyperglycemia, diabetes, and increased blood cholesterol and triglycerides when taking one of these medicines. It is much easier to prevent weight gain than to lose weight later. When your child first starts taking ziprasidone, it is a good idea to be sure that he or she eats a well-balanced diet without "junk food" and with healthy snacks like fruits and vegetables, not sweets or fried foods. He or she should drink water or skim milk, not pop, sodas, soft drinks, or sugary juices. Regular exercise is important for maintaining a healthy weight (and may also help with sleep).

One very rare side effect that may not go away is *tardive dyskinesia* (or TD). Patients with tardive dyskinesia have involuntary movements (movements that they cannot help making) of the body, especially the mouth and tongue. The patient may look as though he or she is making faces over and over again. Jerky movements of the arms, legs, or body may occur. There may be fine, wormlike, or sudden repeated movements of the tongue, or the person may appear to be chewing something or smacking or puckering his or her lips. The fingers may look as though they are rolling something. If you notice any unusual movements, be sure to tell the doctor. The doctor may use the AIMS test to look for these movements.

Neuroleptic malignant syndrome is a very rare side effect that can lead to death. The symptoms are severe muscle stiffness, high fever, increased heart rate and blood pressure, irregular heartbeat (pulse), and sweating. It may lead to unconsciousness. If you suspect this, **call 911 or go to an emergency room right away.**

Some Interactions With Other Medicines or Food

Please note that the following are only the most likely interactions with food or other medicines.

Heart problems are more common if other medicines that affect the heart or antibiotics such as erythromycin are being taken as well. Be sure to tell all your child's doctors and your pharmacist about all medications your child is taking.

Taking ziprasidone with food may decrease stomach upset.

Carbamazepine (Tegretol) and phenytoin (Dilantin) may decrease levels of ziprasidone, making it not work as well.

It is better to limit drinks with caffeine (coffee, tea, soft drinks) because caffeine works in the opposite way from this medicine, and the positive effects might be decreased.

What Could Happen if This Medicine Is Stopped Suddenly?

Involuntary movements, or *withdrawal dyskinesias*, may appear within 1–4 weeks of lowering the dose or stopping the medicine. Usually these go away, but they can last for days to months. If ziprasidone is stopped suddenly, emotional disturbance (such as irritability, nervousness, moodiness, or oppositional behavior) or physical problems (such as stomachache, loss of appetite, nausea, vomiting, diarrhea, sweating, indigestion, trouble sleeping, trembling, or shaking) may appear. These problems usually last only a few days to a few weeks. If they happen, you should tell your child's doctor. The medicine dose may need to be lowered more slowly (tapered). Always check with the doctor before stopping a medicine.

How Long Will This Medicine Be Needed?

How long your child will need to take this medicine depends partly on the reason that it was prescribed. Some problems last for only a few months, whereas others last much longer. It is important to ask the doctor whether the medicine is still needed, especially with medicines as powerful as this one. Every few months, you should discuss with your child's doctor the reasons for using ziprasidone and whether the medicine may be stopped or the dose lowered.

What Else Should I Know About This Medicine?

There are other medicines that are used for the same kinds of problems. If your child is having bad side effects or the medicine does not seem to be working, ask the doctor if another medicine might work as well or better and have fewer side effects for your child. Each person reacts differently to medicines.

Notes

Use this space to take notes or to write down questions you want to ask the doctor.

Medication Information
for Youth

Ziprasidone—Geodon

What the Medicine Is Called and What It Is For

The name of your medicine may be confusing. Most drugs have two names: 1) a scientific name that we call a *generic name* and 2) a trade or *brand name*. The generic name of this medicine is ziprasidone. The brand name is Geodon.

Ziprasidone is called an *atypical* medicine. It helps people who feel very confused and have severe problems thinking clearly. It can lessen hallucinations (seeing or hearing things that are not really there) and delusions (troubling beliefs that other people do not share). The medicine also can improve *negative symptoms*, such as lack of interest in doing things, lack of motivation, loss of interest in friends, and decreased energy. It helps people who have severe depression or mood swings. This medicine also is sometimes used to help young people who have mania or severe depression or who get very angry and hit people or break things.

How You Take the Medicine

It is very important to take the medicine exactly as the doctor or nurse tells you. Do not skip doses or take extra medicine without asking an adult. If you forget a dose, ask your parent(s) what to do.

It is better to limit drinks with caffeine (coffee, tea, soft drinks) because caffeine works in the opposite way from this medicine, and the positive effects might be decreased.

Your doctor will tell you how much medicine to take and how often to take it so that it can help you the most. It is *very important* that you take all the pills you are supposed to take each day. Your doctor will probably recommend that you take your medicine at the same time each day, which may be with meals or at bedtime.

It may be several weeks or longer before you notice the full effect. You may feel discouraged and think the medicine is never going to help. You may want to give up and stop taking the medicine. Talk to your doctor and parent(s) about how you feel, but **do not stop** taking your medicine unless your doctor tells you to. It also is important not to take extra pills hoping that you will feel better faster. Doing that could make you very sick.

If the medicine makes your stomach upset, taking ziprasidone with food may help.

This medicine is prescribed only for you. It should never be shared with anyone else.

You do not have to tell others that you are taking this medicine, but it is not something you should feel ashamed or embarrassed about. Many young people are helped by ziprasidone. This medicine is not habit-forming, and you cannot become "hooked" on it. You should talk to your doctor or nurse about any questions you have about the medicine. It is important to remember that the medicine *helps* you. It cannot *make* you do anything or change you as a person.

711

How Your Doctor Will Follow Your Progress

Before giving you the medicine, your doctor or nurse will talk with you and your parent(s) and may measure your height, weight, heart rate (pulse), and blood pressure. There may be other tests, such as blood tests for sugar, cholesterol, and potassium. Before you start taking the medicine and every so often afterward, the doctor or nurse will look at your tongue, arms, and legs to check for unusual movements. This is called the AIMS (Abnormal Involuntary Movement Scale) test. Before starting ziprasidone, at times of increasing the dose, and every 6 months to a year after that, your doctor will ask for an ECG (electrocardiogram or heart rhythm test) to be done. This test counts your heartbeats through small wires that are taped to your chest. It takes only about 15 minutes.

Be sure to tell your doctor or nurse about any other medicines or supplements you are taking, including vitamins, herbs, or aids to weight loss or bodybuilding. Also be sure to tell the doctor or nurse if you are using alcohol or drugs. Because many medicines may affect babies, it is very important to tell the doctor if you might be pregnant or if you are at risk of becoming pregnant. Tell the doctor if you have ever had very fast heartbeat, chest pain, light-headedness, or fainting.

Your teachers may be asked to fill out a form about your grades and behavior in school. A psychologist may give you some tests to see how you learn best.

Most doctors have regular appointments with young people who are taking medicine. You should use these visits to share any concerns you may have about your medicine and to talk about if it has helped you. From time to time, your physician or nurse may measure your height, weight, heart rate (pulse), and blood pressure to be sure that you are in good health while you are taking the medicine. There may be blood tests, to watch for diabetes or high cholesterol. Your doctor also will ask for regular reports from your parents and maybe from your teachers (with your permission) to see how well the medicine is working.

If the medicine helps you, your doctor will probably want you to take it for several months to a year. Your doctor will decide how long you will need to take the medicine as he or she watches your progress.

How the Medicine Might Affect You

In addition to the ways the medicine can help you, it may have other effects called *side effects*. Different medicines have different side effects. It is helpful to know about some of the most common side effects of your medicine so that you will understand what they are if they happen. Some people do not have any side effects. Some side effects are just uncomfortable, but others may mean a more serious problem with the medicine. Side effects are most common after starting the medicine or after a dose increase. They may go away with time, or the medicine can be adjusted or changed—ask the doctor.

You could have an allergy to any medicine, which might show up as a rash on your skin, swelling, itching, or trouble breathing.

Please tell your parent(s) and doctor or nurse about any changes that you notice after taking the medicine. It is especially important to tell a responsible adult right away if you are feeling depressed or that you may not want to live; if you have thoughts of hurting yourself; or if you begin to feel more irritable, nervous, or restless. Also be sure to tell your parent(s) or doctor if you begin to feel more "speeded up" or have more trouble sleeping.

One of the most common side effects of this medicine is feeling tired or sleepy during the day, even if you have had a full night's sleep. If this medicine is making you sleepy, it is very important not to drive a car or ride a bicycle or motorcycle. After starting the medicine or increasing the dose of medicine, please be extra careful when driving a car, riding a bike, or using machines until you can tell how the medicine affects your alertness, attention, and coordination. After you have been taking the medicine for a few weeks, your body will adjust, and this side effect will likely go away. If you had trouble sleeping at night before taking the medicine, it can help you sleep better, especially if the doctor tells you to take a dose of medicine in the evening.

Another common side effect is dry mouth. You may be more thirsty than usual and find that you are drinking more water or other liquids than usual. Sucking on sugar-free hard candy or cough drops usually helps. You also could try chewing sugar-free gum or sucking on ice chips. Do not chew the ice; you could hurt your teeth. Also, using lip balm will keep your lips from cracking. It is important to be especially good about brushing your teeth.

Sometimes people taking ziprasidone notice that their heart is beating a little faster than normal. Usually this happens within the first few weeks of taking the medicine and gets better or goes away. However, if you notice that your heart is beating very fast for more than a few minutes when you have not been exercising, if you feel light-headed or dizzy when you are sitting or standing still, or if you faint, you should let your parent(s) and doctor know right away. Some people feel dizzy or light-headed when standing up fast. If this happens, try to get up more slowly, especially first thing in the morning when getting out of bed.

Some people become constipated (have hard bowel movements) when taking this medicine. Try drinking more water and eating more fruits, vegetables, and whole grains. If that does not help, tell your parent(s) or doctor—you may need a medicine to help with this side effect.

If you get *very* thirsty, have to go to the bathroom a lot, feel *very* tired, or have dizziness or blurred vision, be sure to tell your parent(s) or doctor.

A few teenagers who take ziprasidone gain weight. The weight gain may be from increased appetite and also from ways that the medicine changes how the body processes food. People who take ziprasidone, especially those who gain a lot of weight, might be at increased risk of developing diabetes and of having increased fats (lipids—cholesterol and triglycerides) in their blood. Over time, both diabetes and increased fats in the blood may lead to heart disease, stroke, and other complications. The U.S. Food and Drug Administration has put warnings about these problems on all medicines like ziprasidone. It is much easier to prevent weight gain than to lose weight later. It is a good idea to eat a well-balanced diet without "junk food" and with healthy snacks like fruits and vegetables, not sweets or fried foods. It is better to drink water or skim milk, not pop, sodas, soft drinks, or sugary juices. Regular exercise is important for maintaining a healthy weight (and may also help with sleep).

This is a very powerful medicine. Some side effects include feeling nervous, restless, or shaky or having stiff muscles. Talk with your doctor about these side effects. They can be helped by adding another medicine, adjusting the dose, or switching to another medicine.

Another, more serious, side effect can be longer lasting and more difficult to treat. This very rare side effect is called *tardive dyskinesia* (or TD). A person taking ziprasidone may develop movements of the mouth, tongue, face, arms, legs, or body that are not being made on purpose. This side effect can go away when the medicine is stopped, but in some people it does not go away. Your doctor will explain this effect to you and your parent(s) and how he or she will watch for any signs that you are developing this problem. Be sure to ask your doctor any questions that you may have about this, but do not worry too much about it. It hardly ever happens to teenagers.

You should tell your parent(s) and doctor if you notice anything different or unusual about how you feel once you start taking the medicine. This includes good things, such as feeling less confused, feeling less sad, not hearing voices anymore, or sleeping better at night.

Notes

Use this space to take notes or to write down questions you want to ask the doctor or nurse.

_____

_____

_____

_____

_____

_____

_____

_____

_____

_____

_____

_____

_____

From Dulcan MK (editor): _Helping Parents, Youth, and Teachers Understand Medications for Behavioral and Emotional Problems: A Resource Book of Medication Information Handouts_, Third Edition. Washington, DC, American Psychiatric Publishing, 2007

Medication Information for Parents and Teachers

Zolpidem—Ambien

General Information About Medication

Each child and adolescent is different. No one has exactly the same combination of medical and psychological problems. It is a good idea to talk with the doctor or nurse about the reasons a medicine is being used. It is very important to keep all appointments and to be in touch by telephone if you have concerns. It is important to communicate with the doctor, nurse, or therapist.

It is very important that the medicine be taken exactly as the doctor instructs. However, once in a while, everyone forgets to give a medicine on time. It is a good idea to ask the doctor or nurse what to do if this happens. Do not stop or change a medicine without asking the doctor or nurse first.

If the medicine seems to stop working, it may be because it is not being taken regularly. The youth may be "cheeking" or hiding the medicine or forgetting to take it. A different dose may be needed. Something at school, at home, or in the neighborhood may be upsetting the youth, or he or she may need special help for learning disabilities or tutoring. Please discuss your concerns with the doctor. **Do not just increase the dose.**

All medicines should be kept in a safe place, out of the reach of children, and should be supervised by an adult. If someone takes too much of a medicine, call the doctor, the poison control center, or a hospital emergency room.

Each medicine has a "generic" or chemical name. Just like laundry detergents or paper towels, some medicines are sold by more than one company under different brand names. The same medicine may be available under a generic name and several brand names. The generic medications are usually less expensive than the brand name ones. The generic medications have the same chemical formula, but they may or may not be exactly the same strength as the brand-name medications. Also, some brands of pills contain dye that can cause allergic reactions. It is a good idea to talk to the doctor and the pharmacist about whether it is important to use a specific brand of medicine.

All medicines can cause an allergic reaction. Examples are hives, itching, rashes, swelling, and trouble breathing. Even a tiny amount of a medicine can cause a reaction in patients who are allergic to that medicine. Be *sure* to talk to the doctor before restarting a medicine that has caused an allergic reaction.

Taking more than one medicine at the same time may cause more side effects or cause one of the medicines to not work as well. Always ask the doctor, nurse, or pharmacist before adding another medicine, whether prescription or over-the-counter. Be sure that each doctor knows about *all* of the medicines your child is taking. Also tell the doctor about any vitamins, herbal medicines, or supplements your child may be taking. Some of these may have side effects alone or when taken with this medication.

Everyone taking medicine should have a physical examination at least once a year.

If you suspect the youth is using drugs or alcohol, please tell the doctor right away.

Pregnancy requires special care in the use of medicine. Please tell the doctor immediately if you suspect the teenager is pregnant or might become pregnant.

Printed information like this applies to children and adolescents in general. If you have questions about the medicine, or if you notice changes or anything unusual, please ask the doctor or nurse. As scientific research advances, knowledge increases and advice changes. Even experts do not always agree. Many medicines have not been approved by the U.S. Food and Drug Administration (FDA) for use in children. For this reason, use of the medicine for a particular problem or age group often is not listed in the *Physicians' Desk Reference*. This does not necessarily mean that the medicine is dangerous or does not work, only that the company that makes the medicine has not received permission to advertise the medicine for use in children. Companies often do not apply for this permission because it is expensive to do the tests needed to apply for approval for use in children. Once a medication is approved by the FDA for any purpose, a doctor is allowed to prescribe it according to research and clinical experience.

Note to Teachers

It is a good idea to talk with the parent(s) about the reason(s) that a medication is being used. If the parent(s) sign consent to release information, it is often helpful to talk with the doctor. If the parent(s) give permission, the doctor may ask you to fill out rating forms about your experience with the student's behavior, feelings, academic performance, and medication side effects. This information is very useful in selecting and monitoring medication treatment. If you have observations that you think are important, do not hesitate to share these with the student's parent(s) and treating clinicians.

All medicines should be kept in a secure place and should be supervised by an adult. If someone takes too much of a medicine, follow your school procedure for an urgent medical problem.

Taking medicine is a private matter and is best managed discreetly and confidentially. It is important to be sensitive to the student's feelings about taking medicine.

If you suspect that the student is using drugs or alcohol, please tell the parent(s) or a school counselor right away.

Please tell the parent(s) or school nurse if you suspect medication side effects.

Any expression of suicidal thoughts or feelings or self-harm by a child or adolescent is a clear signal of distress and should be taken seriously. These behaviors should not be dismissed as "attention seeking."

What Is Zolpidem (Ambien)?

Zolpidem is a *hypnotic* or *sedative-hypnotic* medicine. It is *not* a *benzodiazepine*. It comes in Ambien brand name tablets and Ambien CR (controlled-release) tablets.

How Can This Medicine Help?

Zolpidem is used to treat insomnia—problems falling asleep or staying asleep—when used for a short time along with a behavioral program.

How Does This Medicine Work?

Zolpidem works in certain parts of the brain to help people fall asleep. It works in a different way than other sleep medicines. When Ambien CR is taken, the outer coating of the pill helps the person to fall asleep, and the slow-release medicine inside the pill helps with staying asleep.

How Long Does This Medicine Last?

Zolpidem is taken right before going to bed, because it starts working very quickly. It leaves the body very quickly, so it is less likely to cause daytime sleepiness or memory problems than other kinds of sleep medicines.

How Will the Doctor Monitor This Medicine?

The doctor will review your child's medical history and physical examination before starting zolpidem.

After the medicine is started, the doctor will want to have regular appointments with you and your child to see how the medicine is working, to see if a dose change is needed, to watch for side effects, to see if zolpidem is still needed, and to see if any other treatment is needed.

What Side Effects Can This Medicine Have?

Any medicine can have side effects, including an allergy to the medicine. Because each patient is different, the doctor will monitor the youth closely, especially when the medicine is started. The doctor will work with you to increase the positive effects and decrease the negative effects of the medicine. Please tell the doctor if any of the listed side effects appear or if you think that the medicine is causing any other problems. Not all of the rare or unusual side effects are listed.

Side effects are most common after starting the medicine or after a dose increase. Many side effects can be avoided or lessened by starting with a very low dose and increasing it slowly—ask the doctor.

Allergic Reaction

Tell the doctor in a day or two (if possible, before the next dose of medicine):

- Hives
- Itching
- Rash

Stop the medicine and get *immediate* medical care:

- Trouble breathing or chest tightness
- Swelling of lips, tongue, or throat

Zolpidem is usually very safe when used for short periods as the doctor prescribes.

The most common side effect is daytime sleepiness. Zolpidem can also cause dizziness, feeling "spacey," or decreased coordination. If the medicine is causing any of these problems it is very important not to drive a car, ride a bicycle or motorcycle, or operate machinery.

Zolpidem can cause decreased concentration and memory. These problems, along with daytime sleepiness, may decrease learning and performance in school.

Some children and adolescents who have taken zolpidem have had dreamlike states right before falling asleep in which they see or hear things that are not there. Some of the youth had unusual or bizarre behaviors in between taking zolpidem and falling asleep. If this happens, zolpidem should be stopped and not used again.

People who take zolpidem must not drink alcohol. Severe sleepiness or even loss of consciousness may result.

It is possible to become psychologically and physically dependent on zolpidem, but that is not a common problem for patients who see their doctors regularly. It is less common for zolpidem than for other types of sleep medicines.

Some Interactions With Other Medicines or Food

Please note that the following are only the most likely interactions with food or other medicines.

Caffeine may cause trouble sleeping and make zolpidem less effective. If caffeine is eliminated, less zolpidem may be needed, or zolpidem may not be needed at all.

It is important not to use other sedatives, tranquilizers, or sleeping pills or antihistamines (such as Benadryl) when taking zolpidem because of greatly increased side effects.

What Could Happen if This Medicine Is Stopped Suddenly?

Many medicines cause problems if stopped suddenly. Zolpidem must be decreased slowly (tapered) rather than stopped suddenly. When zolpidem is stopped suddenly, there are withdrawal symptoms that are uncomfortable. Problems are more likely in patients taking high doses of zolpidem for 2 months or longer, but even after taking zolpidem for just a few weeks, it is important to stop it slowly. Withdrawal symptoms may include anxiety, irritability, shaking, sweating, aches and pains, muscle cramps, vomiting, confusion, and trouble sleeping.

How Long Will This Medicine Be Needed?

Zolpidem is usually prescribed for only a week or so or for occasional use. A behavioral program, such as regular soothing routines at bedtime and increased exercise in the daytime, should be used along with the medicine, to improve sleep. Finding developmentally appropriate bed- and wake-times and sticking to them is very important. These strategies should be continued after the medicine is tapered (stopped slowly) or when the medicine is used only occasionally.

What Else Should I Know About This Medicine?

Because zolpidem can be abused (especially by people who abuse alcohol or drugs) and can cause psychological dependence or physical dependence (addiction), it is regulated by special state and federal laws as a *controlled substance*. These laws place limitations on telephone prescriptions and refills.

People with sleep apnea (breathing stops while they are asleep) should not take zolpidem. Tell the doctor if your child snores very loudly.

Zolpidem works faster if taken on an empty stomach.

Do not cut or crush the Ambien CR tablet—it should be swallowed whole.

Notes

Use this space to take notes or to write down questions you want to ask the doctor.

_____

_____

_____

_____

_____

_____

_____

_____

_____

_____

_____

_____

From Dulcan MK (editor): _Helping Parents, Youth, and Teachers Understand Medications for Behavioral and Emotional Problems: A Resource Book of Medication Information Handouts,_ Third Edition. Washington, DC, American Psychiatric Publishing, 2007

Medication Information
for Youth

Zolpidem—Ambien

What the Medicine Is Called and What It Is For

The name of your medicine may be confusing. Most drugs have two names: 1) a scientific name that we call a *generic name* and 2) a trade or *brand name*. The generic name of this medicine is zolpidem. The brand name is Ambien.

Zolpidem works by calming the parts of the brain that are too excitable. Zolpidem can help with insomnia (difficulty falling asleep or staying asleep) when used for a short time along with routines that help you to relax and fall asleep.

How You Take the Medicine

It is very important to take the medicine exactly as the doctor or nurse tells you. Do not skip doses or take extra medicine without asking an adult. If you forget a dose, ask your parent(s) what to do.

Do not chew, cut, or crush the tablet—swallow it whole.

Zolpidem works best if combined with a regular bedtime, calming routines before bedtime, and physical exercise during the day. Getting up on time is also important in keeping a regular sleep schedule.

Zolpidem works faster if you do not eat for a few hours before taking it.

It is better to limit drinks with caffeine (coffee, tea, soft drinks) because caffeine works in the opposite way from zolpidem, and the positive effects might be decreased.

This medicine is prescribed only for you. It should never be shared with anyone else.

You do not have to tell others that you are taking this medicine, but it is not something you should feel ashamed or embarrassed about. Many young people are helped by zolpidem. You should talk to your doctor or nurse about any questions you have about the medicine. It is important to remember that the medicine *helps* you. It cannot *make* you do anything or change you as a person.

Many medicines cause problems if stopped suddenly. Always ask your doctor before stopping a medicine. Problems are more likely to happen in patients taking high doses of zolpidem for 2 months or longer, but it is important to decrease the medicine slowly (taper) even after a few weeks. If you notice anxiety, irritability, shaking, sweating, aches and pains, muscle cramps, vomiting, or trouble sleeping, you may need to decrease the medicine more slowly.

How Your Doctor Will Follow Your Progress

Before giving you the medicine, your doctor or nurse will talk with you and your parent(s) and may measure your height, weight, heart rate (pulse), and blood pressure.

Be sure to tell your doctor or nurse about any other medicines or supplements you are taking, including vitamins, herbs, or aids to weight loss or bodybuilding. Also be sure to tell the doctor or nurse if you are using alcohol or drugs. Because many medicines may affect babies, it is very important to tell the doctor if you might be pregnant or if you are at risk of becoming pregnant.

Most doctors have regular appointments with young people who are taking medicine. You should use these visits to share any concerns you may have about your medicine and to talk about if it has helped you. From time to time, your physician or nurse may measure your height, weight, heart rate (pulse), and blood pressure to be sure that you are in good health while you are taking the medicine. Your doctor also will ask for regular reports from your parents to see how well the medicine is working.

Zolpidem is usually prescribed for only a week or so to allow you to develop better sleep habits. A regular bedtime, a relaxing routine before bedtime, and physical exercise in the daytime usually help with sleep at night.

Each person is unique, and some people may need this medicine for months or years.

How the Medicine Might Affect You

In addition to the ways the medicine can help you, it may have other effects called *side effects*. Different medicines have different side effects. It is helpful to know about some of the most common side effects of your medicine so that you will understand what they are if they happen. Some people do not have any side effects. Some side effects are just uncomfortable, but others may mean a more serious problem with the medicine. Side effects are most common after starting the medicine or after a dose increase. They may go away with time, or the medicine can be adjusted or changed—ask the doctor.

You could have an allergy to any medicine, which might show up as a rash on your skin, swelling, itching, or trouble breathing.

Please tell your parent(s) and doctor or nurse about any changes that you notice after taking the medicine. It is especially important to tell a responsible adult if you are feeling depressed or that you may not want to live; if you have thoughts of hurting yourself; or if you begin to feel more irritable, nervous, or restless.

The most common side effect of zolpidem is daytime sleepiness. If this medicine is making you sleepy during the day, it is very important not to drive a car or ride a bicycle or motorcycle. After starting zolpidem or increasing the dose, please be extra careful when driving a car, riding a bike, or using machines until you can tell how the medicine affects your alertness, attention, and coordination.

Sometimes sleep medicines seem to work in the opposite way, causing more trouble sleeping, nightmares, excitement, irritability, anger, aggression, or other problems. If this happens, tell your parent(s) or your doctor.

Some people feel dizzy, clumsy, or "spacey" or have more trouble remembering things when taking this medicine. Some people have "waking dreams" as they are falling asleep and see or hear things that are not there. Some people get up at night after taking the medicine and eat a lot or do things as if they were sleepwalking. Be sure to tell your parent(s) or doctor right away if any of these happen.

Drinking alcohol while taking this medicine can cause severe drowsiness or even passing out. **Don't do it!** Do not use marijuana or street drugs while taking this medicine. They can cause serious side effects. Skipping your medicine to take drugs does not work because many medicines stay in your body for a long time.

Zolpidem can be habit-forming, but that is not a common problem for people who take their medicine as the doctor says.

Notes

Use this space to take notes or to write down questions you want to ask the doctor or nurse.

_____

_____

_____

_____

_____

_____

_____

_____

_____

_____

_____

_____

From Dulcan MK (editor): *Helping Parents, Youth, and Teachers Understand Medications for Behavioral and Emotional Problems: A Resource Book of Medication Information Handouts*, Third Edition. Washington, DC, American Psychiatric Publishing, 2007

Appendix 1

FDA-Approved Medicines Used for Attention-Deficit/Hyperactivity Disorder (ADHD)

Methylphenidate	
Generic (IR; 3–4 hours)	Tablet
Methylin (IR; 3–4 hours)	Tablet
	Chewable tablet
	Oral solution (grape)
Ritalin (IR; 3–4 hours)	Tablet
Methylin ER (6–8 hours)	Wax matrix
Ritalin SR (6–8 hours)	Wax matrix
Metadate ER (6–8 hours)	Wax matrix
Ritalin LA (8–10 hours)	Capsule with beads (sprinkle)
Metadate CD (8 hours)	Capsule Diffucap with beads (sprinkle)
Concerta (10–12 hours)	Oros osmotic controlled-release tablet
Daytrana	Transdermal system (skin patch)

Dexmethylphenidate	
Focalin (IR; 3–4 hours)	Tablet
Focalin XR (8–10 hours)	Capsule with beads (sprinkle)

Dextroamphetamine	
DextroStat (IR; 3–5 hours)	Tablet
Dexedrine (IR; 3–5 hours)	Tablet
Generic (IR; 3–5 hours)	Tablet
Dexedrine Spansule (6–8 hours)	Capsule with particles
Dextroamphetamine ER (6–8 hours)	Capsule

Mixed Salts Amphetamine	
Adderall (IR; 3–5 hours)	Tablet
Generic (IR; 3–5 hours)	Tablet
Adderall XR (10–12 hours)	Capsule with beads (sprinkle)

Atomoxetine	
Strattera (24 hours)	Capsule

Note. ER=extended-release; IR=immediate-release; LA=long-acting; SR=sustained-release; XR=extended-release

Appendix 2

Medicines Typically Used for
Anxiety and Depression

Generic name	Brand name(s)
Alprazolam*	Xanax
Buspirone*	BuSpar
Citalopram	Celexa
Clomipramine[†]	Anafranil
Clonazepam*	Klonopin
Diazepam*	Valium
Duloxetine	Cymbalta
Escitalopram	Lexapro
Fluoxetine	Prozac
Fluvoxamine	Luvox
Lorazepam*	Ativan
Mirtazapine	Remeron
Nortriptyline	Pamelor
Paroxetine	Paxil, Pexeva
Sertraline	Zoloft
Venlafaxine	Effexor

*Anxiety only
[†]Obsessive-compulsive disorder only

Appendix 3

Medicines Typically Used for Psychosis

Generic name	Brand name
Aripiprazole	Abilify
Chlorpromazine	Thorazine
Clozapine	Clozaril
Fluphenazine	Prolixin
Haloperidol	Haldol
Loxapine	Loxitane
Olanzapine	Zyprexa
Perphenazine	Trilafon
Quetiapine	Seroquel
Risperidone	Risperdal
Thiothixene	Navane
Trifluoperazine	Stelazine
Ziprasidone	Geodon

Appendix 4

Medicines Typically Used for
Mood Stabilization or Reducing Aggression

Generic name	Brand name(s)
Aripiprazole	Abilify
Carbamazepine	Carbatrol, Tegretol
Gabapentin	Neurontin
Lamotrigine	Lamictal
Lithium	Eskalith, Lithobid, Lithotab
Olanzapine	Zyprexa
Oxcarbazepine	Trileptal
Quetiapine	Seroquel
Risperidone	Risperdal
Topiramate	Topamax
Valproic acid, Divalproex sodium	Depakene, Depakote
Ziprasidone	Geocon

Index of Medicines
by Brand Name